Concepts in
Biochemistry
with Clinical Approach
for undergraduate Medical Students

As per the latest competency-based curriculum prescribed by Medical Council of India

W0235490

Concepts in
Biochemistry
with Clinical Approach
for undergraduate Medical Students

As per the latest competency-based curriculum prescribed by Medical Council of India

Poonam Agrawal MBBS, MD

Professor
Department of Biochemistry
Dr Baba Saheb Ambedkar Medical College and Hospital
New Delhi

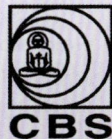

CBS Publishers & Distributors Pvt Ltd

New Delhi • Bengaluru • Chennai • Kochi • Kolkata • Mumbai
Bhopal • Bhubaneswar • Hyderabad • Jharkhand • Nagpur • Patna • Pune • Uttarakhand • Dhaka (Bangladesh)

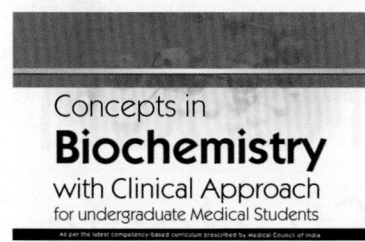

Concepts in
Biochemistry
with Clinical Approach
for undergraduate Medical Students

ISBN: 978-93-89261-85-1

First Edition: 2020

Published by Satish Kumar Jain and produced by Varun Jain for

CBS Publishers & Distributors Pvt Ltd

4819/XI Prahlad Street, 24 Ansari Road, Daryaganj, New Delhi 110 002, India.
Ph: 011-23289259, 23266861, 23266867   Fax: 011-23243014
Website: www.cbspd.com   e-mail: delhi@cbspd.com; cbspubs@airtelmail.in

Corporate Office: 204 FIE, Industrial Area, Patparganj, Delhi 110 092, India
Ph: 011-4934 4934   Fax: 011-4934 4935   e-mail: publishing@cbspd.com; publicity@cbspd.com

Branches

- **Bengaluru:** Seema House 2975, 17th Cross, K.R. Road, Banasankari 2nd Stage, Bengaluru 560 070, Karnataka, India
  Ph: +91-80-26771678/79   Fax: +91-80-26771680   e-mail: bangalore@cbspd.com

- **Chennai:** 7, Subbaraya Street, Shenoy Nagar, Chennai 600 030, Tamil Nadu, India.
  Ph: +91-44-26680620, 26681266   Fax: +91-44-42032115   e-mail: chennai@cbspd.com

- **Kochi:** 42/1325, 1326, Power House Road, Opposite KSEB Power House, Ernakulam 682 018, Kochi, Kerala, India.
  Ph: +91-484-4059061-65   Fax: +91-484-4059065   e-mail: kochi@cbspd.com

- **Kolkata:** 6/B, Ground Floor, Rameswar Shaw Road, Kolkata-700 014, West Bengal, India
  Ph: +91-33-22891126, 22891127, 22891128   e-mail: kolkata@cbspd.com

- **Mumbai:** 83-C, Dr E Moses Road, Worli, Mumbai-400018, Maharashtra, India
  Ph: +91-22-24902340/41   Fax: +91-22-24902342   e-mail: mumbai@cbspd.com

Representatives

• **Bhopal**	0-8319310552	• **Bhubaneswar**	0-9911037372	• **Hyderabad**	0-9885175004
• **Jharkhand**	0-9811541605	• **Nagpur**	0-9421945513	• **Patna**	0-9334159340
• **Pune**	0-9623451994	• **Uttarakhand**	0-9716462459	• **Dhaka (Bangladesh)**	01912-003485

Printed at: EIH Limited, India.

_to_
_____
the medical students who are learning to
reduce the suffering of
humanity

Foreword

There was always a need of a biochemistry book, which could provide all the topics to be learned by medical undergraduates in a concise, relevant and organized fashion blended with clinical correlations.

Finally, we have this book *Concepts in Biochemistry with Clinical Approach* written by an excellent teacher who is well known for her unique simplified approach towards the subject. Her style of teaching is well reflected in various chapters and student community will largely benefit from her insight into the subject.

This book explains all the topics in a simple and reproducible manner with the help of innumerable illustrations and flowcharts which are easily imprinted in learners mind, making the learning of biochemistry easy.

I wish ma'am all the very best for this enthusiastic work.

Katyani Sharma
MBBS, Phase II, ACMS, New Delhi
GGSIPU University Batch Topper (2017–2018)

Preface

Medical undergraduates face a special challenge of time constraint in first year of 4½ years MBBS curriculum, as they have to learn three important subjects — biochemistry, anatomy and physiology in limited time frame with good detail. As an author, every effort is made to deliver relevant and 'to the point information' in a simple and lucid manner with precise clinical correlation.

While describing the clinical connections, special precaution has been taken to keep the discussion simple, keeping in mind that first year medical undergraduate student who is reading this book has no exposure to patients or hospital settings in the real world. Every effort is made to help the student learn the subject in an easy and reproducible manner with the help of a plenty of diagrams and flowcharts.

This book is written keeping in the mind the latest MCI guidelines on competencies based medical education (CBME) and the competencies covered in a chapter are mentioned at the beginning of the chapter itself.

I wish learner find this book useful for their learning of biochemistry with its relevance in clinical setting.

Feedback and comments are most welcomed and will be duly acknowledged in the next edition.

Poonam Agrawal
drpoonam24agrawal@yahoo.com

Acknowledgment

First of all, I thank Almighty for giving me the dream and then the courage to work hard to best of my abilities to fulfil that dream.

I owe my sincere thanks and gratitude to Dr Achal Gulati, Director and Principal, Dr Baba Saheb Ambedkar Medical College and Hospital, New Delhi and Dr J M Kaul, Academic Coordinator, Dr Baba Saheb Ambedkar Medical College and Hospital, New Delhi for their invaluable guidance and support all the time.

My respected teachers who have always encouraged me to do the best and have guided me throughout deserve special mention here, as their valuable contribution cannot be thanked in words:

Dr S K Gupta: Director Professor and Head, NDMC, New Delhi

Dr Dinesh Puri: Director Professor and Head, UCMS, New Delhi

Dr Alpana Saxena: Director Professor, Dr BSAMCH, New Delhi

Dr Anju Jain: Director Professor and Head, LHMC, New Delhi

Dr T K Mishra: Ex-Director Professor and Head, MAMC, New Delhi

All my students who approach me for discussions, doubt clarification, deserve special thanks, as their interaction enlightens me of their difficulties, give an insight to the subject and help me grow as a teacher.

My friends Dr Sumita Sethi, Associate Professor BPSGMC; Dr Binita Goswami, Professor, MAMC; Dr Niket Verma, Assistant Professor, AIMS, New Delhi; Dr R Shanti, Professor and HOD, GMC Omandurar, deserve thanks from bottom of my heart as their association has made my life more meaningful.

It has been a long and challenging journey with many editing, rewritings and reframing. I thank my husband **Dr Mohit Agrawal**, who has been a constant guide and motivator throughout the preparation of this book. It is not an exaggeration to say that this work is the result of his belief in my abilities, which kept me going non-stop in this roller coaster journey.

I am obliged to my little angel '**Misti**' for her understanding and full cooperation, when at times I was totally engrossed in writing chapters for this book, even on her Sundays and holidays. Blessings of my parents 'Dr. Shri Prakash Agarwal' and 'Mrs. Manju Agarwal' and my parent-in-laws 'Mr. Ram Baboo Agarwal' and 'Late Smt. Aadesh Agarwal' are most valuable asset, which support me through all walks of life.

I expressed special gratitude to Mr Satish Jain, CMD, CBS Publishers & Distributors Pvt Ltd., for his endeavour in multifarious ways to publish this book.

I would like to offer my special thanks to Mr YN Arjuna (Senior Vice-President, Publishing, Editorial and Publicity) and his entire team comprising Ms Ritu Chawla (AGM Production), Mr Manish Raj (graphic artist) Ms Hemlata (DTP operator), and Mr Neeraj Sharma (editor) for their excellent work to bring out this edition. I am really obliged to all of them.

Poonam Agrawal

Contents

Section 4
METABOLISM OF LIPIDS

Section 5
METABOLISM OF AMINO ACIDS

Section 6
INTEGRATED PATHWAYS

Section 7
NUTRITION, VITAMINS AND MINERALS

Section 8
MISCELLANEOUS TOPICS

Section 9

NUCLEIC ACIDS: CHEMISTRY, METABOLISM AND APPLIED ASPECTS

Section 10

HEME AND HEMOPROTEINS

Section 11

OXIDATIVE STRESS AND CANCER

Cell and its Biomolecules

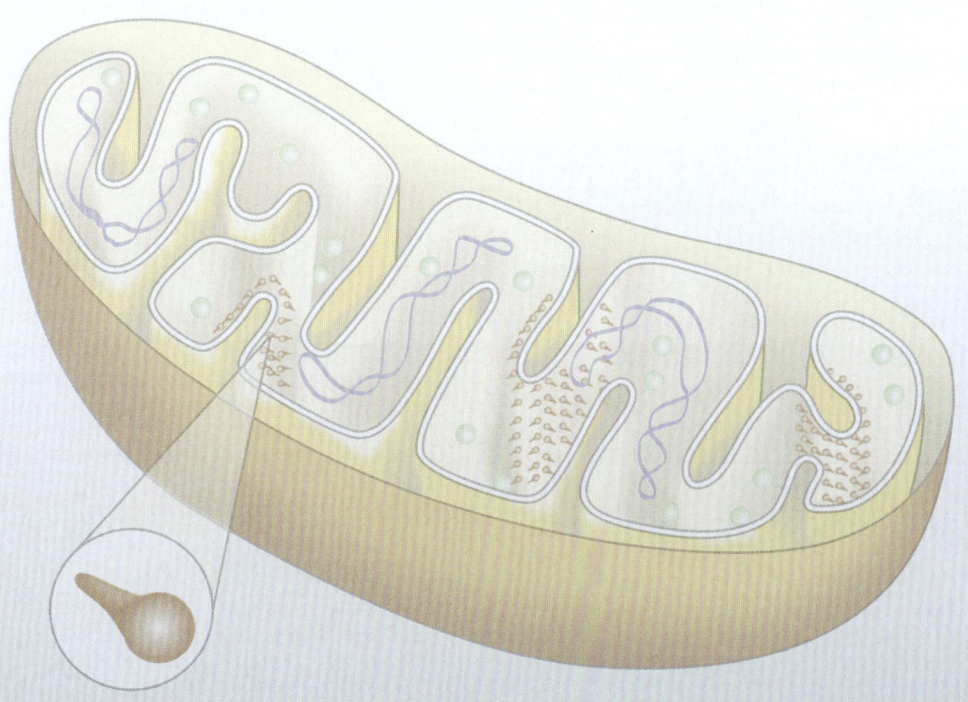

1

Cell and its Biomolecules

1

Cell and its Organelles

All living cell may be classified into two broad categories: Prokaryote and Eukaryote.

Prokaryotes

Prokaryotic cells are characterized by lack of well defined nucleus and internal membranous structures like mitochondria, peroxisomes, etc. They are mostly unicellular. They have dense area in the cell known as nucleoid, where single strand DNA is segregated in discrete mass (Fig. 1.1).

Eukaryotes

Eukaryotic cell may be single cell (yeast, fungi) or may be multicellular (plants, animals). Eukaryotic cell is characterized by well defined nucleus, and other well defined organelles like mitochondria, lysosomes, peroxisomes surrounded by membranes. Membrane system is well defined in eukaryotic cells. This membrane meshwork is organized in important systems like endoplasmic reticulum and Golgi apparatus. Major advantage of presence of organelles in eukaryotes is that the concentration of chemical intermediates can be maximized locally and relatively lower amount of reactants will be desired to get the same outcome (Fig. 1.2).

Basic composition and fundamental chemical reaction is same in both prokaryotic and eukaryotic cells. They do have remarkable differences, e.g. histone protein is found in eukaryotic cells but prokaryotic cells do not contain histone proteins.

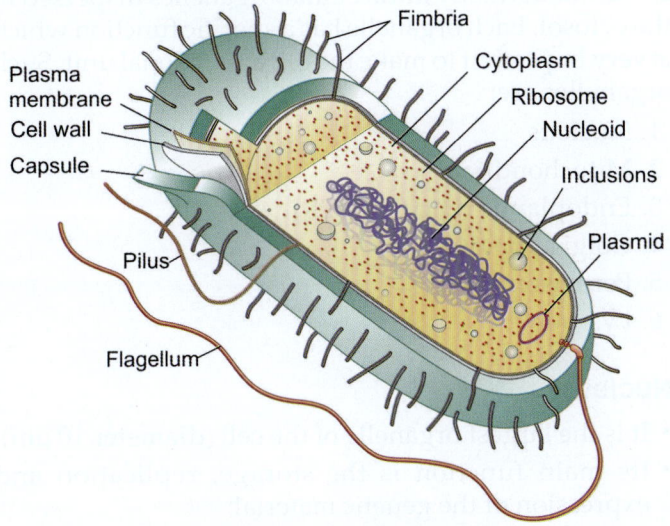

Fig. 1.1: A prokaryotic cell

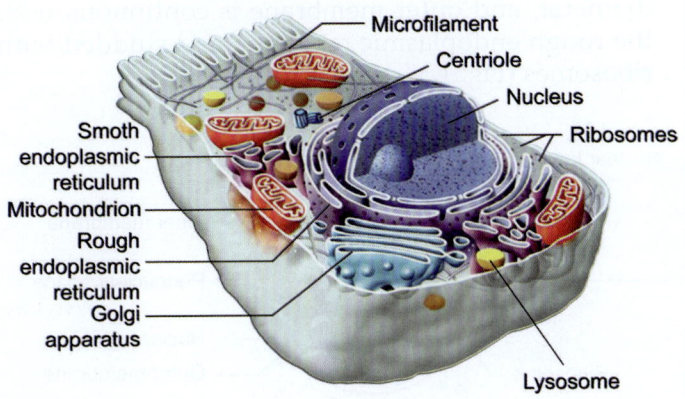

Fig. 1.2: Basic structure of an eukaryotic cell

PLASMA MEMBRANE

Outermost covering of the cell is plasma membrane which consists of mainly lipid and protein. It has numerous functions like

a. Cell morphology and movement
b. Transportation of small molecule and ions
c. Cell-to-cell interaction
d. Recognition
e. Receptor for small molecule.

Detail of structure and function of plasma membrane will be dealt separately in Chapter 2.

DESCRIPTION OF INDIVIDUAL ORGANELLE IN THE EUKARYOTIC CELL

Cell contains many intracellular organelles dispersed in the cytosol. Each organelle has a specific function which is very important to make the cell a functional unit. Such organelles are:

1. Nucleus
2. Mitochondria
3. Endoplamic reticulum (ER)
4. Golgi apparatus
5. Peroxisome
6. Lysosome

Nucleus

- It is the largest organelle of the cell (diameter 10 μm).
- Its main function is the storage, replication and expression of the genetic material.
- Nucleus is surrounded by an envelop which contains outer and inner nuclear membranes. Inner membrane contains a number of pores of approximately 90 Å diameter, and outer membrane is continuous with the rough endoplasmic reticulum and studded with ribosomes (Fig. 1.3).

- Perinuclear space (the space between outer and inner membrane of the nucleus) is continuous with the lumen of rough endoplasmic reticulum.
- In eukaryotic cell, nucleus contains DNA which together with the histone and other structural proteins form chromatin. During cell divison chromatin further condenses to form chromosome.
- Nucleus sometimes contains one or more electron dense region known as nucleolus. DNA in nucleolar area contains gene for rRNA.
- Nucleus is responsible for DNA replication and transcription of various RNA.
- Nucleus also carry a special metabolic task where NAD^+ is synthesized in the nucleolus from its precursor NMN^+ (nicotinamide mononucleotide). NMN^+ is transported to nucleolus from the cytosol where it is converted to NAD^+. Finally, NAD^+ from nucleus is transported to the cytosol. Protein synthesis does not take place in the nucleus. Histone and nonhistone proteins, which are needed in the nucleus are, synthesized in cytosol and are transported to the nucleus.

Mitochondria

- Size of the mitochondria is about 0.5–1.0 μm in diameter and 7 μm in length. Each cell contains a large number of mitochondria (approx. 2000), which constitute 25% of total cell volume.
- In an electron micrograph, mitochondria appear as a rod, sphere or filamentous body which is surrounded by an outer and an inner membrane (OMM and IMM).
- Outer membrane is smooth, but inner membrane contains a number of folds or cristae.
- Between outer and inner membranes, there is intermembranous space (Fig. 1.4). Inner membrane is rich in cardiolipin, but has no cholesterol.

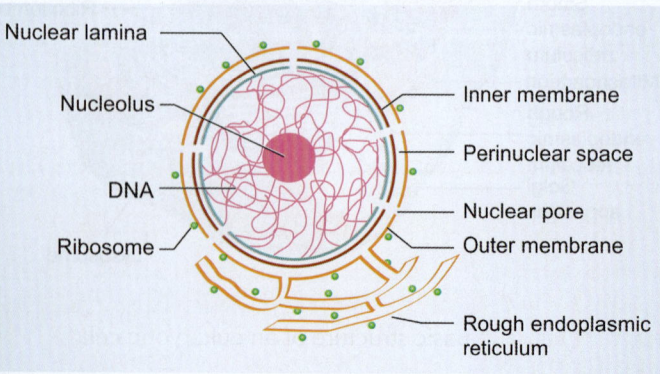

Fig. 1.3: Nucleus

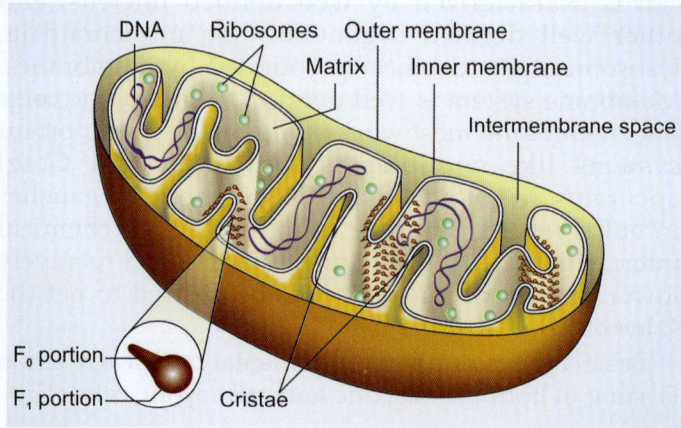

Fig. 1.4: Mitochondrion

- Human mitochondria contain small circular DNA which has code for two rRNA, 22 tRNA and 13 proteins. Outer membrane allows particle less than 10 kDa to pass through it, but inner membrane is completely impermeable, even to small molecule. Inner membrane of mitochondria contains numerous transporters, which allow transportation of many metabolites.
- IMM is the host for many enzymes including enzymes of ETC, which are involved in the process of oxidative phosphorylation.
- Mitochondria are involved in various biochemical processes which are summarized in Table 1.1.

TABLE 1.1	Biochemical processes in which mitochondria are involved	
Inner membrane	Mitosol (matrix)
Oxidative phosphorylation	Fatty acid oxidation
	Heme biosynthesis
	Gluconeogenesis
	Urea synthesis
	TCA cycle
	Amino acid oxidases

- In addition to the roles described above, mitochondria also play a very important role in the process of apoptosis. Cytochrome *c* (a component of ETC) is an initiator of apoptosis.
- Mitochondria also possess 2–10 copies of double stranded circular DNA, which are maternally transmitted.
- Replication of mitochondrial DNA occurs without proofreading, hence it is very much prone for mutation. There are many diseases associated with mitochondrial DNA mutation (Table 1.2).

Endoplasmic Reticulum (ER)

- It is a membrane-bound tubular organelle, which is continuous with the outer membrane of the nucleus. It is a structure which looks like interconnected mesh of membrane-bound tubules.
- There are two types of ER in a cell.
  - a. **Rough endoplasmic reticulum (RER):** These are studded with multiple ribosomes on its outer surface, giving it a rough appearance.
  - b. **Smooth endoplasmic reticulum (SER):** These are devoid of ribosome on the outer surface and hence it is a smooth structure.

Rough Endoplasmic Reticulum (RER)

This is the site of protein synthesis. Those proteins which are destined for lysosome, membrane and for export from the cell (secretory proteins) are synthesized in the ribosome of the rough endoplasmic reticulum. Other proteins are synthesized on the ribosome which are lying free in the cytosol. ER is also involved in protein folding (Fig. 1.5).

Smooth Endoplasmic Reticulum (SER)

These are not studded with the ribosome and are not involved in the biosynthesis of the protein, rather they are involved in lipid synthesis and detoxification reactions (Fig. 1.5).

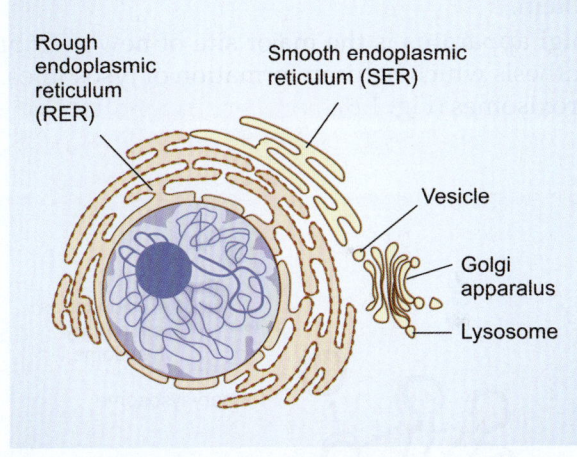

Fig. 1.5: Rough and smooth endoplasmic reticulum

Generally, number of SER is small in a cell, but in cells like hepatocyte and Leydig cell it is abundant. Membrane-bound enzyme of the SER is responsible for phospholipid, cholesterol and steroid hormone synthesis. This also contains enzyme cytochrome P450 which is involved in hydroxylation reactions during biotransformation.

ER and Golgi apparatus are concurrently involved in formation of lysosome and peroxisome and Ca^{++} signaling.

TABLE 1.2	Diseases associated with mitochondrial DNA gene mutation
Laber hereditary optic neuropathy (LHON)	Single base change in mitochondrial gene encoding three subunits (ND1, ND4, ND6) of complex I (ubiquinone oxidoreductase), which lowers the activity of NADH.
MERRF	Myoclonic epilepsy and ragged red fiber
MELAS	Mitochondrial encephalopathy, lactic acidosis and stroke like activity.

ER meshwork is fragmented during cell fractionation and small vesicles called *microsomes* are produced. These microsomes are not present in intact cell.

Golgi Apparatus

- Golgi apparatus is also known as Golgi complex. They are network of flattened smooth membrane stacks-cistern-vesicles.
- They are involved in modification and sorting of various proteins which are to be incorporated into various membranes and organelles or have to be secreted out.
- They also have enzymes which are involved in the process of transfer of carbohydrate residues on newly synthesized protein (glycoconjugation as a post-translational modification). This process of conjugation of carbohydrate on the protein is important in deciding the ultimate destination of the protein.
- Golgi apparatus is the major site of new membrane synthesis which helps in formation of lysosomes and peroxisomes (Fig. 1.6).

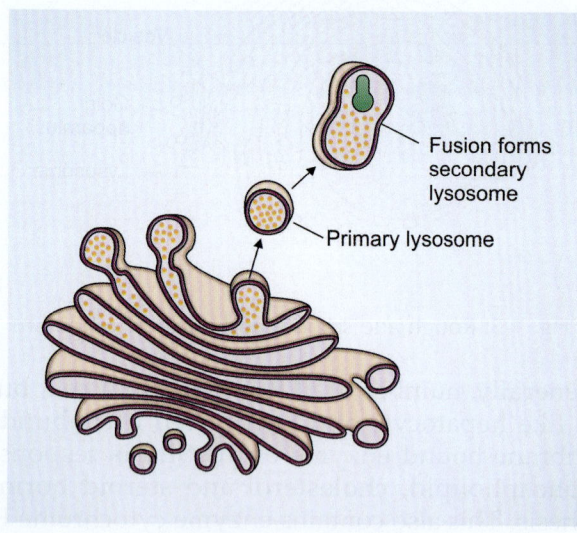

Fig. 1.6: Golgi apparatus

Peroxisome

It is also called microbodies (not to be confused with microsome, which is produced due to fragmentation of ER during cell fractionation) (Fig. 1.7).

As the name implies, these organelles are involved in the production or utilization of hydrogen peroxide. Peroxisomes are spherical as well as oval in shape and surrounded by a single layer of membrane. Their size is small (0.3–1.5 μm).

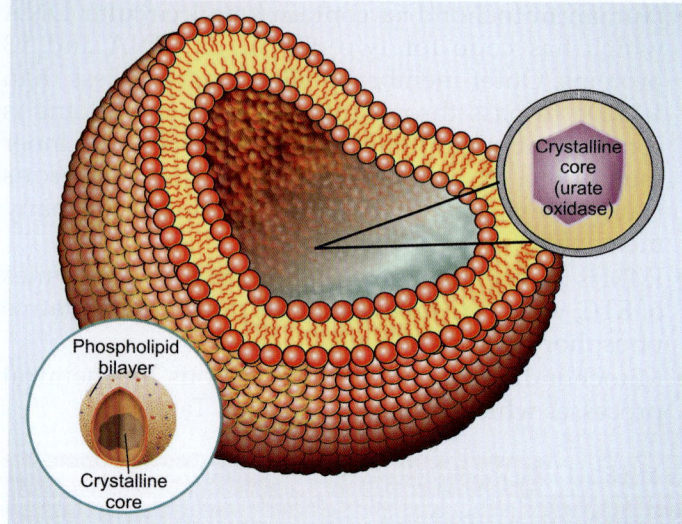

Fig. 1.7: Peroxisome

They play a very important role in

1. Very long chain fatty acid (VLCFA) oxidation
2. Synthesis of glycerolipid
3. Synthesis of glycerol ether lipid (plasmalogen)
4. Synthesis of isoprenoid

Catalase enzyme is found in peroxisome which is involved in conversion of H_2O_2 to H_2O and O_2 molecules.

Zellweger syndrome: This is a severe neurological disorder which is due to absence of functional peroxisome in various cells of the body. Death occurs by age of 6 months. Underlying problem in this disorder is the *defect of mechanism of protein import in the lumen of the peroxisome*. It is an autosomal recessive disorder.

Lysosome

- These organelles are rich in hydrolase class of enzymes (class III) which cleave the carbon-oxygen, carbon-nitrogen, carbon-sulphur, oxygen-phosphorous bonds in lipids, protein, carbohydrate and nucleic acid. The enzymes of lysosome act best at acidic pH, hence intralysosomal pH is 5.
- Primary lysosome fuses with vesicle containing external material which may have been ingested in the cell by phagocytosis, pinocytosis or endocytosis. This creates secondary lysosome in the cell which has both the material as well as the hydrolase enzyme to digest them.
- Lysosomes are involved in the process called autophagy whereby they hydrolyse cellular components like proteins, nucleic acids, lipids and organelles like mitochondria (Fig. 1.6).

I CELL DISEASE (INCLUSION CELL DISEASE)

Here, the defect lies in the targeting of newly synthesised lysosomal enzymes to the lysosome which is due to lack of enzyme 'N-acetyl D-glucosamine phosphotransferase'. This enzyme is responsible for transfer of N-acetylo glucosamine phosphate to high mannose type oligosaccharide of the proteins destined for lysosome.

Fibroblast of affected individual shows dense inclusion bodies (I cell) and lack phosphotransferase activity.

This disease is characterized by severe psychomotor retardation, skeletal abnormality, coarse facial features, and restricted joint movement.

Symptoms are present at birth and death occurs by 8 years of age (Fig. 1.8).

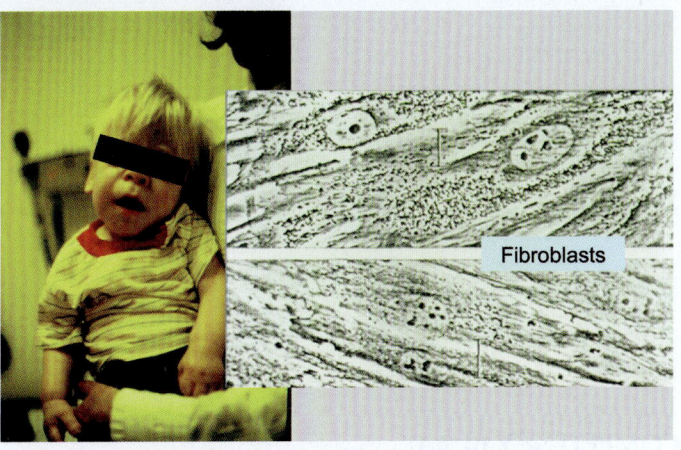

Fig. 1.8: I cell disease (Inclusion cell disease)

2
Enzymes

COMPETENCY BI 2.1

At the end of this chapter learner should be able to explain fundamental concepts of enzyme, isoenzyme, alloenzyme, coenzyme and cofactors. Enumerate the main classes of IUBMB nomenclature.

COMPETENCY BI 2.3

At the end of this chapter learner should be able to describe and explain the basic principles of enzyme activity.

COMPETENCY BI 2.4

At the end of this chapter learner should be able to describe and discuss enzyme inhibitors as poisons and drugs and as therapeutic enzymes.

COMPETENCY BI 2.5

At the end of this chapter learner should be able to describe and discuss the clinical utility of various serum enzymes as markers of pathological conditions.

COMPETENCY BI 2.6

At the end of this chapter learner should be able to discuss use of enzymes in laboratory investigations (enzyme-based assays).

Specific Learning Objectives

BI 2.1.1	Define enzymes, isoenzymes, coenzyme, alloenzymes, cofactors.
BI 2.1.2	Describe functions of isoenzymes, alloenzymes, and coenzymes.
BI 2.3.1	Describe mechanism of action of different enzymes.
BI 2.3.2	Describe 'lock and key' hypothesis.
BI 2.3.3	Describe Koshland's induced fit theory.
BI 2.3.4	Describe Michelis Menten theory.

Contd.

Specific Learning Objectives (*Contd.*)

BI 2.4.1	Describe competitive inhibition.
BI 2.4.2	Describe noncompetitive inhibition.
BI 2.4.3	Describe uncompetitive inhibition.
BI 2.4.4	Describe therapeutic action of enzyme inhibition.
BI 2.5.1	Describe various enzymes used as diagnostic markers of pathological condition.
BI 2.6.1	Enumerate important enzyme based assays used in lab investigation.

Frederich W. Kühne coined the term 'enzyme'.

What is an Enzyme?

- Enzymes are biocatalysts which enhance the rate of a biochemical reaction which otherwise progress very slowly in absence of enzyme.
- Enzymes are neither changed nor lost during or after the reaction and are recovered intact at the end of reaction.

What is the Biochemical Nature of the Enzyme?

Enzymes are mostly proteins. There are certain RNAs which are known to possess enzymatic activity. Such type of RNAs which have catalytic activity, are known as ribozymes.

GENERAL CHARACTERISTIC OF ENZYMES

Enzymes are mostly proteins which are generally heat labile and are water soluble.

CLASSIFICATION OF ENZYMES

According to International Union of Biochemistry and Molecular Biology, 1964 (IUBMB) enzymes are divided into six major classes:

i. Oxidoreductase   iv. Lyase
ii. Transferase   v. Isomerase
iii. Hydrolase   vi. Ligase

Oxidoreductase

Enzymes in this class are involved in transfer of hydrogen ion from one substrate to other. The substrate which is donating the hydrogen is oxidized and the one which is accepting the hydrogen is reduced.

Transferase

Enzymes in this class are involved in transfer of groups other than hydrogen. Various examples of such enzymes are:
- Transminase/aminotransferase
- Methyltransferase
- Transaldolase
- Transketolase
- Kinase
- Pyruvate dehydrogenase complex
- Branching enzyme

Hydrolase

Enzymes of this class use water and cleave the bonds so that the substrate is cleaved into simpler products. These enzymes act in irreversible manner.

All digestive enzymes belong to this class.

Following are the examples of such enzymes:
1. Lipase (cleaves the ester bond)
2. Amylase (cleaves the glycosidic bond)
3. Pepsin (cleaves the peptide bond)
4. Urease (cleaves C–N bond other than peptide bond)

Lyase

Enzymes of this class are involved in cleavage of C–C, C–O and C–N bonds. These bonds are cleaved due to atom elimination. At times the bond is not even cleaved after the atoms are eliminated, rather double bond is left at that place. Nature of enzyme may be reversible or irreversible. Important examples of such enzymes are:
- Aldolase
- Fumarase
- Arginosuccinate lyase
- HMG-CoA lyase
- ATP citrate lyase

Isomerase

This class of enzymes rearranges the atoms within the same molecule. This results in synthesis of isomeric form of the original molecule. Important examples of such enzymes are:
- Methyl malonyl CoA mutase
- Triose phosphate isomerase
- Retinene isomerase
- Epimerase
- Phosphohexose isomerase

Ligase

This class of enzymes catalyzes the joining together of two molecules coupled to the hydrolysis of ATP. Important examples of such enzymes are:
- Acetyl CoA carboxylase (all carboxylases)
- PRPP synthetase
- Glutamine synthetase
- Aminoacyl-tRNA synthetase
- Arginosuccinate synthetase
- Carbamoyl phosphate synthetase I and II

■ MODE OF ACTION OF ENZYME

Enzymes act via lowering the 'activation energy'.

What is 'Activation Energy' and how Enzyme Facilitates its Lowering?

Whenever a substrate is converted to a product, a transient intermediate is produced which is known as transition state.

Difference of energy of the substrate and the transition state is known as activation energy (Fig. 2.1).

Enzyme Lowers Activation Energy.

It is said that whenever the substrate is binding the active site of the enzyme, certain amount of energy known as binding energy is released, which lowers the activation energy.

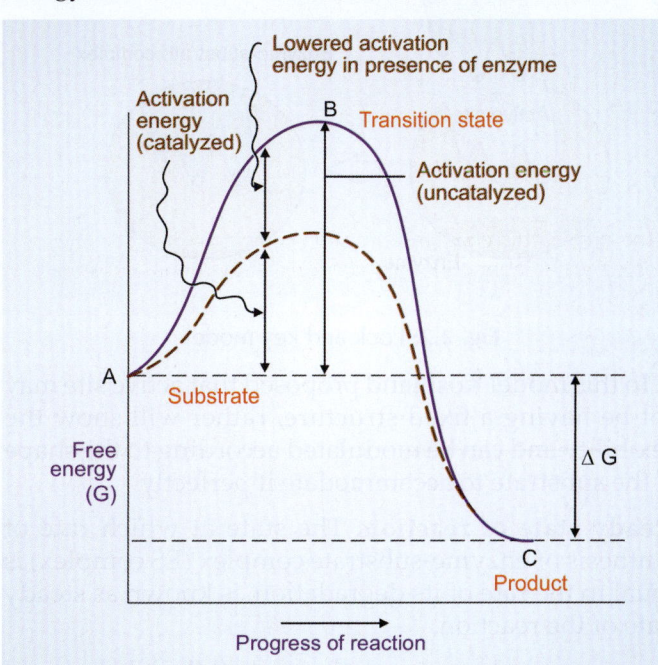

Fig. 2.1: Lowering of activation energy by enzyme

2

What is the Advantage of Lowering of Activation Energy?

In the presence of enzyme when the activation energy is lowered, the reaction proceeds faster and substrate is quickly converted to product.

Models to Explain the Binding of Substrate to the Active Site of the Enzyme

Substrate binds the enzyme at its active site. To explain the binding of substrate to the active site of the enzyme, there are two theories.

1. **Lock and key model (rigid template model):** By Emil Fisher (1890) (Fig. 2.2)
2. **Induced fit model (hand in glove model):** By Daniel E. Koshland (1958) (Fig. 2.3)

In 'lock and key model', it was proposed that the active site of the enzyme has predetermined shape which correctly fits the substrate into it, facilitating the reaction. This was compared to lock and key where key correctly fits into rigid groove in the lock.

This model could explain the specificity with which the enzyme functions, but could not explain the the action of allosteric modifiers on to the enzyme.

Emil Fisher's 'lock and key model' was undebated till 1958, when Daniel E. Koshland proposed 'induced fit model' to explain the binding of the substrate to the enzyme.

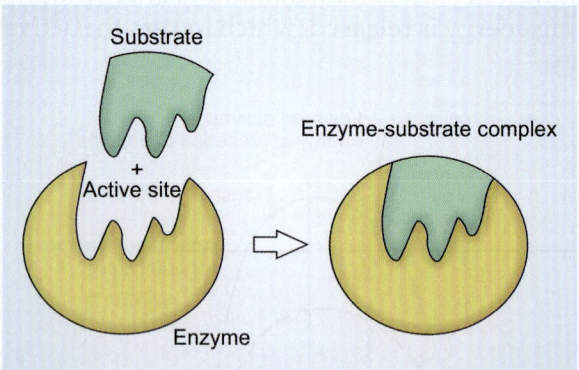

Fig. 2.2: Lock and key model

In this model Koshland proposed that active site may not be having a fixed structure, rather will show the flexibility and can be modulated according to the shape of the substrate to accommodate it perfectly.

Steady state of reaction: The state at which rate of synthesis of enzyme-substrate complex (ES complex) is equal to the rate of its degradation, is known as steady state of the reaction.

Turnover number or catalytic constant (k_{cat}): Number of substrate molecules converted to product by an enzyme

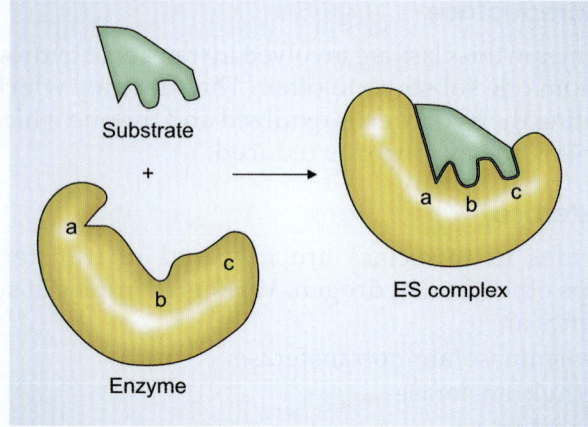

Fig. 2.3: Induced fit model

in unit time is called as turnover number or catalytic constant (k_{cat}).

ENZYME KINETICS

Enzyme kinetics is the study of reaction rate and their response to the changes of experimental parameters.

There are many factors which affect the enzyme kinetics. They are:

1. Substrate concentration
2. Temperature
3. pH
4. Enzyme concentration
5. Product concentration
6. Inhibitors

Effect of Substrate Concentration on Enzyme Kinetics

The effect of substrate concentration on velocity of reaction in a fixed concentration of enzyme is shown in Fig. 2.4.

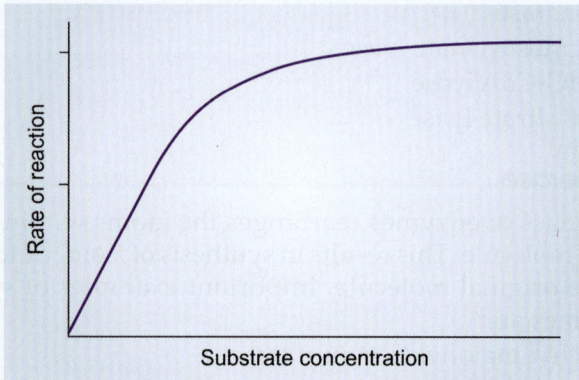

Fig. 2.4: Effect of substrate concentration on reaction velocity

Fig. 2.4 shows, when the substrate concentration is increased, initially the velocity is increased in direct proportion (linear part of the graph/first order kinetics) till all the active site of the enzyme is saturated with the substrate.

Further increase of substrate no more increases the velocity (hyperbolic part of the graph/zero order kinetics), as all the active site of the enzyme is already saturated with the substrate.

Michaelis Constant (K_m)

- It is the substrate concentration at which the velocity of reaction is half of the maximum velocity (Fig. 2.5).
- K_m is the measure of substrate concentration which is required for significant catalysis to occur.
- K_m signifies that half of the active sites of the enzyme is saturated with the substrate.
- K_m also signifies the affinity of substrate to the enzyme. Numerically K_m value is inversely proportional to the affinity of the substrate.

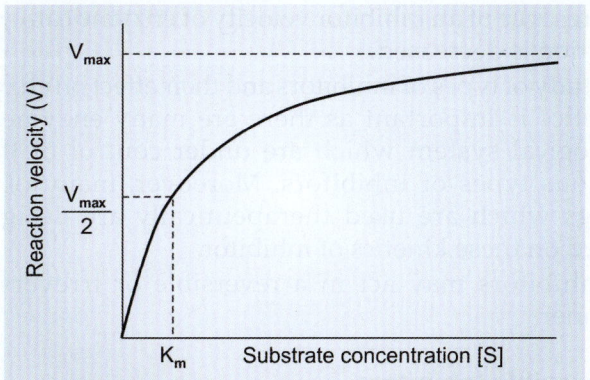

Fig. 2.5: Plot to show K_m value (Michaelis Menten constant)

- K_m is the numerical value which has a unit. Unit of K_m is same as that of substrate concentration.
- K_m is said to be the 'signature of enzyme' as it is used to identify the unknown enzyme which is separated from a protein mixture.
- K_m is sensitive to pH, temperature and ionic strength of the solution.
- Isoenzymes of an enzyme may have different substrate affinity and hence different K_m values.

Lineweaver-Burk Plot (Double Reciprocal Plot)

When 1/S concentration and 1/V is plotted on X- and Y-axes, respectively, we get Lineweaver-Burk plot (double reciprocal plot). The point at which line intersects the X-axis represents $-1/K_m$ numerically and the point at which line intersects the Y-axis represents $1/V_{max}$ numerically (Fig. 2.6).

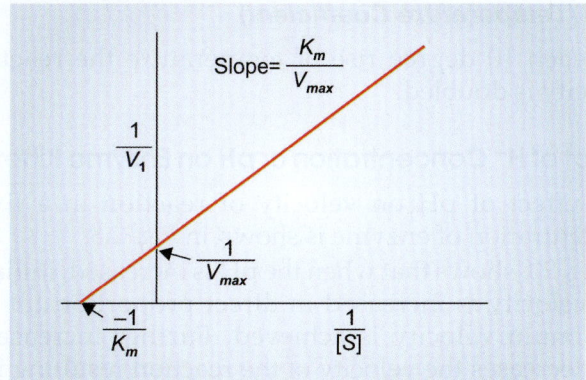

Fig. 2.6: Lineweaver-Burk plot (double reciprocal plot)

Major use of this plot resides in the fact that kinetic mechanism of enzyme inhibitor can be determined with greater ease using this plot compared to Michaelis Menten graph.

Effect of Temperature on Enzyme Kinetics (Bell Shaped)

The effect of temperature on velocity of reaction in a fixed concentration of enzyme is shown in Fig. 2.7.

Fig. 2.7 shows that when the temperature is increased, initially the velocity is increased in direct proportion till the maximum velocity is achieved. Further increase of temperature decreases the velocity of the reaction resulting in a bell-shaped curve.

The temperature at which the velocity of the reaction is maximum is known as optimum temperature. Rise of temperature initially increases the velocity of reaction due to the fact that this temperature overcomes the energy barrier, but further increase of temperature denatures the active site of the enzyme which leads to lowering of the velocity of enzyme catalyzed reaction.

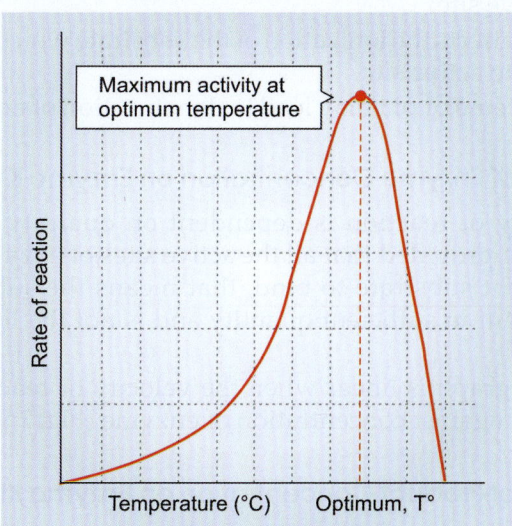

Fig. 2.7: Bell-shaped curve to show optimum T°

Section 1 ■ Cell and its Biomolecules

2

Q10 (Temperature Coefficient)

For each 10 degree rise of temperature the reaction velocity is doubled.

Effect of H⁺ Concentration or pH on Enzyme Kinetics

The effect of pH on velocity of reaction in a fixed concentration of enzyme is shown in Fig. 2.8.

Fig. 2.8 shows that when the pH is increased, initially the velocity is increased in direct proportion till the maximum velocity is achieved. Further increase of pH decreases the velocity of the reaction resulting in a bell-shaped curve. The pH at which the velocity of the reaction is maximum is known as optimum pH.

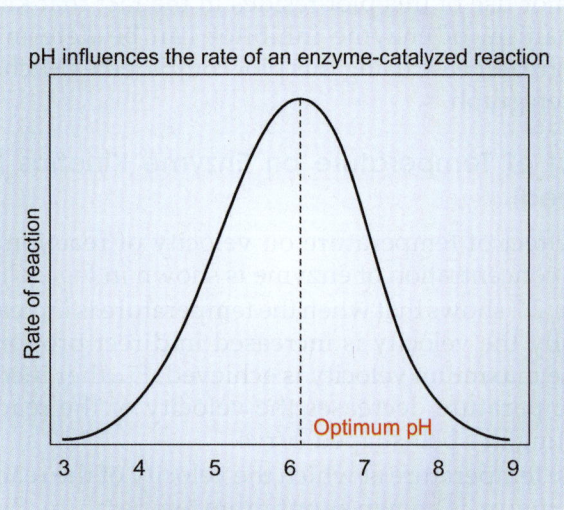

Fig. 2.8: Bell-shaped curve to show optimum pH

Changing H⁺ concentration and so the pH, affects the enzyme activity in many ways:
a. pH affects the ionization of the amino acids at the active site.
b. pH affects the ionization of the substrate which binds at the active site.
c. Extreme of pH may lead to denaturation of enzyme.

Effect of Enzyme Concentration on Enzyme Kinetics

Velocity of reaction is dependent on quantity of the enzyme provided that all the active sites of enzyme get sufficient substrate to bind, that means the substrate is present in sufficient quantity and is not the limiting factor.

The graph is linear when the velocity of reaction is plotted against concentration of enzyme (Fig. 2.9).

Effect of Product Concentration on Enzyme Kinetics

Product imparts inhibitory affect on the activity of the enzyme. This is called product inhibition. This type of

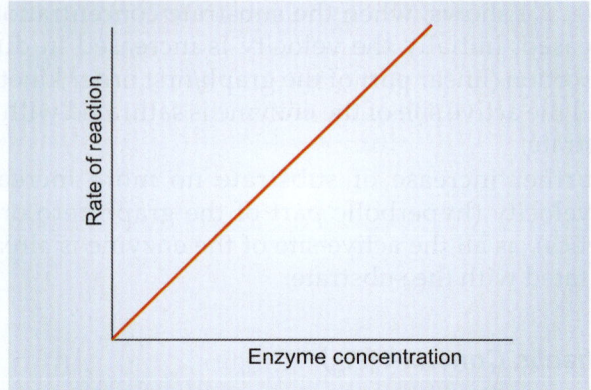

Fig. 2.9: Effect of enzyme concentration on reaction velocity

inhibition is not generally observed as the product of one enzymatic reaction acts as a substrate for another enzymatic reaction.

Effect of Inhibitors on Enzyme Kinetics

An inhibitor is any substance which decreases the velocity of an enzyme catalyzed reaction. In other words in presence of an inhibitor velocity of enzyme catalyzed reaction is decreased.

Study of types of inhibitors and their effect on enzyme kinetics is important as there are many enzymes in biological system which are under control of these various types of inhibitors. Moreover, many of the drugs which are used therapeutically are designed based on these kinetics of inhibitor.

Inhibitors may act in a reversible or irreversible manner.

Reversible Inhibitors

Such type of inhibitors bind the enzyme in a reversible fashion mostly in noncovalent bond.

Full function of enzyme is restored once the inhibitor is dissociated from the enzyme.

There are various types of inhibitors which act in a reversible fashion:
1. Competitive inhibitor
2. Noncompetitive inhibitors
3. Uncompetitive inhibitors

▣ Competitive inhibitors

- Such type of inhibitors are structurally similar to the substrate and hence they compete with the substrate to bind at the active site.
- The binding of such inhibitors at the active site is through noncovalent bond.
- Inhibitors may get dissociated at the active site as the noncovalent bond is weak and hence it is a reversible type of inhibition.

- In this type of inhibition when the inhibitor binds the active site, no product is formed.
- At very high concentration of substrate the effect of inhibitor will be negligible as practically all the substrate will get the opportunity to bind the active site resulting in the achievement of maximum velocity which is possible for that enzyme.

> New maximum velocity and new K_m value in the presence of inhibitor is known as apparent V_{max} and apparent K_m value respectively (V'_{max} and K'_m).

Following is the effect of competitive inhibitors on the kinetics of enzyme:

1. *Effect on V_{max}:* The effect of a competitive inhibitor is reversed by increasing [S]. At a sufficiently high substrate concentration, the reaction velocity reaches the V_{max} observed in the absence of inhibitor.
2. *Effect on K_m:* A competitive inhibitor increases the apparent K_m for a given substrate. This means that in the presence of a competitive inhibitor more substrate is needed to achieve ½ V_{max}.
3. *Effect on Lineweaver-Burk plot:* Competitive inhibition shows a characteristic Lineweaver-Burk plot in which the plots of the inhibited and uninhibited reactions intersect on the Y-axis at $1/V_{max}$ (V_{max} is unchanged). The inhibited and uninhibited reactions show different X-axis intercepts, indicating that the apparent K_m is increased in the presence of the competitive inhibitor (Fig. 2.10).

Examples of competitive inhibitors:
1. Sulphonamide as para-aminobenzoic acid analogue
2. Methotrexate as dihydrofolate reductase inhibitor
3. Dicumarol as vitamin K analogue
4. Statins as HMG-CoA reductase analogue
5. Ethanol in methanol poisoning
6. 5-Fluorouracil as an inhibitor of thiamidylate synthase.
7. Isoniazid (INH) as vitamin B_6 analogue

◪ Noncompetitive inhibition (Mixed type of inhibition)
This type of inhibition is recognized by its characteristic effect on V_{max} and occurs when the inhibitor and substrate bind at different sites on the enzyme. The noncompetitive inhibitor can bind either free enzyme or the ES complex, thereby preventing the reaction from occurring.

1. *Effect on V_{max}:* Noncompetitive inhibition cannot be overcome by increasing the concentration of

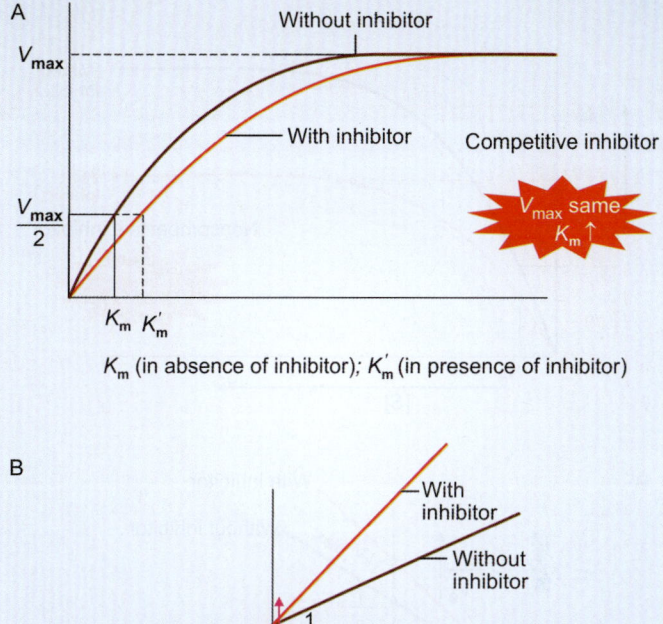

Fig. 2.10: Effect of competitive inhibitors (A = effect shown on Michaelis Mentem plot, B = effect shown on Lineweaver-Burk plot

substrate. Thus, noncompetitive inhibitors decrease the V_{max} of the reaction.

2. *Effect on K_m:* Noncompetitive inhibitors do not interfere with the binding of substrate to enzyme. Thus, the enzyme shows the same K_m in the presence or absence of the noncompetitive inhibitor.

3. *Effect on Lineweaver-Burk plot:* Noncompetitive inhibition is readily differentiated from competitive inhibition by plotting $1/V_0$ *vs* $1/[S]$ and noting that V_{max} decreases in the presence of a noncompetitive inhibitor, whereas K_m is unchanged (Fig. 2.11).

Examples of noncompetitive inhibitors:
1. Cyanide as cytochrome oxidase inhibitor
2. Fluoride as enolase inhibitor in glycolysis
3. Iodoacetate as inhibitor of glyceraldehyde-3-phosphate dehydrogenase
4. British anti-Lewisite (BAL) as antidote of heavy metal poisoning
5. Organophosphorus poisoning as an inhibitor of acetylcholinesterase.

Section 1 ■ Cell and its Biomolecules

2

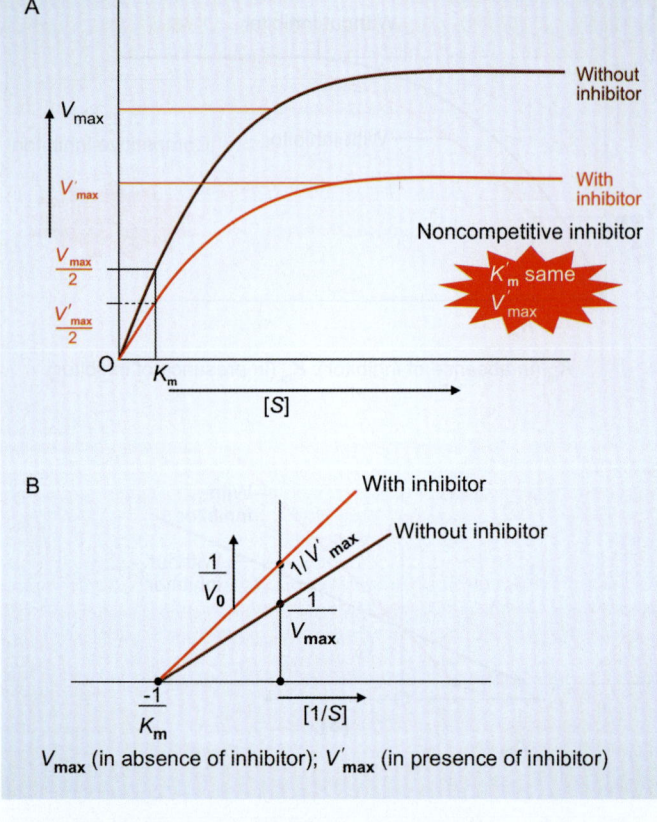

Fig. 2.11: Effect of noncompetitive inhibitors (A = effect shown on Michaelis Menten plot; B = effect shown on Lineweaver-Burk plot

▣ Uncompetitive inhibition

This type of inhibition is recognized by decrease of both V_{max} and K_m value. It is a very rare type of inhibition.

Example: Inhibition of placental ALP by phenyl alanine (Fig. 2.12).

Irreversible Inhibitors

This type of inhibitors bind the enzyme covalently and tightly and are not dissociated from them leading to irreversible type of inhibition.

Irreversible inhibitors may be of following types:

1. Group specific inhibitors
2. Substrate analogue inhibitors (affinity labels)
3. Suicidal inhibitors (mechanism based in-activation)

∎ SUICIDAL INHIBITION

Suicidal inhibition is also called as 'mechanism based inactivation' as in this type of inhibition of enzymes, the enzyme's own activity is utilized first, to convert a less potent inhibitor to more potent inhibitor. This more

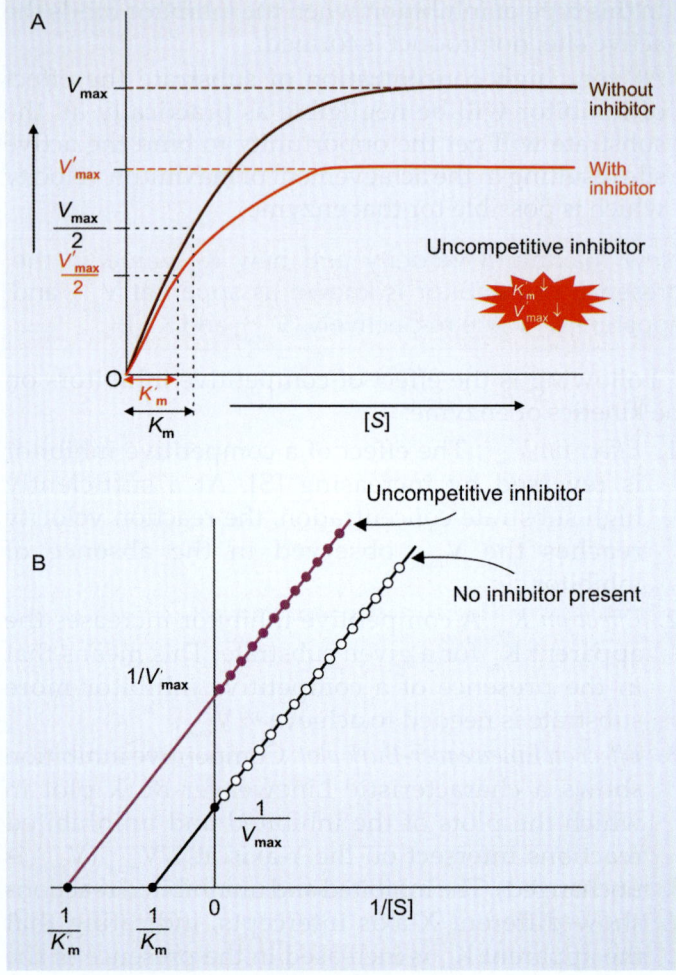

Fig. 2.12: Effect of uncompetitive inhibitors (A = effect shown on Michaelis Menten plot; B = effect shown on Lineweaver-Burk plot

potent inhibitor in turn inactivates the enzyme which actually had synthesized it.

In other words, enzyme synthesizes its own poison.

Allopurinol given to reduce hyperuricemia shows suicidal inhibition of xanthine oxidase.

Xanthine oxidase is the enzyme which converts hypoxanthine to xanthine and xanthine to uric acid (Fig. 2.13).

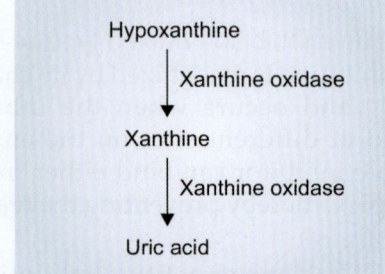

Fig. 2.13: Role of xanthine oxidase in uric acid synthesis

2

Allopurinol as such does not inhibit the action of xanthine oxidase. It is first converted to alloxanthine by action of xanthine oxidate (Fig. 2.14).

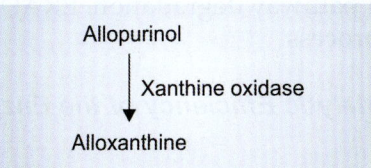

Fig. 2.14: Activation of allopurinol by xanthine oxidase

This alloxanthine now competes with xanthine for xanthine oxidase and inhibits it. It is a classic example of suicidal inhibition.

COFACTOR AND COENZYME

Some enzymes require an additional chemical component for their activity, this additional component is known as cofactor.

Cofactor may be inorganic ions, such as Fe^{++}, Mg^{++}, Mn^{++} or Zn^{++}; or it may be a complex organic or metallo-organic molecule called a coenzyme (Tables 2.1 and 2.2).

Coenzyme may be covalently or noncovalently linked.

Prosthetic group denotes covalently bound cofactor. Example:

1. Biotin as prosthetic group for carboxylase enzymes.
2. Heme as prothestic group for cytochromes.

Serine proteases: These are proteolytic enzymes with serine residue at its active center. Trypsin, chymotrypsin, thrombin and elastin are examples of such enzymes.

TABLE 2.1	Inorganic elements as a cofactor for certain enzymes
Cu^{++}	Superoxide dismutase (SOD) Monoamino oxidase (MAO) Lysyl oxidase Cytochrome oxidase ALA synthase Tyrosinase
Fe^{++}/Fe^{+++}	Cytochrome oxidase Catalase Peroxidase Proline hydroxylase
K^+	Pyruvate kinase
Mg^{++}	Hexokinase Glucose-6-phosphatase Pyruvate kinase
Mn^{++}	Arginase Superoxide dismutase (SOD) Ribonucleotide reductase
Se	Glutathione peroxidase (GPO) Deiodinase
Zn^{++}	Carbonic anhydrase Alcohol dehydrogenase Carboxypeptidase A and B ALA synthase Superoxide dismutase (SOD) RNA polymerase ALP LDH
Mo (molybdenum)	Xanthine oxidase Sulphite oxidase Aldehyde oxidase

TABLE 2.2	Coenzymes and the group they transfer	
Coenzyme	*Group they transfer*	*Dietary precursor*
Biocytin	CO_2	Biotin
Coenzyme A	Acyl group	Pantothenic acid and other compound
FAD	Electron	Riboflavin (vit. B_2)
Lipoate	Electron and acyl group	Not required in diet
NAD	Hydride ion (H^-)	Nicotinic acid (niacin)
Pyridoxal phosphate (PLP)	Amino group	Pyridoxine (B_6)
THF	1 carbon group	Folate
TPP	Aldehyde	Thiamine
Coenzyme B_{12} (5'-deoxyadenosylcobalamin)	H atom and alkyl group	Vit. B_{12}

Section 1 ■ Cell and its Biomolecules

2

Regulation of Enzyme Activity

Overall activity of an enzyme in a rate-limiting step of a pathway depends upon two important factors:
  a. Concentration of the enzyme
  b. Intrinsic catalytic efficiency of the enzyme

Concentration of the Enzyme and Regulation of its Level

Enzymes in a biochemical system are constantly undergoing turnover. It means there is constant synthesis and degradation of the enzymes at a particular rate.

The net concentration of enzyme may be altered by changing the rate constant of synthesis (K_s) or degradation (K_{deg}) or both.

Induction of enzyme synthesis: Enzyme transcription from its gene may be enhanced by an inducer which may be its own substrate, structurally related compound or totally irrelevant molecule.

There are many enzymes which are inducible in human. They are:
  • HMG CoA reductase
  • Tryptophan pyrrolase
  • ALA (aminolevulinic acid) synthase
  • Cytochrome P450
  • Threonine dehydratase
  • Urea cycle enzymes

Repression of enzyme synthesis: Many enzymes are under repression by many factors. Gene of ALA synthase (the rate limiting enzyme of heme biosynthesis) is under repression by heme.

When the gene is derepressed in lack of heme then only the enzyme ALA synthase is synthesized and the heme synthesis can take place (Fig. 2.15).

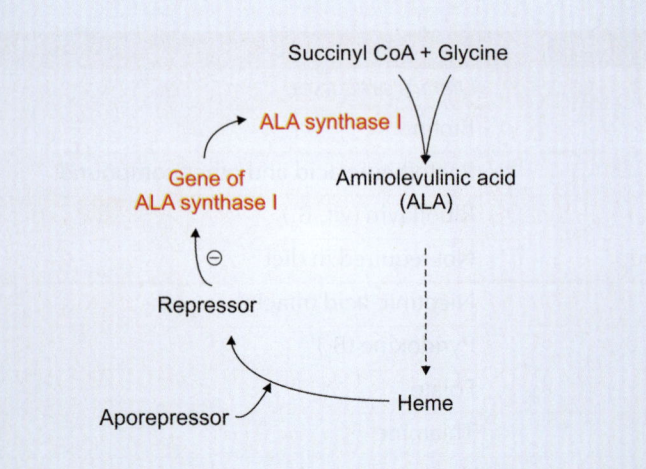

Fig. 2.15: Repression and derepression of enzyme

Degradation of enzyme by endoplasmic reticulum associated degradation (ERAD) (ubiquitin-mediated degradation): Regulatory enzymes having short half-life are important substrate for ubiquitin-mediated proteasomal pathway degradation. ERAD is an energy dependent process.

Intrinsic Catalytic Efficiency of the Enzyme and its Regulation

Two important ways by which intrinsic catalytic efficiency of an enzyme may be altered are:
  (a) Allosteric regulation
  (b) Covalent modification.

In contrast to hours/days needed for changing the concentration of enzyme by regulating its synthesis and degradation, the time duration needed for changing the intrinsic catalytic activity by allosteric or covalent regulation of the enzyme is quite less (seconds/minutes).

Regulation of intrinsic catalytic efficiency is a short term rapid response while regulation of enzyme concentration is a long-term adaptive response.

Allosteric Regulation of Enzyme Activity

• All enzymes have active site where substrate binds.
• Some enzymes have other sites in addition to active site where allosteric modifier bind and change the activity of active site.
• Allosteric modifier do not have any structural resemblence to substrate.
• The activity of enzymes that catalyzes key regulatory reactions (committed steps) of metabolic pathways are often subject to allosteric regulation. Their activity can be modulated by the binding of allosteric effectors to a site on the enzyme that is distinct from the active site (i.e. allosteric site). Effectors are positive, if they enhance the rate of a reaction (i.e. activators) and negative, if they decrease the rate of reaction (i.e. inhibitors).
• Allosteric modifier may be positive or negative depending upon whether they are increasing the activity of active site or decreasing the activity of active site.
• Allosteric modifier may be homotropic or heterotropic. when substrate itself acts as an allosteric modifier, it is called *homotropic effect*, and when allosteric effectors are different from substrate, it is called *heterotropic effect*.
• Allosteric enzymes do not obey Michaelis Menten behavior. They do not produce hyperbolic substrate saturation curve rather they produce sigmoidal saturation kinetic curve.

- Allosteric enzymes may be classified into *k series* enzyme and *v series enzyme*.

 k series: Here substrate saturation kinetics is like competitive inhibition (*V_{max}* same but *K_m* increased).

 v series: Here substrate sturation kinetics is like noncompetitive inhibition (*V_{max}* decreased but *K_m* same).

What is feed-forward reaction?

ATP synthesized in purine nucleotide biosynthesis stimulates pyrimidine nucleotide biosynthesis by allosteric activation of aspartate transcarbamoylase (ATC) enzyme. It is an example of feed-forward reaction.

Regulation of Enzyme Activity by Covalent Modification

- May be reversible or irreversible
- To regulate the catalytic activity of enzyme the types of covalent modification which are observed, are:
  a. Partial proteolysis
  b. Phosphorylation
- Histone and other DNA binding protein undergo various covalent modifications like methylation, acetylation, phosphorylation, ADP-ribosylation. Such modification of histone protein changes their interaction with DNA and hence chromatin structure (euchromatin *vs* heterochromatin). This certainly has effect on gene transcription and DNA replication.
- Phosphorylation of protein occurs at specific amino acid like serinyl, threonyl or tyrosyl by protein kinase. Such phosphate group may be removed by protein phosphatase enzyme. In certain enzymes, the addition of a phosphate group to a specific amino acid residue dramatically enhances or depresses the enzymatic activity.
- Other residues which may be target for phosphorylation may be histidyl, lysyl, arginyl and aspartyl residue.

 List of enzymes where catalytic activity is altered by phosphorylation/dephosphorylation is given in Table 2.3.

TABLE 2.3	List of enzymes active in phosphorylated and dephosphorylated states	
Active in phosphorylated state	*Active in dephosphorylated state*	
Glycogen phosphorylase	Acetyl CoA carboxylase	
Citrate lyase	Glycogen synthase	
Phosphorylase β kinase	PDH	
HMG-CoA reductase kinase	HMG CoA reductase	
Fructose-2,6-bisphosphatase	PFK-2	
Hormone sensitive lipase	Pyruvate kinase	

- Most common types of covalent modification are phosphorylation, dephosphorylation and acetylation and deacetylation. Other types are glycosylation, hydroxylation and prenylation.
- Protein phosphorylation may have following effect on effect of protein:
  - Catalytic efficiency of the enzyme may get effected.
  - Alteration of protein location in the cell
  - Susceptibility of protein for degradation
  - Response to allosteric regulator may vary.

Compartmentalization

Sometimes the various enzymes of a pathway are distributed in different compartments of the cell. For example, enzymes of urea biosynthesis, heme biosynthesis and gluconeogenesis are distributed both in mitochondria and cytosol. Such kind of physical barrier which separates the enzyme of a pathway in different compartments of the cell helps in better regulation of enzymes.

ISOENZYMES

Isoenzymes are different molecular forms of enzymes that may be isolated from the same or different tissues.

 Isoenzymes are physically distinct and separable forms of given enzymes.

Types of Isoenzymes

a. **True isoenzymes:** Here the genes of isoenzymes are different which may be located on same or different chromosomes.
  - Malate dehydrogenase isoenzymes (cytosolic and mitochondrial), are derived from different genes located on the same chromosome.
  - Salivary and pancreatic amylase are derived from different genes located on different chromosomes.

TABLE 2.4	Hybrid isoenzymes
LDH1	HHHH
LDH2	HHHM
LDH3	HHMM
LDH4	HMMM
LDH5	MMMM
CPK-1	BB
CPK-2	MB
CPK-3	MM

Section 1 ■ Cell and its Biomolecules

2

b. **Hybrid isoenzymes:** Here isoenzymes are made up of more than two subunits which are different. It is a varied subunit combination which gives rise to different isoenzymes, e.g. LDH isoenzymes, CPK isoenzymes (LDH is made up of four subunits either of all H, or all M or HM in varied combination) (Table 2.4).

c. **Allozymes/Allelozymes:** Here isoenzymes are derived from different alleles of the same gene, e.g. G6PD. There are more than 300 alleles known for G6PD of human species.

d. **Isoforms:** These isoforms are derived after different post-translational modifications, e.g. sialic acid content of ALP in various isoenzymes is different.

Characteristics of Isoenzymes

1. Same function/biochemical role
2. Different structure
3. Different electrophoretic mobility
4. Different immunological characteristics
5. Different affinity to substrate
6. Different K_m value.

Certain Definitions

1. **Specific activity of enzyme:** On separation of enzyme from a protein mixture it is important to assess the purity of preparation. This is assessed by 'specific activity of enzyme'.
   'Specific activity of enzyme' is defined as 'number of enzyme units in each mg of separated protein'. Its unit is IU/mg. Higher the specific activity of the enzyme, purer the preparation is.

2. **Katal:** One katal is defined as 'amount of enzyme which is required to convert one mole of substrate to its product in one second time'.

3. **International unit:** One IU is defined as amount of enzyme required to convert one mole of substrate to its product in one minute duration.

Relation between IU and Katal
1 IU = 60 millikatal (m kat)

We need to have lesser amount of enzyme in one IU compared to amount of enzyme required to make one Katal unit.

ENZYMES IN DIAGNOSTICS AND THERAPEUTICS

In addition to their role in enhancing the rate of reaction, enzymes also are used in diagnosis and therapeutics (Table 2.5).

TABLE 2.5	Enzymes in diagnostics and therapeutics
Enzymes in diagnostics	*Used for*
Alanine aminotransferase (ALT)	• Hepatocyte damage
Aspartate aminotransferase (AST)	• Hepatocyte damage • Myocardial infarction
Amylase	• Pancreatic disease
Alkaline phosphatase (ALP)	• Hepatobilliary disorder • Bone disease
Acid phosphatase	• Prostate cancer
Prostate specific antigen (PSA)	• Prostate cancer
Creative kinase	• MI muscle dystrophy
Enzymes in therapeutics	*Used for*
Streptokinase • Bacterial asparginase	To lyse blood clot In treatment of leukemia
Enzymes in analysis	*Used for*
GDD-POD	Glucose estimation
Uricase	Uric acid estimation
Urease	Urea estimation
CHOD and POD	Cholesterol estimation

EXERCISE

LONG QUESTIONS (10 MARKS EACH)

Q 1. Describe different types of inhibition of enzymes. Show their effect on enzyme kinetics with the help of double reciprocal graph.

Q 2. What are isoenzymes? How many varieties of isoenzymes you know? Describe the diagnostic significance of the isoenzymes of lactate dehydrogenase.

SHORT NOTES (5 MARKS EACH)

Q 1. Profile of serum enzymes in diagnosis of myocardial infarction

Q 2. Classification of enzymes (IUPAC system) with two examples in each class

Q 3. Diagrams of double reciprocal plot (Lineweaver-Burk plot) of enzyme activity *vs* substrate concentration in presence and absence of a noncompetitive inhibitor of an enzyme and mark $1/V_{max}$ and $-1/K_m$ on the diagrams

Q 4. Michaelis Menten equation and its importance

Q 5. Isoenzymes and their importance in the diagnosis of myocardial infarction

Q 6. Differences between cofactors and coenzymes

Q 7. Covalent modification of enzymes and its metabolic significance, using glycogen turnover as an example

Q 8. Factors affecting rate of enzyme catalysed reaction

Q 9. Role of metal ions in enzyme catalysis

Q 10. Enzyme inhibition, two examples of competitive inhibition and any two drugs which are based on competitive inhibition

Q 11. General properties of an allosteric enzyme and one example of the reaction catalysed by an allosteric enzyme

MULTIPLE CHOICE QUESTIONS

2.1 The substrate saturation curve given below is the characteristic of allosteric enzyme. True statement is:

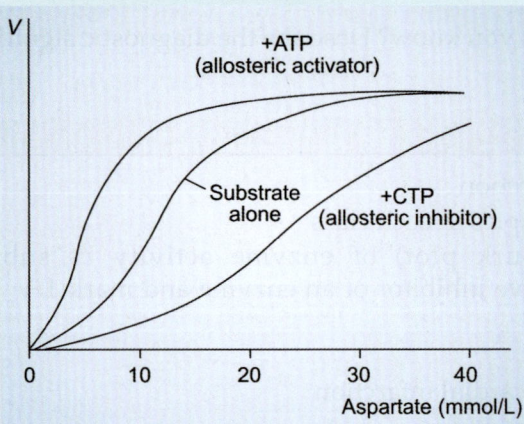

a. Allosteric modifier binds in a concentration dependent manner
b. Modifier can affect the catalytic site by binding to the allosteric site
c. Adding more substrate to the enzyme can displace the allosteric modifier
d. Allosteric modifiers change the binding constant of the enzyme but not the velocity of reaction

2.2 Activator of sulphite oxidase is:
    a. Molybdenum
    b. Copper
    c. Selenium
    d. Zinc

2.3 Treatment of multiple carboxylase deficiency is:
    a. Biotin
    b. Pyridoxine
    c. Thiamine
    d. Folic acid

2.4 All are true about oxygenase enzymes, except:
    a. Incorporate one oxygen atom in the substrate
    b. Incorporate two oxygen atoms in the substrate

    c. Involved in hydroxylation reaction
    d. Involved in carboxylation of drugs

2.5 All of the following enzymes are regulated by calcium or calmodulin, except:
    a. Adenylate cyclase
    b. Glycogen synthase
    c. Guanylyl cyclase
    d. Hexokinase

2.6 The predominant isoenzyme of LDH in the cardiac muscle is:
    a. LDH-1
    b. LDH-2
    c. LDH-3
    d. LDH-5

2.7 All are nonfunctional enzymes, except:
    a. Alkaline phosphatase
    b. Acid phosphatase
    c. Lipoprotein lipase
    d. Gamma glutamyl transpeptidase

2.8 Refsum's disease is due to deficiency of which of the following enzymes?
    a. Malonate dehydrogenase
    b. Thiophorase
    c. Succinate thiokinase
    d. Phytanic acid alpha oxidase

2.9 Which of the following enzymes is active in dephosphorylated state?
    a. HMG-CoA reductase
    b. Glycogen phosphorylase
    c. Glycogen phosphorylase kinase
    d. Citrate lyase
    e. Glycogen synthase

2.10 Zinc is a cofactor for:
    a. Pyruvate dehydrogenase
    b. Pyruvate decarboxylase
    c. α-ketoglutarate dehydrogenase
    d. Alcohol dehydrogenase

ANSWERS

2.1 (b) Modifier can affect the catalytic site by binding to the allosteric site

- Allosteric enzyme does not bind the modifier in concentration dependent manner as exemplified by sigmoidal shape of such curve.
- Allosteric modifier binds the allosteric site and addition of more substrate as such does not displaces the allosteric modifier from allosteric sites.
- Allosteric modifier changes both the binding constant of the enzyme and velocity of reaction.

2.2 (a) Molybdenum

2.3 (a) Biotin

Biotin is a water-soluble vitamin and acts as a coenzyme for carboxylase group of enzymes.

2.4 (d) Involved in carboxylation of drugs

- Oxygenases are oxidoreductase class of enzymes where, oxygen is incorporated into the substrate.
- Mono-oxygenase incorporates one atom of the oxygen into the substrate.
- Addition of hydroxyl group is catalysed by mono-oxygenase enzymes.
- Dioxygenase incorporates two atoms of the oxygen into the substrate.
- Carboxylation is catalysed by carboxylase group of enzyme which incorporates CO_2 into the substrate.

2.5 (d) Hexokinase

Following is the list of enzymes which are regulated by calcium or calmodulin:
1. Adenylyl cyclase
2. Guanylyl cyclase
3. Glycogen synthase
4. Phospholipase A2
5. Pyruvate carboxylase
6. Pyruvate dehydrogenase
7. Pyruvate kinase
8. Phosphodiesterase
9. Glycerol-3-phosphate dehydrogenase

2.6 (a) LDH-1

In normal plasma, LDH-2 is more in concentration than LDH-1.

In myocardial infarction level of LDH-1 increases and this leads to altered ratio of LDH isoenzymes. It means LDH-1 becomes more than LDH-2 (LDH-1 > LDH-2).

This altered ratio of the LDH is known as **flipped pattern**.

2.7 (c) Lipoprotein lipase

Nonfunctional plasma enzymes are those which normally do not function/reside in the plasma, rather they come to plasma only due to damage of respective cell where they are normally reside.

Example:
- Lipoprotein lipase
- Clotting factor
- 5'-nucleotidase

2.8 (d) Phytanic acid alpha oxidase

2.9 (a) HMG-CoA reductase and (e) Glycogen synthase

Enzymes active in dephosphorylated state
- Glycogen synthase
- Glucokinase
- Phosphofructokinase
- Pyruvate kinase
- HMG-CoA reductase

Enzymes active in phosphorylated state
- Glycogen phosphorylase
- Phosphorylase kinase
- HMG-CoA reductase kinase
- Hormone sensitive lipase
- Citrate lyase

2.10 (d) Alcohol dehydrogenase

Enzymes requiring Zn are:
a. Carbonic anhydrase
b. Alcohol dehydrogenase
c. Carboxypeptidase A and B
d. ALA synthase
e. Superoxide dismutase (SOD)
f. RNA polymerase
g. ALP
h. LDH

Section 1 ■ Cell and its Biomolecules

2

Chapter

3

Carbohydrates and their Chemistry

COMPETENCY BI 3.1

At the end of this chapter learner should be able to discuss and differentiate monosaccharides, disaccharides and polysaccharides giving examples of main carbohydrates as energy fuel, structural element and storage in the human body.

Specific Learning Objectives

BI 3.1.1	Describe the classification of carbohydrates.
BI 3.1.2	Discuss and differentiate monosaccharides, disaccharides and polysaccharides.
BI 3.1.3	Enumerate various carbohydrates which play structural role.
BI 3.1.4	Enumerate various carbohydrates which play role in energy production.
BI 3.1.5	Enumerate various carbohydrates which play storage role.

▌CARBOHYDRATE

Carbohydrates are aldehyde or keto derivatives of polyhydroxy alcohols or substances which yield such compounds on hydrolysis.

Glycerol having three hydroxyl groups is the parent alcohol from which carbohydrates are derived.

Classification

Carbohydrates are classified based on number of individual monosaccharide units derived from complete hydrolysis of the carbohydrate compound.

Accordingly they are classified into following four major groups:

1. **Monosaccharides [Cn(H$_2$O)n]:** They are carbohydrates which cannot be further hydrolyzed into simple carbohydrates. Monosaccharides are subdivided further depending on (i) number of carbon atoms and (ii) presence of aldehyde/ketone group (Table 3.1).

TABLE 3.1	Monosaccharides	
General formula	*Aldosugar*	*Ketosugar*
Trioses	Glyceraldehyde	Dihydroxyacetone
Tetroses	Erythrose	Erythrulose
Pentoses	Ribose	Ribulose
Hexoses	Glucose	Fructose
Heptoses	Glucoheptose	Sedoheptulose
Nanoses	Sialic acid (NANA)	—

2. **Disaccharides [Cn(H$_2$O)n–1]:** Yield two molecules of same/different monosaccharides on hydrolysis (Fig. 3.1 and Table 3.2).

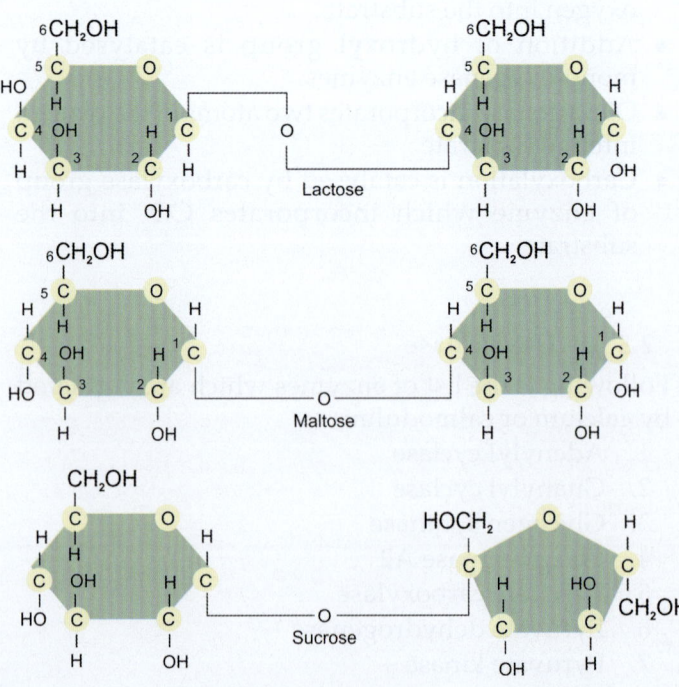

Fig. 3.1: Disaccharides

TABLE 3.2	List of disaccharides		
Disaccharides	Reducing (R) or nonreducing (NR)	Individual monosaccharide units	Bonds
Sucrose	NR	Glucose + Fructose	α-D-glucopyranosyl β-D-fructofuranoside
Trehalose	NR	Glucose + Glucose	α-1,1-glycosidic
Maltose	R	Glucose + Glucose	α-1,4-glycosidic
Isomaltose	R	Glucose + Glucose	α-1,6-glycosidic
Lactose	R	Glucose + Galactose	β-1,4-glycosidic
Lactulose	R	Fructose + Galactose	β-1,4-glycosidic

3. **Oligosaccharides:** Yield 3–10 molecules of monosaccharide units on hydrolysis.

4. **Polysaccharides:** Yield more than 10 molecules of monosaccharides on hydrolysis.

Polysaccharides may be classified as homopolysaccharides or heteropolysaccharides depending on whether the same or different individual monosaccharides are produced on complete hydrolysis of the compound.

a. **Homopolysaccharides (homoglycans):** Polymers of same monosaccharide units, e.g. starch, glycogen, inulin, cellulose, etc. (Table 3.3).

b. **Heteropolysaccharides:** Mucopolysaccharides are important example of heteropolysaccharides (HPS). They are also known as glycosaminoglycans (GAG).

Other examples of heteropolysaccharides are:
1. Heparin
2. Heparan sulphate
3. Chondroitin sulphate
4. Dermatan sulphate
5. Keratan sulphate I and II
6. Hyaluronic acid

Important characteristics of various heteropolysaccharides are given in Table 3.4.

ISOMERS

Compounds which have same chemical formula but differ in their spatial configuration are known as stereoisomers. Number of possible isomers depends on number of asymmetric carbon atoms (n). If a compound has 'n' number of asymmetric C-atom, it will have total n^2 stereoisomers.

Types of Isomers

1. **D- and L-isomers:** In this type of isomers the difference in the structure is in the orientation of –H and –OH groups around carbon atom adjacent to terminal primary alcohol group (penultimate carbon/reference carbon atoms). If –OH group on this carbon atom is towards right, carbohydrate is called D-isomer, when –OH group is on left, it is a member of L-series (Fig. 3.2).

Optical activity: Presence of asymmetric carbon atom confers optical activity on the compound. When a

TABLE 3.3	List of homopolysaccharides	
Homopolysaccharides	Units of monosaccharides	Bonds
Starch	Glucose	α-1,4 and α-1,6 glycosidic bond
Glycogen	Glucose	α-1,4 and α-1,6 glycosidic bond
Cellulose	Glucose	β-1,4 glycosidic bond
Inulin	Fructose	β-1,2 glycosidic bond
Dextran	Glucose	α-1,6 glycosidic bond α-1,4 glycosidic bond α-1,3 glycosidic bond
Chitin	N-acetyl D-glucosamine	β-1,4 glycosidic bond

Section 1 ■ Cell and its Biomolecules

3

beam of plane polarized light is passed through a solution exhibiting optical activity, it will be rotated to right/left:

- If rotated to right, the compound is called dextrorotatory (*d* or + sign),
- When rotated to left, compound is called levorotatory (*l* or –sign).

Racemic mixture: When equal amount of dextrorotatory and levorotatory isomers are present in a mixture, the resulting mixture has no net optical activity, such a mixture is called racemic mixture.

2. **Aldo-keto isomers:** If the reactive group of the carbohydrate is aldehyde, it is an aldose and if the reactive group of the carbohydrate is ketone, it is a ketose (Fig. 3.3).

3. **Pyranose and furanose ring structures:** Pyranose is heterocyclic, hexacyclic ring structure and furanose ring is heterocyclic pentacyclic ring structure. In physiological state 99% of the glucose is in pyranose form, and 99% of the fructose is in furanose form (Fig. 3.4).

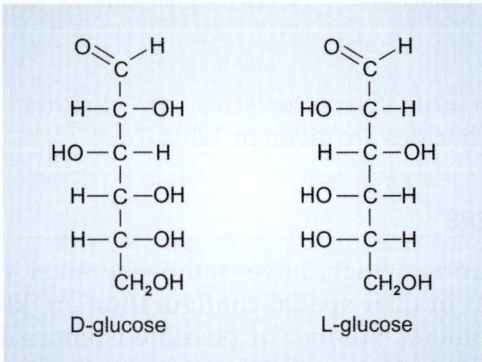

Fig. 3.2: D- and L-isomers of glucose

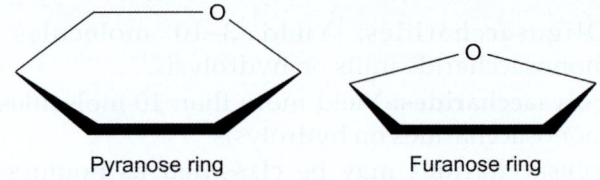

Pyranose ring   Furanose ring

Fig. 3.4: Pyranose and furanose rings

4. **Alpha and beta anomers:** In the ring structure form, if the –OH group on anomeric carbon atom is above the plane of ring, the anomeric form is β and if –OH

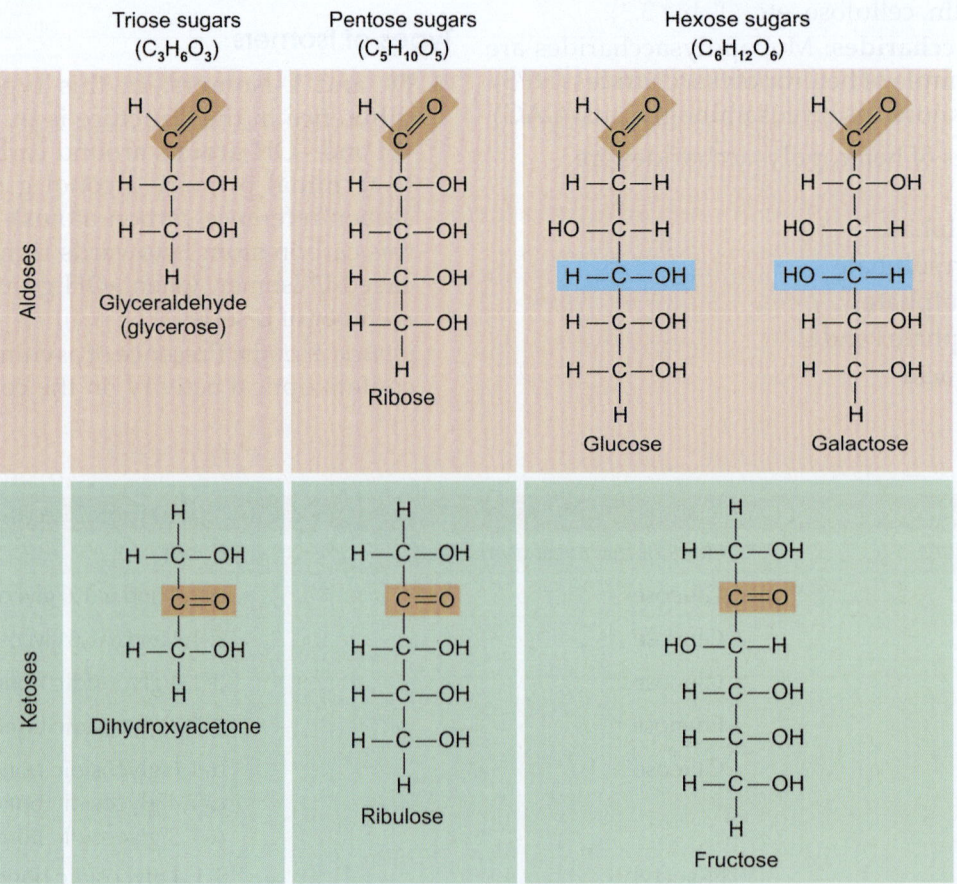

Fig. 3.3: Aldo-keto isomers

TABLE 3.4 | Important characteristics of various glycosaminoglycans

Name	Location	Role they play	Remarks
Hyaluronic acid	Skin, synovial fluid, vitreous humor, bone, cartilage, embryonic tissue	Cell migration during morphogenesis and wound healing	No sulphation
Heparin	Mast cell, liver, lung, skin	Anticoagulant (bind factor IX and XI)	Releases lipoprotein lipase from capillary endothelial wall
Heparan sulphate	Skin, kidney, basement membrane	Cell growth, cell-to-cell communication receptor role	IdUA* is also found
Chondroitin sulphate	Cartilage, bone, CNS	Structure of ECM, cartilage	—
Dermatan sulphate	Skin, wide distribution	Blood coagulation, wound repair, resistance to infection	IdUA* is also found
Keratan sulphate I and II	Cornea, cartilage, loose connective tissue	Corneal transparency	No uronic acid

* IdUA: Iduronic acid (it is 5' epimer of 'D' glucuronic acid)

group on anomeric carbon atom is below the plane of ring, the anomeric form is α. Anomeric carbon atom is the carbon at which hemiacetal or hemiketal group is present.

Mutarotation: Interconversion of α and β forms of D-glucose in aqueous medium is known as mutarotation (Fig. 3.5).

5. **Epimers:** Isomers differing as a result of variation in configuration of the hydroxyl group on only one of the asymmetric carbon atoms (carbon 2, 3, 4 or 5) of glucose are known as epimers.

Glucose and mannose are C2-epimers and glucose and galactose are C4-epimers (Figs 3.6a to c).

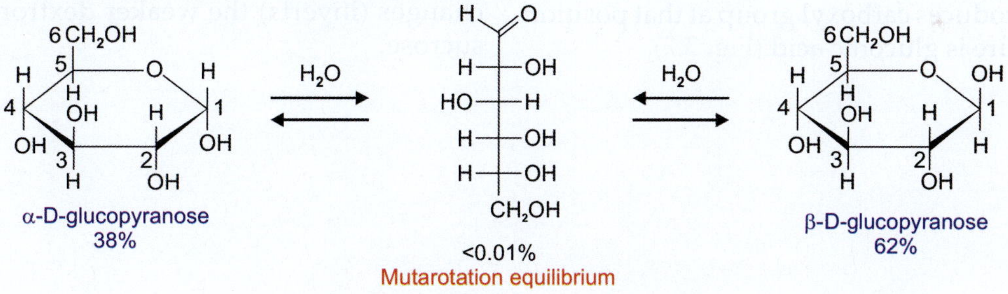

Fig. 3.5: Mutarotation (in glucose)

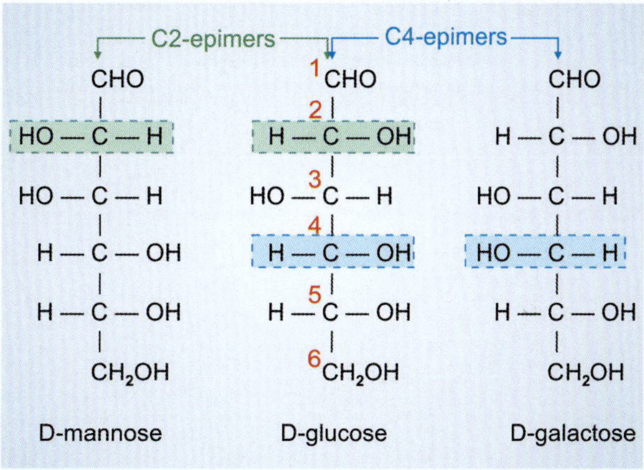

Fig. 3.6a: C2 and C4-epimers of glucose

Section 1 ■ Cell and its Biomolecules

3

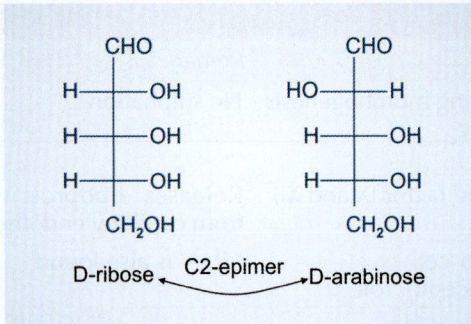

Fig. 3.6b: C2-epimers of ribose

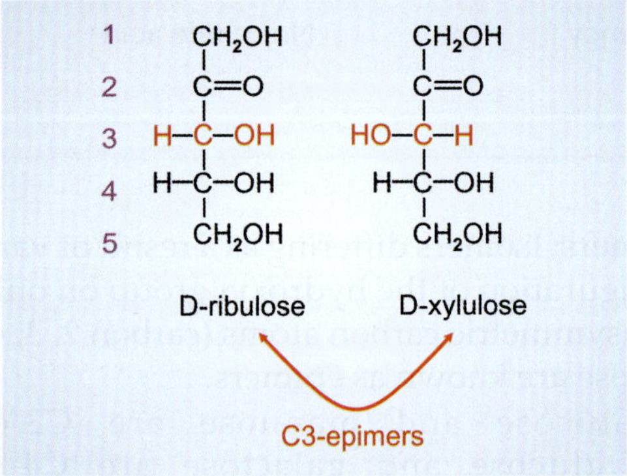

Uronic acid: Oxidation of the last carbon atom of the chain (C6 in case of glucose and other hexoses) produces uronic acid, e.g. glucuronic acid, etc. (Fig. 3.8).

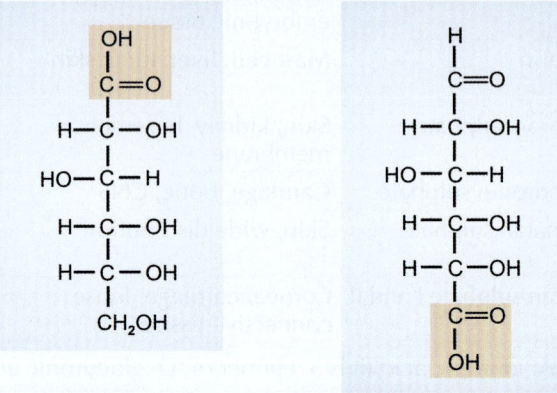

Fig. 3.7: D-gluconic acid   **Fig. 3.8:** D-glucuronic acid
(aldonic acid)   (uronic acid)

Fig. 3.6c: C3-epimers of ribulose

Aldonic acid: Oxidation of carbonyl (aldehyde) carbon of the glucose produces carboxyl group at that position. This new structure is gluconic acid (Fig. 3.7).

Invert sugar: Sucrose is known as invert sugar Sucrose has specific optical rotation of +66.5°. On hydrolysis sucrose solution yields equimolar mixture of D-glucose (specific rotation of +52.5°) and D-fructose (specific rotation of −92°), this results in net levorotation. Hence, sucrose is known as invert sugar.

In other words, fructose is strongly levorotatory and changes (inverts) the weaker dextrorotatory action of sucrose.

4

Amino Acids and their Chemistry

Amino acids are the building blocks of the protein. There are 20 standard amino acids.

The general structure of a standard amino acid contains a central alpha (α) carbon atom to which following groups are attached (Fig. 4.1):

a. Carboxylic group
b. Amino group
c. Hydrogen atom
d. Side chain (R)

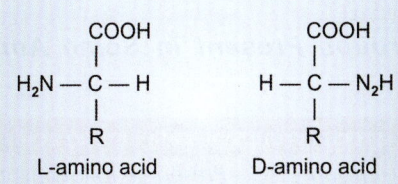

Fig. 4.1: Structure of an amino acid

Proline is the only exception of the above rule where imino group (not the amino group) is attached to the alpha carbon atom.

Stereoisomer of Amino Acid

All amino acids except glycine have two stereoisomers, D and L forms.

In proteins, it is mainly L form of amino acid. D-amino acids are very rare, they are found in bacterial cell wall and antibiotics (Fig. 4.2).

COOH	COOH
H₂N — C — H	H — C — N₂H
R	R
L-amino acid	D-amino acid

Fig. 4.2: Amino acids

Physical and chemical characteristics of stereoisomers are mostly same, but they differ in their optical activity, where D form rotates the optical light in right direction and L form rotates the optical light in left direction.

Peptide bond: Amino acids are linked together through peptide bonds to make a long stretch of protein. It is the α-amino group of one amino acid which is linked with the α-carboxyl group of another amino acid to form a peptide bond (Fig. 4.3).

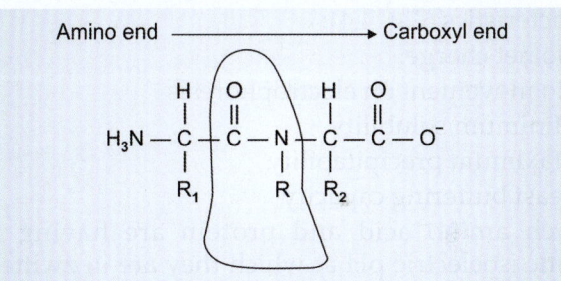

Fig. 4.3: Peptide bond formation

Characteristics of peptide bond

- Partial double bond (distance is 1.32Å)
- Rigid and planar
- The hydrogen of amino group and oxygen of the carbonyl group are *trans* (opposite) in nature, rather than in *cis* (adjacent).
- Uncharged but polar

The free NH_2 group of the terminal amino acids is called N-terminal end and free COOH end is called as C-terminal end.

Ionization of Amino Acids

All standard amino acids have two ionizable groups:

a. α-amino group
b. α-carboxyl group

In addition to above two ionizable groups, most of the amino acids also have ionizable acid or base group in their side chain.

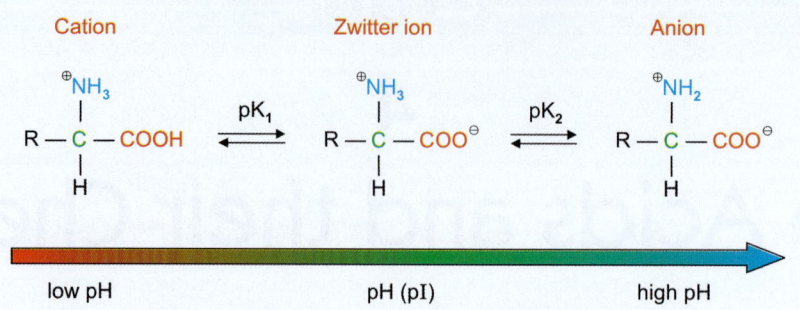

Fig. 4.4: Isoelectric pH (pI) and zwitter ion form

Zwitter ions (ampholyte): Amino acids in solution are predominantly present as dipolar ions (zwitter ions/ampholytes) rather than as unionized molecules. Net charge on the amino acid depends upon the pH of the medium.

pH at which amino acids are electrically neutral (equal positive and negative charges present) is known as isoelectric pH (pI).

At isoelectric pH, amino acids show following characteristics (Fig. 4.4):
1. No net charge.
2. No movement on electrophoresis
3. Minimum solubility
4. Maximum precipitability
5. Least buffering capacity

Each amino acid and protein are having their specific isoelectric pH at which they are in zwitter ion form.

For albumin, isoelectric pH is 4.7. This is the reason of negative charge on albumin at plasma pH (7.4) and at urine pH (6.5).

Structure of a Typical Amino Acid (Fig. 4.5)

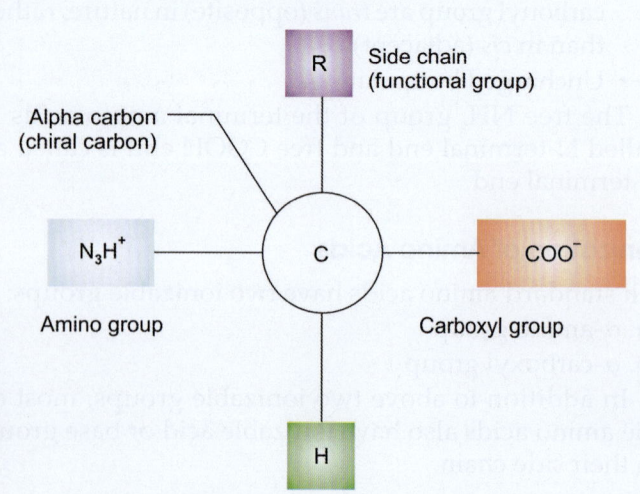

Fig. 4.5: Structure of a typical amino acid

CLASSIFICATION OF AMINO ACIDS (Fig. 4.6)

They are classified based on following four characters:
1. Based on structure
2. Based on side chain character
3. Based on metabolic fate
4. Based on nutritional requirement

1. Classification of Amino Acids Based on Structure

a. **Aliphatic amino acids**
   1. *Monoamino monocarboxylic acid*
      - *Simple:* Glycine, alanine
      - *Branched:* Valine, leucine, isoleucine
      - *Hydroxyl:* Serine, threonine
      - *Sulphur containing:* Cysteine, methionine
      - *Amide group containing:* Glutamine, asparagine
   2. *Monoamino dicarboxylic acid:* Aspartic acid, glutamic acid
   3. *Dibasic monocarboxylic acid:* Arginine, lysine
b. **Aromatic amino acids:** Phenylalanine, tyrosine
c. **Heterocyclic amino acids:** Histidine, tryptophan
d. **Imino amino acid:** Proline
e. **Derived amino acids:** Hydroxyproline, hydroxylysine, ornithine, citrulline, homocysteine.

Special Groups Present in Some Amino Acids (Table 4.1)

TABLE 4.1	Special groups of some amino acids	
Amino acid	*Group*	*Present at following carbon atom*
Arginine	Guanidium	δ carbon
Tryptophan	Indole	β
Histidine	Imidazole	β
Proline	Pyrrolidine	α
Tyrosine	Phenol	β

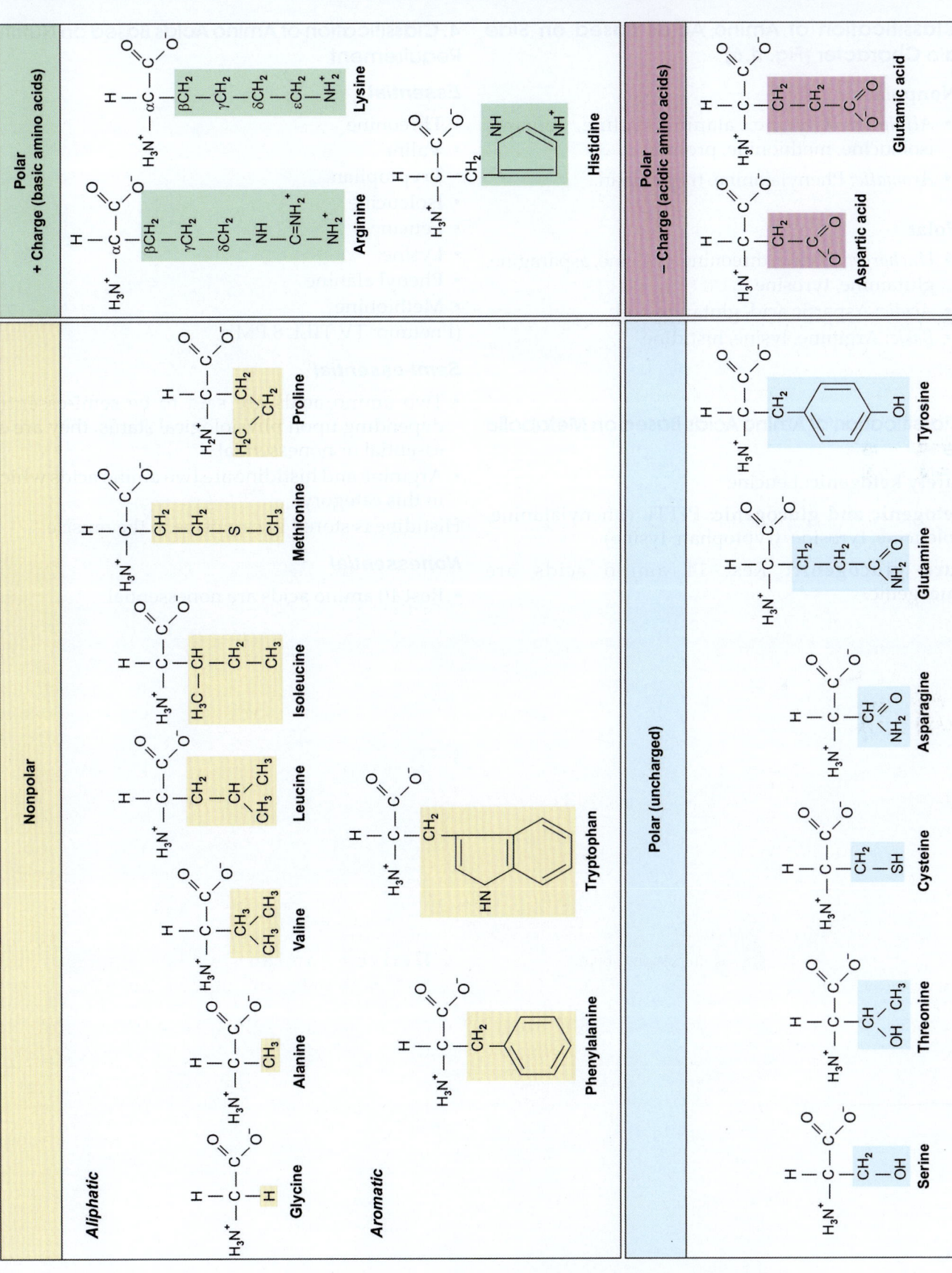

Fig. 4.6: Various amino acids

2. Classification of Amino Acids Based on Side Chain Character (Fig. 4.6)

a. **Nonpolar**
- *Aliphatic:* Glycine, alanine, valine, leucine, isoleucine, methionine, proline.
- *Aromatic:* Phenylalanine, tryptophan.

b. **Polar**
- *Uncharged*: Serine, threonine, cysteine, asparagine, glutamine, tyrosine.
- *Acidic*: Aspartic acid, glutamic acid
- *Basic*: Arginine, lysine, histidine

3. Classification of Amino Acids Based on Metabolic Fate

- **Purely ketogenic:** Leucine
- **Ketogenic and glucogenic:** PITTL (phenylalanine, isoleucine, tyrosine, tryptophan, lysine)
- **Pure glucogenic:** Rest 14 amino acids are glucogenic.

4. Classification of Amino Acids Based on Nutritional Requirement

Essential
- Threonine
- Valine
- Tryptophan
- Isoleucine
- Leucine
- Lysine
- Phenyl alanine
- Methionine

(Pneumo: TV TILL 8 PM)

Semi-essential
- Two amino acids are said to be semi-essential as depending upon physiological status, they are either essential or nonessential.
- Arginine and histidine are two amino acids which fall in this category.

Histidine is stored in carnosine in the muscle.

Nonessential
- Rest 10 amino acids are nonessential.

5

Lipids and their Chemistry

COMPETENCY BI 4.1

At the end of this chapter learner should be able to describe and discuss main classes of lipids (essential/nonessential fatty acids, cholesterol and hormonal steroids, triglycerides, major phospholipids and sphingolipids) relevant to human system and their major functions.

Specific Learning Objectives	
BI 4.1.1	Define lipids.
BI 4.1.2	Discuss the classification of lipids.
BI 4.1.3	Describe biochemical importance of various lipids in human body.

WHAT IS LIPID?

- Lipids are heterogenous groups of compounds which are soluble in nonpolar solvents such as ether, chloroform and benzene and relatively insoluble in water and other polar solvents.
- Lipids are either the esters of fatty acids with the alcohol or are compounds which are capable of forming such esters.

CLASSIFICATION OF LIPIDS

As lipids are heterogenous groups of compounds, classifying them is little challenging. There is no

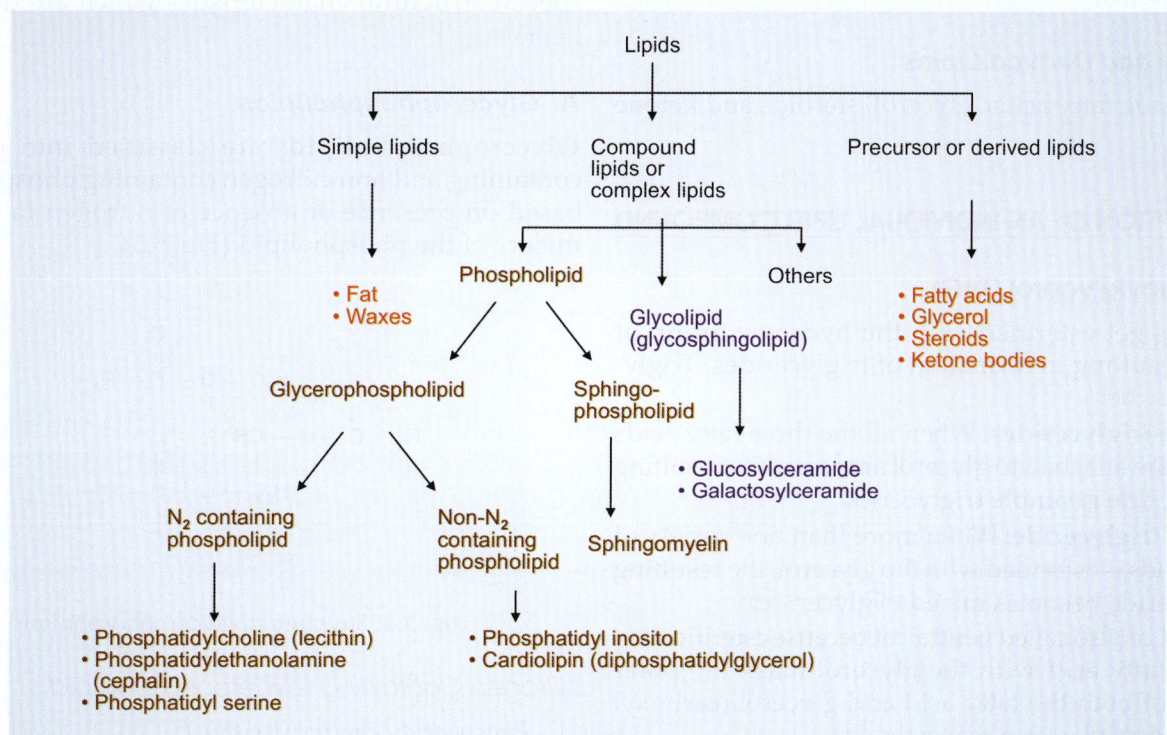

Fig. 5.1: Modified Bloor's classification

internationally accepted classification for the lipid. The most widely accepted classification is Bloor's Classification which is described below:

Modified Bloor's Classification (Fig. 5.1)

Simple Lipids

These are fatty acids esterified with various alcohols. Depending on alcoholic moiety, they are known as either fat or wax.

a. *Fats or triacylglycerol:* Esters of fatty acids with glycerol. A fat in the liquid state is known as oil.

b. *Waxes:* Esters of fatty acids with higher molecular weight monohydric alcohols like sphingosine.

Compound or Complex Lipids

Esters of fatty acids containing 'groups' in addition to an alcohol and fatty acids.

Depending upon additional group, complex lipids are further classified into:

a. *Phospholipids:* Lipids containing a fatty acid, an alcohol and a phosphoric acid residue, e.g. glycerophospholipids and sphingophospholipids.

b. *Glycolipids:* Lipids containing a fatty acid, alcohol and carbohydrates.

c. *Other complex lipids:* Sulpholipids, aminolipids and lipoproteins.

Precursor and Derived Lipids

These include fatty acids, glycerol, steroids and ketone bodies.

■ DESCRIPTION OF AN INDIVIDUAL LIPID COMPOUND

Fat or Triacylglycerol (TAG)

Fatty acids get esterified with the hydroxyl group of glycerol resulting in formation of triglycerides. Triglycerides may be:

a. **Simple triglycerides:** When all the three fatty acids which are attached to glycerol are same, the resulting triglyceride is simple triglyceride.

b. **Mixed triglyceride:** When more than one variety of fatty acids is esterified with the glycerol, the resulting triglyceride becomes mixed triglyceride.

TAG is also called neutral fat because esterification of the fatty acid with the glycerol mask the polar group of both the fatty acid and glycerol (carboxyl and hydroxyl group respectively).

Stored TAG provides energy for longer duration compared to stored glycogen, during period of fasting or starvation (Fig. 5.2).

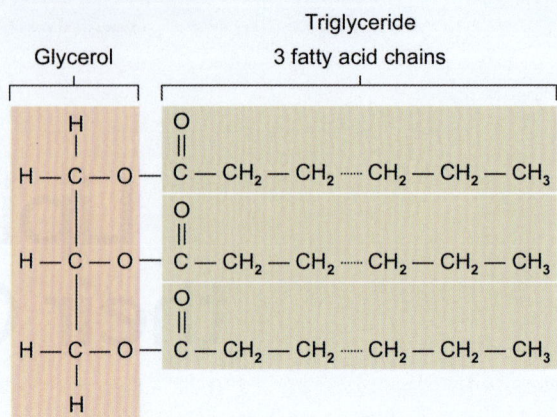

Fig. 5.2: Structure of triacylglycerol

Waxes

Waxes are esters of fatty acids with high molecular weight alcohol like sphingosine. They are also known as ceramide.

Phospholipids

Phospholipids are major constituents of plasma membrane. Phospholipids may be glycerophospholipid or sphingophospholipid depending upon whether they have glycerol or sphingosine as their component alcohol.

Plasmalogens are special types of phospholipids with special structural characteristics which are described later.

A. Glycerophospholipids

Glycerophospholipids are classified into nitrogen containing and non-nitrogen containing phospholipids based on presence or absence of nitrogen in the base moiety of the phospholipid (Fig. 5.3).

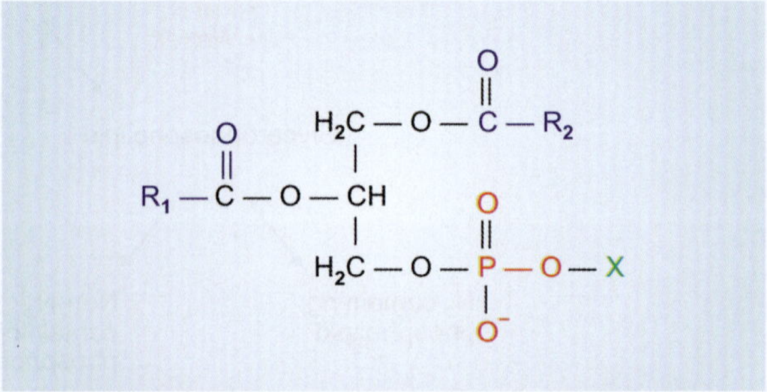

Fig. 5.3: Structure of glycerophospholipid

Nitrogen Containing Glycerophospholipid

1. *Phosphatidylcholine (lecithin):*
   • Most abundant phospholipid of membrane, store of choline (choline is important for nerve transmission and acts as a source of methyl group).

- It is important for lipoprotein synthesis and is also important for esterification of cholesterol.
- Dipalmitoyl lecithin (DPL) acts as lung surfactant.

2. *Phosphatidylethanolamine (cephalin)*
   - Clotting factor III (thromboplastin) is composed mainly of cephalin

3. *Phosphatidylserine*

Non-nitrogen Containing Glycerophospholipid

1. *Phosphatidylinositol:* Acts as a precursor of second messenger. Phospholipase C acts on phosphatidyl inositol to convert it to inositol triphosphate and diacylglycerol.

2. *Cardiolipin (diphosphatidyl glycerol):*
   - Cardiolipin is abundantly found in the inner membrane of mitochondria.
   - This phospholipid has a key role in mitochondrial structure and function.
   - Cardiolipin is antigenic in nature.

- It is thought to be involved in programmed cell death (apoptosis) (Fig. 5.4).

B. Sphingophospholipids
These phospholipids have got sphingosine alcohol, e.g. sphingomyelin. It is further described under the heading sphingolipids.

C. Plasmalogens
Plasmalogens are rare form of phospholipids which are found in brain myelin and cardiac muscle. They have important structural difference compared to a classical glycerophospholipid. Plasmalogens have an unsaturated alcohol linked through ether linkage at S_N1 carbon of glycerol instead of a saturated fatty acid esterified there.

Important examples of plasmalogens are:
- Choline plasmalogen (cardiac muscle)
- Ethanolamine plasmalogens (myelin)
- Platelet activating factor (PAF)

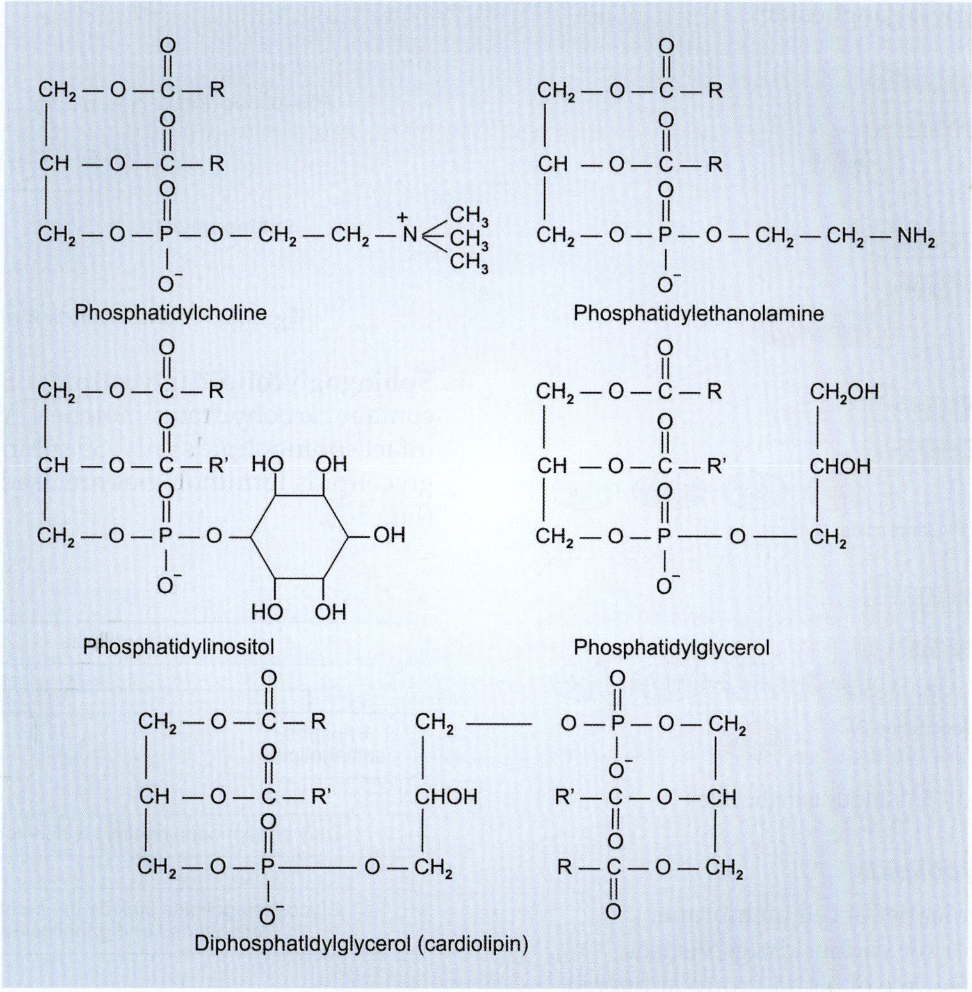

Fig. 5.4: Various phospholipids

Section 1 ■ Cell and its Biomolecules

5

Glycolipid (Glycosphingolipid)

Lipids with carbohydrate component are called glycolipids (Fig. 5.5).

They are:

i. **Cerebrosides** are ceramide monohexosides (e.g. galactocerebroside and glucocerebroside).
- *Galactosylceramide* abundant in brain and nervous system.
- *Glucosylceramide* abundant in extraneural tissue.
- *Sulphatidated cerebroside* that contains sulphated sugars, e.g. sulphogalactocerebroside.

ii. **Globosides** are ceramide oligosaccharides that contain two or more sugar molecules, most often galactose, glucose or N-acetylgalactosamine, attached to ceramide.

iii. **Gangliosides** are glycosphingolipids that contain one or more sialic acid residue mainly N-acetyl derivative of neuraminic acid (Fig. 5.5).

GM1 is the receptor of cholera toxin.

GM3 is the simplest ganglioside.

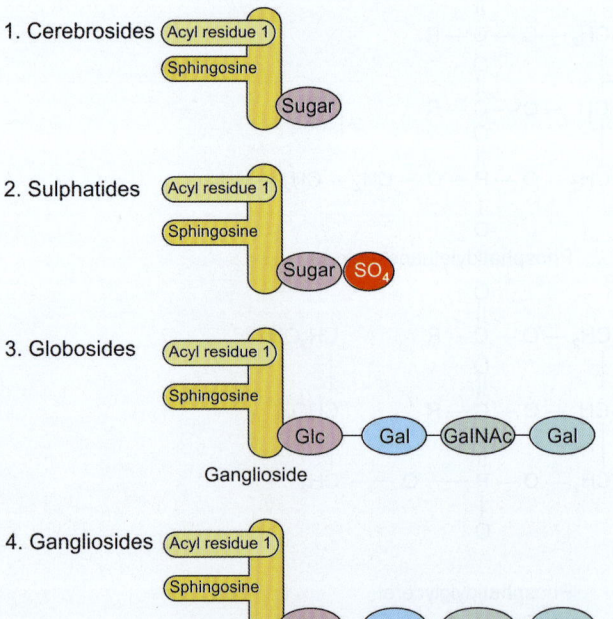

Fig. 5.5: Various gangliosides

Functions of Glycolipids

1. Found at outer leaflet of cell membrane.
2. It is the receptor for various drugs/viruses.
3. It is antigenic (source of blood group antigens).
4. Immunological reaction determinant.

▌ SPHINGOLIPIDS

Sphingolipids are found in central nervous system and specially in white matter. They are those compound lipids which have sphingosine alcohol in them. They are:

a. **Sphingophospholipids:** Important example is sphingomyelin which on hydrolysis yields a fatty acid, phosphoric acid, choline and a complex amino alcohol, sphingosine (Fig. 5.6).
- The combination of sphingosine plus fatty acids is known as ceramide.
- Fatty acid component of sphingomyelin may be:
  - Lignoceric acid
  - Nervonic acid
  - Stearic acid

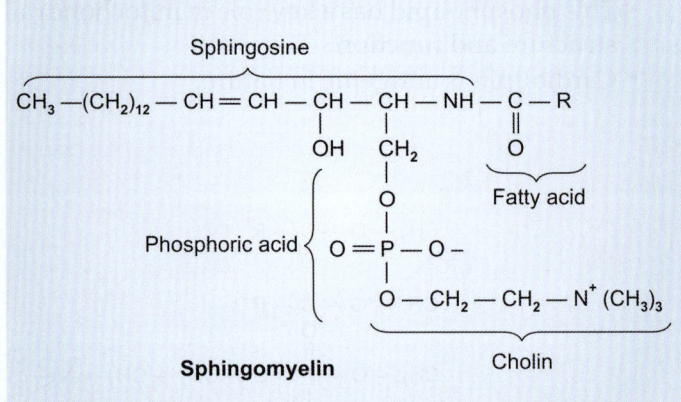

Fig. 5.6: A sphingophospholipid

b. **Sphingoglycolipid (glycolipids):** Sphingolipids that contain carbohydrates moieties. All glycolipids are infact sphingolipids only. So sphingoglycolipid and glycolipids terminologies are used interchangeably (Fig. 5.7).

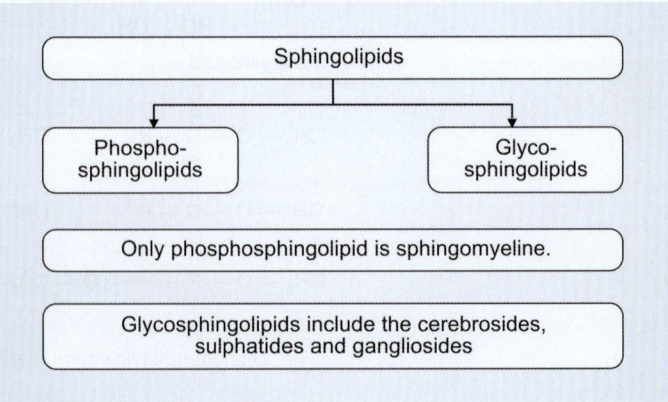

Fig. 5.7: Classification of sphingolipids

Sterols

- Sterols are structural lipids of the membrane.
- Cholesterol is an important sterol in the animal tissue.
- Cholesterol has cyclo-pentano-perhydro-phenan-therene ring (CPPP) (Fig. 5.8).
- Cholesterol is found in animal lipid but not in plant lipid.

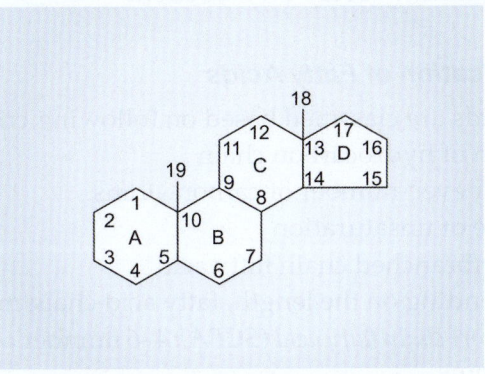

Fig. 5.8: Cyclo-pentano-perhydro-phenantherene ring

Functions of the Cholesterol

1. Formation of cell membrane
2. Cholesterol is the precursor of steroids (progesterone, androgens, estrogens, mineralocorticoids, glucocorticoids)
3. Cholesterol is the precursor of bile acid.
4. Cholesterol is the precursor of vitamin D.

LIPOPROTEINS

Lipoprotein is an important macromolecular complex which acts as vehicle for transport of various lipids in the plasma from one place to other.

It is a water soluble structure having amphipathic shell and nonpolar core (Fig. 5.9).

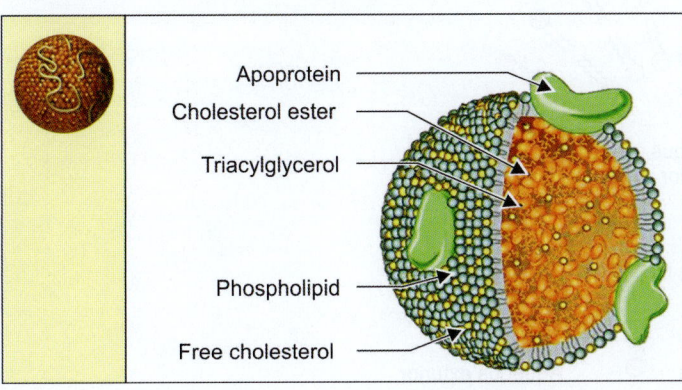

Fig. 5.9: Structure of a typical lipoprotein

Phospholipids and free cholesterol are lipid components of shell which also contain certain protein known as apoprotein or apolipoprotein. Apoproteins may be integrated or peripheral depending upon whether they are embedded in the shell or simply sitting on the surface of the lipoprotein just like a cap.

Core has nonpolar lipids like triacylglycerol and cholesterol ester in varied proportion among various lipoproteins. Some lipoproteins like chylomicron and VLDL have excess quantity of triacylglycerol and others like LDL have excess amount of cholesterol ester in the core section.

Role of Phospholipids in formation of Micelles, Lipid Bilayers and Liposomes

Micelle

Phospholipids are amphipathic molecules having a polar head and a nonpolar tail. These phospholipids tend to aggregate in the aqueous medium as to make a structure which has a polar head exposed to the surface and a nonpolar tail sandwiched in the center of the structure (Fig. 5.10).

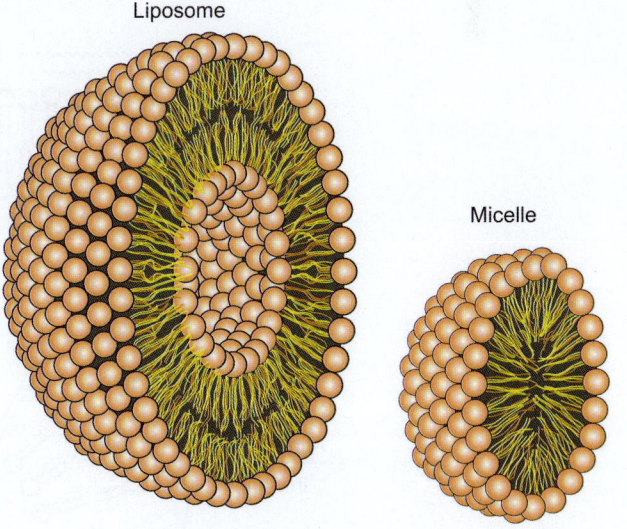

Fig. 5.10: Micelle structure

Lipid Bilayer

Phospholipids are capable of forming lipid bilayers. In this bilayer hydrophobic tail is approximated and polar head is exposed outwards as to face the aqueous media (Fig. 5.11).

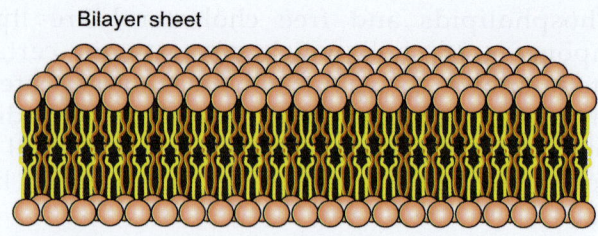

Fig. 5.11: Lipid bilayer

Liposomes

Liposomes are artificial structures which are produced in the laboratories when phospholipids are suspended in the aqueous media and are sonicated (high frequency sound waves are applied) (Fig. 5.12).

These liposomes act as vehicle for transportation of drugs for therapeutic use and DNA for gene therapy. They are injected in patients where lipid bilayer is metabolized by reticuloendothelial cell and the material in the vesicles are delivered locally.

Liposomes are used for following:
- To study the membrane permeability
- To deliver the drugs
- To deliver the DNA for gene therapy

Liposomes are coated sometimes with the specific material as to deliver its content at the precise location.

Fatty Acids

- Fatty acids are aliphatic carboxylic acid which is represented as RCOOH.
- They are amphipathic lipids which means they have both polar (hydrophilic) and nonpolar (hydrophobic) moeity in them.
- Fatty acids are good source of energy as they generate good number of ATP on oxidation.

Classification of Fatty Acids

Fatty acids are classified based on following criteria:
- Length of hydrocarbon chain
- Odd or even number of carbon atoms
- Degree of unsaturation
- Linear/branched chain fatty acid
1. Depending on the length, fatty acid chain may be:
   - *Short chain fatty acid (SCFA):* 4–6 number of carbon atoms.
   - *Medium chain fatty acid (MCFA):* 8–14 number of carbon atoms.
   - *Long chain fatty acid (LCFA):* 16–22 number of carbon atoms.
   - *Very long chain fatty acid (VLCFA):* >24 number of carbon atoms.

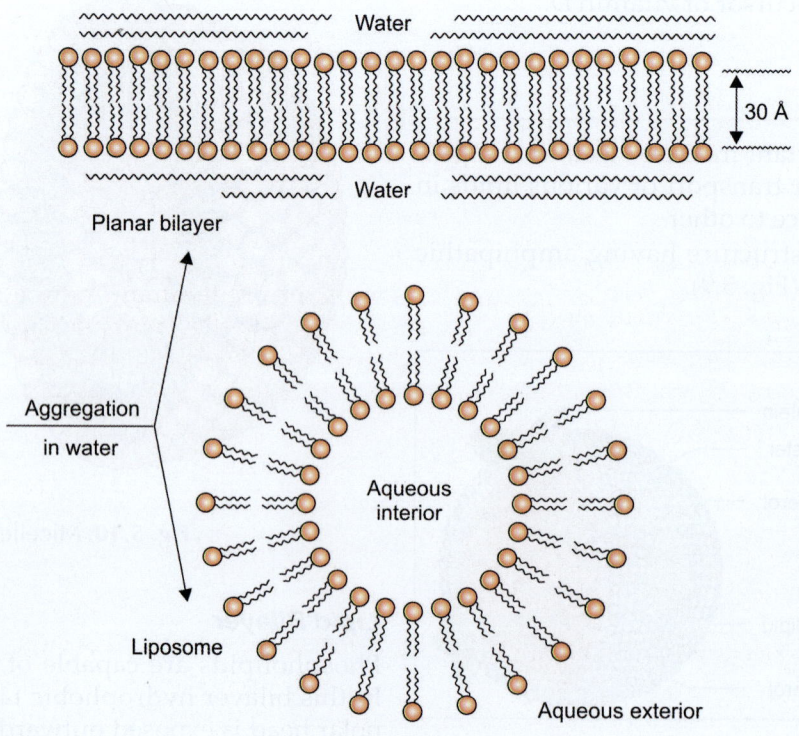

Fig. 5.12: Liposome

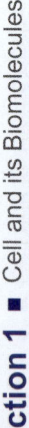

2. Depending on odd or even number of carbon atoms, fatty acid chain may be:
   - Odd chain fatty acid
   - Even chain fatty acid
3. Depending on the degree of unsaturation the fatty acid chain may be:
   - *Saturated fatty acids:* They do not contain double bond in the chain. Suffix is—anoic acid.
   - *Unsaturated fatty acids:* They have one or more double bonds. Suffix is—enoic acid.
4. Depending upon presence or absence of branching, the fatty acid chain may be:
   - Linear
   - Branched
   - Cyclic

Isomers of Fatty Acids

Unsaturated fatty acids may be *cis* or *trans* depending on the configuration of hydrocarbon chain beyond the double bond (Fig. 5.13).
   - *Cis:* When the fatty acid tail beyond the double bond is organized in the same direction. Naturally occurring fatty acids in human, bacteria and plants are mainly *cis* type.
   - *Trans:* When the fatty acid tail beyond the double bond is oriented in the extended fashion.

Trans fatty acids are not naturally found, rather they are produced due to artificial hydrogenation of vegetable oil to make margarine.

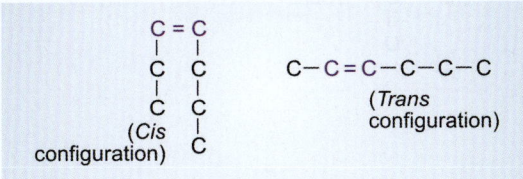

Fig. 5.13: *Cis* and *trans* fatty acids

Numbering System of Carbon in Fatty Acids

Numbering of carbon atom of fatty acid chain is important to delineate the number and the position of double bond in an unsaturated fatty acid. There are two ways described as follows:

1. **C numbering system:** The carbon atoms are numbered from the carboxyl carbon. Carboxyl carbon is given number 1, further upward the carbon atoms are given number in sequential order 2, 3, 4, 5, 6, etc.
2. **Omega (Ω) or n numbering system:** The carbon adjacent to carboxyl carbon is known as α-carbon. Carbon atom numbers 3 and 4 are the β and γ, respectively.

- The terminal methyl carbon is known as ω-carbon (Fig. 5.14).

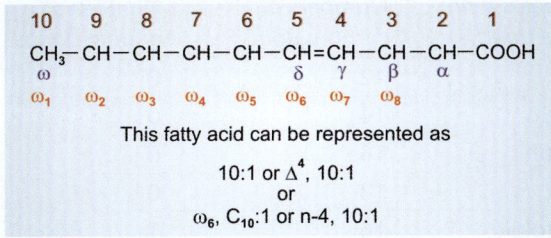

This fatty acid can be represented as

$10:1$ or $\Delta^4, 10:1$
or
$\omega_6, C_{10}:1$ or n-4, $10:1$

Fig. 5.14: Δ and ω systems of nomenclature

To nomenclate the fatty acid both the systems are utilized.

Delta system: This system of numbering not only tells the position of double bond but also indicates the number of double bonds in a fatty acid, e.g. $\Delta 7$ fatty acid means, there is a single double bond present between carbon atoms 7 and 8.

Omega system: This system of numbering shows position of first double bond starting from ω end. $\omega 3$ family means that the first double bond is between $\omega 3$ and $\omega 4$ carbon atoms, $\omega 7$ family means that the first double bond is between $\omega 7$ and $\omega 8$ carbon atoms.

ω system of numbering does not give idea about total number of double bonds present in a fatty acid chain.

Some important fatty acids and the ω family they belong to are as follows:

ω9	ω6	ω3	ω7
Oleic acid	Linoleic acid	α-linolenic acid	Palmitoleic acid
Elaidic acid	γ-linolenic acid	Timnodonic acid	
	Arachidonic acid	Cervonic acid	

List of predominant fatty acids of the mammalian system, with their number of carbon atoms and double bonds is shown in Table 5.1.

Important dietary sources of linoleic acid are (decreasing order of predominance):
- Safflower oil
- Corn oil
- Sunflower oil
- Soya bean oil

Functions of the Fatty Acids

- From building blocks of phospholipids and glycolipids
- Fatty acid produces prostaglandin.
- Fatty acid is an important source of energy.

5

TABLE 5.1	List of important fatty acids (with their number of carbon atoms and double bonds)	
Fatty acids with double bond(s)	*Numbers of carbon atoms*	*Number of double bonds*
Lauric	12	0
Myristic	14	0
Palmitic	16	0
Stearic	18	0
Palmitoleic	16	1
Oleic	18	1
Linoleic	18	2
Linolenic	18	3
Arachidonic	20	4
Timnodonic	20	5
Cervonic	22	6

Essential Fatty Acids

They are essential fatty acids as they can not be synthesized in the human cell. They are:
- Linoleic acid
- Alpha linolenic acid

Semi-essential Fatty Acid

- Arachidonic acid is a semi-essential fatty acid. It is important to know why arachidonic acid is called semi-essential fatty acid. Dietary linoleic acid is capable of synthesizing arachidonic acid by following a pathway in human cell (Fig. 5.15). When a person is taking an adequate quantity of linoleic acid in the diet, arachidonic acid becomes nonessential, but when a person is deprived of dietary linoleic acid, arachidonic acid becomes essential. Hence, it is called semi-essential fatty acid.

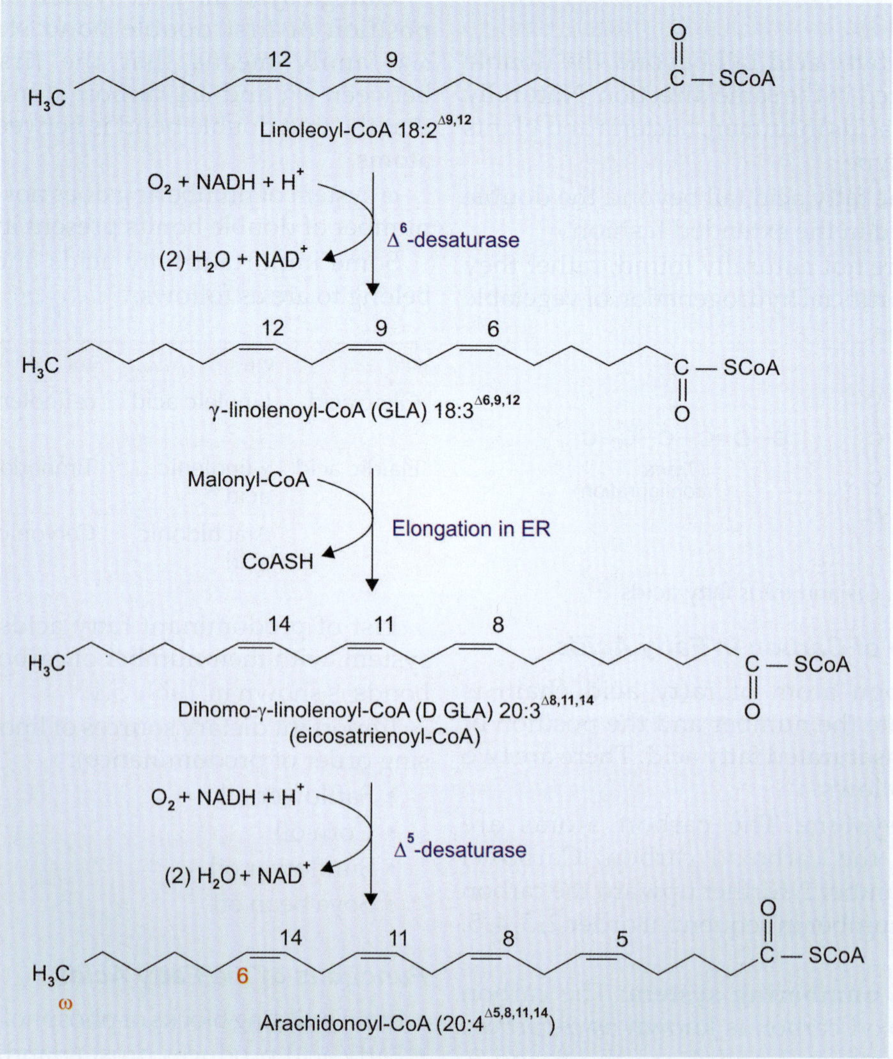

Fig. 5.15: Pathway in human cell to synthesize arachidonic acid from linoleic acid

Functions of Essential and Semi-essential Fatty Acids

- *Important for synthesis of phospholipid of the membrane:* Arachidonic acid constitutes 15% of total fatty acid which may be there in phospholipids.
- *Important for retina and brain development:* Docosahexaenoic acid is derived from fish oil or is synthesized from linoleic acid and is very important for retina and brain development.
- *Important for cholesterol esterification:* Polyunsaturated fatty acid is involved in esterification of cholesterol which helps in its excretion from the body.
- *Precursors for prostaglandins:* Arachidonic acid is an important fatty acid which help in prostaglandin synthesis.

Deficiency of Essential Fatty Acid

Deficiency of essential fatty acid is associated with
- Poor wound healing
- Dermatitis
  ω3 fatty acid is good for health.

Eicosanoids

Eicosanoids are group of 20 carbon compounds. Various compounds which are collectively named as eicosanoids are (Fig. 5.16):
1. Prostaglandins (PG)
2. Prostacyclins (PGI)
3. Thromboxanes (TX)
4. Leukotrienes (LT)
5. Lipoxins (LX)

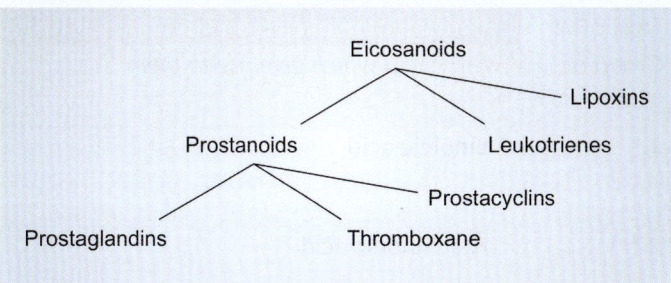

Fig. 5.16: Classification of eicosanoids

There are three groups of eicosanoids which are derived from different fatty acids. For example, group 1 eicosanoids are derived from linoleic acid. Group 2 eicosanoids are derived from arachidonic acid and group 3 eicosanoids are derived from α-linolenic acid.

Collectively eicosanoids play a very important role in human health and disease. For example, in blood clotting, maintenance of blood pressure, muscle contraction, inflammation, pain, asthma, fever, etc. (Table 5.2).

Synthesis of Group 2 Eicosanoids

Arachidonic acid is released from membrane phospholipid by action of phospholipase A2. Arachidonic acid may enter in cyclo-oxygenase pathway where it undergoes oxidative-cyclization to produce various prostanoids or it may enter in lipoxygenase pathway to produce various leukotrienes and lipoxins (Fig. 5.17).

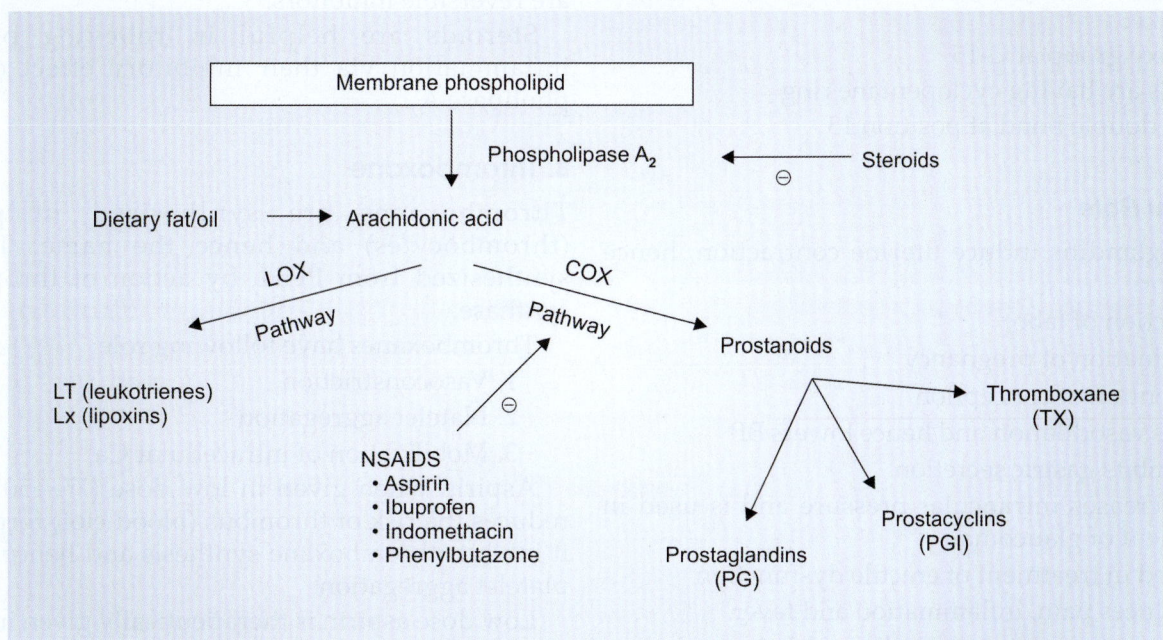

Fig. 5.17: Phospholipase A$_2$ releasing arachidonic acid from membrane phospholipid

Section 1 ■ Cell and its Biomolecules

5

TABLE 5.2	Different groups of eicosanoids and their members			
Group of eicosanoids	Fatty acid which give rise to them	Members		
		Prostanoids	Leukotrienes	Lipoxin**
1.	Linoleic acid	PGE_1 PGF_1 TXA_1	LTA_3 LTC_3 LTD_3	Nil
2.*	Arachidonic acid	PGD_2 PGE_2 PGF_2 PGI_2 TXA_2	LTA_4 LTB_4 LTC_4 LTD_4 LTE_4	LXA_4 LXB_4 LXC_4 LXD_4 LXE_4
3.	α-linolenic acid	PGD_3 PGE_3 PGF_3 PGI_3 TXA_3	LTA_5 LTB_5 LTL_5	Nil

* Group 2 eicosanoids are biologically most important group of eicosanoids in human.

** Lipoxins are produced only by arachidonic acid.

COX and LOX Pathways of Arachidonic Acid

These pathways are shown in Fig. 5.18.

IMPORTANT CHARACTERISTICS AND BIOLOGICAL ROLE OF VARIOUS EICOSANOIDS

A. Prostaglandin

Though originally isolated from human seminal fluid, prostaglandin now is isolated from all the mammalian tissues. Various prostaglandins (PGs) though differ in their structures, they have certain common structural features like:

1. Hydroxy group at C-15
2. All PGs are having cyclopentane ring
3. 'Trans' double bond at position 13.

Biological Role

1. Prostaglandins induce uterine contraction, hence used for:
   • Induction of labor
   • Termination of pregnancy
   • Prevention of conception
2. Causes vasodilation and hence lowers BP
3. PG inhibits gastric secretion
4. PG decreases intraocular pressure and is used in treatment of glaucoma
5. PG used in treatment of erectile dysfunction
6. PG induces pain, inflammation and fever.
7. Daily excretion of prostaglandin and their metabolites is 1 mg.

COX inhibtors inhibit prostaglandin synthesis and help relieving pain, inflammation and fever.

COX inhibitors are NSAIDS (nonsteroidal anti-inflammatory drugs) like:

• Aspirin (acetylsalicylic acid)
• Ibuprofen
• Indomethacin
• Phenylbutazone
• Naproxen

Aspirin is irreversible inhibitor while other NSAIDS are reversible inhibitors.

Steroids are helpful in relieving pain and inflammation via their inhibitory effect on phospholipase A_2.

B. Thromboxane

Thromboxanes are synthesised in platelets (thrombocytes) and hence the name. They are synthesized from PGH_2 by action of thromboxane synthase.

Thromboxanes have following role:

1. Vasoconstriction
2. Platelet aggregation
3. Mobilization of intracellular Ca^{++}.

Aspirin when given in low dose (75–150 mg/day) reduces the risk of thrombus (blood clot) formation as it inhibits thromboxane synthesis and hence prevents platelet aggregation.

Low dose aspirin is therapeutically given in patients of cardiovascular disease to reduce the risk of myocardial infarction.

C. Prostacyclins

Enzyme prostacyclin synthase produces prostacyclins from PGH_2 in vascular endothelial cells.

Prostacyclins inhibit platelet aggregation and leads to vasodilatation.

D. Leukotrienes and Lipoxins (LT and LX)

LT and LX play role in vasoconstriction, broncho-constriction, vascular permeability, smooth muscle contraction, WBC chemotaxis, etc. and are important in hypersensitivity and inflammation.

▌LIPIDS AND THEIR DIVERSE ROLE

Lipids play diverse role in biological system ranging from storage form of energy to being a component of plasma membrane.

Following Table 5.3 represents important functions of various members of lipids.

TABLE 5.3	Important lipids and their functions in human body
Lipid(s)	Function(s)
Triacylglycerol	Storage of energy
Phospholipids, glycolipids, sterols	Structural role
Cholesterol	Precursor of steroid hormone, precursor of vitamin D
Myelin	Electroinsulator
Phospholipids	Activator of enzymes
Phospholipids, bile salts	Absorption of fat soluble vitamins
Bile acid	Digestion of lipid
Bile acid	Absorption of lipid
Phospholipids	Precursor of second messenger

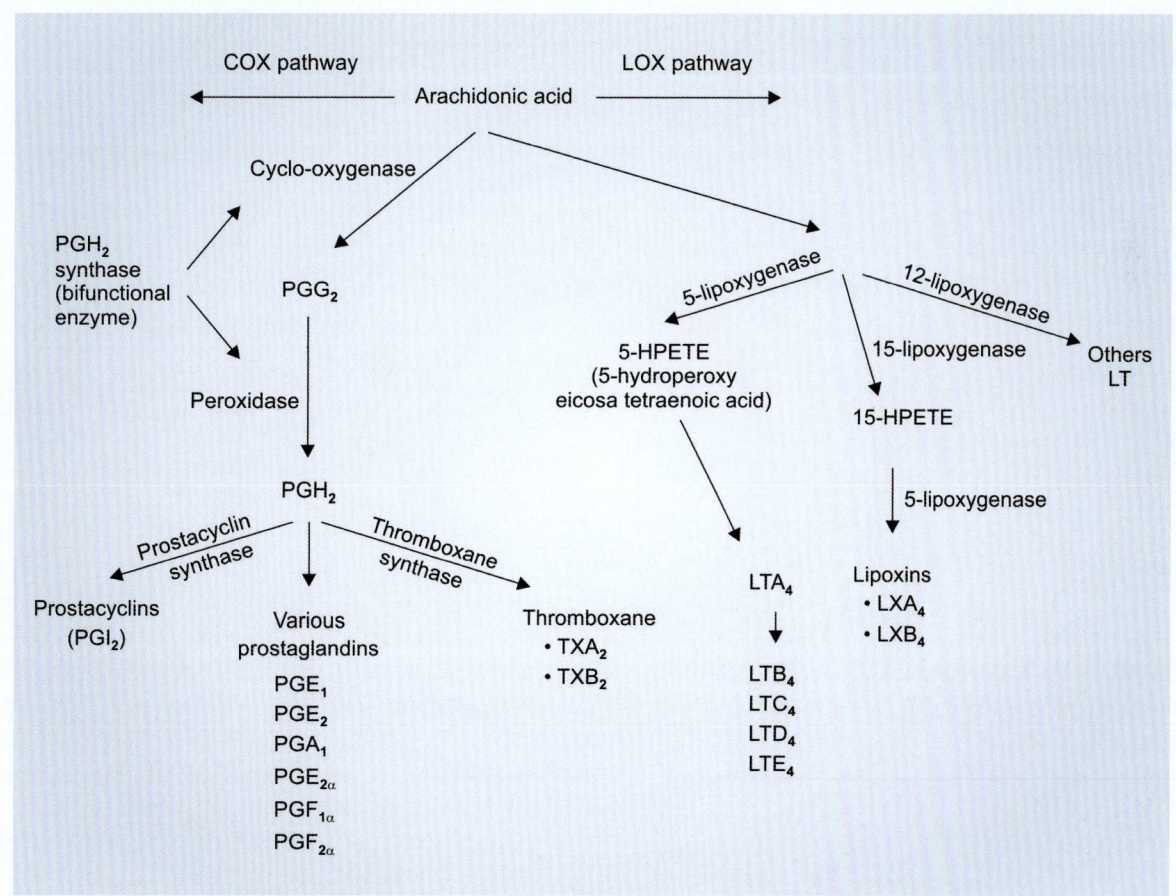

Fig. 5.18: COX and LOX pathways of arachidonic acid

Section 1 ■ Cell and its Biomolecules

5

Proteins, Membrane and Extracellular Matrix

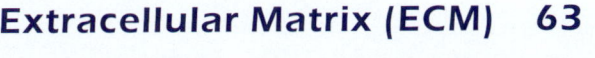
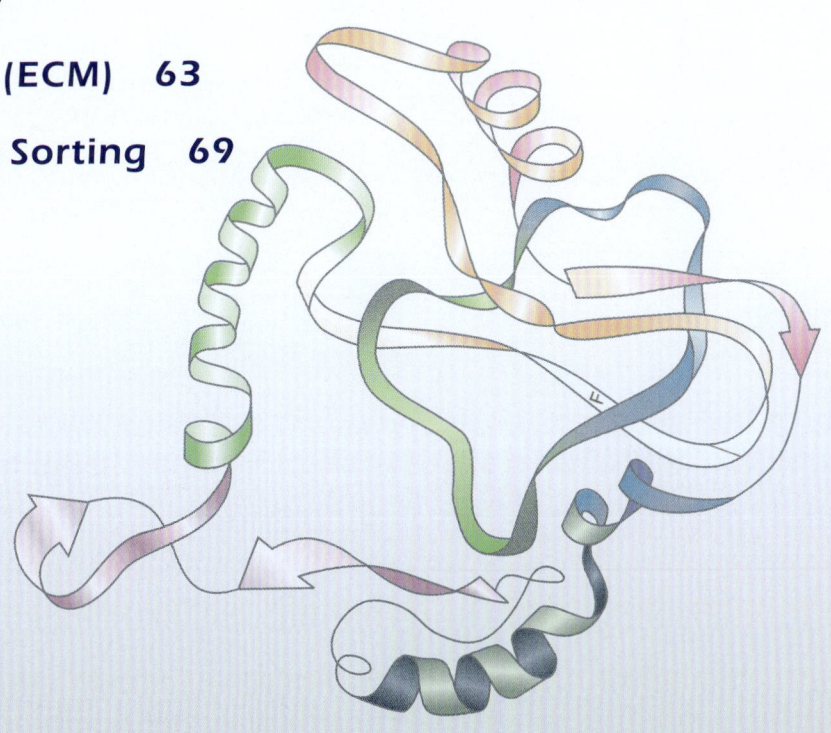

6

Proteins:
Structure and Properties

COMPETENCY BI 5.1

At the end of this chapter learner should be able to describe and discuss structural organization of proteins.

COMPETENCY BI 5.2

At the end of this chapter learner should be able to describe and discuss functions of proteins and structure-function relationships in relevant areas, e.g. hemoglobin and selected hemoglobinopathies.

Specific Learning Objectives	
BI 5.1.1	Describe various levels of protein structure.
BI 5.1.2	Discuss alpha helix structure of protein.
BI 5.1.3	Discuss beta pleated structure of protein.
BI 5.1.4	Define tertiary and quaternary structure of protein.
BI 5.2.1	Discuss important functions of proteins.
BI 5.2.2	Describe how structure helps protein to perform specific function.
BI 5.2.3	Discuss various hemoglobinopathies.

The term protein was coined by J J Berzelius in 1838. This term is derived from Greek word 'Protos' which means 'primary'.

Proteins are polypeptides. They are made up of number of amino acids which are bonded together by peptide bond.

Protein is an important biomolecule in a living system. Their important biological roles are mentioned below:
1. They are building blocks of the cell, they help in formation of cell membrane.
2. They are involved in formation of various ion channels and transporters.
3. They act as enzyme, hormone, clotting factor, etc.
4. They help in transportation of O_2 and other gases (hemoglobin).

5. They play important role in immunity (immuno-globulin).
6. They play role in receptor activity.

STRUCTURAL ORGANIZATION OF THE PROTEIN

There are three (in monomeric proteins) and at times four (in multimeric proteins) levels of protein structure which decide final conformation of the protein in the cell/extracellular space.

These various levels of protein structure are described below.

Primary Structure

It is the sequence of amino acid in the polypeptide chain (Fig. 6.1). The amino acids are held together by peptide bonds in the polypeptide chain.

Peptide bond is formed by condensation of α amino group of one amino acid and α-carboxyl group of another amino acid. Formation of this bond is associated with removal of a single molecule of water (Fig. 6.2).

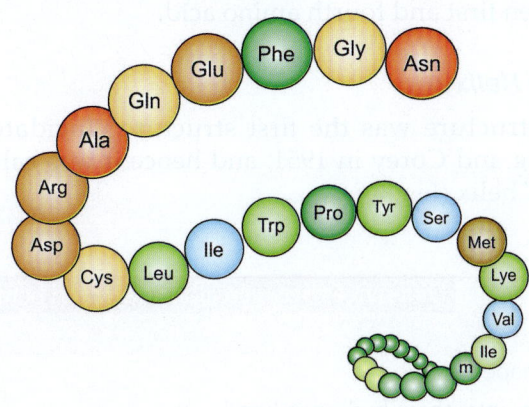

Fig. 6.1: Primary structure of proteins

Characteristics of peptide bonds are as follows:

  a. It is an amide linkage.

  b. It is partially double bond.

  c. It is rigid.

  d. The H atom of 'NH' and O atom of 'CO' are in *trans* configuration.

  e. It is uncharged but polar.

The sequence of the amino acid in a polypeptide chain is decided by the codons present in the mRNA. The mRNA brings this information from the gene.

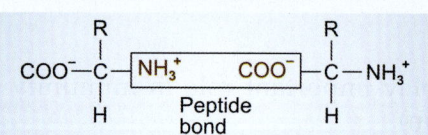

Fig. 6.2: Peptide bond formation

Secondary Structure

Folding and coiling of the protein give rise to secondary structure.

Following are the important varieties of secondary structures seen in various proteins:

  1. Alpha-helix

  2. Beta-pleated sheet

  3. Beta bends (also known as beta-turns)

  4. Beta loop

To stabilize above secondary structure noncovalent (hydrogen) bonds are utilized.

Hydrogen bonds: It is formed by sharing of a single hydrogen atom between electronegative oxygen atom of the carbonyl group (–CO) of one peptide bond and electronegative nitrogen atom of amide group (–NH) of another peptide bond. This hydrogen bond is formed between first and fourth amino acid.

Alpha Helix

This structure was the first structure elucidated by Pauling and Corey in 1951, and hence it was called as 'alpha' helix (Fig. 6.3).

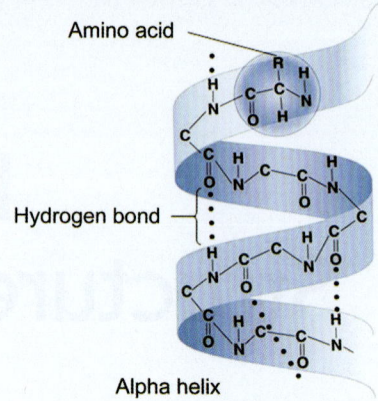

Fig. 6.3: Alpha helix

Folding of polypeptide on its own axis in a helical fashion give rise to alpha helix for most of the protein alpha helix is right handed.

Multiple hydrogen bonds which are formed between carbonyl 'oxygen' (–CO) and amide 'Nitrogen' stabilize alpha helix.

Characteristics of Alpha Helix

  a. Most common and stable form of the protein structure

  b. Right handed helix (mostly)

  c. 3.6 amino acid per turn

  d. Hydrogen bond is parallel to the axis of the α-helix.

  e. Found in both fibrous as well as in globular proteins.

    • *Fibrous proteins where alpha helix is found:* Keratin, myosin, fibrin

    • *Globular protein where alpha helix is found:* Hemoglobin

Beta-pleated Sheet

This was the second structure (after alpha) which was elucidated by Pauling and Corey, and hence they called it 'beta'.

It is more extended configuration compare to alpha helix.

Comparison of alpha helix and beta-pleated sheet is shown in Table 6.1

TABLE 6.1	Differences between alpha helix and beta-pleated sheet
Alpha helix	*Beta-pleated sheet*
Rod shaped	Sheet shaped
Exhibits intrachain hydrogen bond	Exhibits interchain hydrogen bond
Hydrogen bond is parallel to axis	Hydrogen bond is perpendicular to axis
Coiled structure	Extended structure
Formed between single polypeptide	Formed between two or more polypeptides

Section 2 ■ Proteins, Membrane and Extracellular Matrix

6

Here two or more polypeptide chain lie side by side either in parallel or anti-parallel fashion. Parallel sheets are more common.

They are stabilized due to formation of multiple interchain hydrogen bonds between carbonyl oxygen (–CO) and amide nitrogen (–NH) of the peptide bonds of the adjacent chain.

Beta-pleated sheet can also be formed by single polypeptide chain which is folded on itself in a pleated fashion (Fig. 6.4). Examples:
- Silk fibroin consists of beta keratin which has antiparallel beta-pleated sheet.
- Amyloid protein in human.

Globular protein like hemoglobin, immunoglobulin, fibrinogen have both alpha helix and beta-pleated structure.

Beta Bend/Turn

It is an abrupt turn seen in polypeptide chain which changes the direction of polypeptide. This turn or bend area is a narrow region which at the most consists of four amino acids. Proline and glycine are most abundant amino acids in this narrow region. This bend is stabilized by formation of hydrogen bond between first amino acid and fourth amino acid (Fig. 6.5).

Beta Loop/Coil

These are extended configuration which connect two adjacent secondary structures.

Supersecondary Structure

A typical protein has got various types of arrangements in its different regions. Some of the region is having alpha helix which is followed by beta-pleated sheet (parallel or antiparallel). Yet some other region may have beta bend/turn or loop structure. Collectively this type of configuration is called supersecondary structure. It is also called as motif/domain (Figs 6.6 and 6.7).

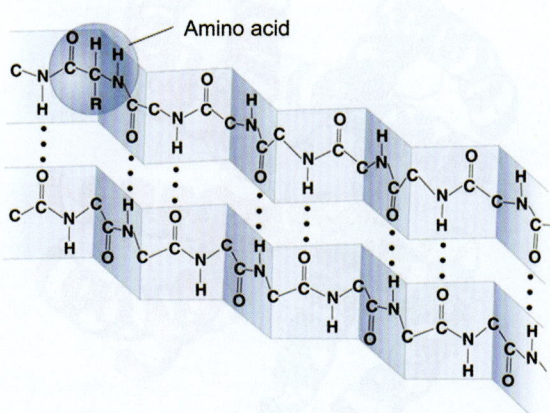

Fig. 6.4: Beta-pleated sheet

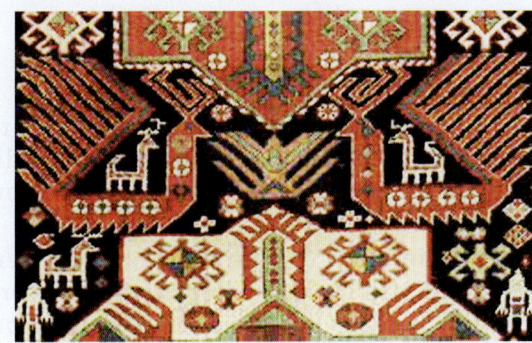

Fig. 6.6: A motif

☐ Also known as beta bends or tight turns.

☐ In a beta turn, a tight loop is formed when the carbonyl oxygen of one residue forms a hydrogen bond with the amide proton of an amino acid, three residues down the chain. This hydrogen bond stabilizes the beta bend structure.

☐ Proline and glycine are frequently found in beta turns, proline because of its cyclic structure, is ideally suited for the beta turn, and glycine, because with the smallest side chain of all the amino acids, it is the most sterically flexible.

☐ A beta turn is a measure by which the protein can reverse the direction of its peptide chain.

☐ Beta turns often promote the formation of antiparallel beta sheets.

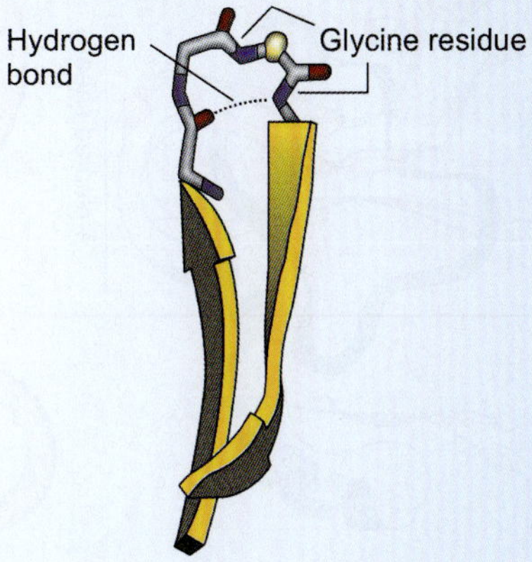

Hydrogen bond   Glycine residue

Fig. 6.5: Beta turns

Section 2 ■ Proteins, Membrane and Extracellular Matrix

6

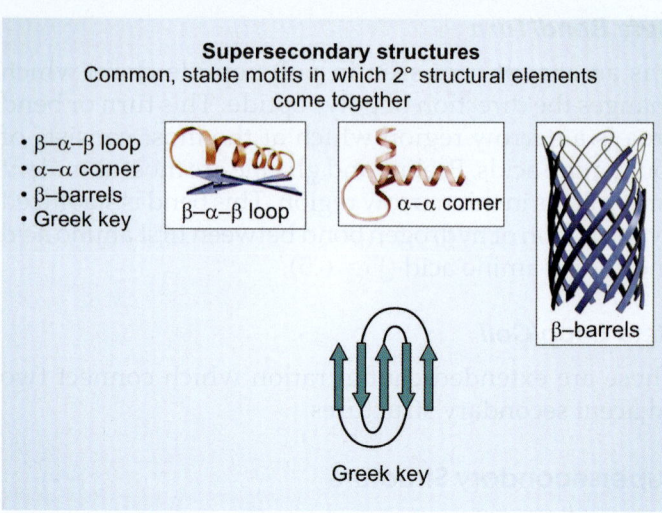

Fig. 6.7: Supersecondary structure

Motif/Domain

1. Helix turn helix
2. Helix loop helix
3. Zinc finger motif
4. Leucine zipper motif

Tertiary Structure

Further folding of secondary structure as to give rise to a condensed three-dimensional structure where distant amino acid of polypeptide interacts, is called tertiary structure.

This approximation of amino acids in the tertiary structure gives rise to regions or area in the protein structure which plays very important role in proper functioning of the protein (Fig. 6.8a).

Both noncovalent and covalent bonds are involved in stabilization of tertiary structure.

Bonds Involved in Tertiary Structure

- *Noncovalent bonds:* Hydrogen bond, hydrophobic interactions, ionic or electrostatic interactions, van der Waals' forces (Fig. 6.8b).
- *Covalent bonds:* Disulphide bonds (Fig. 6.8b).

Quaternary Structure

- It refers to spatial relation between individual sub-unit/monomer of an oligomeric/multimeric protein.
- This type of structure is not seen in all the proteins. Only those proteins which have more than one subunits show quaternary structure (Fig. 6.9).

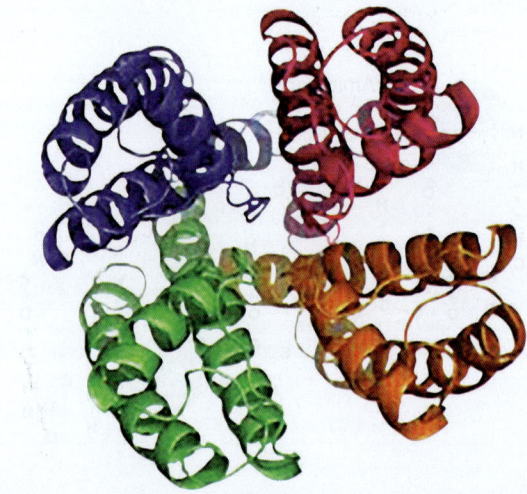

Fig. 6.9: Quaternary structure of protein: Subunit's interaction

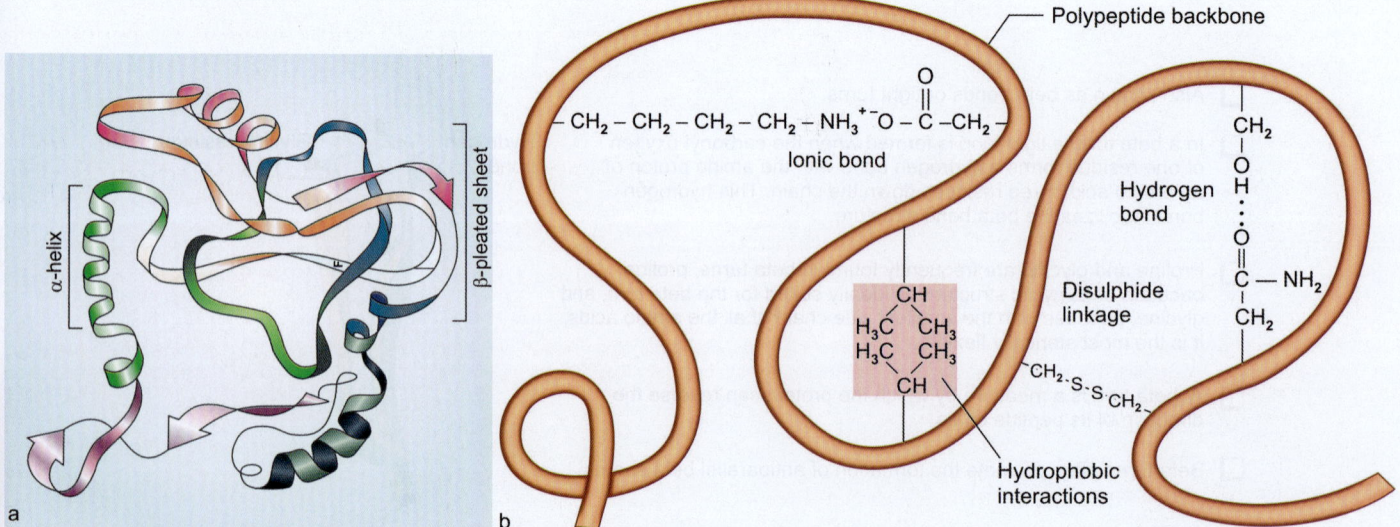

Figs 6.8a and b: (a) Tertiary structure of protein showing 'α-helix', 'β-pleated sheets' in various regions of it; (b) Tertiary structure of protein—various bonds (hydrogen, hydrophobic, ionic, disulphide bonds)

- Bonds involved in quaternary structures are hydrogen bonds, hydrophobic interactions, ionic or electrostatic interactions.

Following proteins show quaternary structure as they have more than one subunits:

1. CPK—it is a dimer.
2. Aldolase
3. Hemoglobin—it is a tetramer.
4. LDH—it is a tetramer.
5. ATC (aspartate transcarbamoylase)

SEPARATION, PURIFICATION AND IDENTIFICATION OF PROTEINS

Separation of a specific protein from a mixture of other proteins or biomolecules is based on the following characteristics:

1. Solubility
2. Molecular size
3. Molecular charge
4. Affinity binding
5. Hydrophobicity

1. **Solubility:** For separation of a specific protein based on solubility, following methods may be adopted:
   a. Salting in/salting out
   b. Isoelectric pH
   c. Organic solvent
   d. Heavy metal ions
   e. Precipitation by alkaloidal reagent
2. **Molecular size:** For separation of a specific protein based on size, following methods may be adopted:
   a. Dialysis
   b. Gel filtration
   c. Ultracentrifugation
   d. SDS-PAGE
3. **Molecular charge:** For separation of a specific protein based on charge, following methods may be adopted:
   a. Ion-exchange chromatography
   b. Electrophoresis
   c. Isoelectric focussing
4. **Affinity binding:** For separation of a specific protein based on affinity binding, following methods may be adopted:
   a. Affinity chromatography
   b. Precipitation by antibody interaction
5. **Hydrophobicity:** For separation of a specific protein based on hydrophobicity, following method may be adopted:
   - Chromatography

SEQUENCING OF PROTEIN

a. Sanger's Approach

Sanger used 1-fluoro-2,4-dinitrobenzene (FDNB, Sanger reagent) to remove and identify the N-terminal amino acid residues of the polypeptide chain.

Dansyl chloride may also be used for identifying the N-terminal of a polypeptide.

b. Edman Degradation

Edman introduced a procedure for automated sequencing of amino acids beginning at the N terminal in a polypeptide, using Edman reagent phenyl-iso-thiocyanate (PIT).

The reaction sequence releases the terminal amino acid as a phenyl-thio-hydantoin (PTH) derivative, which is then identified by HPCL.

DNA sequencing as a method of detecting primary structure of proteins.

Protein's primary structure can also be determined by DNA sequencing, but this method has got following limitations:

a. Not able to detect the disulphide bond in the folded chain.
b. Not able to predict the post-translational modification of the amino acid.

GENERAL CHARACTERISTICS OF PROTEINS

1. **Colloidal osmotic pressure:** Colloids are particles of size 1–100 μm. Protein exist in the form of colloid particle in the plasma and are responsible for osmotic pressure. Plasma albumin is responsible for 75–80% of osmotic pressure in the plasma.
2. **Amphoteric biomolecules:** Proteins may accept the protons in acidic media or may donate the proton in alkali media, hence they are called amphoteric biomolecules.
3. **Isoelectric pH (pI):** pH at which ampholytes have equal positive and negative charge are called as pI. At pI ampholytes are in zwitter ion form.

Important characteristics of zwitter ion at pI (isoelectric pH)
   a. No net change
   b. No electrophoretic movement
   c. Least solubility
   d. Maximum precipitability
   e. Least buffering capacity

Section 2 ■ Proteins, Membrane and Extracellular Matrix

6

Following are the pI of some important proteins:
   a. Pepsin: 1.1
   b. Casein: 4.6
   c. Albumin: 4.7
   d. Globulin: 6.4

CLASSIFICATION OF PROTEINS

The classification of proteins based on various criteria is shown in Flowchart 6.1.

DENATURATION OF PROTEINS

Denaturation of proteins may be defined as 'loss of secondary and tertiary structures of the protein accompanied by loss of their functions'.

It is important to note that 1° structure is intact in protein after denaturation.

Characteristic Features of the Denaturation

- Primary structure of molecules, i.e. peptide bonds are not affected.
- Denatured proteins are generally less soluble and thus precipitate more easily.
- Denaturation is caused by physical and chemical agents, e.g. heat, UV light, organic solvents, acids, urea, sodium docedyl sulphate (SDS) and various detergents.
- Denaturation is a reversible phenomenon.

Prion disease: Prion protein (PrP) is held responsible for occurrence of transmissible spongiform encephalopathies (TSE) (Fig. 6.10).

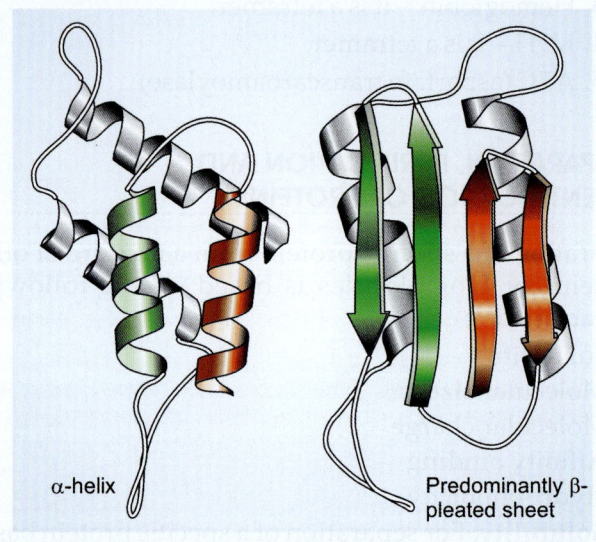

Fig. 6.10: Prion disease (conversion of 'α-helix' to β-pleated sheet)

Flowchart 6.1: Classification of proteins

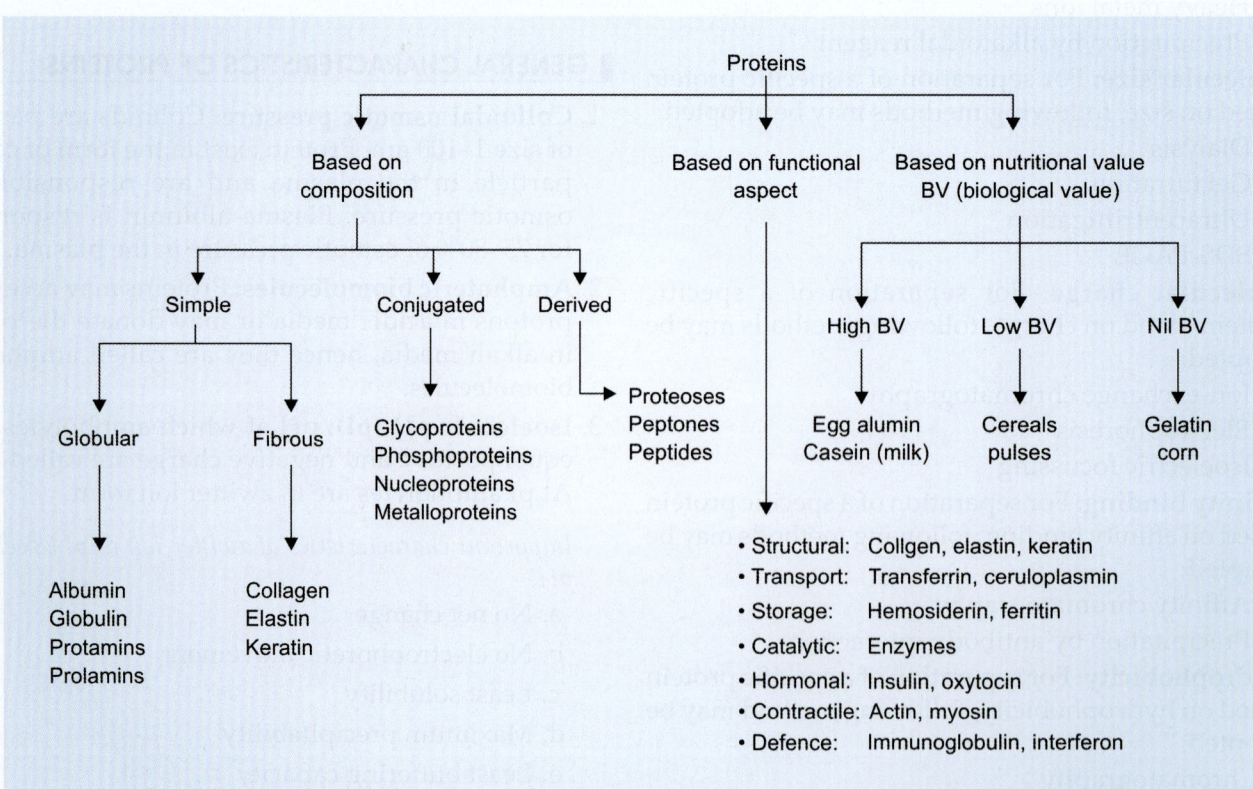

Examples of TSE are:
- Creutzfeldt-Jakob disease
- Scrapie
- Bovine spongiform encephalopathy (mad cow disease)

PrP is an infectious protein, the noninfectious form of PrP has the same amino acid and the gene sequence as that of the infectious form of the protein, and it is found in normal mammalian brains on surface of neurons and glial cell. PrP is thus a **host protein**.

Key of conversion of noninfectious form of PrP to the infectious form lies in the fact that number of alpha-helix present in the noninfectious form is **replaced by beta-sheet** in the infectious form.

This abnormally configured PrP acts as a template which induces other proteins also to take the infectious configuration (i.e. α-helix is replaced by β-sheet).

Collagen (Fibrous Protein)

- Collagen is the most abundant protein of animal world. It is a structural protein with unique amino acid composition—glycine, proline, hydroxyproline and hydroxylysine.
- Collagen has a triple helical structure.
- Each alpha polypeptide or subunit is twisted in left-handed helix, then three of such subunits are twisted in a right-handed superhelical pattern. Next, these triple helix is arranged in the staggered pattern

where there occurs overlapping of the bundles in the pattern given in Figs 6.11 and 6.12.

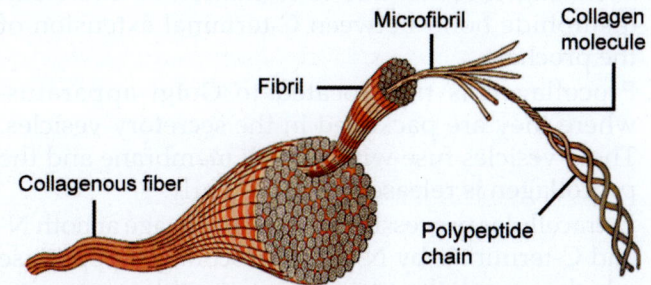

Fig. 6.11: Structure of collagen—collagen fiber and collagen molecule

Biosynthesis

a. Collagen chain contains a signal sequence at the N-terminal end. This signal sequence facilitates the binding of the ribosome to the RER and directs the passage of the nascent chain to the lumen of the RER.

b. After removal of the signal sequence, the collagen chain is known as pro α-collagen chain.

c. There in the lumen of RER, proline and lysine are converted into hydroxyproline and hydroxylysine respectively.

d. Some of the hydroxylysine residues are modified by glycosylation by glucose or galactose residue.

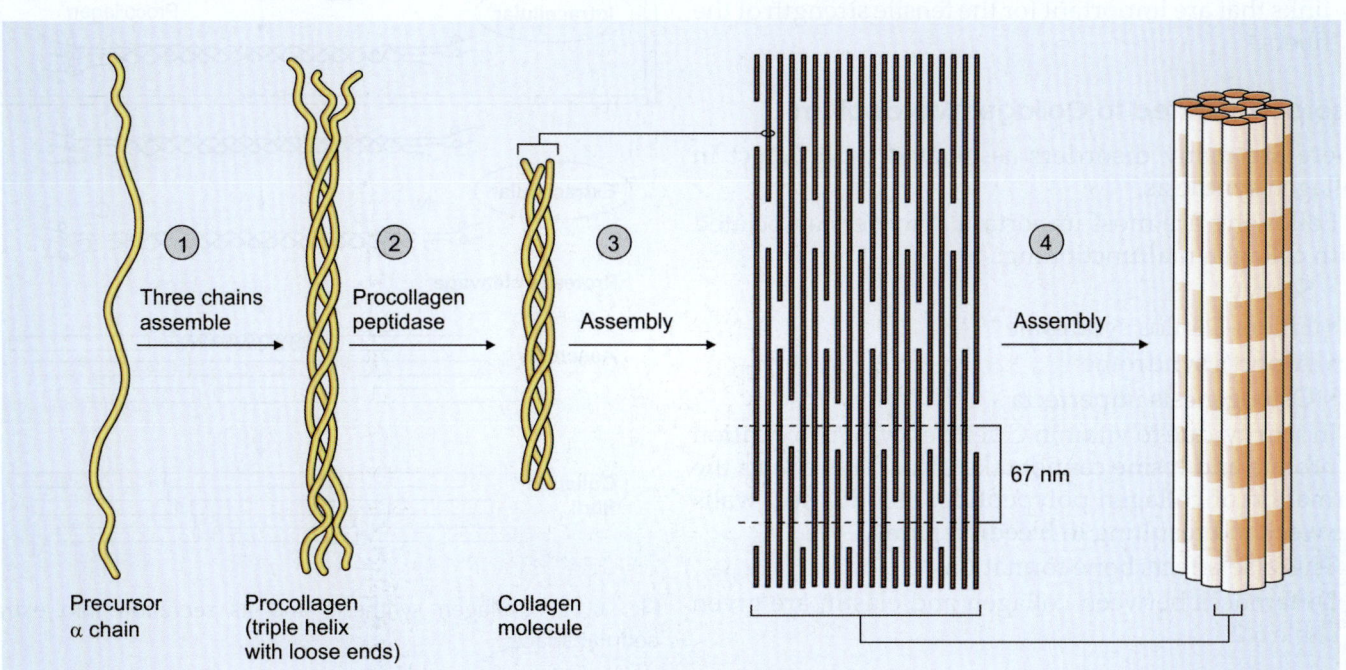

Fig. 6.12: Arrangement of collagen

Section 2 ■ Proteins, Membrane and Extracellular Matrix

6

e. After hydroxylation and glycosylation, prochain forms procollagen.

f. Procollagen forms due to formation of interchain disulphide bond between C-terminal extension of the prochain.

g. Procollagen is translocated to Golgi apparatus, where they are packaged in the secretory vesicles. These vesicles fuse with the cell membrane and the procollagen is released extracellularly.

h. Extracellular processing involves cleavage at both N- and C-terminals by N and C procollagen peptidase which remove the terminal propeptides, releasing triple helical collagen molecule.

i. These triple helical collagen molecules are now assembled in the form of collagen fibril.

j. Collagen fibers are further stabilized by the formation of covalent cross-links, both within and between the triple helical units. These cross-links form through the action of lysyl oxidase, a copper-dependent enzyme that oxidatively deaminates the amino groups of certain lysine and hydroxylysine residues, yielding reactive aldehydes (allysine and hydroxyallysine). Such aldehydes can form aldol condensation products with other lysine- or hydroxylysine-derived aldehydes.

k. Aldehyde derivative of lysine and hydroxylysine may also form Schiff bases with the amino groups of unoxidized lysines or hydroxylysines.

l. These reactions, after further chemical rearrangements, result in the stable covalent cross-links that are important for the tensile strength of the fibers.

Disorders Related to Collagen Metabolism

There are many disorders associated with defect in collagen synthesis.

Following are most important disorders associated with collagen malfunctioning:

- Scurvy
- Ehlers-Danlos syndrome
- Alport's syndrome
- Osteogenesis imperfecta

In scurvy, due to vitamin C deficiency, hydroxylation of proline and lysine cannot take place. This effects the formation of collagen polypeptide. Blood vessel walls are weekend resulting in bleeding gums.

This also affects bone formation.

Differences between collagen and elastin are given in Table 6.2.

TABLE 6.2	Differences between collagen and elastin
Collagen	Elastin
Many different genetic types	One genetic type
Triple helix	No triple helix
(Gly-X-Y)$_n$ repeats	No (Gly-X-Y)$_n$ repeats
Presence of hydroxylysine	No hydroxylysine
Carbohydrate containing	No carbohydrate
Intramolecular aldol cross-links	Intramolecular desmosine cross-links
Presence of extension peptide	No extension peptide

Collagen synthesis and its secretion into extracellular space is shown in Fig. 6.13.

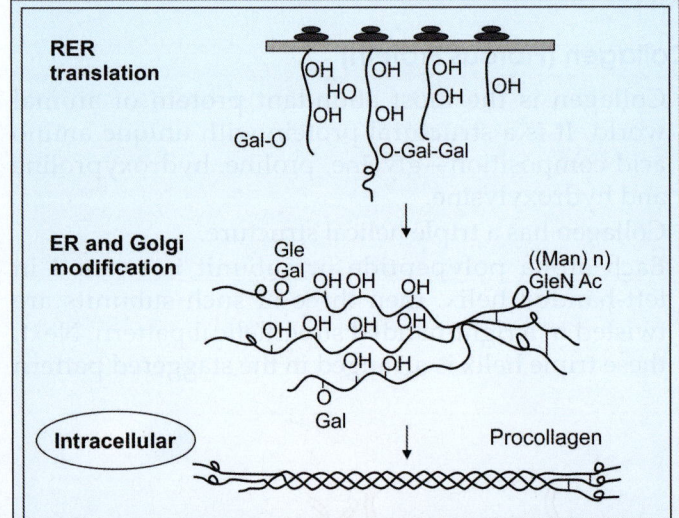

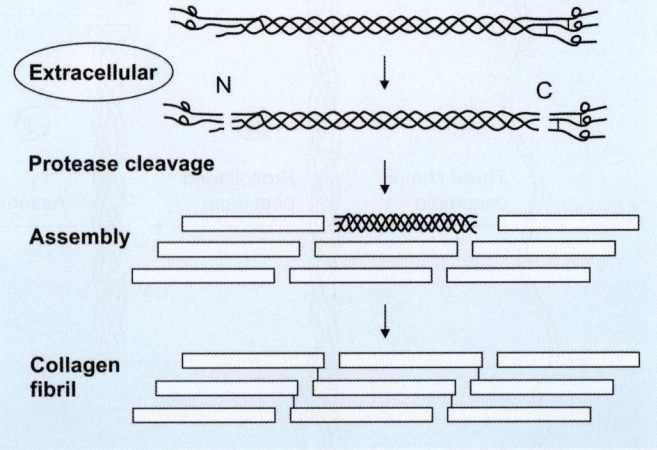

Fig. 6.13: Collagen synthesis and its secretion into extracellular space

6

EXERCISE

LONG QUESTION (10 MARKS)

Q 1. Describe the various levels of organisation of protein structure. Illustrate your answer with suitable example.

SHORT NOTES (5 MARKS EACH)

Q 1. Secondary structure of proteins.
Q 2. Denaturation of protein
Q 3. Methods of purification of proteins
Q 4. Protein sequencing
Q 5. Sanger reagent

Plasma Membrane

COMPETENCY BI 1.1

At the end of this chapter learner should be able to describe the molecular and functional organization of a cell and its subcellular components.

Specific Learning Objectives	
BI 1.1.3	Describe the organization of cell membrane.
BI 1.1.4	Discuss functions of protein and lipid of cell membrane.
BI 1.1.5	Describe protein–lipid ratio of various membranes.

Plasma membrane also called cell membrane is the outermost covering of the cell, which separates content of the cell from external environment. This membrane can be differentiated by other membranes which enclose various organelles like mitochondria, lysosome, peroxisome, Golgi apparatus, endoplasmic reticulum, etc. in the eukaryotic cell, by its composition and function.

All the membranes are made up of lipids, proteins and carbohydrates. Relative concentration of these components vary in various membranes. Plasma membrane and its components are discussed in detail in this chapter.

Plasma membrane is made up of following components (Fig. 7.1):

1. Lipids
2. Proteins
3. Carbohydrates

1. **Lipids:** *Phospholipids* are the main lipid of membrane. Other lipids in membrane are *glycolipid* and *cholesterol*.
2. **Proteins** in the membrane may be
   a. Intrinsic (integral)
   b. Extrinsic (peripheral)
3. **Carbohydrates:** Carbohydrates are not found in prokaryotic cell membrane. Finding of carbohydrate is the characteristic feature of eukaryotic cell membrane, where it is not found in the free

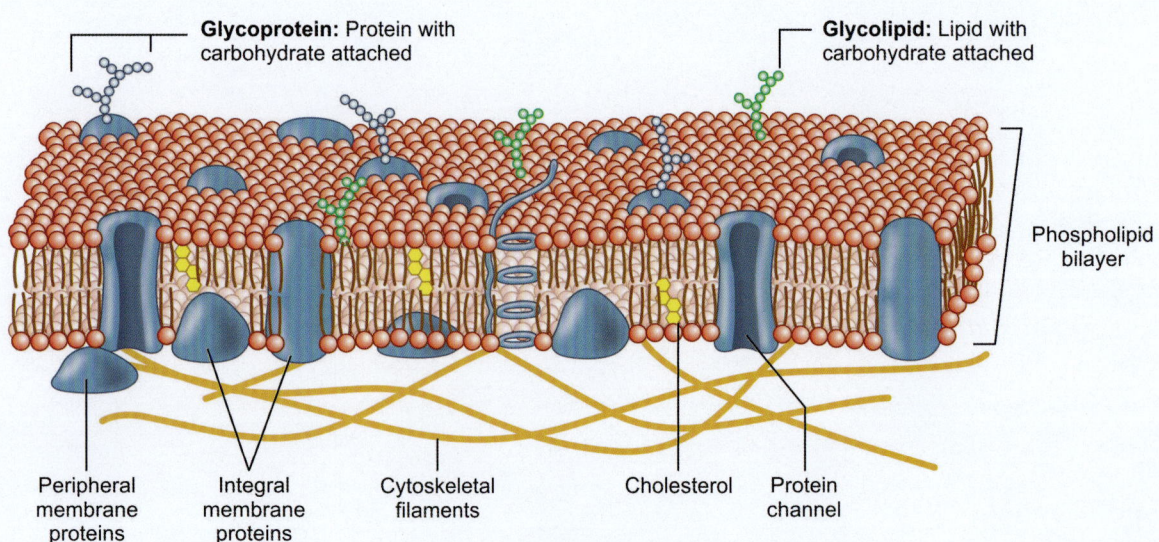

Glycoprotein: Protein with carbohydrate attached

Glycolipid: Lipid with carbohydrate attached

Phospholipid bilayer

Peripheral membrane proteins

Integral membrane proteins

Cytoskeletal filaments

Cholesterol

Protein channel

Fig. 7.1: Plasma membrane

form, rather it is always seen in conjugated form (glycoconjugates like glycolipid and glycoprotein).

LIPIDS OF MEMBRANE

Various lipids found in membrane are phospholipids, glycolipids and cholesterol.
- All the lipids in the membrane are amphipathic in nature.
- Major lipid of the membrane is phospholipid which is arranged in bimolecular layer such that polar group of phospholipid is towards cytosol and also towards ECF.

Phospholipids

Phospholipids are amphipathic molecule, having a polar head and a nonpolar tail (Figs 7.2 and 7.3).

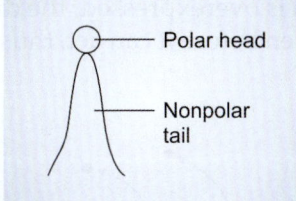

Fig. 7.2: Phospholipid (an amphipathic lipid)

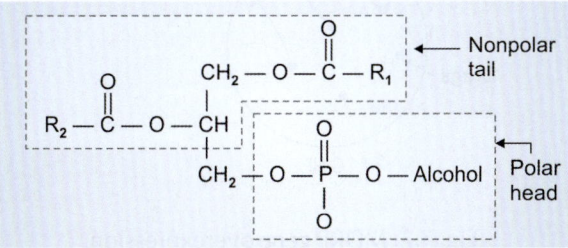

Fig. 7.3: Molecular form of phospholipid

- Polar head of phospholipid is made up of phosphoric and alcohol moiety attached to it.
- Nonpolar tail consists of fatty acid chains which may be unsaturated or saturated.
- Two classes of phospholipids are found in membrane.
  a. Glycerophospholipid
  b. Sphingophospholipid

Glycerophospholipds may be:
- Phosphatidyl choline
- Phosphatidyl ethanolamine
- Phosphatidyl serine
- Phosphatidyl inositol
- Diphosphatidyl glycerol (cardiolipin)

Sphingophospholipid may be:
- Sphingomyelin

- There is noncovalent interaction between phospholipids in the membrane, so slight lateral movement is possible.

Glycolipid

- Carbohydrate portion of glycolipid projects out of the cell membrane and interacts with polar portion of the phospholipid.
- Glycoproteins are present only on the outer surface of the cell membrane.

Cholesterol

Cholesterol is an amphipathic lipid. Its third hydroxyl group is polar in nature which is directed towards aqueous interface and rest of the portion is nonpolar which is embedded in hydrophobic interior of cell membrane (Figs 7.4 and 7.5).

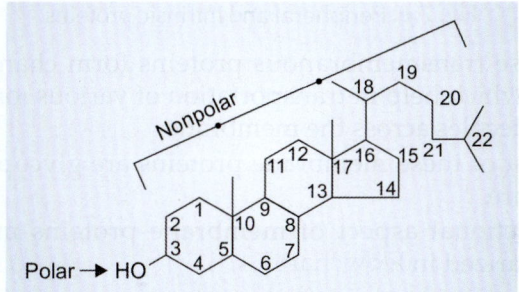

Fig. 7.4: Cholesterol

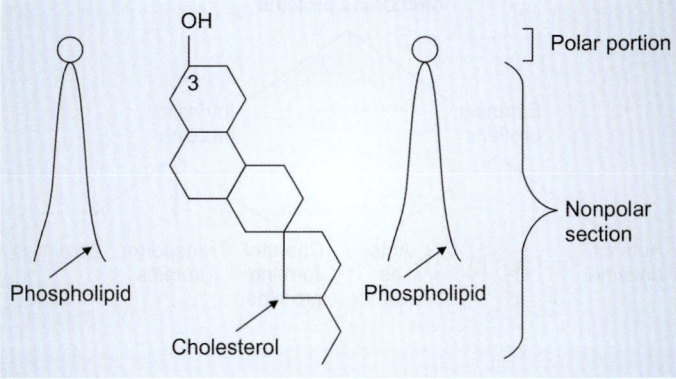

Fig. 7.5: Distribution of lipid in plasma membrane

PROTEINS OF MEMBRANE

Depending upon their location in the membrane, proteins in the membrane may be classified into:
1. 'Integral or integrated proteins' (trans-membraneous or intrinsic)
2. Peripheral or extrinsic proteins

Peripheral or extrinsic proteins are found at the surface of lipid bilayer, while integrated or intrinsic

Section 2 ■ Proteins, Membrane and Extracellular Matrix

7

proteins are partially or completely embedded in lipid bilayer.

Integrated proteins which traverse the whole lipid bilayer is known as transmembrane protein (Fig. 7.6).

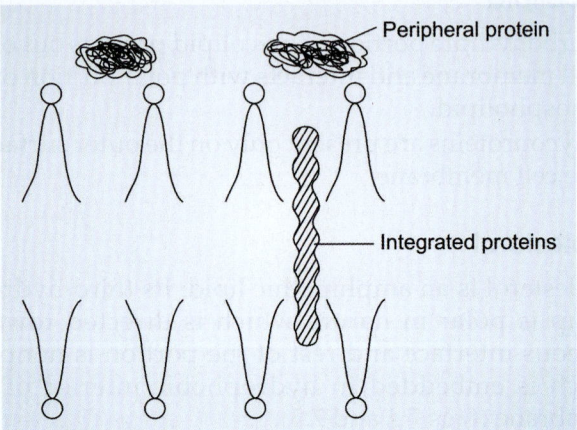

Fig. 7.6: Peripheral and intrinsic proteins

These transmembranous proteins form channel or pores which help in transportation of various ions and biomolecules across the membrane.

Most of these membrane proteins are glycoprotein in nature.

Functional aspect of membrane proteins may be summarized in Flowchart 7.1.

Flowchart 7.1: Functional aspect of membrane proteins

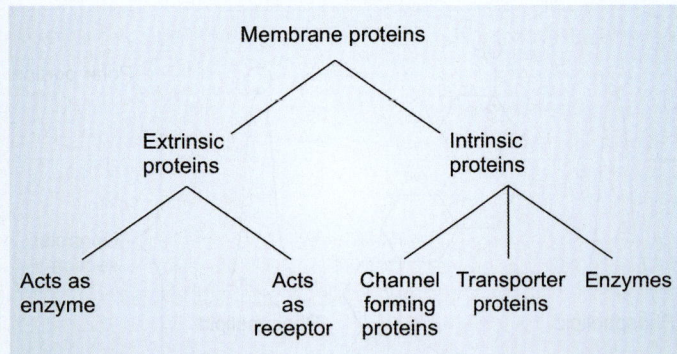

Clinical Correlation

A. Cystic Fibrosis

- Cystic fibrosis (CF) is an autosomal recessive disorder characterized by thick mucus.
- It is due to mutation of gene for Cystic Fibrosis Transmembrane conductance Regulator protein (CFTR).
- Defect in CFTR results in decreased chloride secretion and increased sodium and water reabsorption, resulting in thick mucus secretion by exocine glands.

This affects pancreatic secretion, liver and gallbladder secretion and respiratory tract secretion.

Diagnosis

1. Sweat chloride assessment
2. Prenatal genetic diagnosis can be done by chorionic villus sampling at 8–10 weeks of gestation.

Enzyme replacement therapy (ERT) with pancreatic enzymes has been tried in this disorder and has shown promising result.

B. Multidrug Resistance (MDR)

This is due to over-expression of a gene responsible for transcription of a membrane protein multidrug resistant protein (MDRP) (Fig. 7.7).

MDRP is a glycoprotein, which is responsible for export of wide range of small molecules from the cell. In case this protein is overexpressed, the drug is exported out of the cell even before it can act, thus reducing drug toxicity.

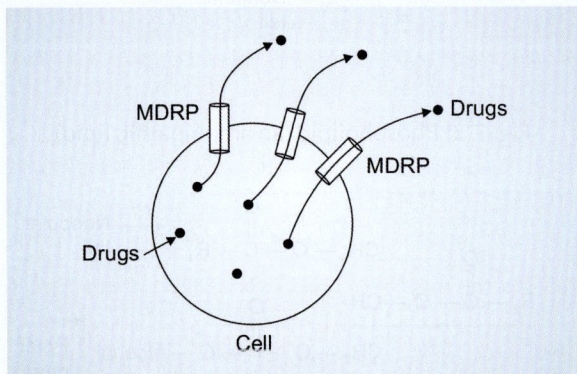

Fig. 7.7: MDRP gene overexpression

CARBOHYDRATE OF MEMBRANE

- In the plasma membrane, carbohydrates are found in bound form, bound either to lipid (glycolipid) or to protein (glycoprotein).
- Proteoglycan is a complex substance which is having glycosaminoglycan as its major component. This proteoglycan sometimes is found at outer layer of membrane forming a structure called 'glycocalyx'.

Functional aspect of membrane carbohydrates:

1. Carbohydrate portion in the cell membrane imparts negative charge to the membrane.
2. 'Glycocalyx' helps in cell attachment.
3. Many of the glycoproteins act as receptor molecules, e.g. insulin receptor.

Fluid Mosaic Model of Cell Membrane

Singer and Nicolson in 1972 proposed a theory for defining membrane structure which is widely accepted now and is known as 'Fluid Mosaic Model'.

Key features of this model are as follows:

- Plasma membrane is composed of many heterogenous molecules like
  1. Phospholipid
  2. Glycolipid
  3. Cholesterol
  4. Integrated proteins
  5. Peripheral proteins

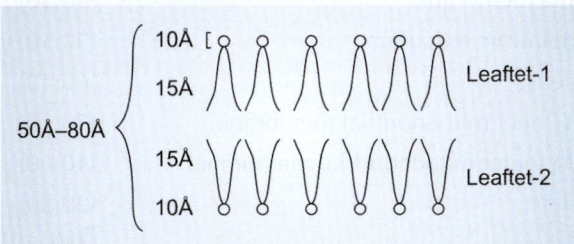

Fig. 7.8: Bilayer leaflet of plasma membrane

Above compounds gives plasma membrane a mosaic appearance.

- Plasma membrane is a lipid bilayer where phospholipids are arranged in two layers with their polar heads towards aqueous media and nonpolar tail sandwiched between the two polar heads.
- Each leaflet is ~25Å, where head portion is 10Å and tail is 15Å thick. Total thickness is about 50Å–80Å (Fig. 7.8).
- Due to presence of appropriate mixture of saturated and unsaturated fatty acids in tail portion of phospholipid, the lipid bilayer is fluid at room temperature.
- This lipid bilayer provides a medium in which integral proteins are interspread.
- This lipid bilayer also acts as permeability barrier.
- This model have proposed that portion of the protein which traverses hydrophobic tail portion of lipid bilayer is having rich amount of hydrophobic amino acids like valine and leucine, and the portion of protein which is peripheral is having polar amino acid like serine, glutamate, etc (Fig. 7.9).
- There is no covalent bond between lipid-lipid or lipid-protein in bilayer.
- Peripheral proteins float in the sea of lipid bilayer, while integral proteins are seen as an iceberg (almost completely submerged in sea).
- Membrane proteins can float in lipid bilayer bidirectionally, but flip-flop movement is not possible (Figs 7.10 and 7.11).
- *Membrane fluidity* is decided by cholesterol content of the membrane and also by nature of fatty acid in tail portion of phospholipid.

  a. **Role of cholesterol in deciding the membrane fluidity:** Cholesterol play dual role in deciding the membrane fluidity.

  Below transition temperature* cholesterol increases the membrane fluidity and **above transition temperature** cholesterol reduces the membrane fluidity.

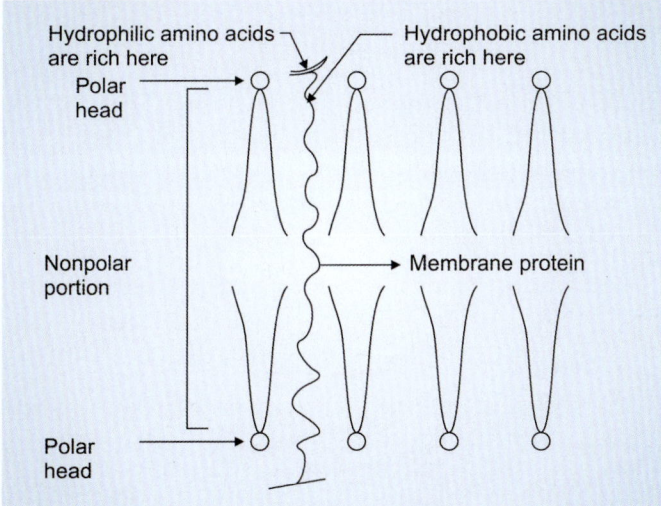

Fig. 7.9: Membrane protein traversing the lipid bilayer

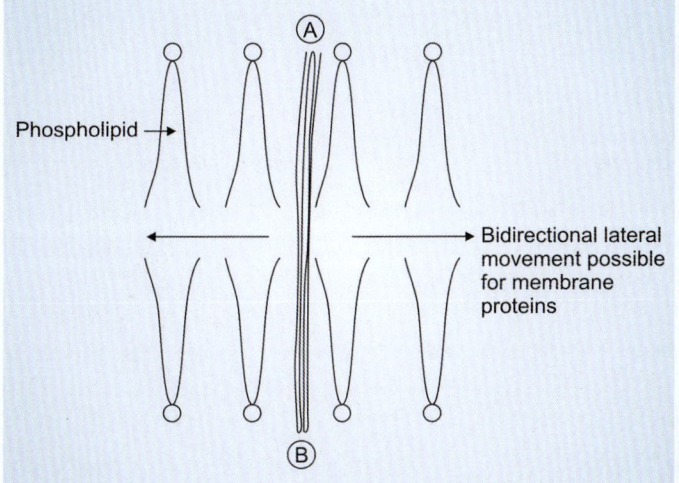

Fig. 7.10: Bidirectional movement for membrane proteins

*Transition temperature: It is the temperature at which membrane transforms into fluid state from more cystalline state.

Section 2 ■ Proteins, Membrane and Extracellular Matrix

7

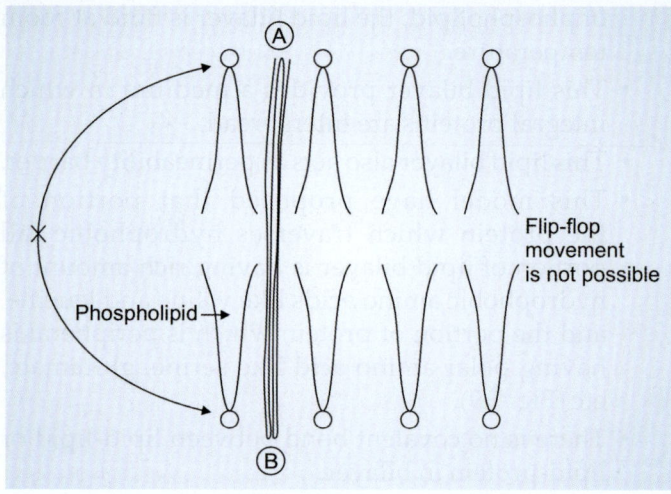

Fig. 7.11: Flip-flop movement of membrane protein is not allowed

b. **Role of fatty acid in deciding the membrane fluidity**

- Unsaturated fatty acid increases and saturated fatty acid decreases membrane fluidity.
- 'Cis' type of unsaturated fatty acid increases the fluidity to larger extent compared to 'trans' type of unsaturated fatty acid which has lesser impact on increasing the membrane fluidity.

Functions of Plasma Membrane

In addition to protecting the internal organelles, plasma membrane has multiple other roles to play:

1. Role in transportation of biomolecules (provides channels and pores)
2. Receptor role

Protein–Lipid Ratio of Different Membranes

See Table 7.1.

TABLE 7.1	Difference in composition of various membranes
Membrane	Protein–lipid ratio
Plasma membrane	[50:50]
Endoplasmic reticulum	[50:50]
Nucleus	[60:40]
IMM (inner mitochondial membrane)	[70:30]
OMM (outer mitochondial membrane)	[40:60]
Myelin	[20:80]
RBC	[45:55]
Golgi apparatus	[45:55]

Different membranes have different ratios for protein and lipid. For example, myelin sheath has more lipid compared to protein (protein–lipid ratio—20:80) and IMM has more protein compared to lipid (protein–lipid ratio—70:30).

Plasma Proteins

There are number of proteins which circulate in plasma in various concentrations and perform diverse roles.

In an attempt to seggregate them by electrophoresis, we get following bands (Fig. 8.1):

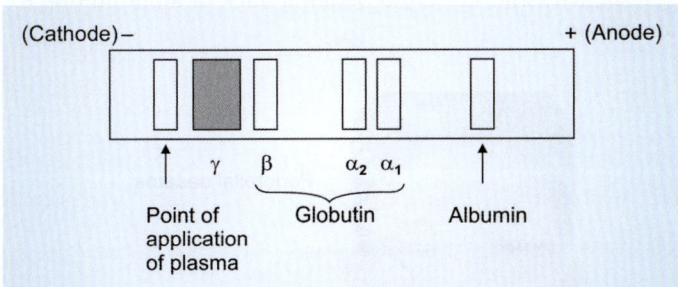

Fig. 8.1: Bands developed on protein electrophoresis

▌ PLASMA VS SERUM

Supernatant received on centrifugation of blood which contains some anticoagulant is plasma, and the one which is received on centrifugation of blood which is clotted is serum (Fig. 8.2).

So, serum is devoid of fibrinogen and other clotting factors as they are utilized in clotting process, while plasma contains fibrinogen and clotting factors.

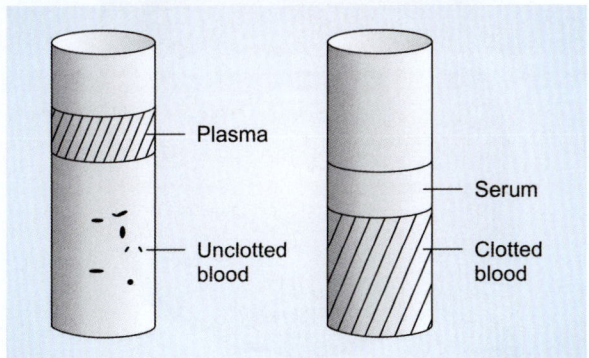

Fig. 8.2: Plasma *vs* serum

Description of Important Plasma Proteins

▶ Albumin

- Albumin is the major protein of plasma.
- Total protein concentration in the plasma is 7.0–7.5 g/dl out of which 3.5–5 g/dl is albumin.
- Albumin is exclusively synthesized by liver, which secretes 12 grams of albumin per day (25% of total hepatic proteins synthesis).
- Half-life of albumin is 20 days.

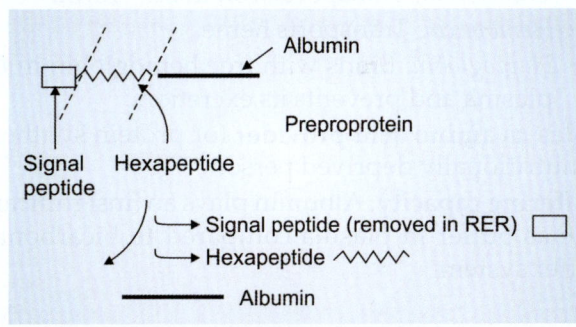

Fig. 8.3: Maturation of albumin

- Albumin is secreted as preproprotein. After removal of its signal peptide and hexapeptide from amino terminal end, it is converted to albumin which is 585 amino acid long (Fig. 8.3).
- Albumin has 17 intrachain disulphide bonds.

Role of Albumin

Albumin has diverse roles to play.

1. **Albumin is mainly responsible for plasma oncotic pressure.**
   - Total plasma oncotic pressure is 25 mmHg. Because of relatively low molecular mass (69 kDa) and high concentration, albumin is considered as important protein responsble for plasma oncotic

pressure (75–80% of total plasma oncotic pressure is because of albumin).

2. **Role of albumin as transporter protein for number of biologically important compounds:**
   - Numerous ligands tend to bind with albumin, which helps in their transportation.
   - Biomolecules which bind albumin are:
     1. Free fatty acid
     2. Bilirubin
     3. Calcium
     4. Copper
     5. Steroid hormones
     6. Tryptophan
     7. Drugs like sulphonamide, penicillin G, dicu-manol, aspirin.
   - *Other transporter proteins other than albumin in the plasma are:*
     - *Prealbumin:* Transports thyroxine.
     - *Retinol binding protein:* Transports vitamin A.
     - *Thyroxine binding protein:* Transports thyroid hormone.
     - *Transcortin:* Transports steroid hormone (cortisol binding protein).
     - *Transferrin:* Transports iron in Fe^{+++} form.
     - *Hemopexin:* Transports heme.
     - *Haptoglobin:* Binds with free hemoglobin in the plasma and prevents its excretion.

3. **Roles as amino acid provider** for protein synthesis in nutritionally deprived person.

4. **Buffering capacity:** Albumin plays an 'insignificant' role as buffer in plasma compared to bicarbonate buffer system.

Clinical Correlation

Albumin is mainly responsible for oncotic pressure of the plasma which prevents oozing of plasma into the interstitial space. In conditions where there is deficiency of albumin, either because of malnutrition (Kwashiorkor) or in cases when there is loss of albumin through urine (nephrotic syndrome) or cases of liver cirrhosis when this organ is not able to produce albumin, the affected person develops oedema (Figs 8.4a, b, c).
- Microalbuminuria (MAU) is the term applied when urine shows very small amount of albumin (30–300 mg/day)
  - MAU denotes high risk of incipient nephropathy, hence corrective action should be started on finding of MAU.
  - *Prealbumin (transthyretin):* Binds T4 and form a complex with RBP.

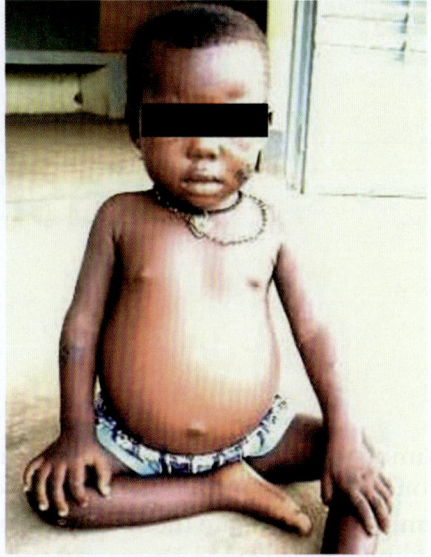

Fig. 8.4a: Kwashiorkor child oedema (lack of albumin due to malnutrition)

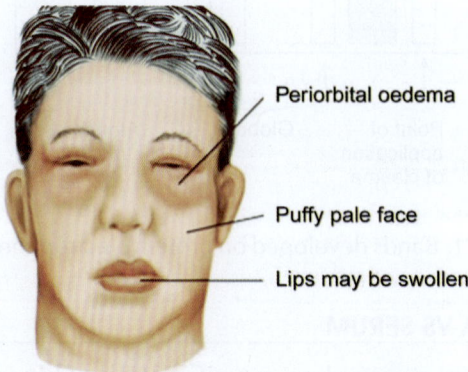

Periorbital oedema

Puffy pale face

Lips may be swollen

Fig. 8.4b: Nephrotic syndrome oedema (deficiency of albumin due to loss through urine)

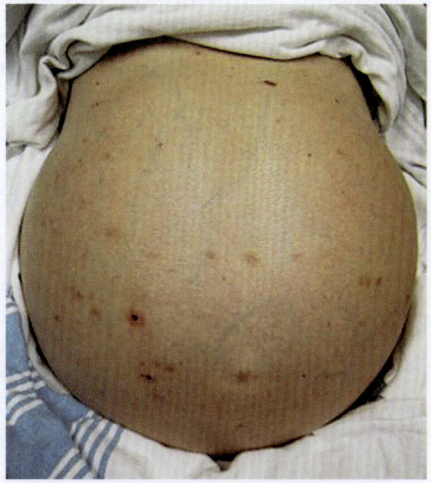

Fig. 8.4c: Liver cirrhosis oedema (deficiency of albumin due to less/no production of albumin)

TABLE 8.1	Components of various globin bands on protein electrophoresis			
α₁-band		α₂-band	β-band	γ-band
• α₁-antitrypsin		• α₂-macroglobulin		Immunoglobulin
		• Haptoglobin	• Transferrin	
• Retinol binding protein (RBP)		• Prothrombin	• Hemopexin	
• Transcortin or cortisol binding globulin (CBG)		• Ceruloplasmin	• Plasminogen	
• Thyroxin binding globulin (TBG)				

▶ Globulin

Under this heading, number of proteins are included.

On electrophoresis, various globulins are seggregated into α₁, α₂, β and γ-bands.

Important globulins in each of these bands are summarized below (Table 8.1).

α₁-Globulin

a. **α₁-antitrypsin (now called α₁-antiproteinase):** It is 394 amino acid long glycoprotein which constitutes >90% of α₁-band.

It is *serpin* (**ser**ine **p**rotease **in**hibitor) which inhibits action of not only trypsin but also elastase and other serine proteases.

α₁-antitrypsin deficiency is associated with following two disorders:

1. Emphysema
2. α₁-antitrypsin deficiency liver disease

Approximately 5% of emphysema (a disorder where abnormal dilatation of alveoli occurs) is due to deficiency of α₁-antiproteinase (Fig. 8.5).

Smoking and Emphysema

• Burning tobacco produces smoke which oxidizes methionine residue at protease binding domain of α₁-antiproteinase.
• The oxidized α₁-antiproteinase can no longer bind the serine proteases.

• Unchecked elastase and other serine proteases damage the lung tissues, contributing to emphysema.

b. **Retinol binding protein (RBP):** It transports vitamin A.

c. **Transcortin or cortisol binding globulin (CBG):** It transports steroid hormone.

d. **Thyroxine binding globulin (TBG):** It transports thyroid hormone.

α₂-Globulin

a. **α₂-macroglobulin**
   • Synthesized by monocyte, hepatocyte and astrocyte.
   • It is homotetrameric glycoprotein.
   • Level of α₂-macroglobulin is increased in plasma in nephrotic syndrome. This is due to increase of its synthesis by liver which is seen as a compensatory mechanism to counterbalance the lost protein in nephrotic syndrome.

b. **Haptoglobin (Hp):** It is a glycoprotein which binds the free Hb (extracorpuscular Hb) to make Hp-Hb complex. Hp-Hb complex cannot cross glomerulus while free Hb can pass through the glomeruli. Half-life of free Hp is 5 days while that of Hp-Hb complex is 90 minutes.

c. **Prothrombin:** It is a blood clotting factor.

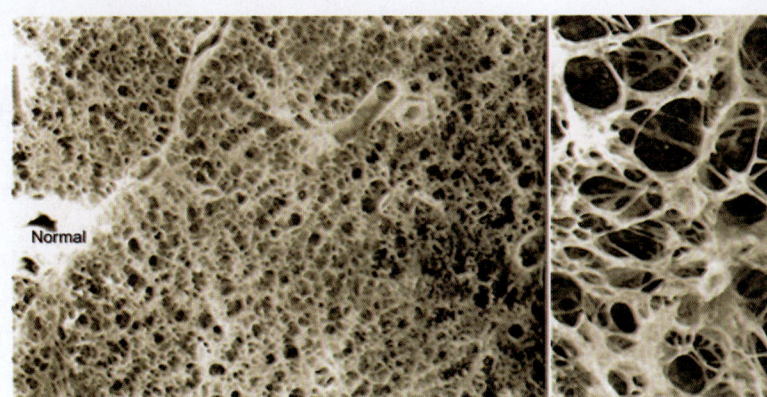

Fig. 8.5: Normal and emphysematous lung tissues

Section 2 ■ Proteins, Membrane and Extracellular Matrix

8

d. Ceruloplasmin

- 90% of plasma Cu is bound to ceruloplasmin and it is not readily distributed to tissues due to tight binding.
- 10% of plasma Cu is bound to albumin which is readily dissociable form and is available to tissues.
- Ceruloplasmin is α_2-globulin with the molecular weight 1,50,000 Da.
- Ceruloplasmin posses ferroxidase activity which converts Fe^{++} to Fe^{+++}.
- Apoceruloplasmin binds with 6 atoms of Cu to form ceruloplasmin.
- Level of ceruloplasmin in the plasma is decreased in Wilson's disease and Menke-Kinky hair disease.

β-Globulin

a. Transferrin (Tf)

- It is a glycoprotein with molecular weight of 76,000 Da (76 kDa).
- Transferrin is synthesized by liver.
- Transferrin transports iron in ferric form (Fe^{+++}).
- One transferrin binds two Fe^{+++} (holotransferrin).
- Plasma level of transferrin is 300 mg/dl.
- Only 30% of transferrin iron binding site is saturated with iron.
- Carbohydrate deficient transferrin (CDT) is a biomarker of chronic alcoholism.

b. **Hemopexin:** Transports heme.

c. **Plasminogen**

γ-Globulin

This contains various immunoglobulins.

ACUTE PHASE PROTEINS

During inflammatory conditions, certain plasma proteins are seen to be increased.

These proteins are called acute phase protein. They are:

- a. CRP (C-reactive protein)
- b. α_1-antiproteinase
- c. α_1-acid glycoprotein
- d. Haptoglobin
- e. Fibrinogen
- f. α_2-macroglobulin
- g. Ceruloplasmin
- h. Complement protein

C-Reactive Protein

During tissue injury, inflammation or infection, level of CRP is increased manyfold (normal plasma level is < 1 mg/dl).

It is called CRP as it interacts with C-polysaccharide of pneumococci.

Negative Acute Phase Reactant

Level of albumin, transferin is seen to be lowered during acute phase and they are known as negative acute phase reactant.

AMYLOIDOSIS

It is a disorder where protein fractions are accumulated between cells, imparing function of the tissues.

Initially, it was thought that insoluble fibrils were starch like structures, hence the name amyloidosis was given to this group of disorder.

Later studies revealed that these fibrils were proteolytic fragments of plasma proteins which were unusually rich in β-pleated sheets (Fig. 8.6).

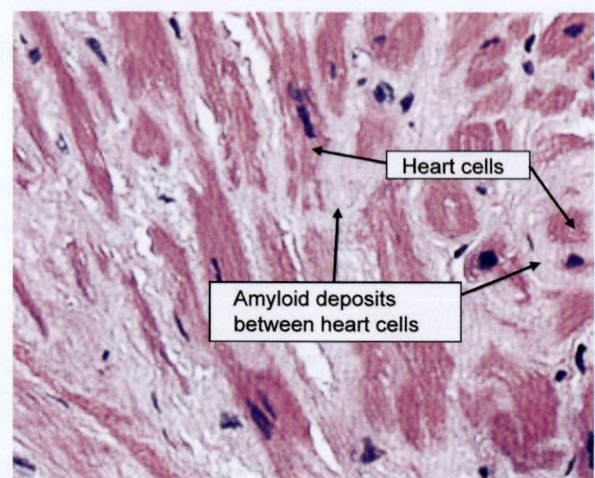

Fig. 8.6: Primary amyloidosis

Types of Amyloidosis

a. **Primary amyloidosis:** Principally light chain of immunoglobulin is deposited.

b. **Secondary amyloidosis:** Fragments of serum amyloid A (SAA) is deposited.

c. **Familial amyloidosis:** Mutated form of transthyretin is deposited.

d. **Alzheimer's disease:** Amyloid β-peptide is deposited.

e. **Dialysis related amyloidosis:** β_2-microglobulin is deposited.

9

Extracellular Matrix (ECM)

Specific Learning Objectives	
BI 9.1.1	Describe the three major components of ECM.
BI9.1.2	Describe the functional aspect of each component of ECM.
BI9.1.3	Describe the role of vitamin C in collagen synthesis.
BI9.2.1	Discuss various collagenopathies with special emphasis on scurvy.

Extracellular matrix (ECM) often called connective tissue, is the structure which surrounds cells in a tissue. It has got protective role and also provides elasticity when required. Three major classes of biomolecules in ECM are:

1. **Structural proteins:**
   - Collagen
   - Elastin
   - Fibrillin
2. **Specialized proteins**
   - Fibronectin
   - Laminin
3. **Proteoglycans**

1. STRUCTURAL PROTEINS

- Collagen is a fibrous protein of ECM just like elastin (collagen is the most abundant protein of animal world) (Fig. 9.1 and Table 9.1).
- There are 28 types of collagen.
- Collagen molecule is a long, rigid structure in which three alpha chains wound around each other in 'right handed fashion' to form rod-like structure. Interchain 'H' bond is present between these three 'α-chains' which stabilizes triple helical structure (Fig. 9.2).

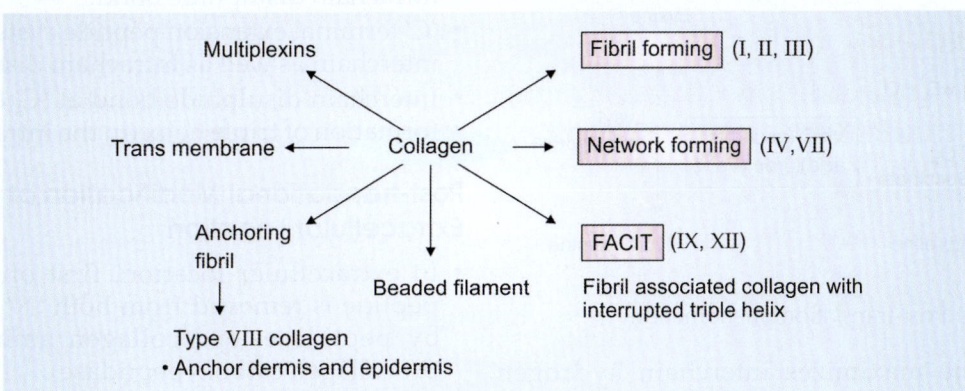

Fig. 9.1: Collagen: Its diverse role

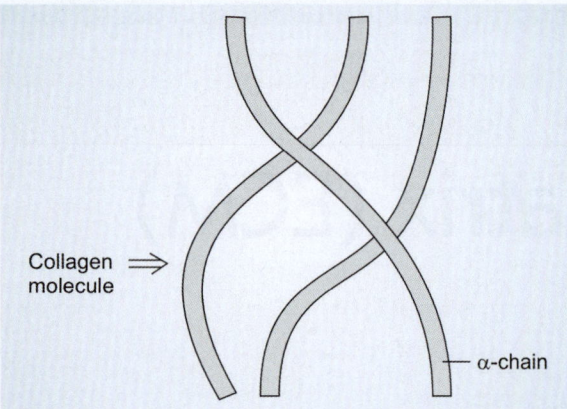

Fig. 9.2: Three α-chains wound around each other in collagen

- Each 'α-chain' is approximately 1000 amino acid long chain which is twisted in left handed polyproline helix.
- Each turn in α-chain consists of three amino acids.
- (Gly-X-Y)n is repeated 333 times to produce collagen α-chain.
- α-chain is not to be confused with 'α helix'.
- Though categorized as fibrous protein, all collagens do not make fibrous structure.
- X and Y may be any other amino acid. 100 of X and 100 of Y are proline and hydroxyproline, respectively.
- Proline favours helical conformation of a chain as it produces 'kink' in the peptide chain.
- Glycine is a small amino acid which fits the narrow space where three polypeptides come together. Hydroxyproline and hydroxylysine in collagen polypeptide are due to post-translation phenomenon, where prolyl hydroxylase and lysyl hydroxylase convert proline and lysine to hydroxyproline and hydroxylysine, respectively. This occurs in lumen of endoplasmic reticulum (Fig. 9.3).

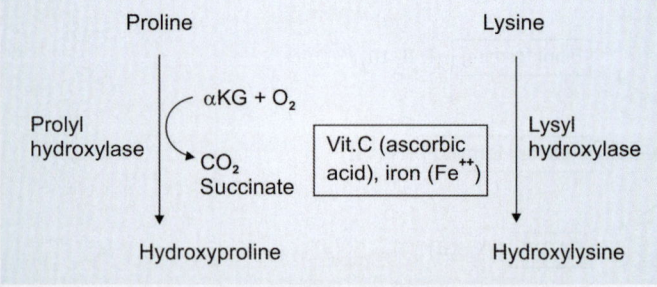

Fig. 9.3: Post-translation phenomenon

- Hydroxyproline maximizes interchain hydrogen bonds that stabilize the triple helical structure.
- Collagen is a glycoprotein. Certain of its hydroxylysine residue is further modified by addition of galactose or galactosyl-glucose in 'O' glycosidic linkage.

- This glycosylation also occurs in ER lumen, prior to triple helix formation.
- Cofactors for both lysyl and prolyl hydroxylases are vitamin C, Fe^{++}, and α-ketoglutarate.

POST-TRANSLATIONAL MODIFICATION OF COLLAGEN

- Collagen is synthesized by polyribosome on rough endoplasmic reticulum (RER) as 'preprocollagen' and is extensively modified post-translationally both intracellularly and extracellularly.
- Like many other proteins synthesized on RER, collagen also contains 'leader' or 'signal' sequence that direct this polypeptide to endoplasmic reticulum (Fig. 9.4).

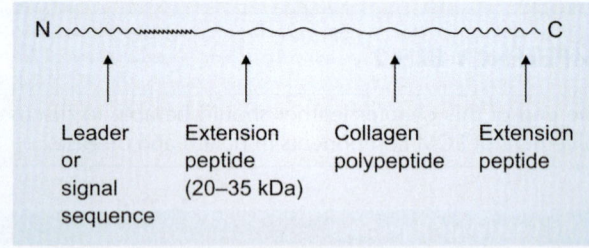

Fig. 9.4: Signal sequence at N terminal of collagen polypeptide

Post-translational Modification of Collagen in Intracellular Location

- Once preprocollagen enters the ER lumen, the leader sequence is enzymatically removed.
- Hydroxylation of proline and lysine and also glycosylation of hydroxylysine occurs at this location in ER lumen.
- Extension peptide is rich in cysteine.
- 'N' terminal extension peptide cysteine residues form intrachain disulphide bond.
- 'C' terminal extension peptide cysteine residue forms interchain as well as intrachain disulphide bond.
- Interchain disulphide bond at 'C' terminal assists in formation of triple helix (in the intracellular location).

Post-translational Modification of Collagen in Extracellular Location

- In extracellular location, first of all the extension peptide is removed from both 'N' and 'C' terminals by peptidases (procollagen aminopeptidase and procollagen carboxypeptidase).
- Next to this collagen fibril is arranged in 'quarter-staggered' alignment.
- The fibrillar array of collagen molecule is an ideal substrate for lysyl oxidase activity.

- There occurs oxidative deamination of lysine and hydroxylysine residue to their aldehyded counterparts (al-lysine and hydroxy-al-lysine) by extracellular enzyme lysyl oxidase.
- Lysyl oxidase is Cu-contaning enzyme.
- Shiff base and aldol condensation produce interchain and intrachain cross-links (Fig. 9.5).

TABLE 9.1 Various types of collagen and their distribution

Type		Distribution
I	Fibril forming	Skin, bone, tendon, blood vessel, cornea
II		Cartilage, intervertebral disc, vitreous body
III		Blood vessel, skin, muscle
IV	Network forming	Basement membrane
VII		Corneal and vascular endothelium
IX	Fibril associated	Cartilage
XII		Tendon, ligaments, some other tissue.

Disorders of Collagen Synthesis (Collagenopathies)

A. Ehlers-Danlos Syndrome (EDS)

- It is a heterogenous group of disorder which is caused by deficiency of collagen processing enzymes.

Villefranche Classification (1997)

1. **Classic form EDS:**
   - Defects in type I and V collagen
   - Characterized by skin extensibility, abnormal tissue fragility and excess joint hypermobility.
   - AD inheritance.
2. **Vascular form EDS:**
   - Due to defect in type III collagen.
   - It is associated with lethal, arterial and bowel rupture.
   - Most lethal type

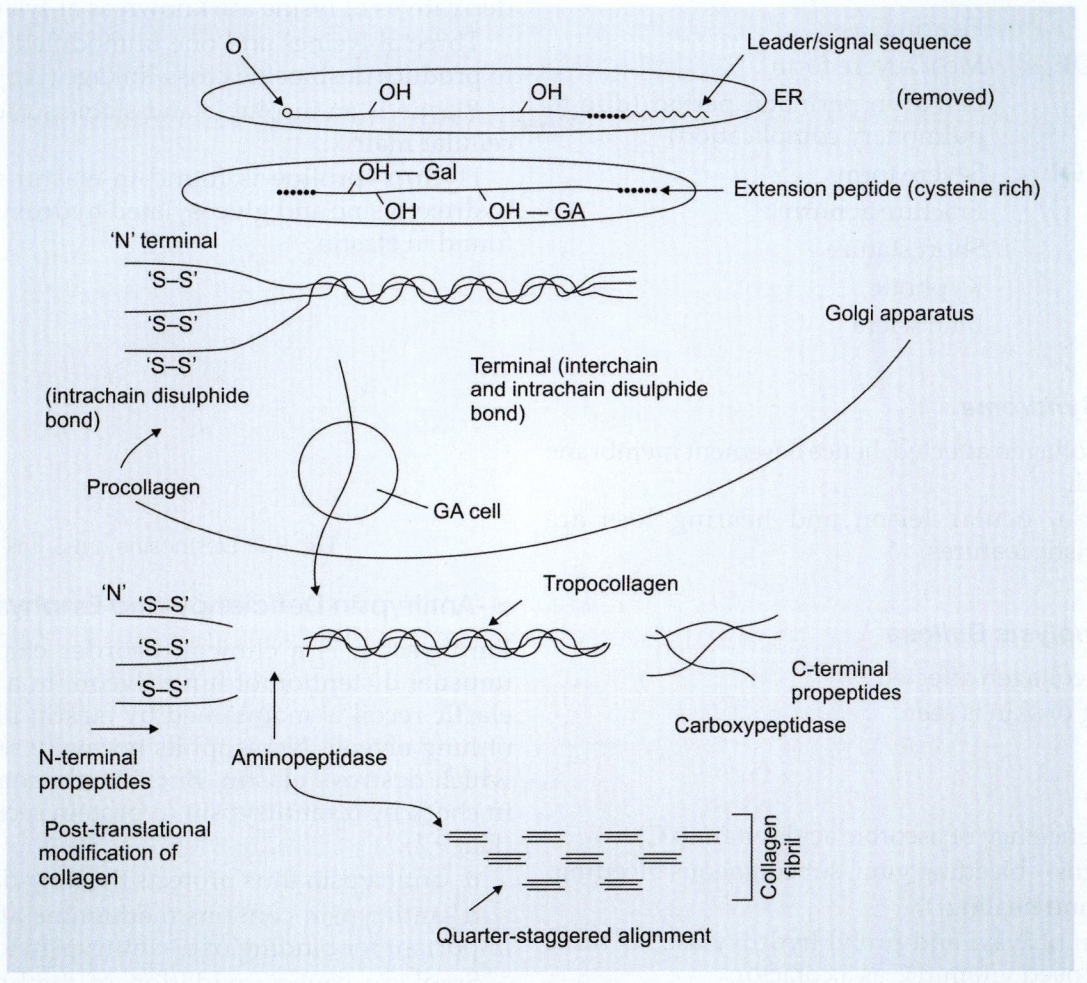

Fig. 9.5: Synthesis of collagen in endoplasmic reticulum and its secretion into extracellular space

Section 2 ■ Proteins, Membrane and Extracellular Matrix

9

3. **Hypermobility**
   • Type III collagen
4. **Kyphoscoliosis**
   • Lysyl hydroxylase
   • Rare defect
   • Kyphoscoliosis and ocular rupture
5. **Arthrochalasis**
   • Type I collagen
   • Rare
6. **Dermatosparaxis**
   • ADAM metalloproteinase with thrombosponds in type I motif.

B. Osteogenesis Imperfecta (OI)

(Brittle Bone Disease)

Bone is fragile in this disorder and breaks easily with minimal or no trauma.

In >80% cases type I collagen is affected.

Type I OI:	Blue sclera
	Mild bone fragility
	Hearing loss
Type II OI:	Most severe form
	Lethal in perinatal period (due to pulmonary complication)
Type III OI:	Severe form
	Fracture at birth
	Short stature
	Kyphotic
	Blue sclera

C. Alport Syndrome

• Type IV collagen affected, hence basement membrane is affected.
• Hematuria, ocular leison and hearing loss are characteristic features.

D. Epidermolysis Bullosa

• Type VII collagen affected
• Blistering of skin is seen.

E. Scurvy

• Due to deficiency of ascorbic acid (vitamin C).
• Major signs—bleeding gum, subcutaneous bleeding.
• Poor wound healing
• No action of lysyl and prolyl hydroxylase, as these enzymes need vitamin C as a cofactor.
  This results in disruption of collagen structure.

F. Menke's Disease

• Deficiency of copper
• Defect in cross-linking due to lack of lysyl oxidase activity.
• It is X-linked recessive disorder, where there is mutation of P type ATPase 7A at gastrointestinal mucosa.

ELASTIN

Compared to collagen, which is a characteristic fibrous protein having high tensile strength; elastin is another fibrous protein which is found in connective tissue characterized by rubber like properties.

Elastin is responsible for extensibility and elastic recoil in tissues. Elastin is found in lung, wall of large arteries, and elastic ligaments. Some amount of elastin is found in skin, ear cartilage and other tissues.

Tropoelastin is 70 kDa, soluble precursor of elastin. Once secreted outside the cell, certain lysine residues of tropoelastin are oxidatively deaminated to their aldehyde forms by lysyl oxidase. These aldehyde derivatives of lysine are known as al-lysine.

Three al-lysines and one unmodified lysine interact to produce desmosine cross-linkage (Fig. 9.6).

Elastin is an insoluble and stable structure in extra-cellular matrix.

Hydroxyproline is found in elastin structure, but hydroxylysine and glycosylated hydroxylysine are not found in elastin.

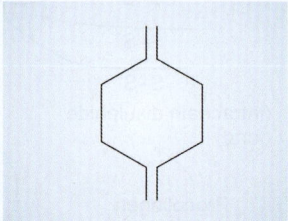

Fig. 9.6: Desmosine cross-link

α_1-Antitrypsin Deficiency and Emphysema

Emphysema is a clinical disorder characterized by unusual distention of lung alveoli. In a healthy lung, elastic recoil is maintained by elastin present in wall of lung alveoli. Neutrophils normally secrete elastase which destroys elastin. But this phenomenon is kept in check by α_1-antitrypsin (a protein secreted by liver) (Fig. 9.7).

α_1-antitrypsin thus protects the lung damage.

α_1-antitrypsin contains methionine at 358 position, important for binding of α_1-antitrypsin to protease.

Smoking causes oxidation of methionine, which inhibits binding of α_1-antitrypsin to protease and thus unimpeded protease activity destroys the lung (refer previous chapter).

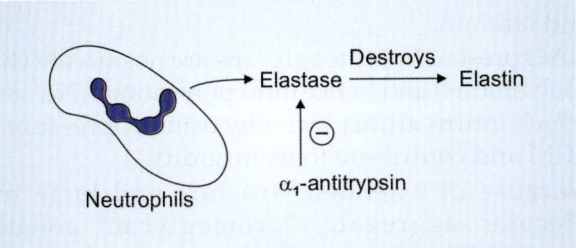

Fig. 9.7: Elastase and its action on elastin

Difference between Collagen and Elastin

See Table 9.2.

TABLE 9.2	Differences between collagen and elastin
Collagen	*Elastin*
28 different genetic types	Only one genetic type
Triple helix	No triple helix
(Gly-X-Y) repeating structure	No (Gly-X-Y) repeating structure
Hydroxylysine is present	No hydroxylysine found
Glycoprotein	Not a glycoprotein
Aldol cross-link	Desmosine cross-link
Extension peptide is present during biosynthesis	No extension peptide present

FIBRILLIN

- Elastin is deposited on fine fiber-like strands of 'microfilaments' which are 10–12 mm in diameter.
- Major structural components of these microfilaments are 'fibrillins'.
- Fibrillins are large glycoproteins (350 kDa) which are secreted by fibroblast in ECM.

Marfan Syndrome

- It is an autosomal dominant disorder.
- There is mutation in fibrillin-1 gene on chromosome-15.
- Fibrillin is abnormal and is deposited in small quantity in ECM.
- It affects the structure of suspensory ligament of eye, the periosteum of the bone and aortic media of blood vessels.
- Affected individual is tall, exhibits long digits (arachanodactyly), hyperextensibility of joints, ectopia lentis (dislocation of lens in eye), dilatation of ascending aorta.

2. SPECIALIZED PROTEINS

A. FIBRONECTIN (FIGS 9.8 AND 9.9)

- It is a glycoprotein found in ECM and also in plasma.
- It is a dimer having two subunits of 230 kDa each.
- Dimer is joined near carboxyl terminal by two disulphide bridges.

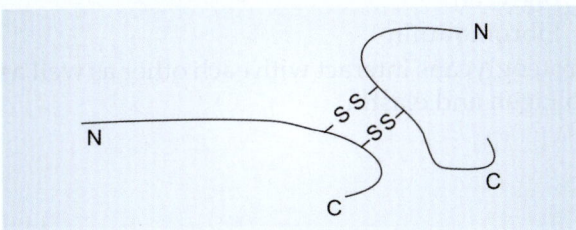

Fig. 9.8: Fibronectin

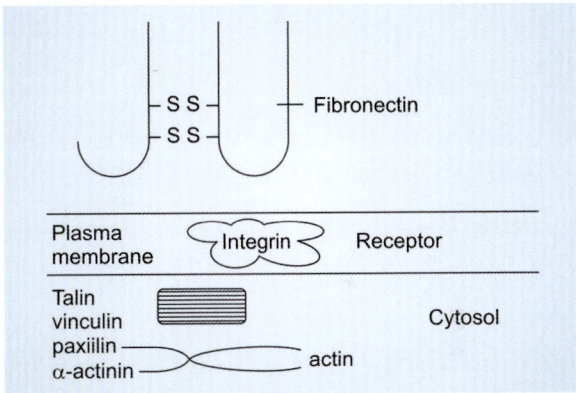

Fig. 9.9: Integrin receptor

- Fibronectin binds to cell via integrin receptors. This interaction of fibronectin with its receptor provides one route whereby the outside of the cell can communicate with the inside.
- Fibronectin is also involved in cell migration.

B. LAMININ

- Laminin is a major protein component of basal lamina.
- Laminin is a glycoprotein of about 850 kDa and 70 nm length.
- Laminin consists of three distinct polypeptides 'α', 'β' and 'γ'.

3. PROTEOGLYCANS

- Proteoglycans are third important component in ECM (ground substance).
- Proteoglycans are proteins that contain covalently-linked glycosaminoglycans (GAG).

- Various proteoglycans are:
  - Syndecan
  - Betaglycan
  - Serglycin
  - Perlecan
  - Aggrecan
  - Versican
  - Decorin
  - Biglycan
  - Fibromodulin
- Proteoglycans interact with each other as well as with collagen and elastin.

- Decorin binds TGF-β and modulates its effect on the cell.
- Some of the proteoglycans interact with fibronectin and laminin.
- GAG present in proteoglycans are negatively charged (polyanions) and hence bind polycations (Na^+ and K^+), which inturn attract water by osmotic pressure in the ECM and contribute to its turgidity.

  Because of extended structure and huge macro-molecular aggregate, 'proteoglycan' constitutes large fraction of extracellular matrix compared to proteins.

10

Intracellular Protein Sorting

At the end of this chapter learner should be able to describe protein targeting and sorting along with its associated disorders.

Specific Learning Objectives

BI 9.3.1	Define protein sorting and mechanism involved in targeting of proteins to different organelles.
BI 9.3.2	Define signal sequence and enlist various signal sequences meant for various organelles.
BI 9.3.3	Describe the pathways of protein import into mitochondria, nuclei, peroxisomes, and the endoplasmic reticulum.
BI 9.3.4	Explain the biochemical mechanism of I cell disease.
BI 9.3.5	Discuss the protein targeting defect in Zellweger's syndrome.

Proteins which are synthesized on 'polyribosome' are destined to either various organelles, cytosol, cell membrane or are being exported out. Blobel in 1970 proposed that protein need signal or coding sequence to target them appropriately.

▌ SIGNAL HYPOTHESIS

- Proposed by Blobel and Sabatini in 1971.
- In this model they proposed that membrane bound polyribosomes and cytosolic free polyribosomes have same structure.
- The difference in them is that the former synthesizes a protein which has N-terminal signal peptide; which is responsible for attachment of such polyribosome to the membrane of endoplasmic reticulum (membrane bound polyribosomes), and also allows such proteins to get into the lumen of ER.
- Cytosolic polyribosomes on other hand synthesize proteins which lack such signal peptides and hence such polyribosomes are not attached to membrane, rather are lying free in cytosol.

A specific signal directs the protein synthesized on free (cytosolic) ribosome to reach mitochondria, nucleus or peroxisome; and the lack of such specific signal allows the protein to stay back in cytosol itself.

Flowchart 10.1: Protein sorting pathway

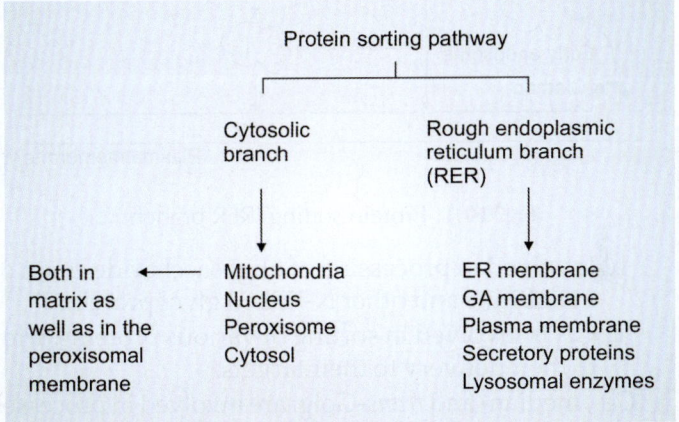

Sorting of Proteins Synthesized on RER

Proteins synthesized on rough endoplasmic reticulum are destined either for membrane (Endoplasmic reticulum, golgi apparatus (Flowchart 10.1). Plasma membrane) or for lysosome or they may be even secretory protein which are secreted outside the cell (Fig. 10.1). For locating these proteins to their destination, two types of vesicles play important roles:

1. Transport vesicles
2. Secretory vesicles

Role of Golgi Apparatus in Protein Synthesis

Golgi apparatus (GA) play following major roles in protein synthesis.

a. GA is involved in 'O' glycosylation of proteins.

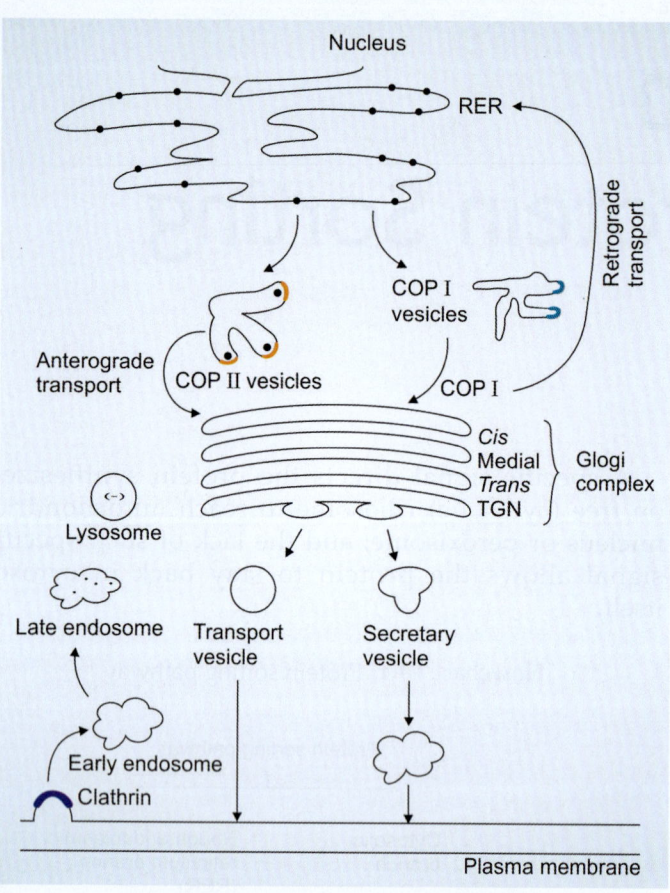

Fig. 10.1: Protein sorting (RER branch)

b. Involved in processing of oligosaccharide chain of membrane and other N-linked glycoproteins.

c. GA is involved in sorting of various proteins prior to their delivery to their targets.

Cis-, median- and *trans-*Golgi are involved in processes (a) and (b) while only *trans-*Golgi is involved in process (c), hence *trans-*golgi is rich in vesicles.

Proteins which are sorted by RER branch have N-terminal signal pepticle. N-terminal signal peptide have approximately 12–35 amino acids, rich hydrophobic core and methionine at 'N' terminal (Fig. 10.1).

Entry of protein in ER lumen may be a cotranslational or post-translational process.

Protein remains in unfolded state and has signal peptide sequence at 'N' terminal.

This process contains following steps:
1. 'N' terminal 70 amino acid chain is recognised by signal recogntion particle (SRP), which contains an RNA molecule in addition to protein components.
2. SRP—ribosome–protein complex traverses through endoplasmic reticulum membrane via SRP receptor and translocons.

Signal peptide in the ER lumen is cleaved by signal peptidase. Secretary proteins or the proteins meant to be distributed to distal organalle are glylcosylated at 'N' terminal and are located in Golgi apparatus lumen.

In Golgi lumen, there occurs further processing of 'N' glycan chain.

ER is rich in number of chaperones and folding enzymes which assist in protein folding.

Chaperones and enzymes present in ER are:
• Calnexin (ER membrane)
• Calreticulin (ER lumen)
• BiP (immunoglobulin heavy chain binding protein)
• GRP94 (glucose regulatory protein)
• PDI (protein disulphide isomerase)
• PPI (peptidyl prolyl *cis-trans* isomerase)

Misfolded and incompletely folded proteins are retained in ER lumen and are prevented from reaching their final destination.

Such misfolded proteins are destroyed by a process called endoplasmic reticulum associated degradation (ERAD) in most of the circumstances.

Endoplasmic Reticulum Associated Degradation (ERAD)

Change in endoplasmic reticulum Ca^{++} status, redox status, exposure to various toxins and viruses, disturb the internal milieu of the ER lumen, leading to accumulation of misfolded proteins. Accumulation of misfolded proteins in ER lumen is known as 'ER stress'.

By a mechanism called unfolded protein response (UPR), the cell senses the level of misfolded protein and initiates intracellular signalling mechanism to restore the ER homeostasis.

Misfolded proteins are transported back from ER membrane or lumen to proteasome in the cytosol (retrotranslocation or dislocation).

Diseases in which ER stress and defective protein folding occurs are listed in Table 10.1.

TABLE 10.1	Diseases and affected proteins
Diseases	*Affected protein*
Tay-Sachs disease	β-hexosaminidase
Gaucher disease	β-glucosidase
Cystic fibrosis	CFTR
I cell disease	N-acetyl glucosamine-1 Phosphotransferase
von Willebrand disease	von Willebrand factor
Hemophilia A and B	Factors VIII and IX
Familial hypercholesterolemia	LDL receptor
α$_1$-antitrypsin deficiency with liver disease	α$_1$-antitrypsin
Hereditary hemochromatosis	HFE

Protein Degradation in Eukaryotes

a. **Lysosomal degradation:** Mediated by lysosomal protease and does not require ATP.

b. **Ubiquitin-mediated degradation:** It is the major route and is ATP dependent. Ubiquitin is 76 amino acid long highly conserved protein which in addition to protein degradation is involved in other physiological processes like

- Cell cycle regulation
- DNA repair
- Inflammation
- Immune response
- Muscle wasting
- Viral infection

Three enzymes play important role in ubiquitation of misfolded proteins:

1. E_1 (activating enzyme)
2. E_2 (conjugating enzyme)
3. E_3 (ligase)

Minimum four ubiquitin proteins need to be attached to a protein to mark it for endoplasmic reticulum associated degradation (ERAD) in proteasome (Fig. 10.2).

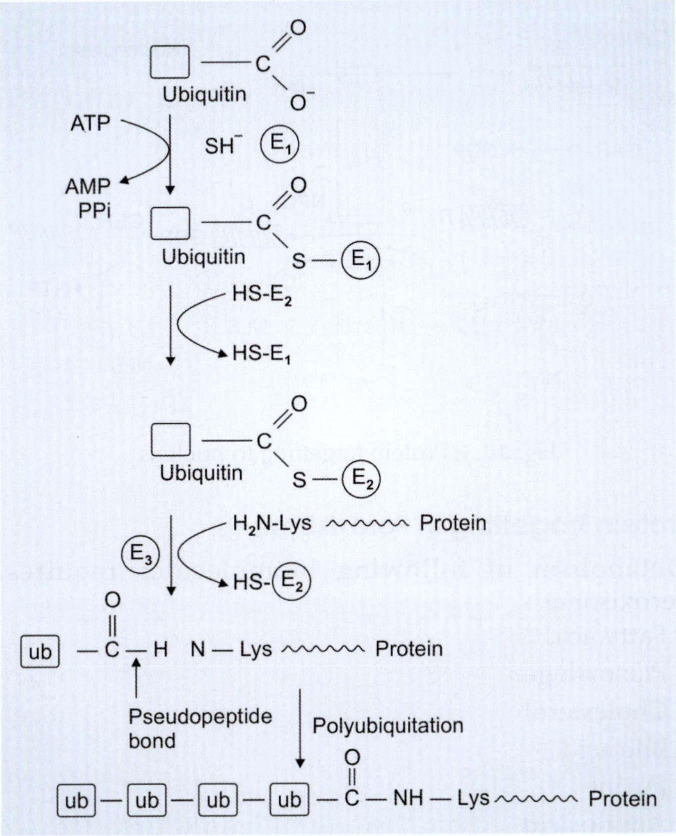

Fig. 10.2: Ubiquitation of proteins

Proteasome: It is a hollow cylindrical structure present in cytosol, made up of four rings. These rings on internal walls have protease like activity (Fig. 10.3).

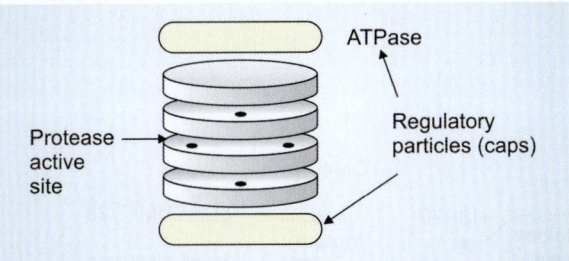

Fig. 10.3: Proteasome

In addition to these ring-like structures, proteasome has two cap-like structures on either end of it. These caps like structures have ATPase activity in them.

ATPase activity present in cap unfold protein first, which then enters in proteasome lumen.

Peptidases in proteasome lumen hydrolyze wide variety of pepticle bond, thus converting large protein into smaller fragments. These smaller fragments are further acted upon by cytosolic peptidases. Liberated ubiquitins are recycled.

Small peptides released by degradation of various viruses and other molecules are represented to MHC class I molecule. Proteasome thus plays important role in antigen presentation to T-lymphocyte.

SORTING OF PROTEINS SYNTHESISED ON FREE RIBOSOMES IN CYTOSOL

Cytosolic ribosomes (free ribosomes) synthesize proteins which are targetted to either mitochondria, nucleus, peroxisome or are retained in cytosol itself.

Uptake of protein by various organelles after its synthesis is complete is known as post-translational translocation.

Protein Targetting to Mitochondria

Though the proteins are located at various sublocations of mitochondria [outer mitochondrial membrane (OMM), inner mitochondrial membrane (IMM), matrix], the process of localization of proteins in mitochondrial matrix is described in detail here (Fig. 10.4).

Proteins destined for mitochondrial matrix have 20–50 amino acid long pre-sequence or leader sequence which is amphipathic in nature.

Translocation (passage through OMM and IMM) occurs post-translationally.

TIM – TOM = Translocase inner membrane (TIM)
Translocase outer membrane (TOM)

Section 2 ▪ Proteins, Membrane and Extracellular Matrix

10

TOM20/22 acts as receptor and TOM40 acts as a component of pore through which these proteins pass through.

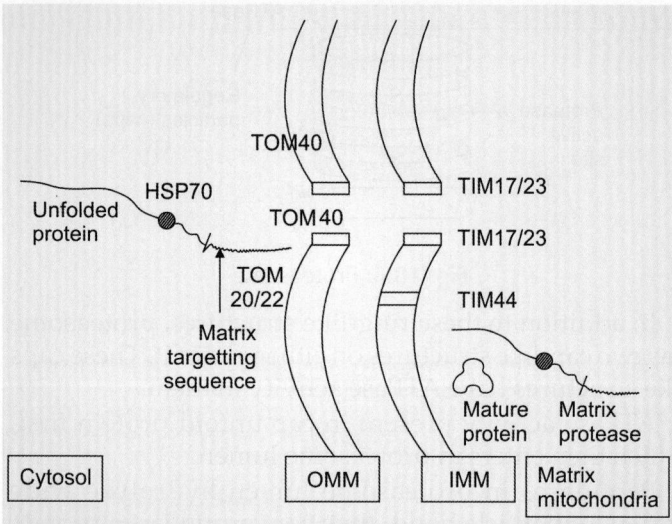

Fig. 10.4: Protein targetting to mitochondria

Similarly on IMM, TIM44 acts as receptor and TIM23/17 layers the channel on IMM.

Matrix protein interacts with HSP70 in the matrix which in turn interacts with TIM44.

- Protein should be maintained in unfolded state for easy passage through the mitochondrial membrane. Unfolded state is maintained by ATP driven chaperones, e.g. HSP70.
- Negatively charged matrix pulls the positively charged leader sequence which helps in entry of protein into the matrix.
- Matrix processing protease (MPP) removes the leader sequence in the matrix.
- Number of chaperones helps in translocation of proteins. For example:
  HSP70 = Prevents misfolding or aggregation
  HSP60 – HSP10 = They help in protein folding inside the mitochondrial matrix.
- Proteins which do not contain pre-sequence (e.g. cytochrome *c*) locate itself in the intermembranous space.
- Number of proteins contains two signal sequence— one to enter the mitochondria matrix and the other for subsequent relocation (into IMM).

Protein Targetting to Nucleus

Number of proteins and other macromolecules are transported between nucleus and cytosol each minute. They include:
- Ribosome subunits

- mRNA
- Ribosomal proteins
- Histone proteins
- Various transcription factors

Nucelar pore complexes (NPCs): These complexes are present on nuclear membrane. They have diameter of 9 nm and made up of 30 different proteins.

Proteins to be imported in nucleus contain NLS (nuclear localization signal) which is amino acid sequence rich in basic residue.

Importins and Ran are important proteins which help in import of protein in GTP dependent manner as described in Fig. 10.5.

Importin and Ran keep on circulating between nucleus and cytosol and help in protein transportation in the nucleus.

Similar to importin, 'exportins' are proteins which are involved in export of various macromolecules.

Ran is involved in the process of import as well as export.

Karyopherins are family of proteins to include importins and exportins.

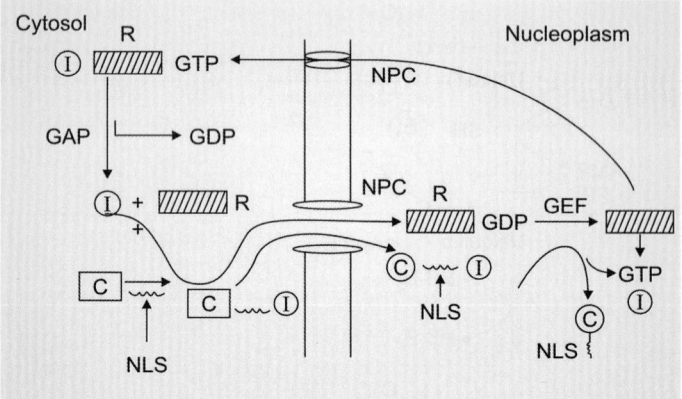

Fig. 10.5: Protein targetting to nucleus

Protein Tragetting in Peroxisome

Metabolism of following biomolecules requires peroxisome.
- Fatty acid
- Plasmalogen
- Cholesterol
- Bile acid
- Purine
- Amino acid
- H_2O_2

Proteins destined to enter in peroxisome have 'Peroxisomal-matrix' targetting sequence (PTS) either on 'C' terminal or 'N' terminal.

PEX5 is cytosolic receptor protein which binds with protein containing PTS-1 sequence (Ser-Lys-Leu).

PEX7 is another cytosolic receptor protein which binds with protein containing PTS-2 sequence.

PEX14 is the receptor on membrane.

PEX2/10/12 is the membrane receptor complex.

Proteins may also be localized in peroxisomal membrane.

ATP is needed for localizing the protein in the matrix but for protein localization in the peroxisomal membrane, ATP is not required.

PEROXISOMAL BIOGENESIS DISORDER (PBD)

PBD is the group of disorders having many overlapping features associated with the dysfunctioning of peroxisome.

- Most severe form of PBD is Zellweger syndrome.
- Intemediate form is neonatal adrenoleukodystrophy.
- Mildest form is infantile Refsum's disease.

Zellweger Syndrome

Zellweger syndrome was described by Dr. Hans Zellweger in 1964. It is most severe form of PBD which is autosomal recessive. In this disorder very long chain fatty acid (VLCFA) tends to accumulate in various organs of the body.

Mutation may be in proteins involved in transportation of protein in the peroxisome (PEX) or in the peroxisomal enzyme itself.

This disease is characterized by low muscle tone (hypotonia), vision and hearing involvment, liver and kidney dysfunction and severe neurological deficit including mental retardation.

Zellweger syndrome often results in life-threating complicant early in infancy.

Bile acid synthesis is abnormal and there is marked reduction in plasmalogen.

3

Metabolism of Carbohydrates

TCA CYCLE

H_2O + H_3C—C=O

Citrate synthase

^-OOC—C—OH (Citrate)

Aconitase

Oxaloacetate

Malate dehydrogenase

$NADH$ + H^+

NAD^+

Malate

Fumarase

H_2O

Fumarate

Succinate dehydrogenase

$FADH_2$

FAD

Succinate

GDP + P_i

GTP

Succinyl CoA synthetase

Succinyl CoA

CoA—S—C=O

α-ketoglutarate dehydrogenase complex

$NADH$ + H^+ + CO_2

NAD^+ + CoA

α-ketoglutarate

Isocitrate dehydrogenase

$NADH$ + H^+ + CO_2

NAD^+

Isocitrate

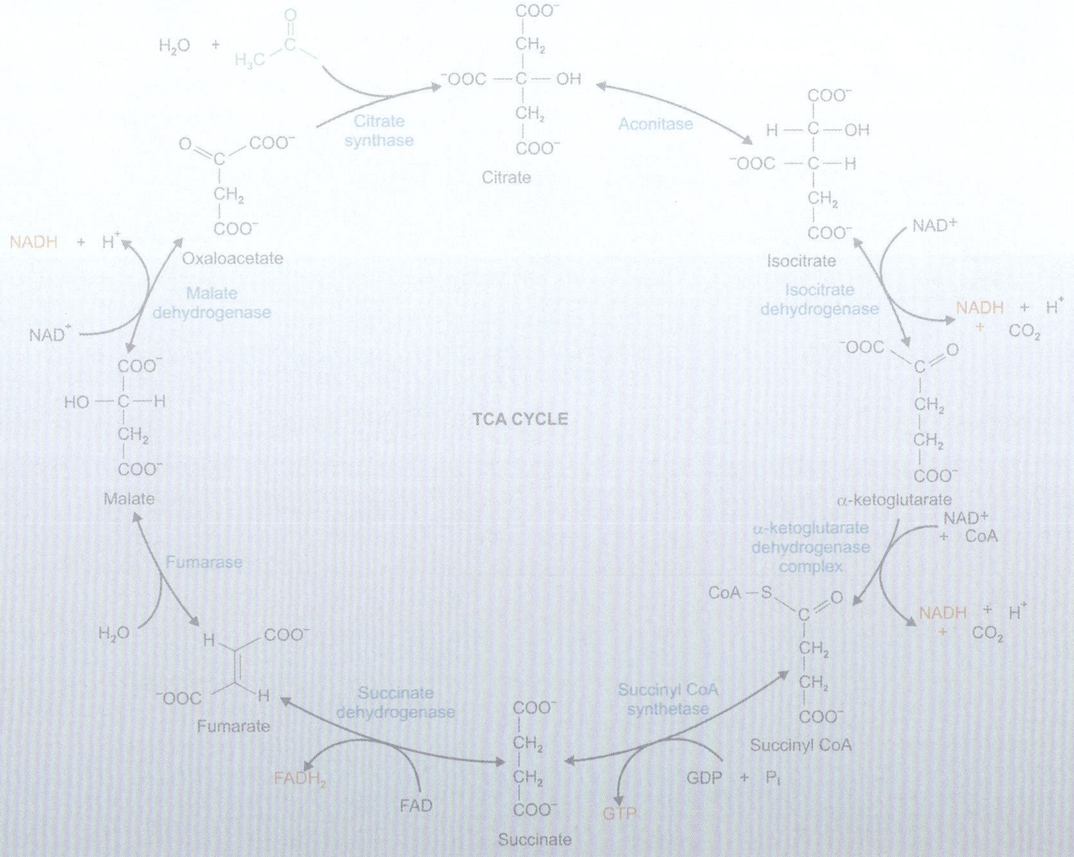

Carbohydrate Metabolism I: Metabolism of Glucose

COMPETENCY BI 3.4

At the end of this chapter learner should be able to define and differentiate the pathways of carbohydrate metabolism, (glycolysis, gluconeogenesis, glycogen metabolism, HMP shunt).

COMPETENCY BI 3.5

At the end of this chapter learner should be able to describe and discuss the regulation, functions and integration of carbohydrate along with associated diseases/disorders.

COMPETENCY BI 3.7

At the end of this chapter learner should be able to describe the common poisons that inhibit crucial enzymes of carbohydrate metabolism (e.g. fluoride, arsenate).

Specific Learning Objectives	
BI 3.4.1	Discuss the steps of glycolysis with special emphasis on rate limiting step.
BI 3.4.2	Discuss the steps of gluconeogenesis with special emphasis on rate limiting step.
BI 3.4.3	Discuss the steps of glycogen metabolism with special emphasis on rate limiting step.
BI 3.4.4	Discuss the steps of HMP shunt with special emphasis on rate limiting step.
BI 3.5.1	Discuss the regulation of various metabolic pathways of carbohydrate.
BI 3.7.1	Discuss the biochemical aspect of fluoride, arsenate as inhibitor of glycolysis.

GLYCOLYSIS

Glycolysis is also known as Embden-Meyerhof Pathway (EMP). It is a cytosolic process by which glucose molecules are metabolised through a series of enzymatic reactions into 2 molecules of pyruvate or 2 lactate (aerobic and anaerobic conditions, respectively).

Main purpose of glycolysis is ATP production. In RBC, its role is beyond sole producer of ATP.

In RBC, the glycolysis intermediate 1,3-BPG is converted to 2,3-BPG in reactions which constitute Rapoport-Luebering shunt (RL shunt).

It is important to mention here that only a fraction of glucose in RBC enters in RL shunt and this percentage which enters RL shunt varies according to physiological state. In conditions like hypoxia, anoxia, high altitute, anemia more percentage of glucose enters in RL shunt.

Net production of ATP in RBC for the glucose which enters the RL shunt is zero.

Steps of Glycolysis (Fig. 11.1)

a. Glucose is converted to glucose-6-phosphate by enzyme hexokinase or glucokinase. One ATP is converted to ADP at this step (Table 11.1).

b. Glucose-6-phosphate is converted to fructose-6-phosphate by phosphohexose isomerase enzyme.

c. Fructose-6-phosphate is converted to fructose 1,6-bisphosphate by enzyme phosphofructokinase-1 (PFK-1). This is the second irreversible step of the glycolysis and this step utilizes one ATP which is converted to ADP.

d. Fructose-1,6-bisphosphate is a hexose (6 carbon) which is cleaved to two trioses (3 carbon)—glyceraldehyde-3-phosphate and dihydroxyacetone phosphate. The enzyme responsible is aldolase (either A or B type of isoenzyme).

e. Glyceraldehyde-3-phosphate and dihydroxyacetone phosphate are interconverted by phosphotriose isomerase enzyme. As glyceraldehyde-3-phosphate is utilized in further reactions of glycolysis, dihydroxyacetone phosphate will ultimately get converted to glyceraldehyde-3-phosphate and will be utilized in similar fashion.

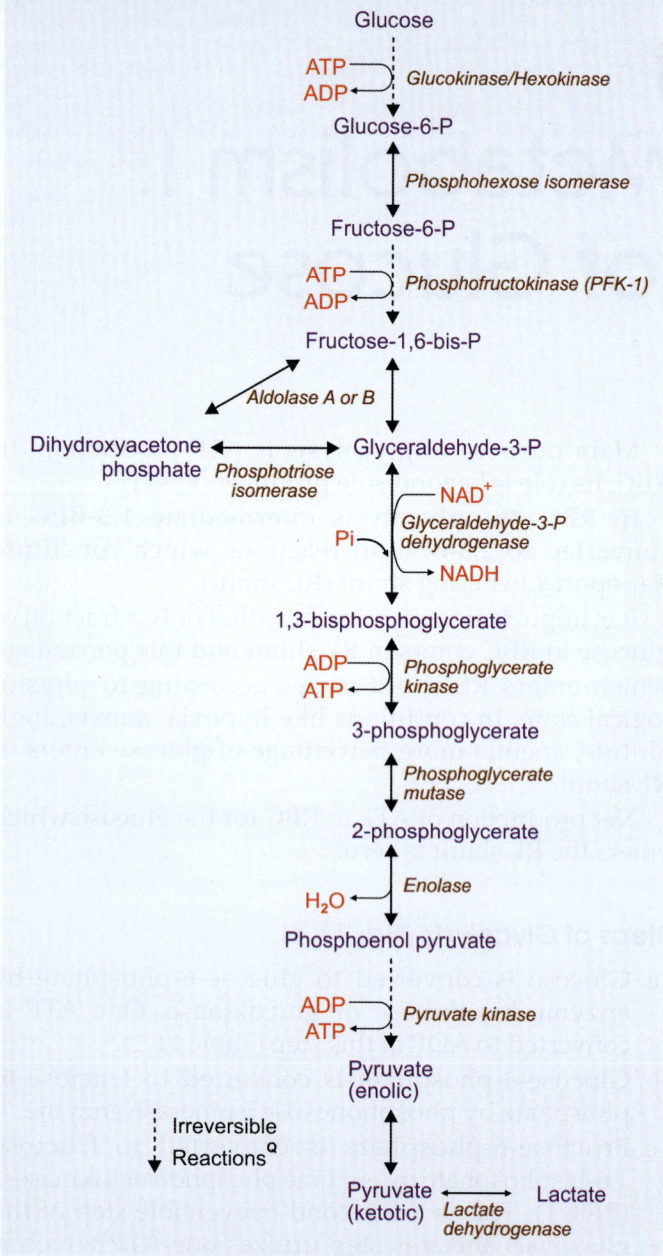

Fig. 11.1: Steps of glycolysis

f. Glyceraldehyde-3-phosphate is converted to 1,3-bisphosphoglycerate by the enzyme glyceraldehyde-3-phosphate dehydrogenase. This enzyme uses NAD^+ which is converted to NADH. One inorganic phosphate is utilized at this step which occupies first position of 1,3-bisphosphoglycerate.

g. High energy phosphate at first position is transferred to ADP to form ATP in the next reaction, which is catalysed by 1,3-bisphosphoglycerate kinase. Product of this reaction is 3-phosphoglycerate.

h. 3-phosphoglycerate is converted to 2-phosphoglycerate by enzyme phosphoglycerate mutase.

i. 2-phosphoglycerate is converted to phosphoenol pyruvate (PEP) after dehydration which is catalysed by enolase enzyme.

j. Phosphoenol pyruvate is next converted to pyruvate by enzyme pyruvate kinase. This reaction produces ATP and is the third irreversible step of the glycolysis.

NOTE: Steps (a) to (e) will occur only once for one glucose, but steps (f) to (j) will occur twice for one glucose molecule.

Site of glycolysis: Cytosol

Purpose of Glycolysis

1. Aerobic glycolysis produces total 9 and net 7 moles of ATP per mole of glucose.
2. Anerobic glycolysis produces total 4 and net 2 moles of ATP per mole of glucose.
3. In addition to ATP production, glycolytic reactions provide important intermediates for number of biosynthetic reactions. For example, acetyl CoA is the precursor molecule for fatty acid synthesis.

Rate limiting and major regulatory enzyme of the glycolysis: It is phosphofructokinase-1.

Phosphofructokinase-1 (PFK-1)

Major regulatory enzyme of glycolysis. It is under both allosteric and hormonal control.

TABLE 11.1	Differences between hexokinase and glucokinase	
	Hexokinase	Glucokinase
Site	All tissues except liver	Only in liver, beta cell of pancreas
Substrate	Glucose, fructose or galactose	Only glucose
Induction	Noninducible	Inducible
K_m for glucose	Low (0.05 mmol/L or 0.9 mg/dl)	High (10 mmol/L or 180 mg/dl)
Inhibition by glucose-6-phosphate	Inhibited	Not inhibited
Effect of feeding and insulin	No change in activity	Increased activity as well as rate of synthesis

Allosteric control of PFK-1

- Positive allosteric modifiers of PFK-1 are AMP, fructose-2,6-bisphosphate.
- Negative allosteric modifiers of PFK-1 are ATP, citrate, H⁺ (Fig. 11.2).

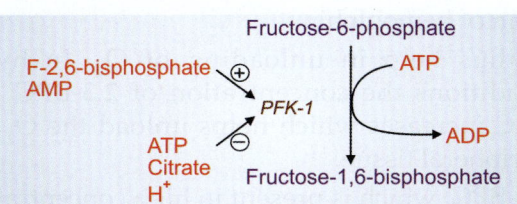

Fig. 11.2: Positive and negative allosteric modifiers of phosphofructokinase enzyme

Hormonal control of PFK-1

Fructose-2,6-bisphosphate plays an important role for hormonal control of the hepatic glycolysis. Fructose-2,6-bisphosphate is synthesized as a side product of the glycolysis.

A bifunctional enzyme named PFK-2/fructose-2, 6- bisphosphatase is responsible for regulating the level of fructose-2,6-bisphosphate in the liver (Fig. 11.3).

In addition to phosphofructokinase enzyme, pyruvate kinase and hexokinase enzyme are also under regulation.

Pyruvate kinase enzyme is activated by fructose-1,6-bisphosphate and is inhibited by ATP and alanine.

Hexokinase enzyme is inhibited by glucose 6-phosphate.

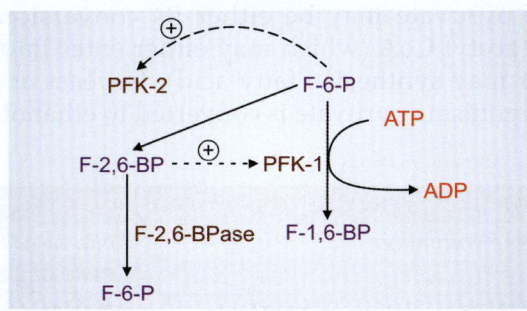

Fig. 11.3: Synthesis and degradation of F-2,6-bisphosphate

Inhibitors of Glycolysis

1. **Fluoride:** Inhibiting enolase enzyme via forming ionic complex with Mg⁺⁺ and Pi. This is an exmple of irreversible inhibition.
2. **Sulphydryl reagents** (mercury containing compounds/ alkylating compounds, e.g. iodoacetate). These compounds bind the active site of glyceraldehyde-3-phosphate dehydrogenase enzyme and inhibits its activity.
3. **Arsenate:** Not a true inhibitor of glycolysis, it acts via competition with inorganic Pi needed at glyceraldehyde-3-phosphate dehydrogenase reaction. In presence of arsenic, glycolysis continues but the net ATP production does not occur. Arsenic prevents formation of 1,3-bisphosphoglycerate and thus the ATP production in subsequent step of BPG kinase is also bypassed in the presence of arsenic (Fig. 11.4).

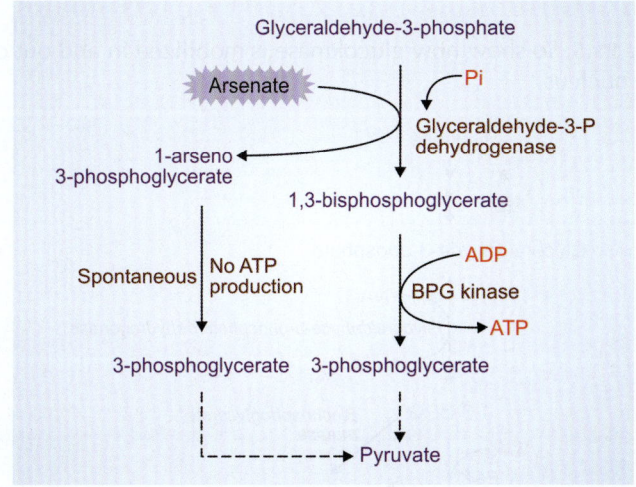

Fig. 11.4: To show how arsenic affects ATP production in glycolysis (it bypasses BPG kinase step)

Glucokinase (GK) is regulated by fructose-6-phosphate by a special mechanism which is explained below:

- *Mechanism by which glucokinase activity is influenced by fructose-6-phosphate:* Fructose-6-phosphate affects compartmentalization of GK enzyme and has inhibitory effect on its activity. Glucokinase is present in the nucleus in the bound state to the glucokinase regulatory protein (GKRP). Whenever glucose enters in the cell, glucokinase is released from this bound protein and is freed into the cytosol. In the presence of fructose-6-phosphate in the cell, glucokinase is translocated back to the nucleus where it binds again with the glucokinase regulatory protein (GKRP), which makes enzyme inactive (Fig. 11.5).
- Energetics of glycolysis (Table 11.2)
- *Rapoport-Luebering cycle or RL shunt:* This pathway occurs exclusively in the RBC. In this cycle shunting of the glycolytic intermediate 1,3-bisphosphoglycerate occurs for the production of 2,3-bisphosphoglycerate (2,3-BPG) (Fig. 11.6).

Section 3 ■ Metabolism of Carbohydrates

11

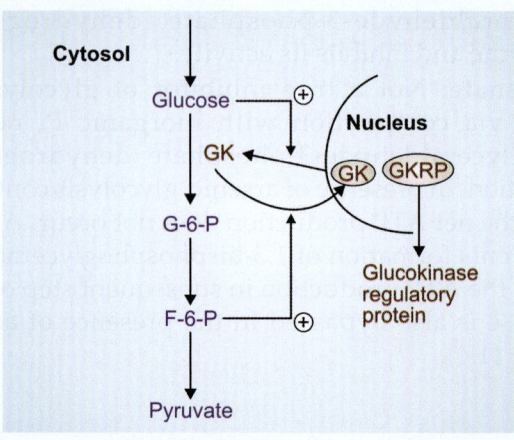

Fig. 11.5: To show how glucokinase is mobilized in and out of the nucleus

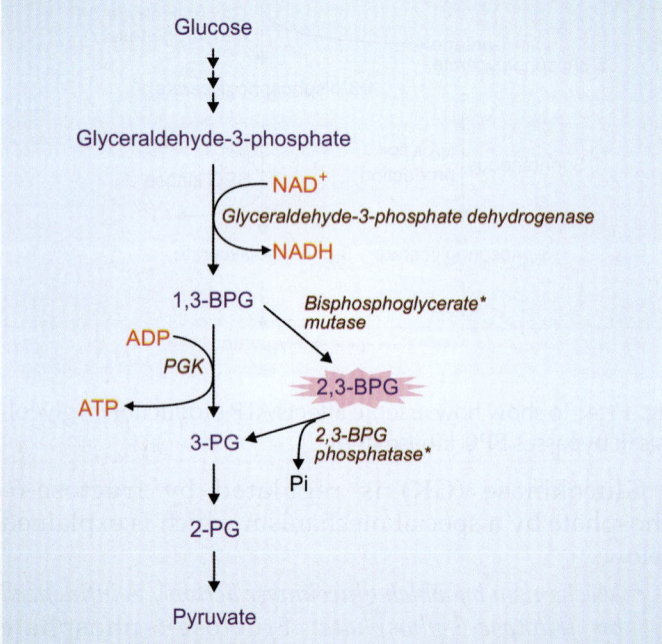

(*BPG mutase and BPG phosphatase are bifunctional enzymes)

Fig. 11.6: Rapoport-Luebering cycle (RL shunt)

- *2,3-bisphosphate glycerate (2,3-BPG):* 2,3-BPG is an important allosteric modifier of oxygenation of hemoglobin.
- Whenever Hb is in the deoxygenated form, one molecule of 2,3-BPG is bound per Hb tetramer in the central cavity, this helps stabilization of deoxy form of hemoglobin.
- It thus help in unloading of O_2. In hypoxic conditions the concentration of 2,3-BPG in the RBC increases which helps unload the O_2 at the peripheral tissue.
- 2,3-BPG, which is present in high concentration in tissues, combines with Hb and causes a decrease in the affinity for oxygen thus helping oxyhemoglobin to unload oxygen and displacing O_2 dissociation curve to the right.
- BPG binds more weakly to fetal Hb than to adult Hb. Thus, BPG has a less profound effect on HbF and is responsible for HbF appearing to have a higher affinity for O_2 than does HbA.

Pasteur effect: Inhibitory effect of O_2 on glycolysis is called Pasteur effect.
- It is due to decreased AMP/ATP ratio.
- AMP has positive effect on PFK and so decreased level of AMP causes inhibition of glycolysis.

Crabtree effect: Relative anaerobiosis produced when glucose concentration is increased in constant supply of oxygen.

Fates of Pyruvate

Fate of pyruvate may be either its conversion into lactate, acetyl CoA (which may either enter into TCA cycle or may synthesize fatty acid). In yeast or other microorganisms pyruvate is converted to ethanol.

TABLE 11.2	Energetics of glycolysis		
Pathway	*Reaction catalyzed by*	*Method of ATP formation*	*No. of ATP per mole of glucose*
Glycolysis	Glyceraldehyde-3-phosphate dehydrogenase	Respiratory chain oxidation of 2 NADH	5 or 3*
	Phosphoglycerate kinase	Substrate level phosphorylation	2
	Pyruvate kinase	Substrate level phosphorylation	2
Total ATP from one glucose during glycolysis in cytosol (aerobic)			**9 or 7***
	Consumption of 1 ATP each for reactions of HK/GK and phosphofructokinase		−2
Net ATP from one glucose during glycolysis in cytosol (aerobic)			**Net 7 or 5***

(*if **malate aspartate shuttle** is used for NADH transfer across mitochondrial membrane, 1 NADH produces 2.5 ATP; and if **glycerophosphate shuttle** is used for NADH transfer across the mitochondrial membrane, 1 NADH produces **1.5 ATP**)

Note: Glucokinase is also called hexokinase D or type IV.

a. Pyruvate to Lactate (in Anaerobic Condition)

Pyruvate is converted to lactate under hypoxic condition in tissues, e.g. skeletal muscle, white fibres, smooth muscles, renal medulla, retina, brain, gastrointestinal tract, cell and skin.

Purpose of this conversion is to regenerate NAD^+ for glyceraldehyde dehydrogenase enzyme which otherwise comes to a halt in absence of NAD^+.

b. Pyruvate to Acetyl CoA (in Aerobic Condition)

Under aerobic condition in the cell, pyruvate enters the mitochondrial matrix, where it is oxidatively decarboxylated by PDH complex enzyme to produce acetyl CoA (Table 11.3).

c. Alcoholic Fermentation

Pyruvate may get converted to alcohol in anaerobic fermentation.

▌PDH COMPLEX

PDH complex is catalysing irreversible oxidative decarboxylation of pyruvate to produce acetyl CoA.

$$Pyruvate + NAD^+ + CoA \rightarrow Acetyl\ CoA + CO_2 + NADH$$

This reaction is irreversible.

PDH complex is a multienzyme complex and contains 3 enzymes and 5 coenzymes (Fig. 11.7).

Enzymes of PDH Complex

a. Pyruvate dehydrogenase (E_1): Also known as pyruvate decarboxylase.
b. Dihydrolipoyl transacetylase (E_2)
c. Dihydrolipoyl dehydrogenase (E_3)

Coenzymes of PDH Complex

• Thiamine pyrophosphate (TPP)
• Lipoate
• CoA-SH (Coenzyme A-SH)
• FAD
• NAD

Energetics

One molecule of pyruvate produces one NADH, while undergoing PDH reaction and thus 2.5 ATP are produced from one pyruvate molecule.

One glucose molecule which produces 2 molecules of pyruvate, produces 5 ATP at this step.

PDH complex is active in dephosphorylated form.

TABLE 11.3	Three fates of pyruvate produced by glycolysis	
Anaerobic (lactic acid fermentation)	*Aerobic oxidation*	*Anaerobic (alcoholic fermentation)*

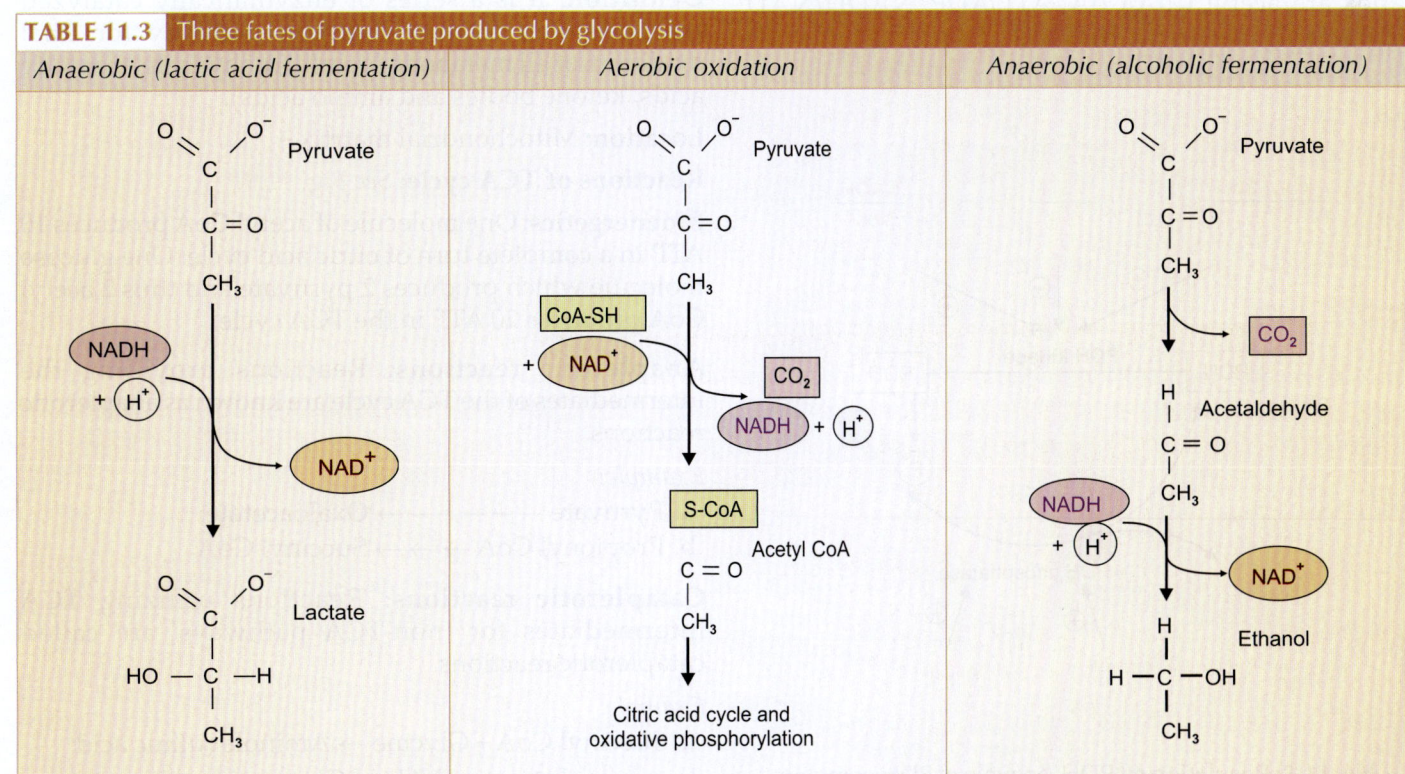

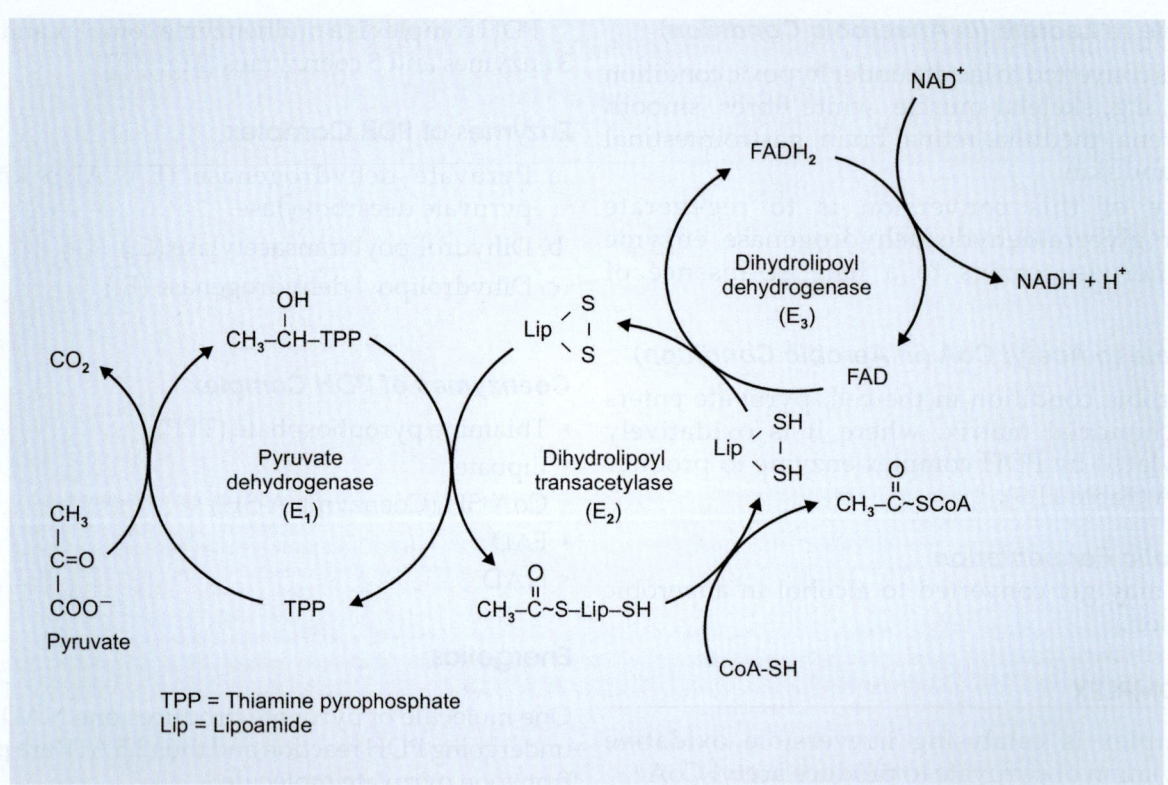

Fig. 11.7: PDH complex

Three ratios are important for converting the PDH to the phosphorylated hence inactivated form. These ratios are acetyl CoA/CoA, ATP/ADP, NADH/NAD+ (Fig. 11.8).

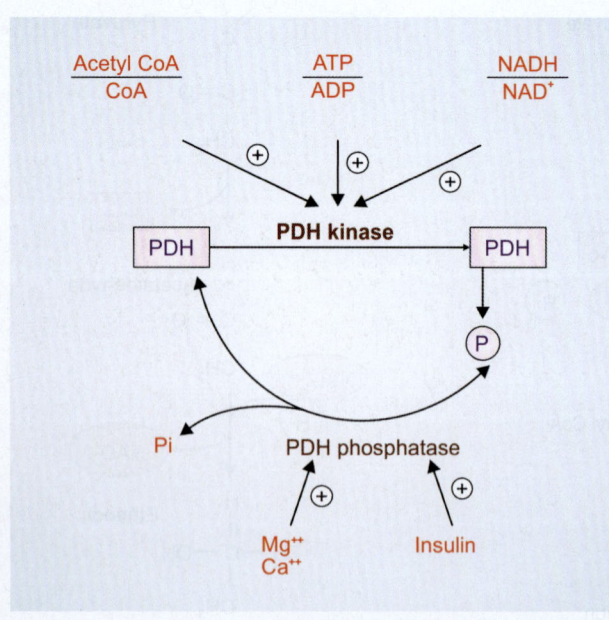

Fig. 11.8: Regulation of 'PDH' enzyme of PDH complex

CITRIC ACID CYCLE (KREBS' CYCLE OR TCA CYCLE)

Definition: It is a series of enzymatically catalyzed reactions that form a common pathway for final oxidation of all metabolic fuels (carbohydrate, free fatty acids, ketone bodies and amino acids).

Location: Mitochondrial matrtix

Reactions of TCA cycle: *See* Fig. 11.9.

Bioenergetics: One molecule of acetyl CoA produces 10 ATP in a complete turn of citric acid cycle. One glucose molecule which produces 2 pyruvate and thus 2 acetyl CoA produces 20 ATP in the TCA cycle.

Anaplerotic reactions: Reactions providing the intermediates of the TCA cycle are known as anaplerotic reactions.

Example:

  a. Pyruvate $-----\rightarrow$ Oxaloacetate

  b. Propionyl CoA $\rightarrow \rightarrow \rightarrow$ Succinyl CoA

Cataplerotic reactions: Reactions utilizing TCA intermediates for 'non-TCA pathways' are called cataplerotic reactions.

Example:

  a. Succinyl CoA + Glycine $\rightarrow$ Aminolevulinic acid

  b. α-ketoglutarate + $NH_3 \rightarrow$ Glutamate

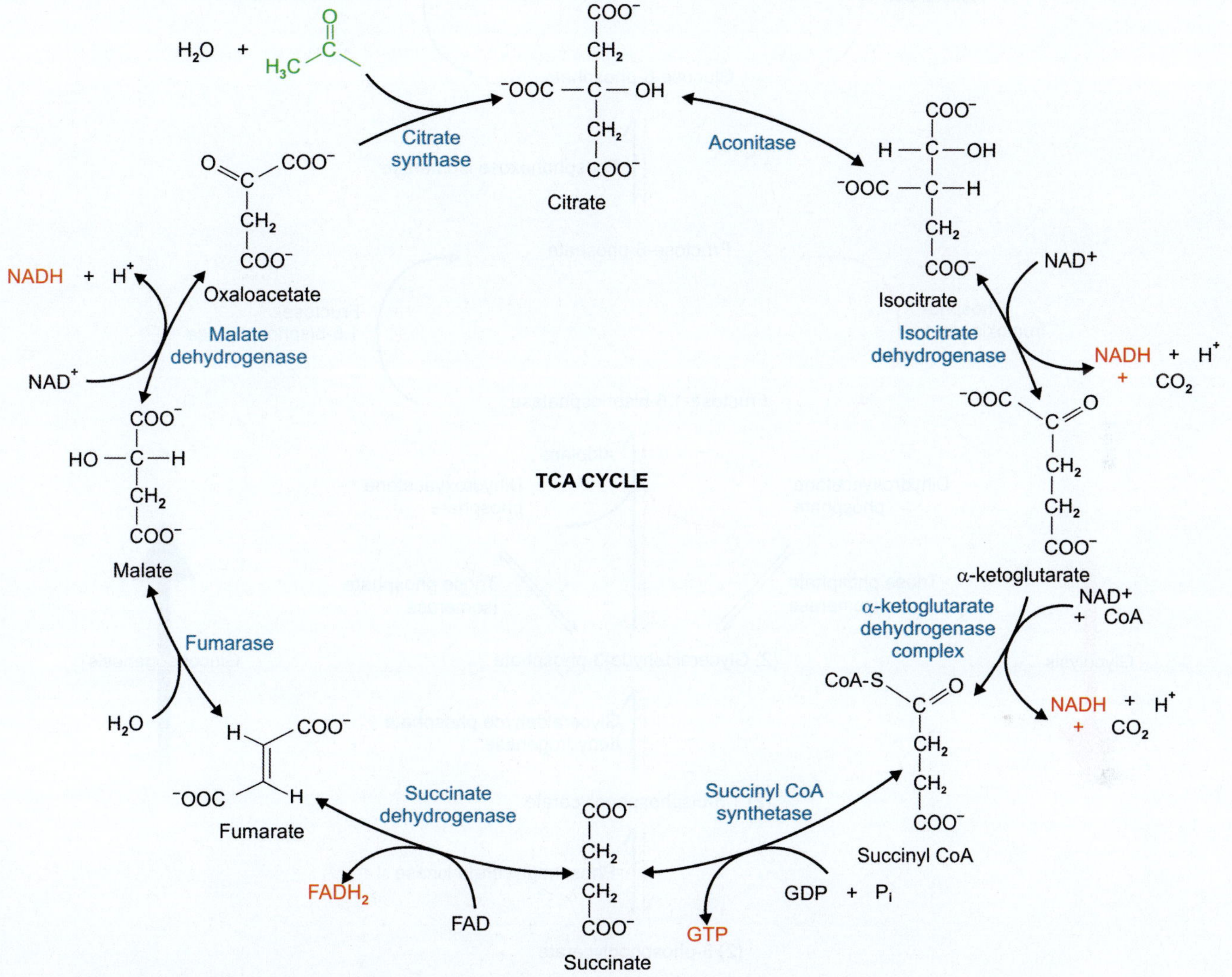

TCA CYCLE

Fig. 11.9: TCA cycle

- Two irreversible reactions of TCA cycle are citrate synthase and α-ketoglutarate dehydrogenese complex.
- Notice the incorporation of water molecule at fumarase step to produce malate.
- Substrate level phosphorylation, occurs at succinyl CoA synthetase step.
- Total 10 ATP are generated from each molecule of acetyl CoA utilized in TCA cycle (Table 11.4).

3 NADH	=	7.5 ATP
1 FADH$_2$	=	1.5 ATP
1 GTP	=	1 ATP
Total		**10 ATP**

Section 3 ■ Metabolism of Carbohydrates

11

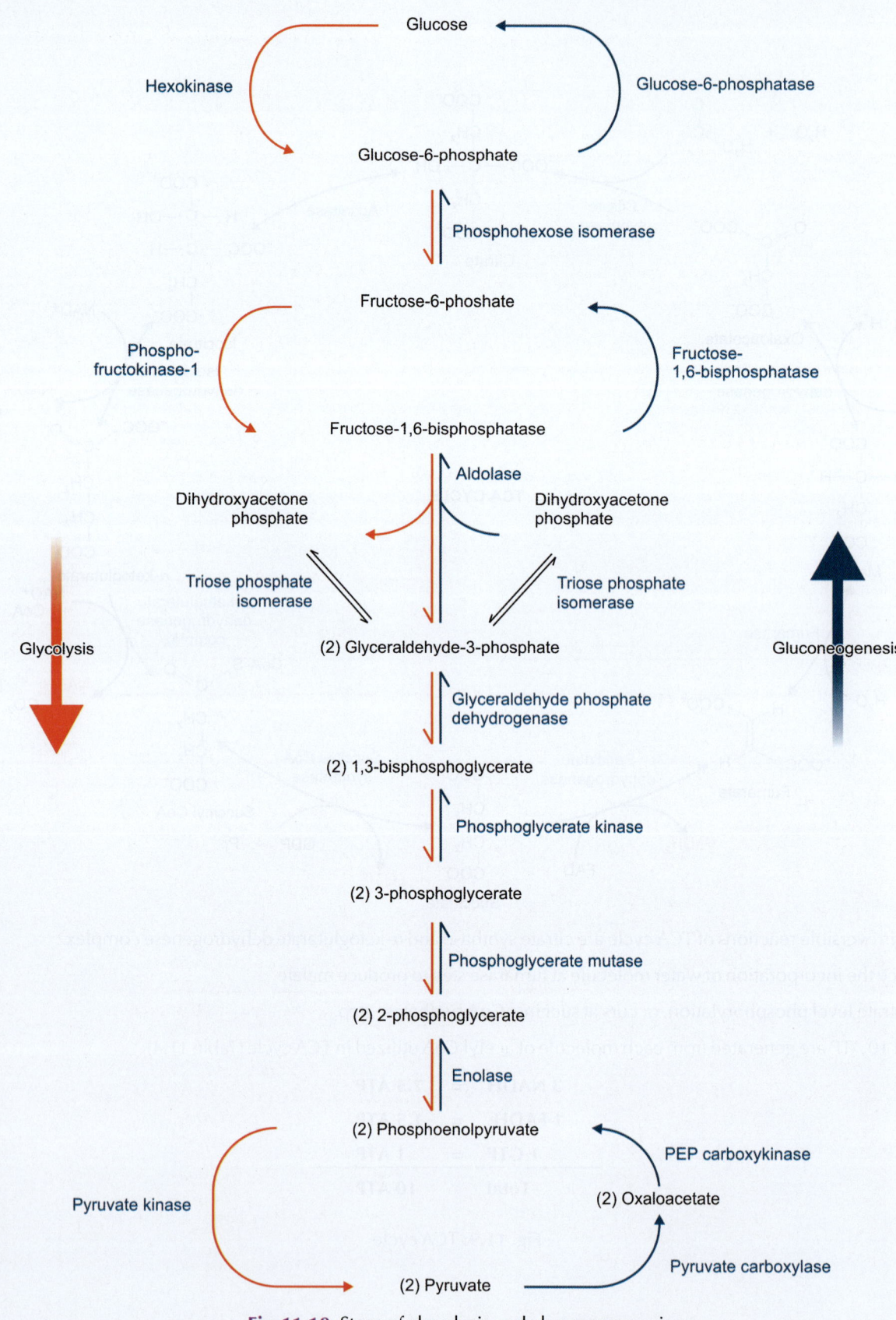

Fig. 11.10: Steps of glycolysis and gluconeogenesis

GLUCONEOGENESIS

This is the process of formation of glucose from noncarbohydrate substances.

TABLE 11.4	ATP calculation in TCA cycle (one acetyl CoA produces 10 ATP in TCA cycle)	
Step catalysed by	Gain from 1 acetyl CoA	ATP
Isocitrate dehydrogenase (ICD)	1 NADH	2.5 ATP
α-ketoglutarate dehydrogenase (α-KGD)	1 NADH	2.5 ATP
Succinate thiokinase	1 ATP	1 ATP
Succinate dehydrogenase (SCD)	1 FADH$_2$	1.5 ATP
Malate dehydrogenase	1 NADH	2.5 ATP
Total	–	10 ATP

Substrate of gluconeogenesis: Glucogenic amino acid, lactate, pyruvate, propionate, glycerol and fumaric acid.

Site of synthesis: Liver, kidney, small intestine.

This pathway of synthesis of glucose utilizes reversible reactions of glycolysis and TCA cycle (Fig. 11.10).

Irreversible steps of glycolysis are bypassed by exclusive reactions of gluconeogenesis.

• *Synthesis of glucose from pyruvate:* Three irreversible/nonequilibrium reactions in glycolysis, catalyzed by hexokinase, phosphofructokinase and pyruvate kinase, prevent simple reversal of glycolysis for glucose synthesis. They are circumvented as follows (Figs 11.11–11.14).

• *Synthesis of glucose from propionate:* Propionyl CoA is converted to succinyl CoA in the reaction as shown in Fig. 11.14.

• *Synthesis of glucose from glycerol:* After synthesizing DHAP (dihydroxyacetone phosphate) glycerol enters gluconeogenic pathway (Fig. 11.15). Glycerol kinase enzyme is found in liver and kidney.

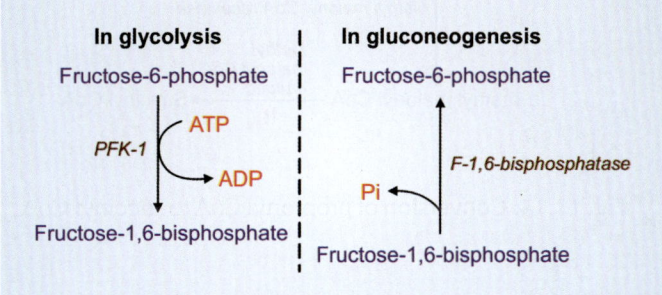

Fig. 11.12: Reversal of PFK-1 reaction

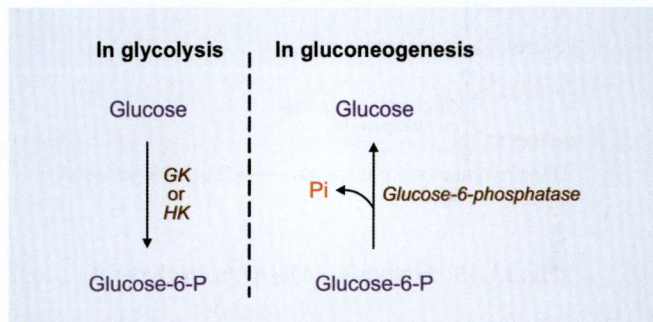

Fig. 11.13: Reversal of glucokinase/hexokinase reaction

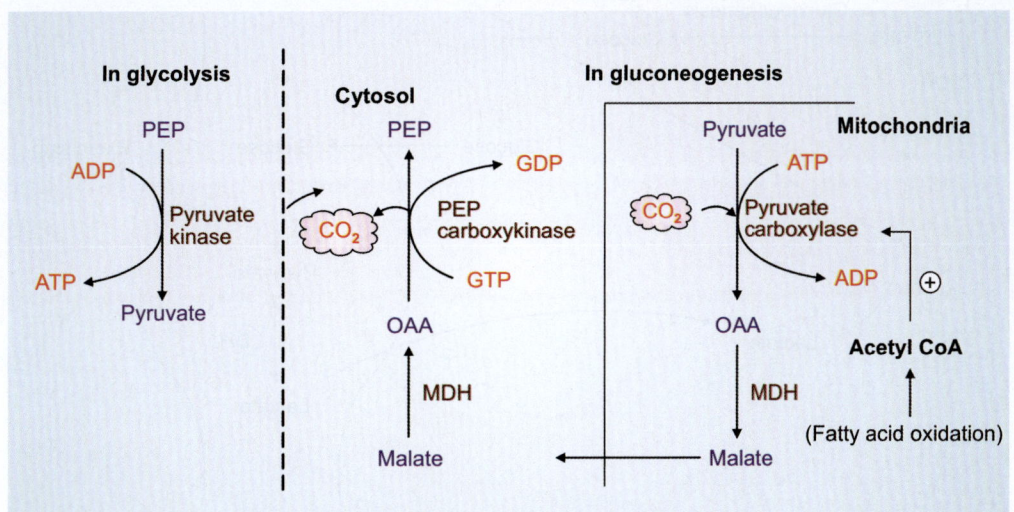

Fig. 11.11: Reversal of pyruvate kinase reaction

Section 3 ■ Metabolism of Carbohydrates

11

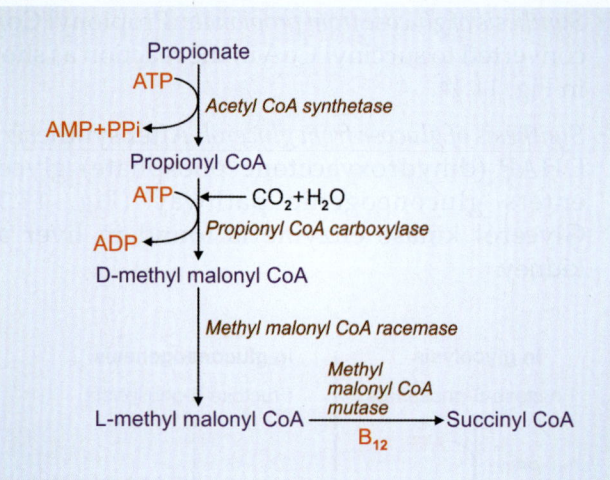

Fig. 11.14: Conversion of propionyl CoA to succinyl CoA

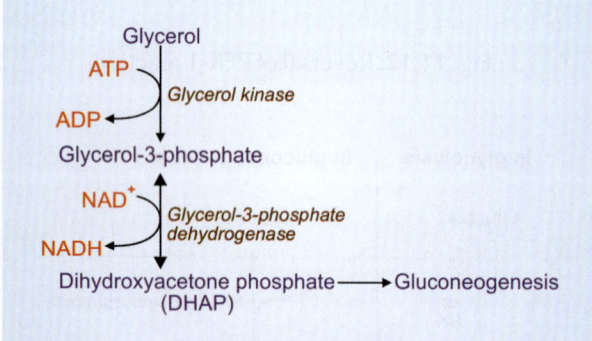

Fig. 11.15: Synthesis of DHAP from glycerol

- *Synthesis of glucose from lactate:* LDH converts lactate to pyruvate after dehydrogenation (Fig. 11.16).

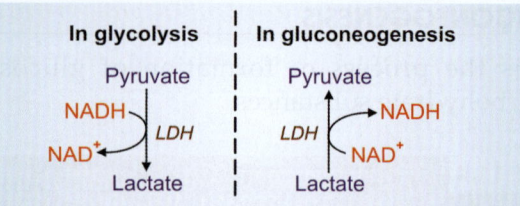

Fig. 11.16: Formation of pyruvate from lactate

Cori's cycle (glucose-lactate cycle): During vigorous exercise rate of glycolysis is enhanced in exercising muscle, which will lead to excess formation of NADH which exceeds the capacity of the electron transport chain to utilize it. This NADH then is utilized to reduce the pyruvate into lactate in the muscle itself.

After getting diffused to blood, this lactate is reached the liver cell where it is converted to glucose by the process of gluconeogenesis. This glucose which is newly synthesized in the liver cell reaches muscle (and brain cell) for utilization through blood circulation. This lactate-pyruvate interconversion which takes place between exercising muscle and the liver cell is known as Cori's cycle (Fig. 11.17).

Regulation of Gluconeogenesis

It occurs in following ways:

A. **Glucagon:** Glucagon stimulates gluconeogenesis by following three mechanisms:
- Decreasing level of fructose-2,6-bisphosphate which is an inhibitor of fructose-1,6-bisphosphatase enzyme, so decreased level of fructose-2,6-bisphosphate in turn stimulate fructose-1,6-bisphosphatase enzyme stimulating the gluconeogenesis (Fig. 11.18).

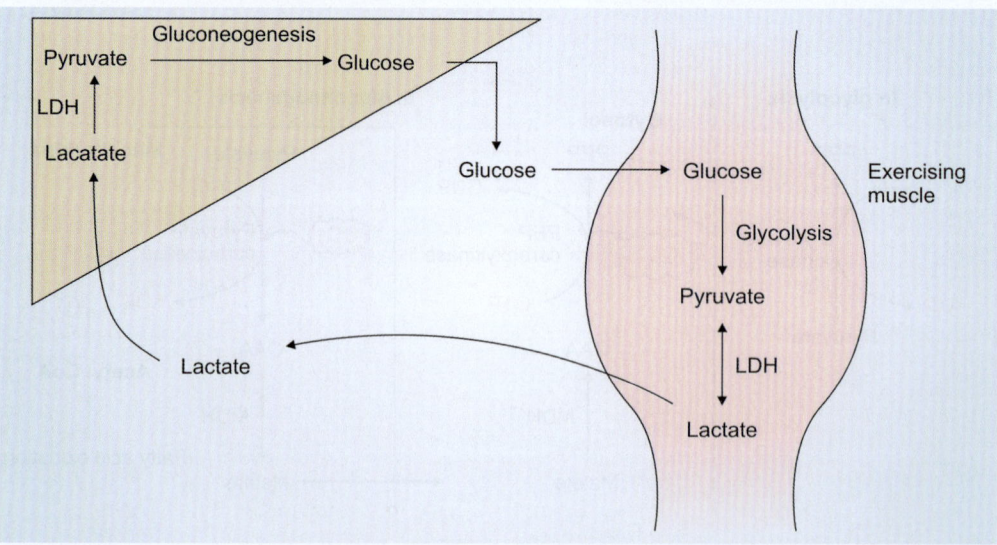

Fig. 11.17: Cori's cycle (glucose-lactate cycle)

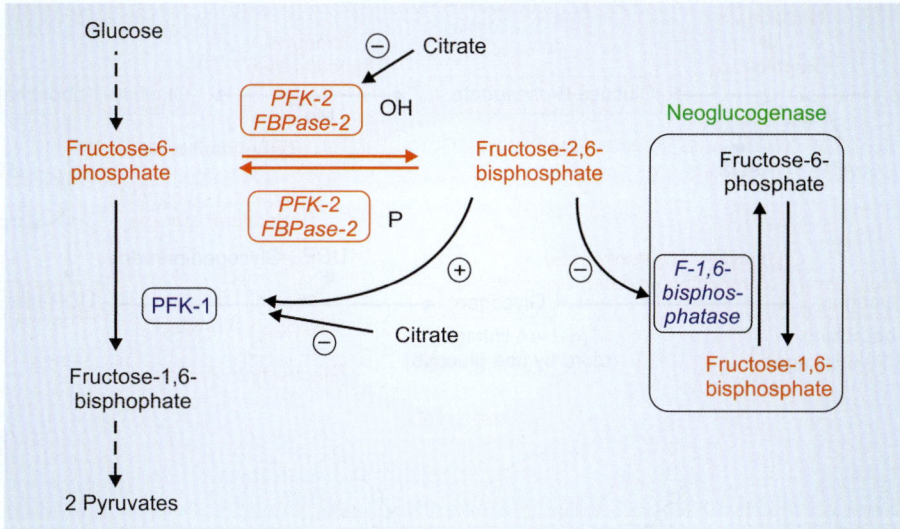

Fig. 11.18: Simultaneous regulation of PFK-1 and F-1,6-bisphosphatase by F-2,6-bisphosphate

- Glucagon elevate the level of cAMP, which phosphorylate pyruvate kinase and thus inactivates it, shunting PEP to gluconeogenesis.
- Glucagon increases the transcription of PEP carboxykinase gene and thus stimulates gluconeogenesis.

B. **Substrate availability:** The amount of oxaloacetate (OAA) in TCA cycle plays an important role in deciding the gluconeogenesis. The source of OAA may be pyruvate imporantly or it may be in any anaplerotic reaction.

C. **Allosteric activation by acetyl CoA:** Acetyl CoA derived from fatty acid oxidation inhibits PDH enzyme and simultaneously stimulates pyruvate carboxylase, thus shunting pyruvate to gluco-neogenesis.

D. **Allosteric inhibition by AMP:** AMP stimulates fructose-1,6-bisphosphatase enzyme and thus stimulates gluconeogenesis.

Energetics of Gluconeogenesis

Conversion of 2 moles of pyruvate into 1 mole of glucose requires 4 moles of ATP, 2 moles GTP and 2 moles of NADH.

GLYCOGEN METABOLISM

Glycogen is a storage form of carbohydrate in animals. It occurs mainly in liver (6%). In muscle, it rarely exceeds 1%, but because of greater muscle mass, muscle represents 3–4 times as much glycogen is stored in liver.

Glycogen is a large branched polymer of glucose molecules linked by α-1,4-glycosidic linkages. Branches arise by α-1,6-glycosidic linkage at approximately every tenth residue (Fig. 11.19).

After 12–18 hours of fasting liver glycogen is depleted almost totally. Muscle glycogen is only depleted significantly after prolonged vigorous exercise.

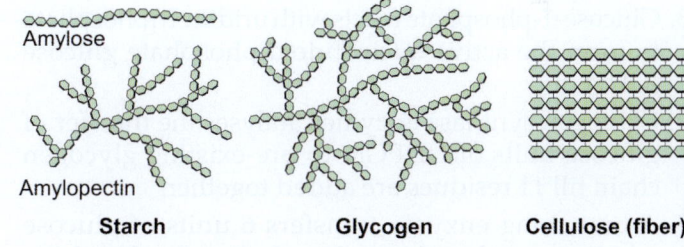

Fig. 11.19: Arrangements of glucogen, starch and cellulose

Glycogenin

It is a protein primer on which are attached a few molecules of glucose to form a glycogen primer.

Glycogenin gets glycosylated at a specifc tyrosine residue. Further glucose residues are attached in 1–4 position to make a short chain of 7 glucose residues, that are further acted upon by glycogen synthase.

Glycogenesis

[Glycogen synthesis (Fig. 11.20)]

1. Glucose is phosphorylated to glucose-6-phosphate by glucokinase enzyme.

Section 3 ■ Metabolism of Carbohydrates

11

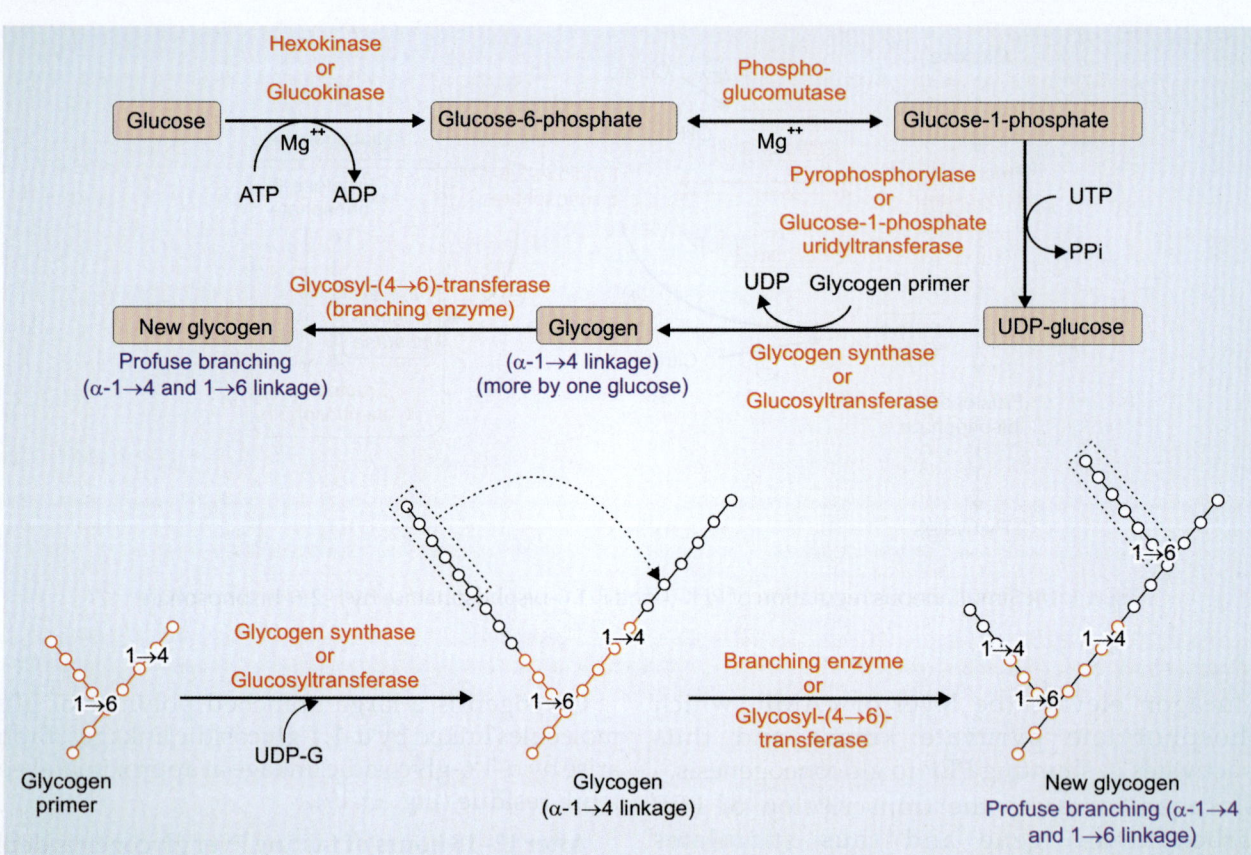

Fig. 11.20: Mechanism of glycogenesis

2. Glucose-6-phosphate is then converted to glucose-1-phosphate by phosphoglucomutase.

3. Glucose-1-phosphate reacts with uridine triphosphate to form the active nucleotide diphosphate glucose (UDPGlu).

4. Glycogen synthase enzyme catalyses the transfer of glucose units of UDPGlu to pre-existing glycogen chain till 11 residues are added together.

5. A branching enzyme transfers 6 units of glucose residue together from this chain after breaking α-1,4-glycosidic bond and forming an α-1,6-linkage, thus establishing the branching points in the molecule.

Glycogenolysis
[Glycogen breakdown (Fig. 11.21)]

1. Phosphorylase enzyme specifically acts on the terminal α-1,4-glycosidic bonds of glycogen molecules resulting in liberation of glucose units as glucose-1-phosphate until four glucose residues remain on either side of branch point. This activity of phosphorylase utilises Pi, which is incorporated in the glucose-1-phosphate.

2. A specific glucantransferase (α-1,4 → α-1,4-glucan tranferase) will then transfer a trisaccharide unit

from one side to the other, thus exposing the branch point.

3. A debranching enzyme (α-1,6-glucosidase) will act on α-1,6-linkage to liberate a free glucose residue (and not glucose-1-phosphate).

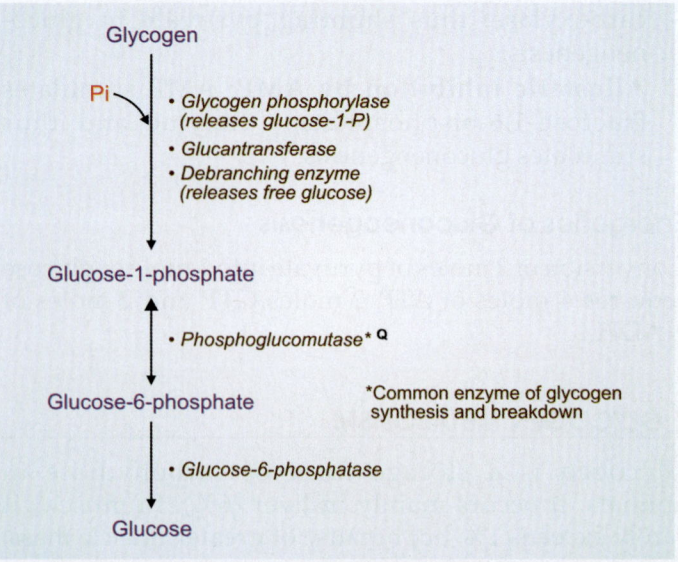

Fig. 11.21: Glycogen degradation (glycogenolysis)

NOTE: Glucantransferase (α-1,4 to α-1,4-glucantransferase) and debranching enzyme (α-1,6-glucosidase) are examples of bifunctional enzymes.

- Glycogenolysis in liver produces glucose as an end-product.
- In muscle, there is no glucose-6-phosphatase enzyme so end-product of glycogenolysis is glucose-6-phosphate (not the free glucose).

Regulatory Enzymes

- Phosphorylase enzyme is the rate-limiting enzyme in the process of glycogenolysis.
- Active phosphorylase in both tissues is allosterically inhibited by ATP and glucose-6-phosphate. In addition, free glucose is also an inhibitor in liver but not in the muscle.
- Muscle phosphorylase differs from the liver isoenzyme in having a binding site for 5'AMP, which acts as an allosteric activator of the (inactive) dephosphorylated 'b' form of the enzyme.
- Muscle phosphorylase kinase, which activates glycogen phosphorylase, is a tetramer of four different subunits, α, β, γ and δ. The α and β subunits contain serine residues that are phosphorylated by cAMP-dependent protein kinase. The δ subunit is identical to the Ca^{++} binding protein calmodulin and binds four Ca^{++}. The binding of Ca^{++} activates the catalytic site of the γ subunit even while the enzyme is in the dephosphorylated 'b' state; the phosphorylated 'a' form is only fully activated in the presence of high concentrations of Ca^{++}.

Glycogen storage diseases are caused by genetic defects that result in deficiency in certain enzymes of glycogen metabolism. The causes and characteristics of several glycogen storage diseases are listed in Table 11.5.

TABLE 11.5	Glycogen storage disorder		
Glyco-genesis	Name	Cause of disorder	Characteristics
Type 0	—	Glycogen synthase	Hypoglycemia, hyperketonemia, early death
Type Ia	von Gierke disease	Deficiency of glucose-6-phosphatase	Hypoglycemia, lactic acidemia, ketosis, hyperlipemia
Type Ib	—	Endoplasmic reticulum glucose-6-phosphate transporter	As type Ia; neutropenia and impaired neutrophil function leading to recurrent infections
Type II*	Pompe's disease	Deficiency of lysosomal α-1,4 and α-1,6-glucosidase	Fatal, accumulation of glycogen in lysosomes. Skeletal and cardiac muscle involved. Liver spared
Type IIIa	Cori's/Forbes' disease/ limit dextrinosis	Absence of debranching enzyme in muscle and liver	Accumulation of characteristic branched polysaccharide in both
Type IIIb	Limit dextrinosis	Liver debranching enzyme is deficient	Accumulation of characteristic branched polysaccharide in liver alone
Type IV	Andersen's disease, amylopectinosis	Absence of branching enzyme	Death due to cardiac or liver failure in the first year of life
Type V*	McArdle's syndrome	Absence of muscle phosphorylase	Diminished exercise tolerance; muscles have abnormally high glycogen content
Type VI	Hers' disease	Deficiency of liver (hepatic)	High glycogen content in liver, tendency towards hypoglycemia
Type VII*	Tarui's disease	Deficiency of muscle and RBC phosphofructokinase	As in type V
Type VIII	—	Liver phosphorylase kinase	Hepatomegaly
Type IX	—	Liver and muscle phosphorylase kinase	Hepatomegaly
Type X	—	cAMP-dependent protein kinase A	Hepatomegaly
Type XI	Fanconi-Bickel disease	GLUT-2 in liver is affected	—

*Liver spared in: GSD type II, V, VII   Muscle spared in: GSD type 0, Ia, Ib, IIIb, VI, VIII, IX, X

Section 3 ■ Metabolism of Carbohydrates

11

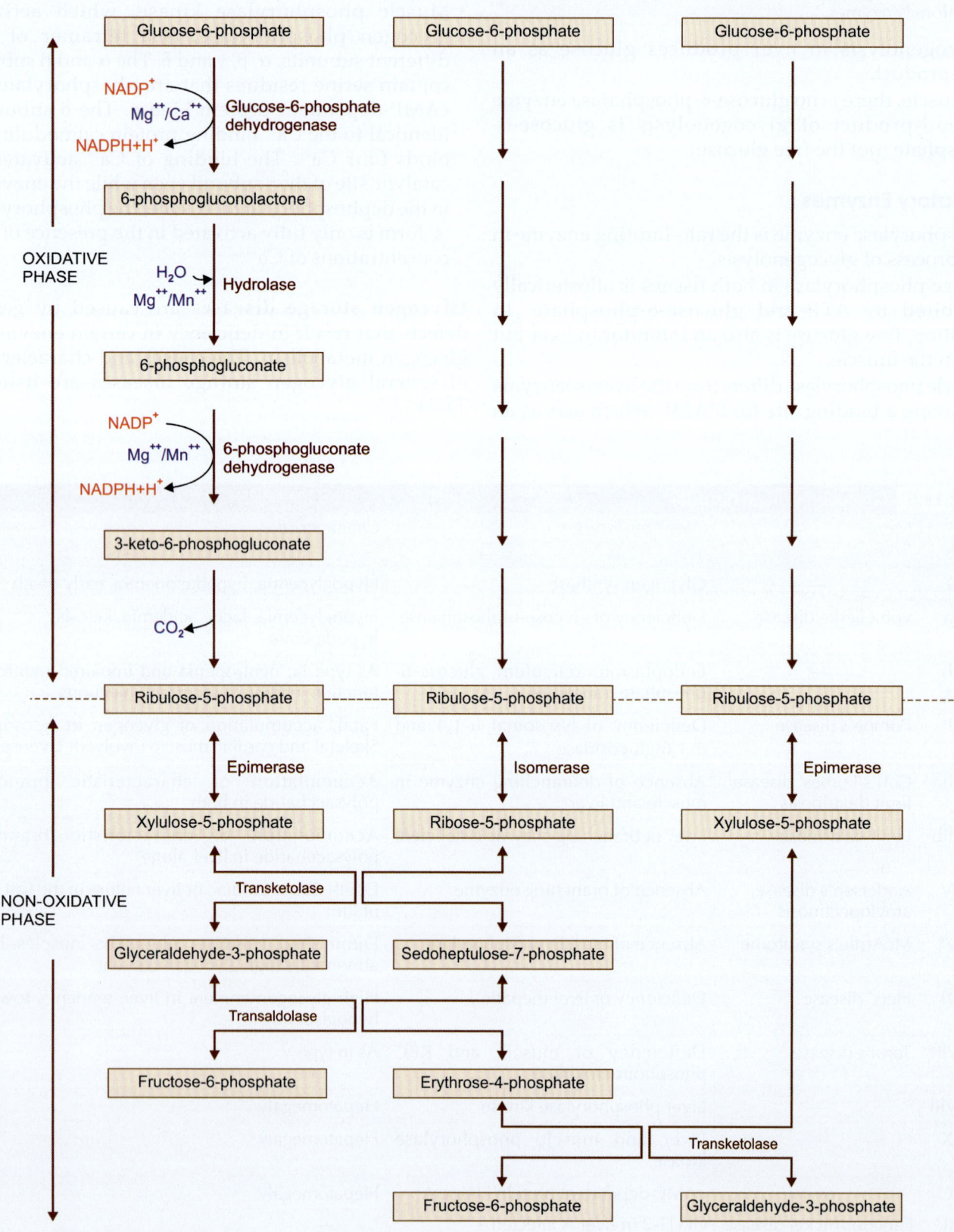

Fig. 11.22: Mechanism of HMP pathway

HEXOSE MONOPHOSPHATE SHUNT

Also known as pentose phosphate pathway (PPP)/Dickens-Horecker pathway/phosphogluconate oxidative pathway (Fig. 11.22).

It is a multicyclic process in which 3 molecules of glucose-6-phosphate give rise to 3 molecules of CO_2 and three 5-carbon residues, the latter are rearranged to generate 2 molecules of glucose-6-phosphate and 1 molecule of glycolytic intermediate glyceraldehyde-3-phosphate.

Functions of HMP Shunt Pathway

1. Generation of NADPH for reductive biosynthesis.
   a. Fatty acid synthesis
   b. Steroid hormones synthesis
   c. Erythrocytes depend on PPP for NADPH, which are required to maintain glutathione in reduced state, which is essential to maintain integrity of RBC membrane.
2. Provides a source of ribose-5-phosphate for nucleic acid biosynthesis.

Location: Erythrocytes, liver, lactating mammary gland, adipose tissue, adrenal cortex (cytosol).

Reactions of Pentose Phosphate Pathway

Reactions of HMP shunt consist of two phases:
1. Oxidative/nonreversible phase
2. Nonoxidative/reversible phase.

Oxidative phase generates NADPH and nonoxidative phase generates various intermediates namely glyceraldehyde-3-phosphate, erythrose-4-phosphate, ribulose-5 phosphate, xylulose-5 phosphate, ribose-5-phosphate, fructose-6-phosphate, sedoheptulose-7-phosphate (Fig. 11.22).

Transketolase: Transfers a 2-carbon unit from a ketose to the aldose sugar. The reaction requires thiamine as TPP along with Mg^{++}.

Transaldolase: Transfers a 3-carbon unit from aldose to ketoses.

Rate-limiting enzyme of HMP shunt pathway is glucose-6-phosphate dehydrogenase (G6PD). Insulin induces it.

Role of Pentose Phosphate in Protecting Erythrocytes against Haemolysis

The pentose phosphate pathway in erythrocytes provides NADPH for reduction of oxidised glutathione to reduced glutathione catalyzed by glutothione reductase. In turn, reduced glutothione removes H_2O_2 from erythrocyte in a reaction catalyzed by glutathione peroxidase, an enzyme that contains the trace element selenium. This reaction is important as GSH removes H_2O_2 from RBC. Accumulation of H_2O_2 may decrease

the lifespan of RBC by increasing the rate of oxidation of heomoglobin to methamoglobin (Fig. 11.23).

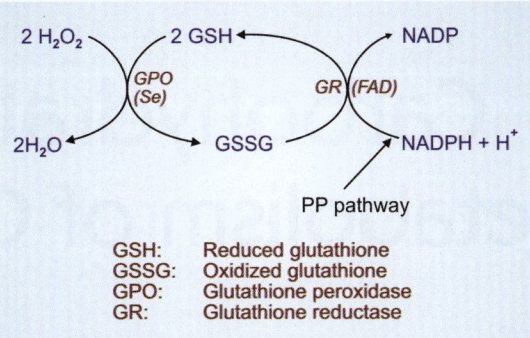

GSH:	Reduced glutathione
GSSG:	Oxidized glutathione
GPO:	Glutathione peroxidase
GR:	Glutathione reductase

Fig. 11.23: Role of NADPH in maintaining integrity of cell membrane by supplying reduced glutathione (GSH)

Uronic Acid Pathway

Significance of Uronic Acid Pathway (Fig. 11.24)

1. Source of UDP glucose that is used for glycogen formation.
2. Formation of glucuronides for bilirubin, steroid hormone and drugs.
3. Pathway integral to formation of ascorbic acid in most animals. (Human, other primates, guinea pigs, bats, fishes and some birds can not synthesise vitamin C due to absence of L-gulonolactone oxidase enzyme).
4. Xylitol dehydrogenase deficiency leads to excretion of L-xylulose in the urine, in the disorder known as essential pentosuria.
5. Alimentary pentosuria: Due to excessive consumption of pears.

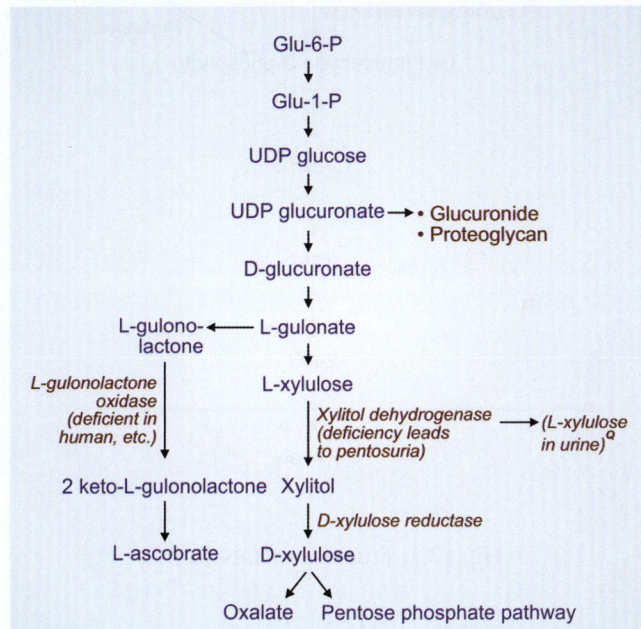

Fig. 11.24: Uronic acid pathway

Carbohydrate Metabolism II: Metabolism of Other Carbohydrates

▌METABOLISM OF FRUCTOSE

Fructose is abundantly found in fruits and honey. Table sugar is sucrose which after hydrolysis gives glucose and fructose (Fig. 12.1).

There are two routes by which fructose is metabolized:
a. In adipose tissue and muscle by hexokinase
b. In liver by fructokinase (fructose-1-phosphate pathway)

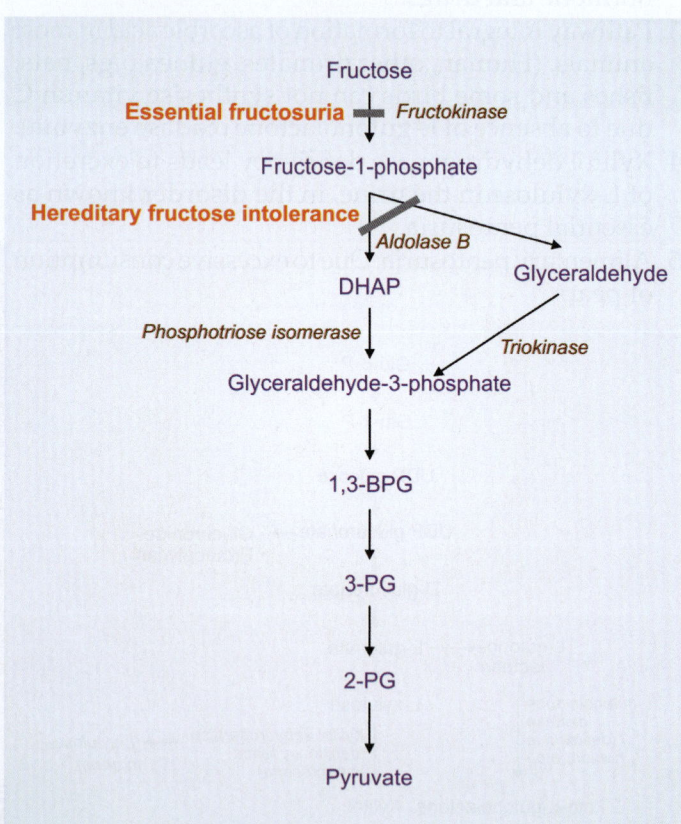

Fig. 12.1: Fructose metabolism

Description of Fructose Metabolic Pathway

a. Fructose is converted to fructose-1-phosphate by fructokinase enzyme.
b. Aldolase B enzyme splits fructose-1-phosphate into glyceraldehydes and dihydroxyacetone phosphate.
c. Dihydroxyacetone phosphate is converted to glyceraldehyde-3-phosphate by phosphotriose-isomerase enzyme.
d. Glyceraldehyde-3-phosphate gets utilized in the glycolytic steps f to j as discussed under glycolytic steps (*see* Chapter 11, page 78).
e. Glyceraldehyde gets converted to glyceraldehyde-3-phosphate by triose isomerase enzyme and enter the glycolysis steps.

Enzyme Defect in Fructose Catabolism

• **Essential fructosuria:** Defect in enzyme fructokinase (benign condition).
• **Hereditory fructose intolerance:** Genetic defect leading to aldolase B deficiency leading to accumulation of fructose-1-phosphate in cell and consequently liver and kidney damage.

▌METABOLISM OF GALACTOSE

Hydrolysis of lactose produces glucose and galactose.

Galactose gets utilized in glycolysis after getting converted to glucose-6-phosphate in the following reactions.
a. Galactokinase catalyses the phosphorylation of galactose to convert it to galactose 1-phosphate using ATP as phosphate donor.
b. Galactose-1-phosphate reacts with uridine diphosphate glucose (UDPGlc) to form uridine diphosphate galactose (UDPGal) and

glucose-1-phosphate, in a reaction catalyzed by galactose-1-phosphate uridyltransferase.

c. UDPGal is converted to UDPGlc in a reaction catalysed by 4 epimerases.

d. Glucose-1-phosphate gained in step b is converted to glucose-6-phosphate by phosphoglucomutase and is utilized in glycolysis.

Since the epimerase reaction is freely reversible, glucose can be converted to galactose making the galactose dietary nonessential.

Galactose is required in the body not only in the formation of lactose but also as a constituent of glycolipids (cerebrosides), proteoglycans, and glycoproteins. In the synthesis of lactose in the mammary gland, UDPGal condenses with glucose to yield lactose, catalyzed by lactose synthase.

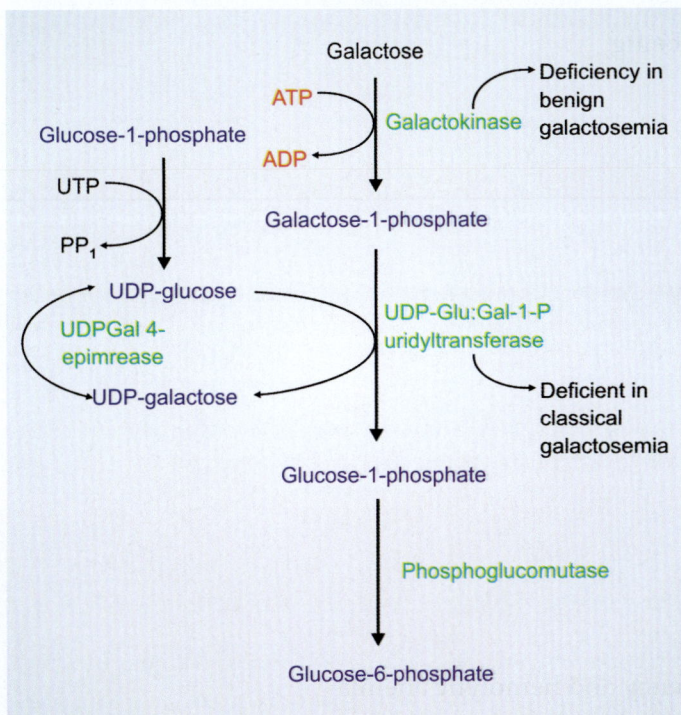

Fig. 12.2: Galactose metabolism

Enzyme Defect in Galactose Metabolism

a. **Classical galactosemia:** This condition is characterised by inability to metabolise dietary galactose due to deficiency of galactose-1-phosphate uridyltransferase. This results in increased level of galactose in blood which produces toxic substances like galactitol after reduction. This leads to cataract, mental disturbance, lethargy, vomiting, liver enlargement and jaundice (Fig. 12.3).

b. **Deficiency of galactokinase** leads to benign galactosemia where cataract is the only feature found. There is no organomegaly or mental retardation in benign galactosemia.

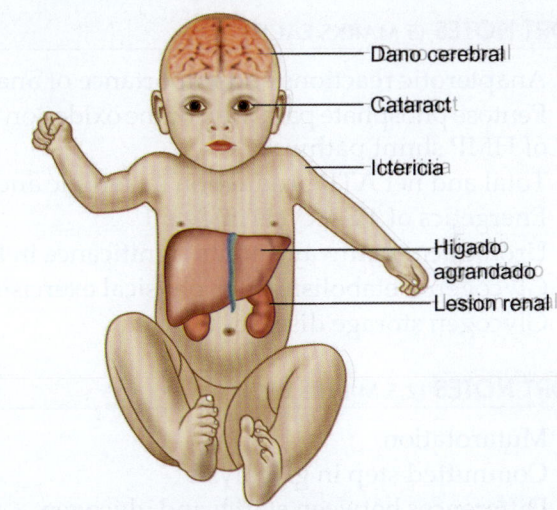

Fig. 12.3

c. **Deficiency of epimerase** if found in association with any of the above two enzymes described, the condition becomes very dangerous and nontreatable.

Treatment of galactosemia is galactose free diet (Fig. 12.4).

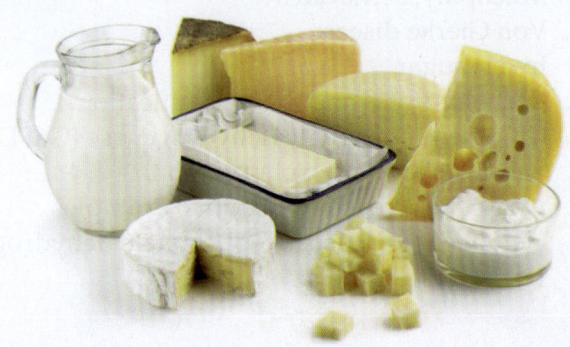

Fig. 12.4: Lactose-containing diet

EXERCISE

LONG QUESTIONS (10 MARKS EACH)

Q 1. Under what conditions, the process of gluconeogenesis is activated in the body? Discuss its important metabolic steps of process of glucose synthesis. How is alanine converted to glucose?

Q 2. Describe the reactions of glycogenolysis with suitable diagram. Also mention salient difference between muscle and liver glycogenolysis.

Q 3. Explain the difference between aerobic and anaerobic glycolysis with suitable flowcharts. Also explain the regulatory role of fructose 2,6-bisphosphate on glycolysis.

SHORT NOTES (5 MARKS EACH)

Q 1. Anaplerotic reactions and importance of anaplerotic reactions of the TCA cycle

Q 2. Pentose phosphate pathway for the oxidation of glucose, tissues it predominate and the metabolic significance of HMP shunt pathway

Q 3. Total and net ATP production in aerobic and anaerobic glycolysis

Q 4. Energetics of TCA cycle in detail

Q 5. Uronic acid pathway and its significance in human being

Q 6. Glycogen metabolism after physical exercise

Q 7. Glycogen storage diseases

SHORT NOTES (2.5 MARKS EACH)

Q 1. Mutarotation

Q 2. Committed step in glycolysis

Q 3. Differences between starch and glycogen

Q 4. Rapport-Leubering cycle

Q 5. Fructose intolerance

Q 6. Lactose intolerance

Q 7. PDH complex

Q 8. Glucose-alanine cycle (Cahill cycle)

Q 9. Glucose-lactate cycle (Cori's cycle)

Q 10. Mucopolysaccharides

Q 11. Von Gierke disease

Q 12. Invert sugar

Q 13. Carbohydrates and their classification

Q 14. Glucose-6-phosphate dehydrogenase (G6PD) deficiency and hemolytic anemia

Q 15. Substrate level phosphorylation

Q 16. Anaplerotic reaction with two examples

Q 17. Hemolysis in glucose-6-phosphate dehydrogenase deficiency

MULTIPLE CHOICE QUESTIONS

12.1 Which of the following is not a gluconeogenic substrate in humans?
a. Lactate
b. Pyruvate
c. Oxaloacetate
d. Acetyl CoA

12.2 What is the total number of ATPs derived from one molecule of Acetyl CoA?
a. 8
b. 9
c. 10
d. 12
e. 10

12.3 Glycosaminoglycans:
a. Are the carbohydrate portion of the glycoprotein
b. Contain large segment of a repeating unit typically consisting of a hexosamine and a uronic acid
c. Always contain sulphate
d. Exist only in two forms

12.4 Which of the following is an anaplerotic reaction?
a. Conversion of pyruvate to acetyl CoA
b. Conversion of pyruvate to acetaldehyde
c. Conversion of pyruvate to lactic acid
d. Conversion of pyruvate to oxaloacetate

12.5 Positive signals for glycogen breakdown include increase in all of the following except:
a. Cyclic AMP
b. Blood glucose
c. Epinephrine
d. Ca^{++}

12.6 During an overnight fast, the major source of blood glucose is:
a. Dietary glucose from the intestine
b. Hepatic glycogenolysis
c. Gluconeogenesis
d. Muscle glycogenolysis

12.7 Which of the following plant components is not fermented by gastrointestinal microorganisms?
a. Lignin
b. Cellulose
c. Hemicellulose
d. Pectin

12.8 A 6-month-old child with hepatomegaly cannot maintain a normal blood glucose either by glycogenolysis or gluconeogenesis. He is very likely suffering from a deficiency of which of the following enzymes?
a. Fructokinase
b. Glucose-6-phosphatase
c. Glucokinase
d. Transketolase

12.9 A genetic disorder renders fructose-1,6-bisphosphatase in the liver less sensitive to regulation by fructose-2,6-bisphosphate. All of the following metabolic changes are observed in this disorder, except:
a. Level of fructose-1,6-bisphosphate is higher than normal
b. Level of fructose-1,6-bisphosphate is lower than normal
c. Less pyruvate will be formed
d. Less ATP will be generated

12.10 The activity of pyruvate carboxylase is dependent upon which positive allosteric effector?
a. Succinate
b. Acetyl CoA
c. AMP
d. Isocitrate

12.11 Fructokinase reaction produces which of the following intermediates?
a. Fructose-1-phosphate
b. Fructose-6-phosphate
c. Fructose-1,6-diphosphate
d. Glyceraldehydes and dihydroxyacetone phosphate

12.12 *In vivo* control of citric acid cycle is effected by:
a. Acetyl CoA
b. Coenzyme A
c. ATP
d. Citrate
e. NADH

Section 3 ■ Metabolism of Carbohydrates

12

12.13 Thiamine requirement increases in excessive intake of:
a. Carbohydrate
b. Fat
c. Lecithin
d. Amino acid

12.14 McArdle's disease is due to the deficiency of:
a. Glucose-1-phosphatase
b. Glucose-1,6-diphosphatase
c. Myophosphorylase
d. Glucose-6-phosphatase

12.15 The first product of glycogenolysis is:
a. Glucose-6-phosphate
b. Glucose-1,3-diphosphate
c. Glucose-1-phosphate
d. Fructose-1-phosphate

12.16 In starvation, nitrogen is carried from muscle to liver and kidney by:
a. Alanine
b. Aspartic acid and sulphate
c. Glycine
d. Asparagine

12.17 Essential pentosuria is due to defect in:
a. HMP pathway
b. Glycolysis
c. Gluconeogenesis
d. Uronic acid pathway

12.18 Hemolytic anemia is seen most commonly due to:
a. Pyruvate kinase
b. Phosphofructokinase 1
c. Phosphoenolpyruvate carboxykinase
d. Glucose-6-phosphate dehydrogenase

12.19 A 7-month-old child develops vomiting after fruit juice feeds. She is diagnosed as hereditary fructose intolerance. The enzyme deficient in this disorder is:
a. Phosphofructokinase
b. Fructose-1,6-bisphosphatase
c. Hexokinase
d. Aldolase B

12.20 Peroxidase enzyme is used in the estimation of:
a. Hemoglobin
b. Ammonia
c. Creatinine
d. Glucose

12.21 In humans, ascorbic acid can not be synthesized because of:
a. Deficiency of G6PD
b. Deficiency of xylulose kinase
c. Deficiency of L-gulonolactone oxidase
d. Deficiency of phosphoglucomutase

12.22 Glucosuria happens when the venous blood glucose fixation exceeds:
a. 100 mmol/L
b. 180 mmol/L
c. 10 mmol/L
d. 18 mmol/L

12.23 Which one of the following statements concerning glycolysis is correct?
a. The conversion of glucose to lactate requires the presence of oxygen.
b. Hexokinase is important in hepatic glucose metabolism only in the absorptive period following consumption of a carbohydrate-containing meal.
c. Fructose-2,6-bisphosphate is a potent inhibitor of phosphofructokinase.
d. The regulated reactions are also the irreversible reactions.

12.24 After a 72-hour fast the substance likely to involved in the formation of energy would be:
a. Muscle glycogen
b. Liver glycogen
c. Amino acid
d. Acetoacetate

12.25 Which of the following is not seen in low insulin-glucagon ratio?
a. Gluconeogenesis
b. Glycogen storage
c. Glycogen breakdown
d. Ketogenesis

12.26 Pancreatic amylase acts on:
a. Terminal α-1,4-glycosidic bond
b. Terminal α-1,6-glycosidic bond
c. Internal α-1,4-glycosidic bond

12.27 An infant with an enlarged liver has a glucose 6-phosphatase deficiency. This infant
a. Cannot maintain blood glucose levels either by glycogenolysis or by gluconeogenesis
b. Can use liver glycogen to maintain blood glucose levels

c. Can use muscle glycogen to maintain blood glucose levels

d. Can convert both alanine and glycerol to glucose to maintain blood glucose levels

12.28 **Which of the following statements about liver phosphorylase kinase is true?**

a. It is present in an inactive form when epinephrine is elevated

b. It phosphorylates phosphorylase to an inactive form

c. It catalyzes a reaction that requires ATP

d. It is phosphorylated in response to elevated insulin

12.29 **Which of the following statements about glycolysis and gluconeogenesis is correct?**

a. All the reactions in glycolysis are freely reversible for gluconeogenesis.

b. Fructose cannot be used for gluconeogenesis in the liver because it cannot be phophorylated to fructose-6-phosphate.

c. Glycolysis can proceed in absence of oxygen only if pyruvate is formed from lactate in muscle.

d. Red blood cells only metabolize glucose by anaerobic glycolysis (and the pentose phosphate pathway).

12.30 **Which of the following events does not occur when concentration of glucose in the liver decreases?**

a. Inactivation of phosphofructokinase-2 (PFK-2)

b. Activation of fructose bisphosphatase-2 (fructose-2,6-bisphosphatase)

c. Increased levels of fructose-2,6-bisphosphate

d. Increased levels of glucagon

12.31 **Glucose-6-phosphate is an initial substrate for all the following, except:**

a. Glycolysis

b. HMP shunt

c. Glycogenesis

d. Neoglucogenesis

12.32 **A patient with von Gierke disease can produce excess of ketone bodies due to all of the following, except:**

a. They suffer from hypoglycemia

b. Lack of insulin is the trigger for ketogenesis

c. Oxaloacetate is needed for gluconeogenesis

d. The mobilization of fat is low

12.33 **A baby is having hypoglycaemia, specially early morning hypoglycaemia. Glucagon raises blood glucose when given in fed state, but same glucagon does not raise blood glucose when given during fasting state. Liver biopsy shows accumulation of glycogen in the liver. What is the enzyme deficiency?**

a. Muscle phosphorylase

b. Glucose-6-phosphorylase

c. Branching enzyme

d. Debranching enzyme

12.34 **The adenylate cyclase system is mediated by:**

a. cAMP

b. Phosphodiesterase

c. GTP regulating proteins

d. Nuclear receptors

12.35 **Which one of the following is not a second messenger?**

a. Cyclic AMP

b. Guanylyl cyclase

c. Diacylglycerol

d. Inositol triphosphate

12.36 **True about G protein coupled receptor is:**

a. G protein bind to hormone on the cell surface

b. All the three subunits of G protein should bind together for G protein to act

c. G protein acts as inhibitory and excitatory because of difference in the alpha subunit

d. G protein bound to the GTP in resting state

12.37 **In which one of the following tissues, glucose transport in the cell is enhanced by insulin?**

a. Brain   c. RBC

b. Lens   d. Adipose tissue

12.38 **Glucose transporter in myocyte stimulated by insulin is:**

a. GLUT-1

b. GLUT-2

c. GLUT-3

d. GLUT-4

12.39 **True about G protein coupled receptors is:**

a. G proteins bind to hormones on the cell surface

b. All the three subunits alpha, beta and gamma should bind to each other for G protein to act

c. G protein is both inhibitory and excitatory

d. G protein is bound to GTP in resting state

ANSWERS

12.1 (d) Acetyl CoA

Acetyl CoA is not capable of synthesizing glucose as it cannot form pyruvate.

PDH complex catalyses irreversible conversion of pyruvate to acetyl CoA.

Following substrates may be gluconeogenic:

- Pyruvate
- Lactate
- Oxaloacetate
- Fumarate
- Gluconeogenic amino acid
- Glycerol
- Propionic acid

12.2 (c) Energetics of TCA cycle : From 1 molecule of acetyl CoA

Enzyme	Method of ATP formation	No. of ATPs	No. of ATPs
Isocitrate dehydrogenase	1 NADH respiratory chain oxidation	2.5	2.5
Alpha ketoglutarate dehydrogenase	1 NADH respiratory chain oxidation	2.5	2.5
Succinate thiokinase	Substrate level phosphorylation	1	1
Succinate dehydrogenase	Respiratory chain oxidation of 1 FADH2	1.5	1.5
Malate dehydrogenase	Respiratory chain oxidation of 1 NADH	2.5	2.5
	Total	10	10

12.3 (b) Contain large segment of a repeating unit typically consisting of a hexosamine and a uronic acid

- This is a major distinction from the glycoprotein, which by definition does not have repeating units of hexosamine and uronic acid.
- They are carbohydrate portions of the proteoglycan, not the glycoprotein.
- Hyaluronate does not contain sulphate.
- Exist in 6 different classes, e.g. heparin, heparan sulphate, keratan sulphate I and II, dermatan sulphate, chondroitin sulphate.

12.4 (d) Conversion of pyruvate to oxaloacetate

- Anaplerotic reactions are chemical reactions that form intermediates of a metabolic pathway.

- Anaplerotic flux must balance cataplerotic flux in order to retain homeostasis of cellular metabolism.

12.5 (b) Blood glucose

- Rate-limiting enzyme in glycogenolysis is glycogen phosphorylase and in glycogenesis is glycogen synthetase. The two processes are reciprocally regulated.
- Phosphorylation makes the enzyme glycogen phosphorylase active whereas phosphorylation of glycogen synthetase results in its inactivation.
- Epinephrine (in both muscle and liver) and glucagons (in liver only) acts in receptors to increase cAMP production.
- Cyclic AMP results in phosphorylation and thus stimulates glycogenolysis (remember that phosphorylated glycogen phosphorylase, also known as phosphorylase, is active) and inhibits glycogenesis (phosphoryl glycogen synthetase is inactive).
- ATP and glucose-6-phosphate act as inhibitors of phosphorylase enzyme.
- Since the two processes are reciprocally regulated, it functions like a negative feedback system where obviously increase in blood glucose will not cause breakdown of glycogen and increase blood glucose further.

12.6 (b) Hepatic glycogenolysis

- During this period, the major source of blood glucose is hepatic glycogen. Through the effects of glycogenolysis, which are mediated by glucagon, hepatic glycogen is slowly parceled out as glucose to the bloodstream, keeping blood glucose levels normal.
- In contrast, muscle glycogenolysis has no effect on blood glucose levels because no glucose-6-phosphatase exists in muscle and hence phosphorylated glucose cannot be released from muscle into the bloodstream.
- Following a more prolonged fast or in the early stages of starvation, gluconeogenesis is needed to produce glucose from glucogenic amino acids and the glycerol released by lipolysis of triacylglycerides in adipocytes.

12.7 (a) Lignin

- Lignin resists attack by most microorganisms, and anaerobic processes tend not to attack the aromatic rings at all.

12

- Aerobic breakdown of lignin is slow and may take many days.
- Lignin is nature's cement along with hemicellulose to exploit the strength of cellulose while conferring flexibility.
- Lignin is found in all vascular plants, mostly between the cells, but also within the cells, and in the cell walls. It makes vegetables firm and crunchy, and gives us what we call 'fiber' in our food.
- Lignin is an insoluble fiber, so it is not fermented. Pectin is a soluble fiber. Soluble fiber is acted on by the microflora and fermented to produce a short chain volatile fatty acid, which improves the colonic environment, regulates immune response, involved in synthesis of some vitamins, helps to lower down the colonization of pathogenic bacteria.

12.8 (b) Glucose-6-phosphatase

Deficiency of glucose-6-phosphatase affects the conversion of glucose-6-phosphate to free glucose both during gluconeogenesis and glycogenolysis in the liver. This leads to frequent hypoglycemic episodes.

This deficiency of glucose-6-phosphatase enzyme is seen in von Gierke disease (GSD type 1).

Manifestations of von Gierke disease are:
- Hypoglycemia
- Lactic acidosis
- Ketosis
- Hepatomegaly
- Hyperuricemia

12.9 (a) Level of fructose-1,6-bisphosphate is higher than normal

Refer to the following diagram

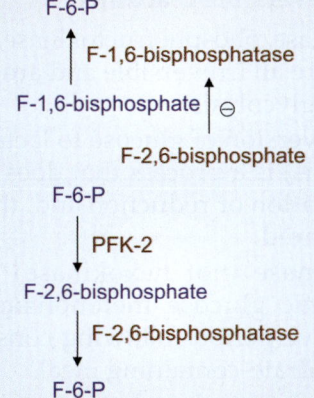

Fructose-2,6-bisphosphate has inhibitory effect on fructose-1,6-bisphosphatase enzyme. If the genetic

disease is rendering fructose-1,6-bisphosphatase enzyme less sensitive by fructose-2,6-bisphosphate, in that case fructose-1,6-bisphosphatase enzyme will act more, reducing level of fructose-1,6-bisphosphate molecule. So,

Option a: Will not be seen, and hence it is the answer of the question.

Option b: Fructose-1,6-bisphosphate level is going to be lower than normal.

Option c: Gluconeogenesis will be upregulated so, pyruvate will be less.

Option d: Gluconeogenesis is the energy consuming process and so ATP will be consumed in this case and level of ATP will be reduced.

12.10 (b) Acetyl CoA

Acetyl CoA derived from fatty acid oxidation is an important positive allosteric activator of pyruvate carboxylase enzyme. So, in condition of starvation when there is excessive fatty acid oxidation, the acetyl CoA produced by fatty acid oxidation acts as a stimulator of pyruvate carboxylase enzyme, stimulating gluconeogenesis.

12.11 (a) Fructose-1-phosphate

First step of fructose metabolism is catalysed by fructokinase and the product is fructose-1-phosphate.

12.12 (a) Acetyl CoA, (b) Coenzyme A, (c) ATP, (d) Citrate, (e) NADH

TCA cycle is tightly regulated at two levels:
- PDH complex reaction
- Citrate synthase reaction

Other places of control:
- ICD
- Alpha-ketoglutarate dehydrogenase

Level of control of TCA cycle		
Enzyme	*Activator*	*Inhibitor*
PDH complex	AMP CoA NAD$^+$ Ca^{++}	ATP Acetyl CoA NADH Fatty acid
Citrate synthase	ADP	NADH Succinyl CoA Citrate ATP
ICD	ADP Ca^{++}	ATP
α-ketoglutarate dehydrogenase	Ca^{++}	Succinyl CoA, NADH

Section 3 ■ Metabolism of Carbohydrates

12

12.13 (a) Carbohydrate

Thiamine is required for oxidation of glucose, so excess consumption of the glucose leads to increased demand of the thiamine. In a similar fashion requirement of vitamin B_6 (pyridoxine) increases with increase in protein content of the food.

12.14 (c) Myophosphorylase

This disease is characterized by poor exercise tolerance, abnormal high glycogen (2.5–4%), low level of blood lactate even after exercise.

12.15 (c) Glucose-1-phosphate

12.16 (a) Alanine

During starvation, in the muscle major keto acid which accepts the amino group is the pyruvate. This results in the formation of alanine.

12.17 (d) Uronic acid pathway

Essential pentosuria is due to xylitol dehydrogenase deficiency.

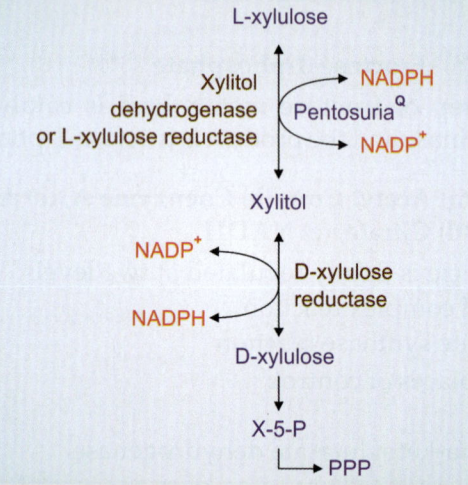

12.18 (d) Glucose-6-phosphate dehydrogenase

Hemolytic anemia due to enzyme deficiency
- G6PD
- Pyruvate kinase deficiency
- Phosphoglucomutase deficiency

12.19 (d) Aldolase B

Hereditary Fructose Intolerance

Deficiency of aldolase B is a severe condition of infants that appears with the ingestion of fructose-containing food and is caused by a deficiency of aldolase B activity in the liver, kidney and intestine.

The enzyme catalyzes the hydrolysis of fructose-1,6-bisphosphate into triose phosphate and glyceraldehyde phosphate.

The same enzyme also hydrolyzes fructose-1-phosphate.

Deficiency of this enzyme activity causes a rapid accumulation of fructose-1-phosphate and initiates severe toxic symptoms when exposed to fructose.

12.20 (d) Glucose

GOD-POD (glucose oxidase-peroxidase) method is the commonly used method for estimation of glucose in biological fluid. Principle of this test is as follows:

(i) $\text{D-glucose} + H_2O + O_2 \xrightarrow{\text{GOD}}$
$\text{D-gluconic acid} + H_2O_2$

(ii) $H_2O_2 + \text{4-aminoantipyrine} + \text{Phenol} \xrightarrow{\text{POD}}$
$\text{Quinoneimine dye} + H_2O$

12.21 (c) Deficiency of L-gulonolactone oxidase

In man, other primates and guinea pigs, ascorbic acid cannot be synthesized due to absence of L-gluconolactone oxidase, an enzyme used in lower animals to synthesize ascorbic acid as a byproduct of uronic acid pathway (glucuronic acid cycle).

12.22 (c) 10 mmol/L

- The limit of **the tubular framework to reabsorb glucose is restricted to a rate of nearly 2 mmol/min.**
- The **glomerular filtrate may** contain more glucose that can be reabsorbed in case of hyperglycemia (as happens in ineffectively regulated diabetes mellitus) bringing about glucosuria.

  When the venous blood glucose fixation **surpasses nearly 10 mmol/L, glucosuria occurs and this is termed the renal edge for glucose.**

12.23 (d) The regulated reactions are also the irreversible reactions.

a. Hexokinase, phosphofructokinase, and pyruvate kinase are all irreversible and are the regulated steps in glycolysis.

b. The conversion of glucose to lactate (anaerobic glycolysis) is a process that does not involve a net oxidation or reduction and, thus, oxygen is not required.

c. Glucokinase (not hexokinase) is important in hepatic glucose metabolism only in the absorptive period following consumption of a carbohydrate-containing meal.

d. Fructose-2,6-bisphosphate is a potent activator (not inhibitor) of phosphofructokinase.

e. The conversion of glucose to lactate yields two ATPs, but no net production of NADH.

12.24 (d) Acetoacetate

- The ketone bodies, acetoacetate and β-hydroxybutyrate are acids.
- In starvation, the dietary supply of glucose is decreased. The increased rate of lipolyssis is to provide alternate source of fuel.
- The excess acetyl CoA is converted to ketone bodies.
- The high glucagon–insulin ratio prevailing under conditions of starvation favours ketogenesis.
- The brain derives 75% of energy from ketone bodies under conditions of fasting.
- Hyperemesis in early pregnancy and prolonged labor are other causes for ketosis in clinical practice.

12.25 (b) Glycogen storage

Low insulin-glucagon ratio means low insulin levels and high glucagon levels.

Process	Insulin	Glucagon
Gluconeo-genesis	Inhibited (inhibition of pyruvate carboxylase, phosphoenolpyruvate carboxykinase, glucose-6-phosphatase)	Increased (inhibition of pyruvate kinase, phosphofructo-kinase; activation of fructose-1, 6-bisphosphatase)
Glyco-genolysis	Inhibited (inhibition of glycogen phosphorylase)	Increased (activation of glycogen phosphorylase)
Ketogenesis	Inhibited [less substrate acetyl coenzyme A (CoA); inhibition of 3-hydroxy-3-methyglutaryl-coenzyme A (HMG-CoA) synthetase]	

12.26 (c) Internal α-1,4-glycosidic bond

On contray to glycogen phosphorylase enzyme which acts on external α-1,4-glycosidic linkage (bond), pancreatic amylase acts on internal α-1,4- glycosidic linkage.

12.27 (a) Cannot maintain blood glucose levels either by glycogenolysis or by gluconeogenesis

- Glucose-6-phosphatase deficiency is a glycogen storage disease (von Gierke disease) in which neither liver glycogen nor gluconeogenic precursors (such as alanine and glycerol) can be used to maintain normal blood glucose levels.

- The last step (conversion of glucose-6-phosphate to glucose) is deficient for both glycogenolysis and gluconeogenesis.
- Muscle glycogen cannot be used to maintain blood glucose because muscle naturally does not contain glucose-6-phosphatase.

12.28 (c) It catalyzes a reaction that requires ATP

- Glucagon in the liver and epinephrine in both the liver and muscle cause cAMP to rise, activating protein kinase A. Protein kinase A phosphorylates and activates phosphorylase kinase, which in turn phosphorylates and activates phosphorylase.
- These phosphorylation reactions require ATP.

12.29 (d) Red blood cells only metabolize glucose by anaerobic glycolysis (and the pentose phosphate pathway).

Due to lack of mitochondria, RBC cannot utilize fatty acid and ketone bodies for ATP production. The only source of ATP in the RBC is anaerobic glycolysis.

12.30 (c) Increased levels of fructose-2, 6-bisphosphate

With the fall of glucose glucagon gets secreted. This leads to decreased level of fructose-2,6-bisphosphate.

12.31 (d) Neoglucogenesis

During neoglucogenesis, glucose-6-phosphate is rather the terminal intermediate, which is converted to glucose by glucose-6-phosphatase enzyme.

12.32 (d) The mobilization of fat is low

12.33 (d) debranching enzyme

- This baby is suffering from Cori's disease (type IIIa) where liver and muscle both are affected. Here debranching enzyme is deficient.
- Phosphorylase enzyme is normal in this baby, so fasting of shorter duration is well managed by glycogenolysis.
- In well-fed state, when complete glycogen is present that time glucagon stimulates phosphorylase enzyme which cleaves the glycogen releasing glucose to the blood.
- During fasting state there is limited dextrin and there is no effect of glucagon on debranching enzyme. Hence, the glucagon is not able to raise the blood glucose in fasting state.

12.34 (c) GTP regulating proteins

- Adenylyl cyclase plays a very important role in such cellular communication pathways.
- This enzyme catalyzes the conversion of ATP to cyclic AMP (cAMP). Adenylyl cyclase is an integral membrane protein.

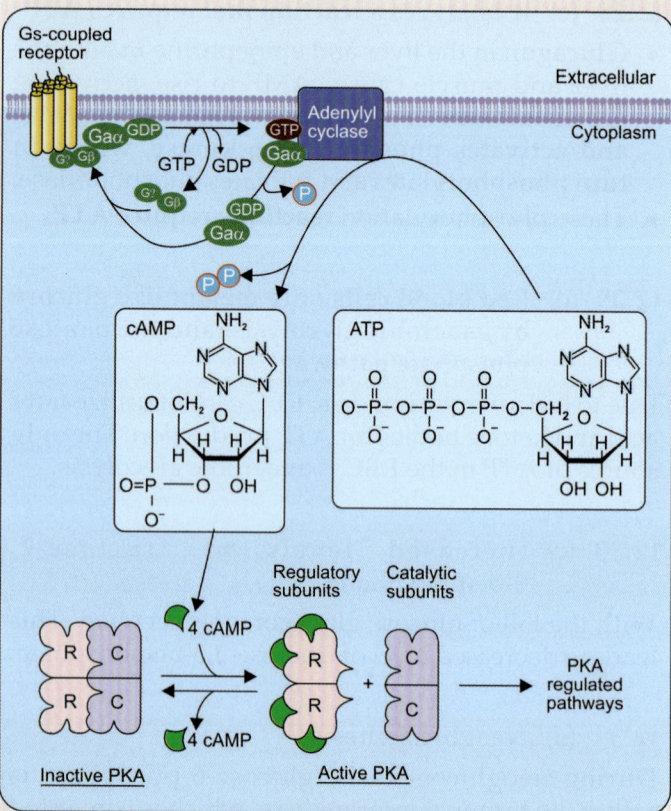

- The extracellular messenger (the hormone) combines with the specific receptor on the plasma membrane forming a complex.
- This complex activates the regulatory component of the protein designated as G protein or nucleotide regulatory protein.
- G proteins are so named, because they are bound to GTP.

12.35 (b) Guanylyl cyclase

Second messenger is the moiety which is responsible for transmitting the message from outside to inside of the the cell. Cyclic AMP, diacylglycerol, inositol triphosphate are examples of the second messenger.

Guanylyl cyclase is the enzyme responsible for the production of cGMP which is also a second messenger, but guanylyl cyclase itself is not a second messenger.

12.36 (c) G protein acts as inhibitory and excitatory because of difference in the alpha subunit.

G protein coupled receptor (GPCR) is a superfamily of cell surface receptor having 7 transmembrane helices.

Cytoplasmic C-terminal of GPCR binds with the G protein. G protein is a heterotrimer having a, b, g-subunits.

In the resting state a-subunit binds with the GDP. Ligandary stimulus of GPCR exchanges GDP for the GTP.

GTP dissociates a-subunit from the b, g-subunits. Now, this GTP-G a complex activates the effector molecule adenylyl cyclase, which synthesizes cAMP.

G protein is having inherent GTPase activity and so GTP is converted to GDP and this leads to reassociation of G a-subunit to Gb and Gg-subunits terminating its function.

12.37 (d) Adipose tissue

Major tissues in which glucose transport requires insulin are muscle and adipose tissues.

The metabolism in the liver responds to insulin, but hepatic glucose transport is determined by blood glucose concentration, and does not require insulin.

12.38 (d) GLUT-4

12.39 (a) G proteins bind to hormones on the cell surface
(c) G protein is both inhibitory and excitatory

Metabolism of Lipids

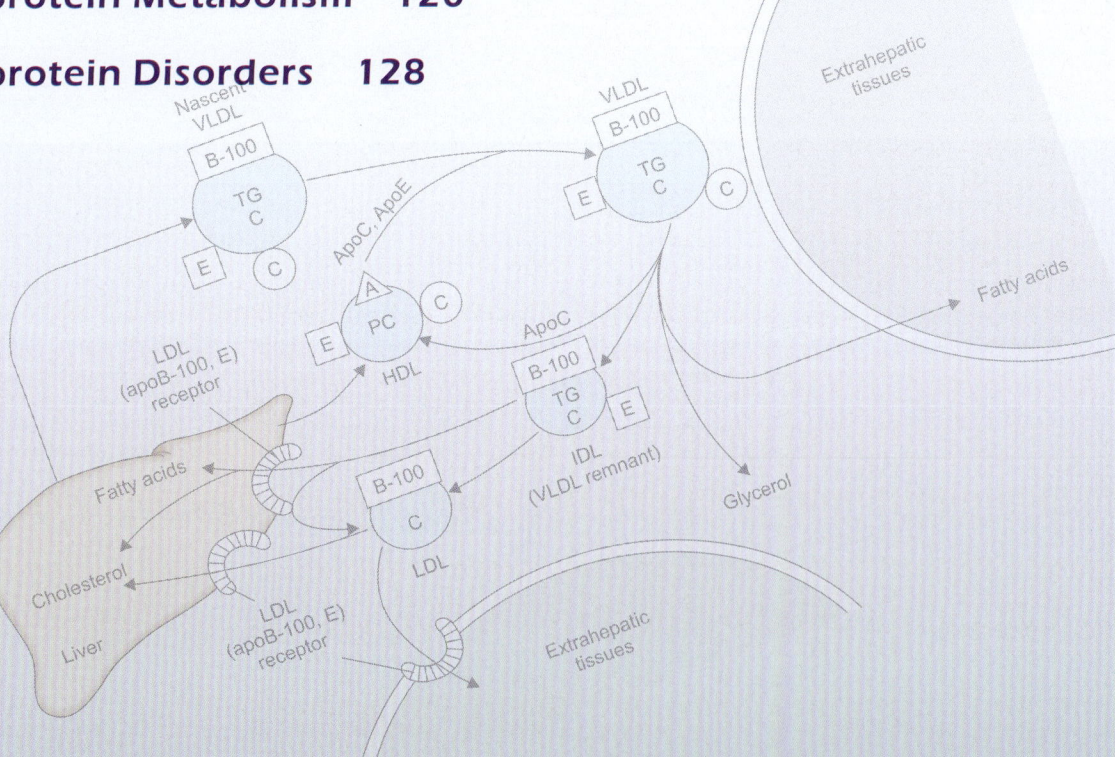

Metabolism of Lipids

4

13

Lipid Metabolism I: Fatty Acid Synthesis

Biosynthesis of fatty acid is the cytosolic process. Whole process of fatty acid synthesis can be learned under two headings.

Conversion of Acetyl CoA to Malonyl CoA

Acetyl CoA is the precursor molecule which is first converted to malonyl CoA in the cytosol by acetyl CoA carboxylase enzyme which is the 'rate-limiting enzyme' for fatty acid synthesis (Fig. 13.1).

Carboxylation of acetyl CoA to produce malonyl CoA occurs in the following two-step process (Fig. 13.2):
   a. CO_2 derived from HCO_3^- is first transformed to biotin in ATP dependent reaction.
   b. This CO_2 then is next transformed to acetyl CoA to produce malonyl CoA.

Synthesis of Fatty Acid Chain in Cyclical Reaction

Cyclical reactions of fatty acid chain synthesis occur on an enzyme complex located in cytosol known as 'fatty acid synthase' complex (FAS complex).

Characteristic Features of FAS Complex

1. It is a dimer having two units of enzyme arranged in head to tail configuration.
2. Each enzyme unit has multiple catalytic domains, so they are multifunction enzyme units.
3. Two active sites are found on FAS complex, each one of which is involved in catalysing the cyclical reation of fatty acid chain synthesis. This results in formation of two fatty acid chains simultaneously on FAS complex (Fig. 13.3).
4. Functional units division line of FAS complex is different from subunit division line (they are perpendicular).
5. Carbon 15 and 16 of palmitic acid are derived from acetyl CoA, remaining carbons of palmitic acid are derived from malonyl CoA.
6. FAS complex in human synthesizes palmitic acid (16C) alone, which is further elongated in endoplamsic retuculum.
7. Final product palmitic acid is produced on Pan-SH site of FAS complex.

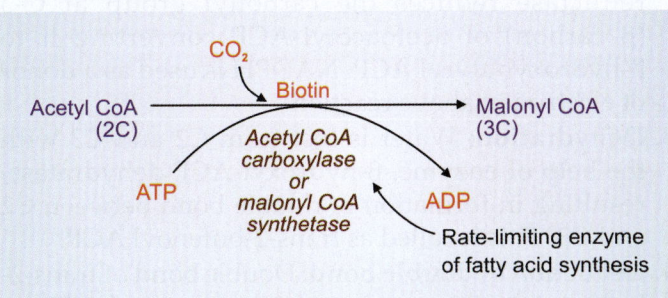

Fig. 13.1: Acetyl CoA carboxylase activity

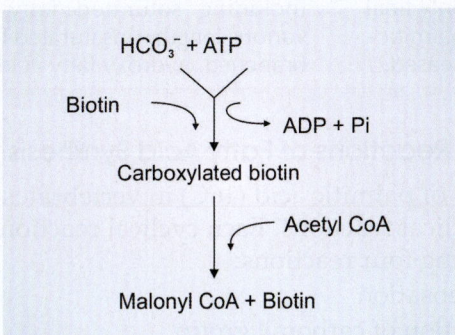

Fig. 13.2: Carboxylation reaction and biotin

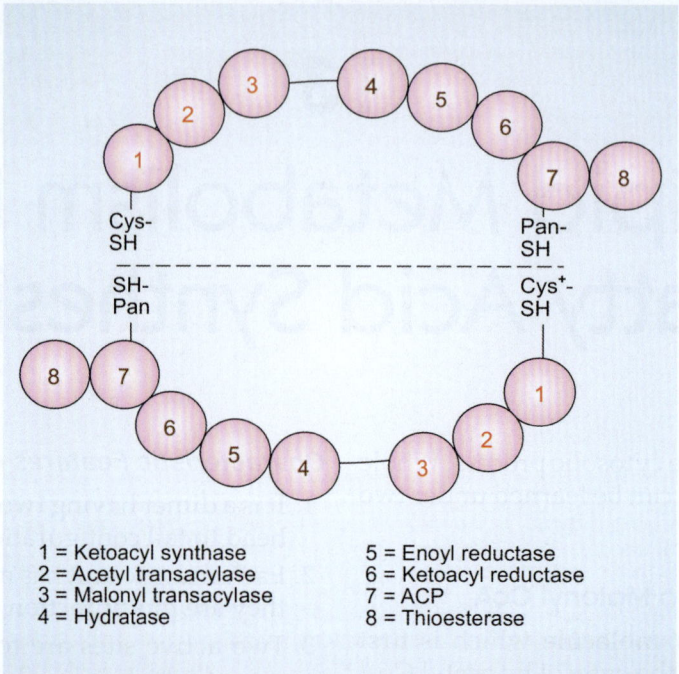

1 = Ketoacyl synthase   5 = Enoyl reductase
2 = Acetyl transacylase   6 = Ketoacyl reductase
3 = Malonyl transacylase   7 = ACP
4 = Hydratase   8 = Thioesterase

Fig. 13.3: Fatty acid synthase complex

FATTY ACID SYNTHASE COMPLEX (FAS COMPLEX)

FAS complex is of two types—FAS I and FAS II. Both of these complexes are different in following ways (Table 13.1):

TABLE 13.1	Comparison of FAS I and FAS II
FAS I	FAS II
Invertebrates and fungi	Plants, vertebrate mitochondria, bacteria
Single multi-functional polypep-tide chain, functional in dimer form.	Here separate enzymes are catalysing each step and intermediates are freely diffusible and may be diverted to other pathways
No intermediate is released only final product 'palmic acid' is released.	FAS II may produce variety of products, including saturated fatty acid of various length, unsaturated fatty acid, branched, hydroxy fatty acid.

Cyclical Reactions of Fatty Acid Synthesis

Synthesis of palmitic acid (16C) in vertebrates requires seven cyclical reactions. Each cyclical reaction consists of following four reactions:

1. Condensation
2. Reduction of carbonyl group
3. Dehydration
4. Reduction of double bond.

But even before the condensation step, the two sulphydryl groups at the active site of FAS should be charged with acetyl CoA and malonyl CoA with the help of enzyme 'MAT' (malonyl/acetyl CoA-ACPtransferase)

Acetyl group of acetyl CoA and malonyl group of malonyl CoA are first transferred to ACP by MAT (malonyl/acetyl CoA-ACPtransferase). This is followed by transfer of acetyl group to Cys-SH and malonyl group remains at –SH group of ACP.

After the placement of acetyl and malonyl residues at respective sites, following cyclical reactions occur:

1. **Condensation:** Acetyl group is condensed with malonyl CoA at –SH of ACP, in this reaction there is loss of CO_2. This results in formation of four carbon acetoacetyl-ACP (Fig. 13.4).

2. **Reduction of carboxyl group:** β-ketoacyl ACP reductase reduces the carbonyl group at C-3 (β carbon) of acetoacetyl-ACP converting it to β-hydroxybutyryl ACP. NADPH is used as a donor of electron in above reaction.

3. **Dehydration:** Water is lost from C2 and C3 with the help of enzyme, β-hydroxyl-ACP dehydratase, resulting in formation of double bond between C2 and C3. This is called as trans-2-butenoyl ACP.

4. **Reduction of double bond:** Double bond of trans-2-butenoyl ACP is saturated to form butyryl-ACP by the action of enoyl-ACP reductase. For this reaction also NADPH acts as a donor of electron.

Above four reactions complete one cycle of fatty acid synthesis.

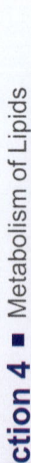

13

Before the start of next cycle, the butaryl group produced at phosphopantethiene SH of ACP is transferred to Cys-SH group of β-ketoacyl ACP synthase.

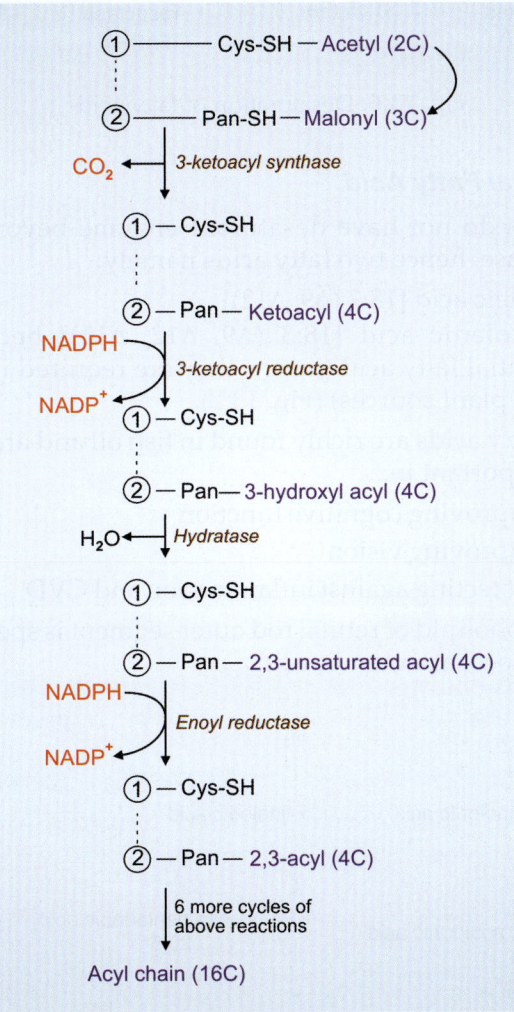

Fig. 13.4: Cyclical reactions of fatty acids chain synthesis

Empty Pan-SH site now accommodates new malonyl CoA and same sets of reactions now give six carbon acyl chain covalently bound to phosphopantethein-SH group.

Total 7 number of such cycles result in formation of 16C saturated palmitoyl chain which is bound to phosphopantetheine-SH covalently (Fig. 13.5). Thioesterase domain of multifunctional protein then releases this free palmitate in a hydrolytic reaction.

Overall reaction can be considered in two parts:

Part 1: 7 acetyl CoA + 7 CO_2 + 7ATP → 7 malonyl CoA + 7ADP + 7 Pi

Part 2: Acetyl CoA + 7 malonyl CoA + 14 NADPH + 14H^+ → 7CO_2 + Palmitate + 8 CoA + 14NADP+ + 6 H_2O

Overall reaction of formation of palmitate from 8 acetyl CoA:

8 acetyl CoA + 7 CO_2 + 14 NADPH + 14 H + 7ATP → Palmitate + 6H_2O + 14 NADP+ + 7ADP + Pi + 8 CoA

For each acetyl CoA transfer from matrix to cytosol, 2ATP are spent.

Further carboxylation of acetyl CoA demands one ATP, hence total of 3 ATP are spent for addition of 2C in the elongating fatty acid chain.

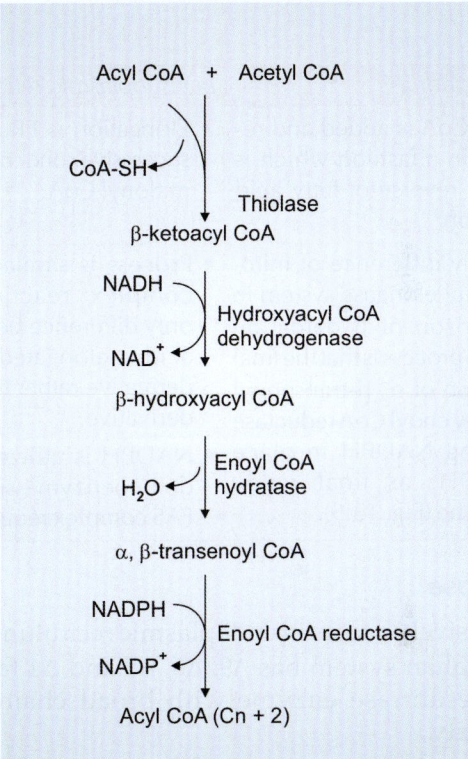

Fig. 13.5: Cyclical reaction of fatty acid synthesis

Regulation

1. *Allosteric and feedback regulation of acetyl CoA carboxylase*
   - Acetyl CoA carboxylase is the rate-limiting enzyme, which is activated by citrate and is inhibited in a feedback manner by palmitoyl CoA.
   - Citrate which acts as positive allosteric factor comes to cytosol in case of excess ATP and acetyl CoA in mitochondrial matrix.
   - Cytosolic citrate not only acts as precursor of acetyl CoA, but it also allosterically regulates the acetyl CoA carboxylase activity, increasing its V_{max}.

2. *Hormonal regulation of acetyl CoA carboxylase:*
   - Acetyl CoA carboxylase is active in dephosphorylated form and is inactive in phosphorylated form.

Section 4 ■ Metabolism of Lipids

13

• Insulin dephosphorylate this enzyme and activates it. Glucagon, epinephrine phosphorylate this enzyme and inactivate it.

FATTY ACID ELONGASE AND DESATURASE

Elongase

Elongase enzyme elongates fatty acid chain and is found in mitochondria as well as in endoplasmic reticulum lumen.

In mitochondria	In endoplasmic reticulum
• Acetyl CoA is added and re-duced in a fashion which is exactly reverse of fatty acid oxidation.	• Elongation is ER involves successive condensation of malonyl CoA.
• The only difference of mito-chondrial elongase system in comparison of β oxidation reversal process is that the final reduction of α, β-transenoyl CoA is by enoyl CoA reductase requiring NADPH in place of FADH$_2$ as final redox coenzyme (Fig. 13.5).	• Process is similar to FAS complex reaction, the only difference being fatty acid is elongated as CoA derivative rather than ACP derivative. • NADPH is utilized as re-dox coenzyme similar to FAS complex requirement.

Desaturase

• It exclusively occurs in endoplasmic recitulum lumen.
• Mammalian system has Δ9, Δ6, Δ5 and Δ4 fatty acyl CoA desaturase enzyme with broad chain length specificity.
• Desaturase enzymes are membrane bound and non heme iron containing enzymes.
• In addition to desaturase enzyme, two other proteins — (a) cytochrome b5 and (b) NADPH cytochrome b5 reductase are required for the process of desaturation in mammalian system (Fig. 13.6).

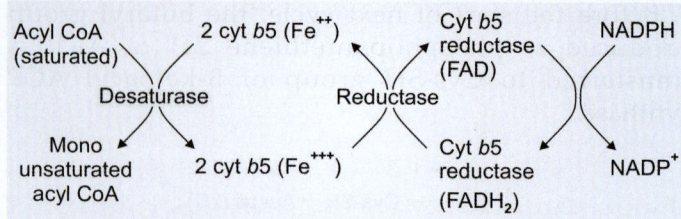

Fig. 13.6: Desaturation of fatty acid

Essential Fatty Acid

Animals do not have desaturase enzyme beyond Δ9 desaturase, hence two fatty acids namely:

a. Linoleic acid [18:2 (Δ9, Δ12)]
b. α-linolenic acid [18:3 (Δ9, Δ12, Δ15)] becomes essential fatty acid (means they are required in diet from plant sources) (Fig. 13.7).

ω3 fatty acids are richly found in fish oil and are seen to be important in:

1. Improving cognitive function
2. Improving vision
3. Protecting against inflammation and CVD

Phospholipid of retinal rod outer segment is specially rich in docosahexaenoic acid.

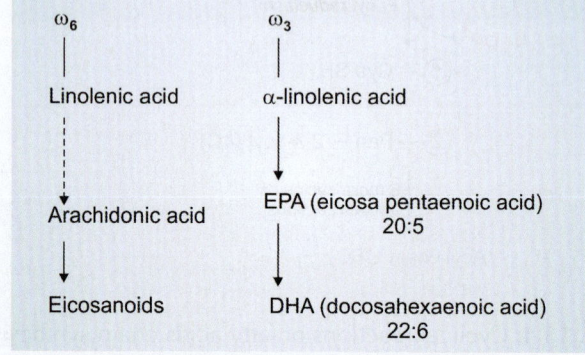

Fig. 13.7: ω$_6$ and ω$_3$ fatty acids

14

Oxidation of Fatty Acid

Fatty acid oxidation can be discussed under following headings:

a. Fatty acid activation (priming of fatty acid in the cytosol)
b. Transport of fatty acid across the mitochondrial membrane.
c. β oxidation occurring in mitochondrial matrix.

A. Fatty Acid Activation

Acyl CoA synthetase is also called thiokinase. It is the enzyme which is responsible for activation process of acyl chain. There are three families of 'acyl CoA synthetase' enzyme which differ according to their fatty acid chain length specificities.

These enzymes are attached with outer mitochondrial membrane and catalyze following reaction:

Fatty acid + CoA + ATP → Fatty acyl CoA + AMP + PPi

The above reaction has an acyl adenylate mixed anhydride intermediate, that is attached by sulphydryl group of CoA to form thioester product.

Hydrolysis of PPi by pyrophosphatase is a highly exergonic reaction.

B. Transport Across the Mitochondrial Membrane

Beta oxidation is the mitochondrial matrix process, hence activated fatty acid (acyl CoA) must be transported across mitochondrial membrane.

Following steps are involved in transportation of acyl CoA across mitochondrial membrane

1. Acyl CoA produced in cytosol by action of thiokinase crosses outer mitochondrial wall and enters the space between the mitochondrial membranes (intermembranous space).
2. Acyl portion of acyl CoA is transferred to carnitine in the intermembranous space. This reaction is catalysed by CPT-I, which is located on outer membrane with the active site directed towards intermembranous space.

3. Resulting acylcarnitine is then transported across inner mitochondrial membrane by a transport system, known as carnitine acyl carnitine translocase (CAT).

4. In the mitochondrial matrix, CoA is transferred to acyl carnitine resulting in formation of acyl CoA and carnitine.

5. Carnitine is exchanged for acyl carnitine by transporter CAT found on inner mitochondrial membrane (Fig. 14.1).

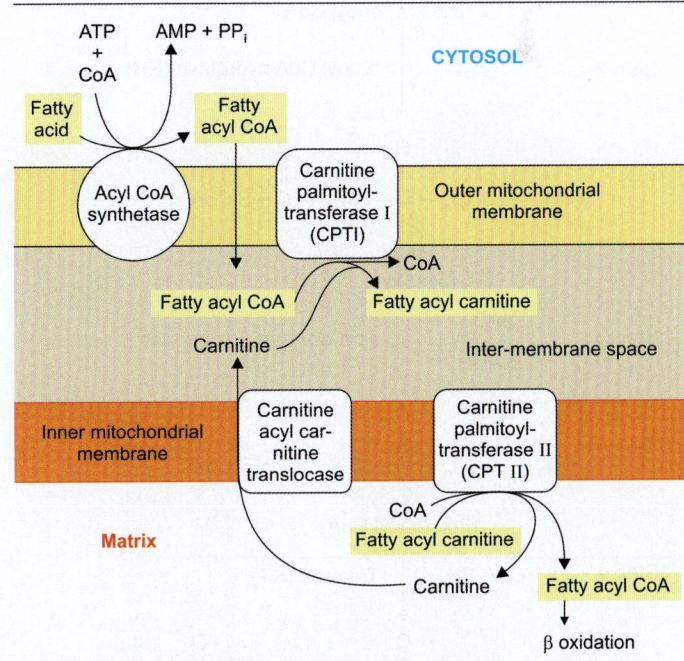

Fig. 14.1: Carnitine shuttle

C. Steps of β Oxidation Process in Mitochondrial Matrix

Beta oxidation is a cyclical process, where sets of four enzymes catalyze each cycle. It is explained below:

1. **Acyl CoA dehydrogenase:** Action of this enzyme removes hydrogen from α and β carbon giving rise to trans Δ2 enoyl CoA (step 1 of Fig. 14.2).
2. Hydration of double bond by enoyl CoA hydratase enzyme to form 3-L-hydroxyacyl CoA (step 2 of Fig. 14.2).
3. NAD^+-dependent dehydrogenation of 3-L- hydroxy acyl CoA by 3-L-hydroxy acyl CoA dehydrogenase (HAD) to form corresponding β-ketoacyl CoA.
4. Breakdown of C_α and C_β in a thiolysis reaction catalyzed by CoA catalyzed by β-ketoacyl CoA thiolase to form acetyl CoA and a new acyl CoA containing 2 carbon less than original one.

Acyl CoA dehydrogenase in mitochondria is of four types:

1. Specific for short chain fatty acid (SCFA)
2. Specific for medium chain fatty acid (MCFA)
3. Specific for long chain fatty acid (LCFA)
4. Specific for very long chain fatty acid (VLCFA)

Acyl CoA Dehydrogenase Deficiency

1. **Sudden infant death syndrome (SIDS):** 10% of such cases are shown to have deficiency of medium chain acyl CoA dehydrogenase (MCAD).
2. **Jamaican vomiting sickness:** Unripe 'ackee fruit' consumption leads to episode of profuse vomiting followed by convulsion, coma and death. This is due to presence of toxin hypoglycin A (an unusual acid) in such fruits, which gets metabolized to produce (MCPA-CoA). MCPA-CoA gets metabolized by acyl CoA dehydrogenase to produce a toxic substance which spoils the enzyme acyl CoA dehydrogenase. MCPA-CoA is said to be a suicidal inhibitor (mechanism based inhibition).

Total and Net ATP Produced during Fatty Acid Complete β Oxidation

Palmitoyl CoA (16 C) complete β oxidation needs 7 cycles which produce following:

- 7 $FADH_2$
- 7 NADH and
- 8 acetyl CoA

Each cycle of β-oxidation produces 1 $FADH_2$ and 1 NADH, thus 7 cycles of β oxidation for 16 carbon fatty acid chain results in formation of 7 $FADH_2$ and 7 NADH. Each cycle releases 1 acetyl CoA, but last cycle releases 2 acetyl CoA as 4 carbon intermediate is cleaved in last cycle resulting in formation of 2 acetyl CoA simultaneously. This results in total 8 acetyl CoA production after complete β oxidation of 16 carbon acyl chain.

$FADH_2$ and NADH produces 1.5 and 2.5 ATP repectively by oxidative-phosphorylation process at ETC and acetyl CoA in TCA cycle also produces 10 ATP. The calculation for ATP production:

7 $FADH_2$	$= 7 \times 1.5$	$= 10.5$ ATP
7 NADH	$= 7 \times 2.5$	$= 17.5$ ATP
8 acetyl CoA	$= 8 \times 10$	$= 80$ ATP
Total ATP		$= 108$ ATP
Net ATP		$= 106$ ATP

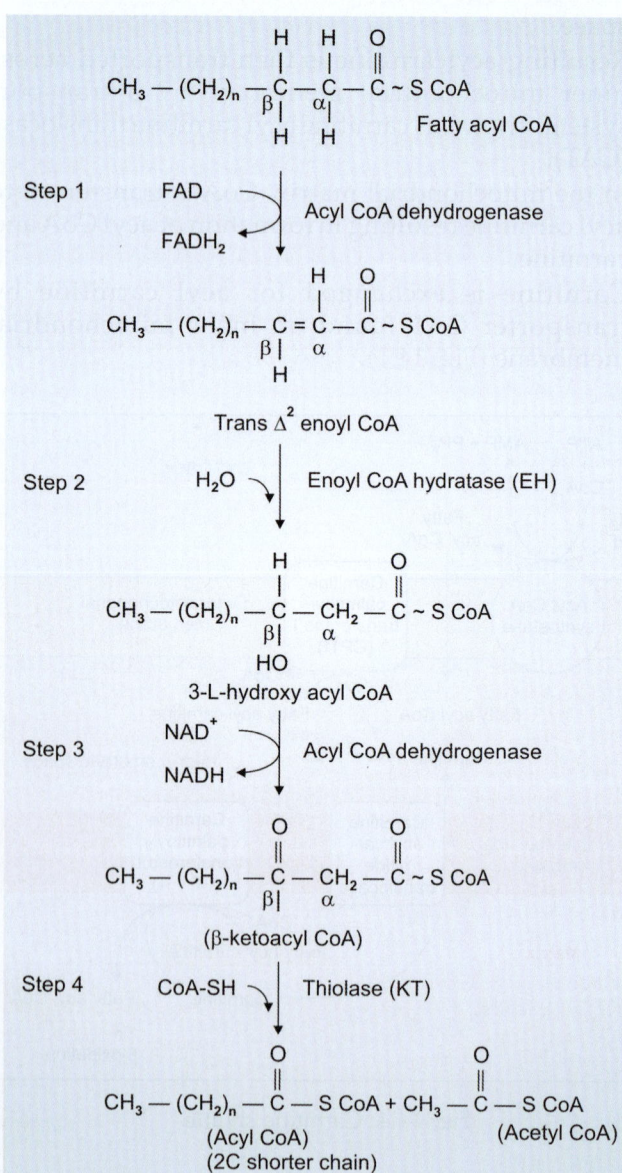

Fig. 14.2: Steps of β oxidation of fatty acid

PEROXISOMAL BETA OXIDATION

Very long chain fatty acid (VLCFA) and branched chain fatty acid undergo β oxidation in peroxisome.

Entry of VLCFA across peroxisome does not require carnitine shuttle, rather a protein called 'ALD protein' is needed for VLCFA transportation across peroxisomal membrane. VLCFA which enters peroxisome is activated by a peroxisomal very long chain acyl CoA synthetase to form their CoA ester, and is oxidized directly.

Adrenoleukodystrophy (ALD)

- Caused by mutation of ALD protein
- X-linked inheritance
- Progressive brain damage and adrenal gland failure.
- Blood has lots of VLCFA, which destroy myelin sheath of axon of many neurons.

Difference of Peroxisomal Beta Oxidation and Mitochondrial Beta Oxidation

1. First enzyme in peroxisomal pathway is acyl CoA oxidase which catalyzes following reaction (Fig. 14.3):

$$\text{Fatty acyl CoA} + O_2 \xrightarrow[\substack{\text{oxidase} \\ (FAD^+)}]{\text{Acyl CoA}} \text{Trans } \Delta^2 \text{ enoyl CoA} + H_2O_2$$

Fig. 14.3: Acyl CoA oxidase

H_2O_2 is converted to H_2O and O_2 by catalase.

2. Peroxisomal enoyl CoA hydratase and 3-L-hydroxy acyl CoA dehydrogenase are enzyme activities that occur on a single common polypeptide and, therefore, are examples of multifunctional enzymes.

3. Peroxisomal thiolase is not active with acyl CoA of length C8 or less, so that fatty acids are incompletely oxidized by peroxisome.

Peroxisome contains carnitine acyltransferases (CAT) which convert shorter acyl chains to their ester forms, which passively diffuse out of the peroxisome to the mitochondria, where they are further oxidized.

---

* ALD: Named after 'adrenal leukodystrophy' disease caused by deficiency of ALD protein.

MINOR PATHWAY OF FATTY ACID OXIDATION

'α' and 'ω' oxidation will be discussed under this heading.

'α' oxidation: This type of oxidation in fatty acid is meant to clear the branch point of branched chain fatty acid like phytanic acid. This is a multistep process catalyzed by multiple enzymes in peroxisome. This type of oxidation does not result in any ATP production.

Phytanic acid: It is a branched chain fatty acid.
Source:
- Dairy products
- Ruminant fats
- Fish
- Chlorophyll (poor source)

Alkyl group present at β carbon of phytanic acid blocks its β oxidation.

Prior to β oxidation, it is important that alkyl group should be cleared from β carbon (Fig. 14.4).

Refsum's Disease (Phytanic Acid Storage Syndrome)

Phytanic acid accumulates throughout the body. It is due to defective phytanyl CoA hydroxylase activity. Affected individual suffers with progressive neurological difficulty.

Following are characteristic findings:
- Tremor
- Unsteady gait
- Poor night vision

ω Oxidation

It is a rare type of fatty acid oxidation. No ATP is generated in this pathway.
- This type of oxidation is meant for medium and long chain fatty acid oxidation.
- ω oxidation results in production of dicarboxylic acid:
- It is an endoplasmic reticulum process.
- Hydroxylation of ω carbon by cytochrome P450 occurs.
- $CH_2OH \rightarrow COOH \rightarrow$ CoA derivative at either end.
- This chain is further oxidized by β oxidation on either end.
- Probably of minor signifance in human.

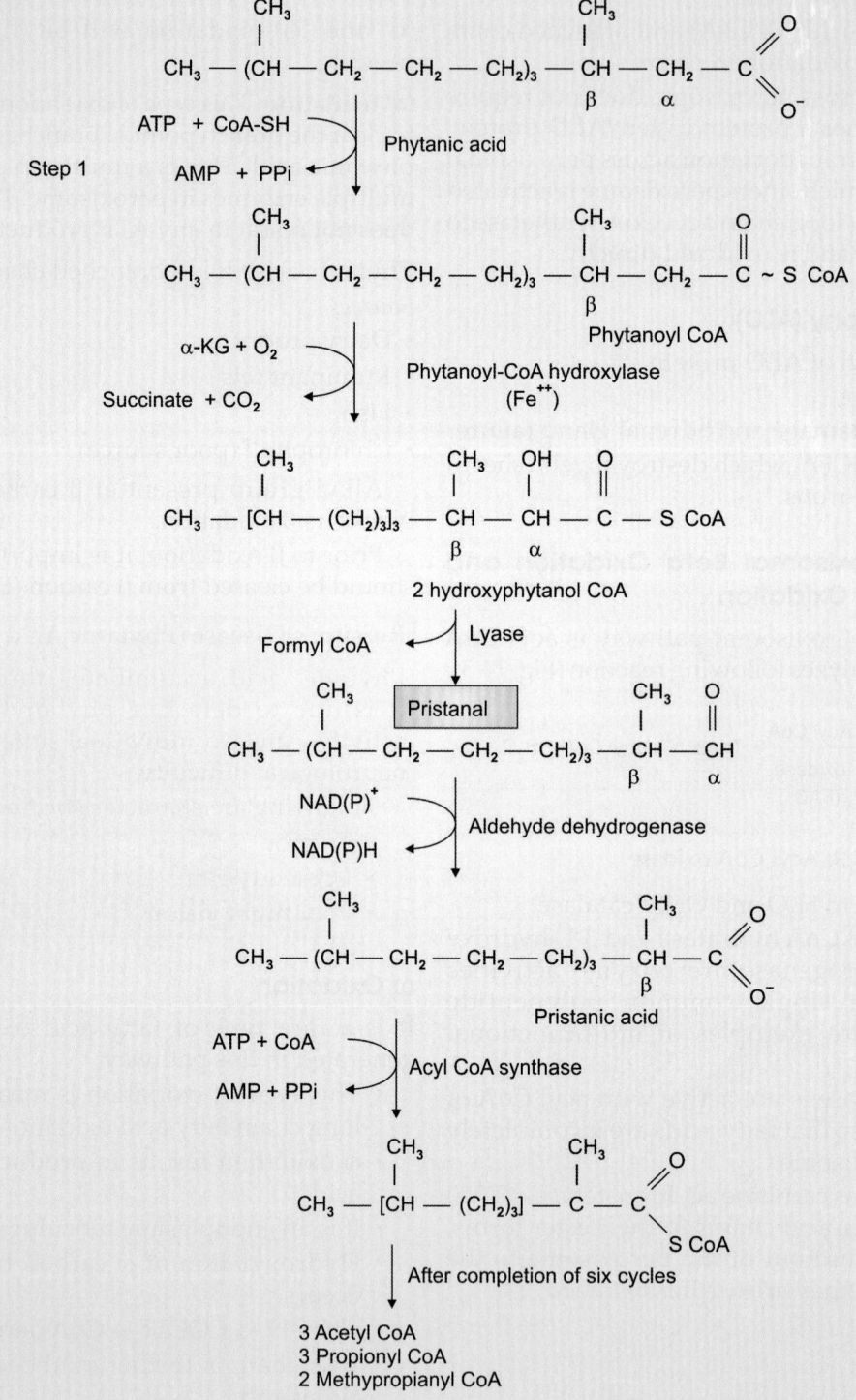

Fig. 14.4: Oxidation of phytanic acid

- *Phytanic acid oxidation occurs in peroxisome.*
- *In Refsum's disease α oxidation is defective, which impairs 'β' oxidation and results in phytanic acid accumulation in various tissues.*

Ketone Body: Synthesis and Utilization

General Points Regarding Ketone Body

- Acetoacetate, β-hydroxybutyrate and acetone are called ketone body. 'Ketone body' is a misnomer, not all the ketone body necessarily should have keto group. For example, acetone and acetoacetate do possess 'keto' group but β-hydroxybutyrate do not have keto group.
- Inability of brain to utilize fatty acid during starvation, makes it mandatory for the biochemical system to produce some alternate fuel which may be easily utilized by the brain cell.
- Ketone body is the fuel which is produced by the liver at the time of excessive fatty acid beta oxidation. Ketone body is permeable to blood brain barrier and hence is easily oxidized in brain cell for ATP production.
- In addition to brain cell, many other cells also use the ketone body for ATP production. These cells possess mitochondria and all enzymes needed to process and utilize ketone bodies.
- Liver and RBC do not use ketone body due to lack of enzyme thiophorase and mitochondria, respectively.

▌KETOGENESIS

Fatty acid β oxidation produces acetyl CoA, majority of which is utilized in TCA cycle for production of ATP. Additionally, significant amount of acetyl CoA is utilized in ketogenesis within the mitochondrial matrix itself.

Following are the steps involved in production of ketone body from acetyl CoA (Fig. 15.1):

1. Condensation of two molecules of acetyl CoA by thiolase enzyme (acetyl CoA—acetyltransferase enzyme) to produce acetoacetyl CoA.
2. Condensation of another molecule of acetyl CoA to acetoacetyl CoA to produce HMG-CoA by HMG-CoA synthase enzyme.
3. HMG-CoA is degraded to acetoacetate and acetyl CoA by HMG-CoA lyase enzyme.
4. Acetoacetate is the common precursor of other two ketone bodies, i.e. β-hydroxybutyrate and acetone.

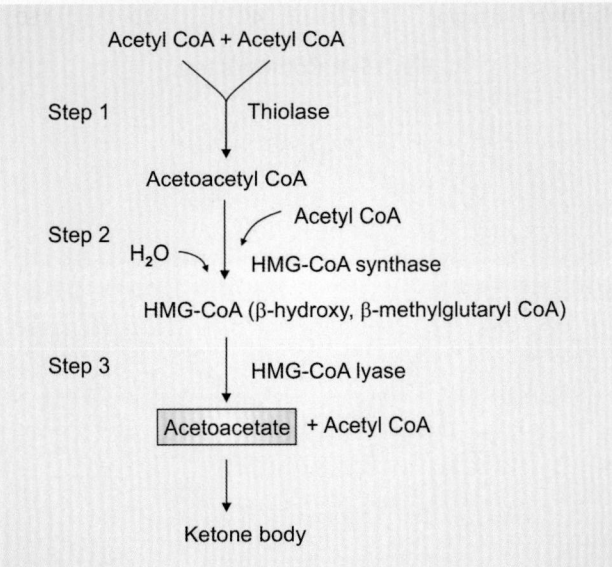

Fig. 15.1: Production of ketone body

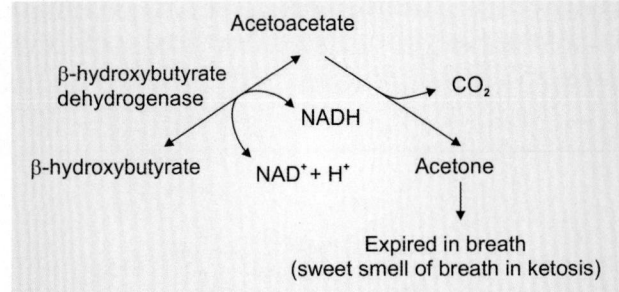

Fig. 15.2: Conversion of acetoacetate to β-hydroxybutyrate and acetone

KETONE BODY UTILIZATION

Ketone bodies (acetoacetate and β-hydroxybutyrate) are released by liver which reach peripheral cells via blood circulation where they are utilized in following enzymatic steps as shown in Fig. 15.3.

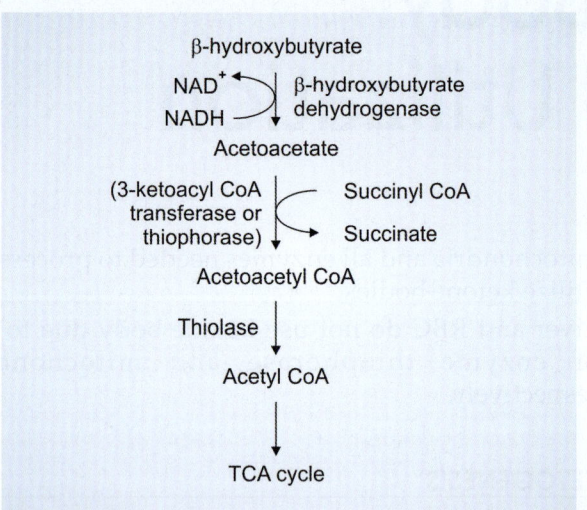

Fig. 15.3: Utilization of acetoacetate and β-hydroxybutyrate at peripheral tissues

Liver and RBC are two such cells which do not utilize ketone body. Liver lacks enzyme thiophorase which is important to convert acetoacetate to acetoacetyl CoA and RBC lacks mitochondria itself which is the site of ketone body utilization.

Clinical Correlation

1. Diabetic ketoacidosis
2. Starvation ketoacidosis

'ROTHERA'S TEST

This test identifies the presence of ketone body (acetone and acetoacetate) in the urine.

Procedure

5 ml of urine is saturated with ammonium sulphate (this precipates the protein in the urine as protein interfers with the test).

Next to this, 2 drops of freshly prepared 2% sodium nitroprusside is added in the urine and mixed thoroughly.

2 ml ammonia is poured from the side of the tube. At the junction of two liquids appearance of purple ring indicates positive test.

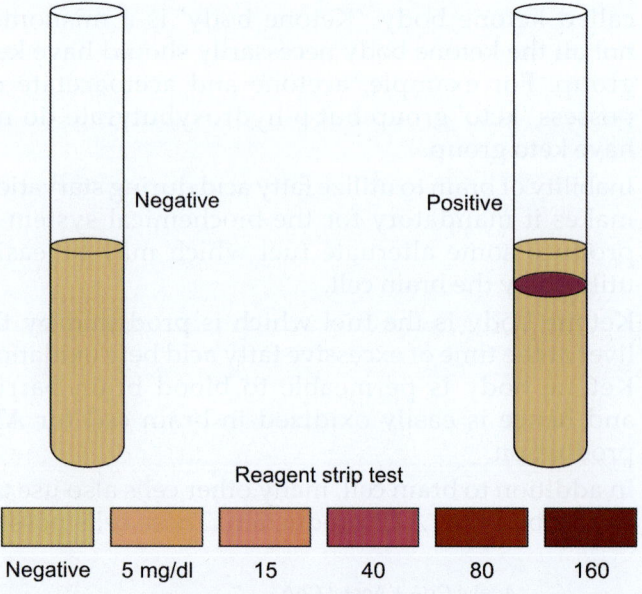

Fig. 15.4: Rothera's test

16

Eicosanoids and Compound Lipids

COMPETENCY BI 4.6

At the end of this chapter learner should be able to describe the therapeutic uses of prostaglandins and inhibitors of eicosanoid synthesis.

Specific Learning Objectives	
BI 4.6.1	Define eicosanoids.
BI 4.6.2	Classify eicosanoids.
BI 4.6.3	Discuss therapeutic role of various eicosanoids.
BI 4.6.4	Enumerate various inhibitors of eicosanoid synthesis.

Eicosanoids are biologically active 20 carbon compounds. They all are derived from arachidonic acid and which is a 20 carbon polyunsaturated fatty acid (PUFA).

Arachidonic acid is released from membrane phospholipid, by action of enzyme phospholipase A2.

Following compounds are categorized under the heading 'eicosanoids' (Fig. 16.1).

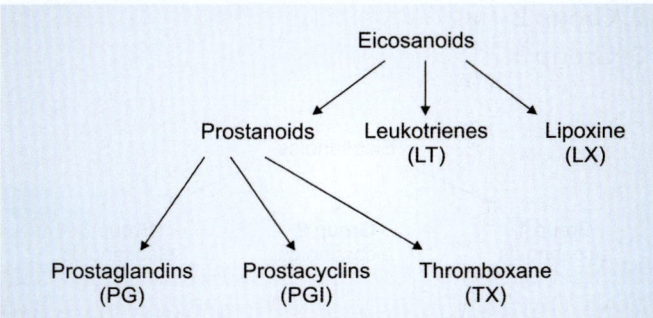

Fig. 16.1: Classification of eicosanoids

1. **Prostanoids:** This include
   • Prostaglandin (PG)
   • Prostacyclin (PGI)
   • Thromboxane
2. **Leukotriens** (LT)
3. **Lipoxin** (LX)

All the above eicosanoids are synthesized from arachidonic acid in following two pathways (Fig. 16.2):
1. Cyclo-oxygenase pathway (COX pathway)
2. Lipo-oxygenase pathway (LOX pathway)
   COX pathway is responsible for synthesis of
   • Prostaglandin (PG)
   • Prostacyclin (PGI)
   • Thromboxane (TX)

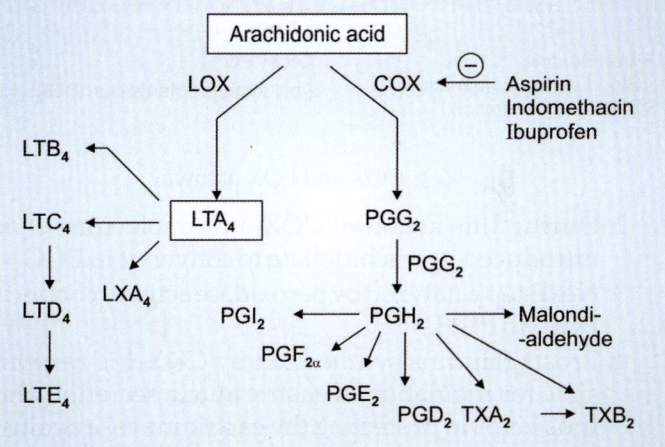

Fig. 16.2: Arachidonic acid and various eicosanoids it produces

LOX pathway is responsible for synthesis of
• Leukotrienes (LT)
• Lipoxins (LX)
COX in mammals have two isoenzymes:
• COX-1
• COX-2
COX-1 produces prostaglandin that regulates gastric mucin.

COX-2 produces prostaglandin that is responsible for pain and fever.

Arachidonate is utilized in either COX pathway or LOX pathway.

A. Following are the steps for conversion of arachidonate to various prostaglandins and thromboxane by COX pathway (Fig. 16.3).
   1. First two steps leading to synthesis of PGH_2 are catalyzed by PGH_2 synthase (a bifunctional enzyme) having two activities:
      a. COX (cyclo-oxygenase)
      b. POD (peroxidase)

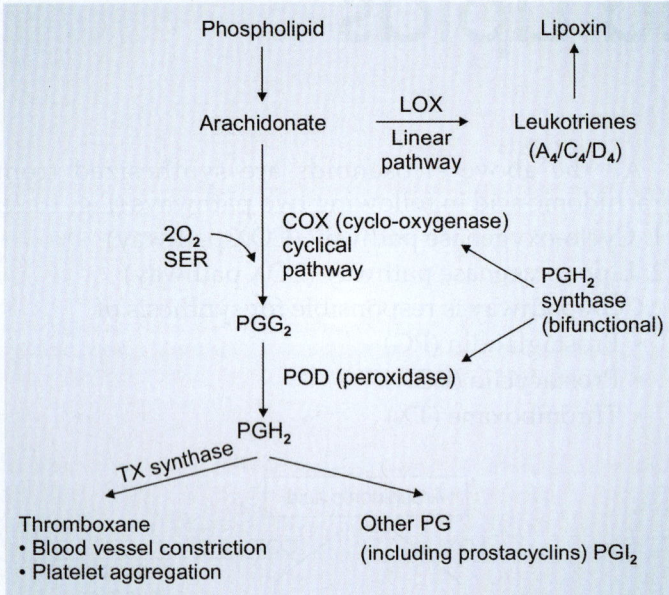

Fig. 16.3: COX and LOX pathway

   2. During this action of COX, first molecular O_2 is introduced to arachidonate to convert it to PGG_2.
   3. Next step catalyzed by peroxidase activity converts PGG_2 to PGH_2.
   4. Prostaglandins synthesized by COX-1 is responsible for regulation of gastric mucin secretion and thus helps in protecting the gastric mucosa against acid erosion.
   5. On the other hand prostaglandins produced by COX-2 mediates inflammatory reaction, pain and fever.
   6. Aspirin is nonselective COX inhibitor inhibitng both COX-1 and COX-2. Thus, aspirin though relieves signs and symptoms of inflammation and acts as antipyretics, by blocking action of COX-2. It also leads to gastric erosion, as it blocks even COX-1 which otherwise helps in protection of gastric mucosa.
      Aspirin acetylates serine residue of active site of COX-1 and COX-2 (irreversible process).

Selective COX-2 inhibitors are:
- Rofecoxib
- Valdecoxib
- Celecoxib

   7. Low dose aspirin reduces thromboxane synthesis and hence is used in heart patients to reduce the chance of vasoconstriction and clot formation.
   8. Nonsteroidal anti-inflammatory drugs (NSAIDS) like ibuprofen also inhibit COX enzyme (both COX-1 and COX-2), but selective COX-2 inhibitors like rofecoxib, valdecoxib do not inhibit COX-1 and thus avoid gastric irritation.
   9. Anti-inflammatory corticosteroids inhibit transcription of COX-1 and COX-2.

B. Now, lets see the steps responsible for synthesis of leukotriences and lipoxins via lipoxygenase pathway (LOX).

The steps involved in LOX pathway may be summarized in Fig. 16.2.

Leukotrienes are family of conjugated trienes. Leukotrienes play important role in immediate hypersensitivity.

LT-C4, D4, E4 cause constriction of bronchial airway muscle and LT-B4, C4, D4 and E4 cause vascular permeability and attraction and activation of WBC.

Lipoxins: Lipoxins are family of conjugated tetraenes.
   Lipoxins are anti-inflammatory.
   There are three groups of eicosanoids (Fig. 16.4):
   1. Group 1
   2. Group 2
   3. Group 3

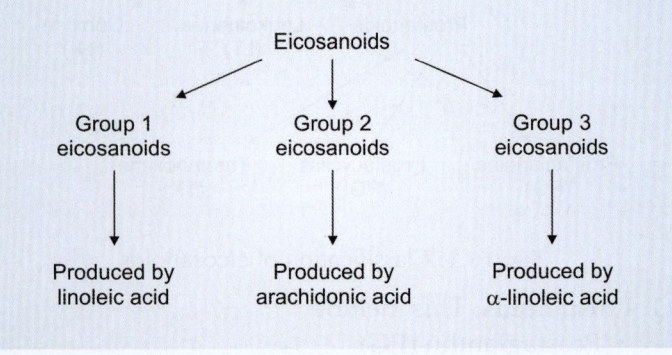

Fig. 16.4: Three groups of eicosanoids and respective fatty acids producing them

Chapter

17

Metabolism of Cholesterol

Cholesterol is a 27 carbon compound which is well known for its association with cardiovascular disease (Fig. 17.1). This compound is important for membrane synthesis, Bile acid and steroid hormone synthesis.

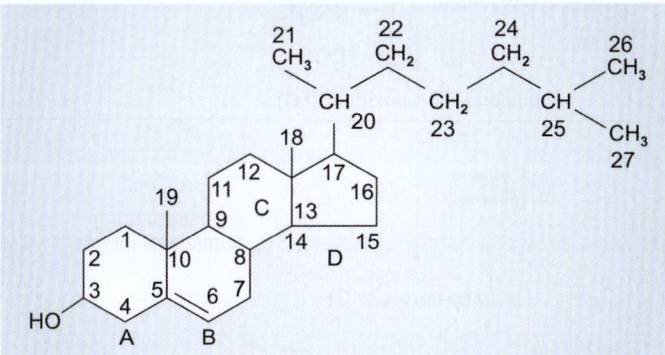

Fig. 17.1: Structure of cholesterol: 27 carbon compound

▌ BIOSYNTHESIS OF CHOLESTEROL (FIG. 17.2)

- Cholesterol is synthesized in all the cells of the body. Major organs being liver, adrenal cortex, testis, ovary and gastrointestinal tract.
- Synthesis of cholesterol is partly cytosolic and partly microsomal process.
- Whole process of cholesterol biogenesis is divided in four stages:
    a. Acetyl CoA producing mevalonate (6 carbon)
    b. Conversion of mevalonate to isoprenoid units (Δ3- isopenteyl pyrophosphate and dimethyl allyl pyrophosphate)
    c. Condensation of 6 isoprenoids to form squalene
    d. Conversion of squalene to cholesterol
  a. **Acetyl CoA producing mevalonate:** In this stage following steps are seen:
    1. Two molecules of acetyl CoA condense to form acetoacetyl CoA in presence of cytosolic thiolase enzyme.
    2. Another molecule of acetyl CoA condenses with acetoacetyl CoA to synthesize HMG-CoA in presence of cytosolic enzyme HMG-CoA synthase.
    3. HMG-CoA reductase is the rate-limiting enzyme of cholesterol biogenesis. HMG-CoA reductase is an integral membrane protein of smooth endoplasmic reticulum. This enzyme converts HMG-CoA to mevalonate.
  b. **Conversion of mevalonate to isoprenoid units:** This stage has following steps:
    1. Phosphorylation of mevalonate with the help of 3 ATP molecules.
  c. **Condensation of six isoprenoids to form squalene:** In this stage total six isoprenoid units condense to produce 30 C compound 'squalene'.
  d. **Conversion of squalene to cholesterol:** It again involves multiple steps which are outlined below.

▌ REGULATION OF CHOLESTEROL BIOGENESIS

Two important factors which regulate cholesterol synthesis are:
1. Level of cholesterol in the cell
2. Hormones: Insulin and glucagon
1. **Level of cholesterol in the cell:** Cellular free cholesterol regulates HMG-CoA reductase gene via sterol regulatory element-binding proteins (SREBPs). Amino terminal domain of SREBP is separated from rest of SREBP by proteolytic cleavage, this amino terminal enters the nucleus, where it plays an important role in activating the gene.

   Amino terminal domain of SREBP has a short half-life and is degraded in the proteasome.

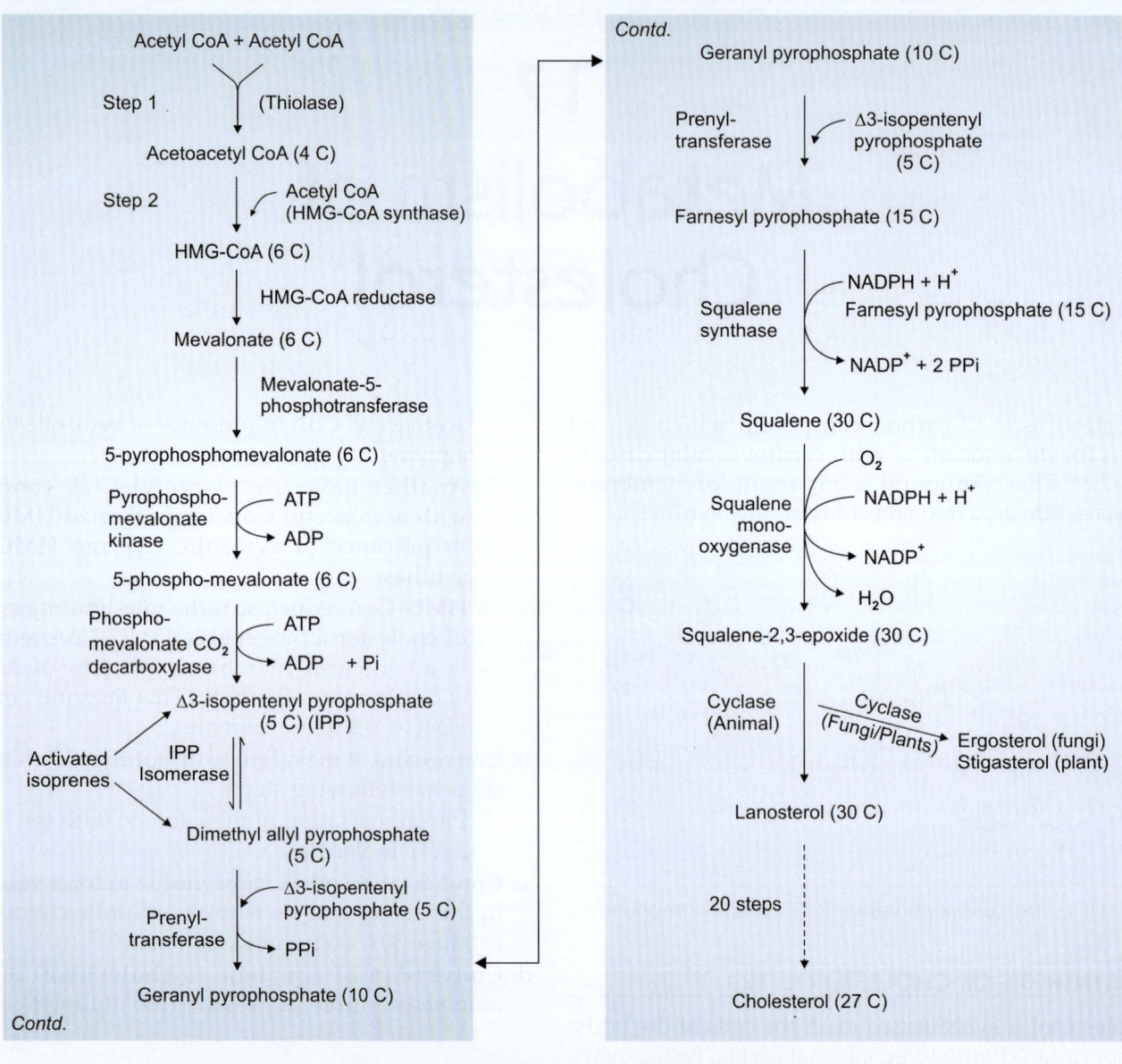

Fig. 17.2: Steps of biosynthesis of cholesterol

When the level of cholesterol is high, SREBP clevage activating protein (SCAP) binds SREBP and retains it in ER lumen; does not allow aminoterminal to be released from SREBP.

When the level of cholesterol declines, SCAP-SREBP complex is released from ER via vesicles, they migrate to Golgi complex. In ER lumen SREBP is cleaved twice and second clevage product (aminoterminal SREBP) enters the cytosol from where it reaches the nucleus to activate HMG-CoA reductase gene transcription.

2. **Hormonal regulation of cholesterol synthesis:** HMG-CoA reductase is active in dephosphorylated form and is inactive in phosphorylated form. Insulin dephosphorylates this enzyme and makes it active, while glucagon phosphorylates it to make it inactive.

In addition to above important factors which regulates cholesterol synthesis in general, level of intracellular cholesterol is maintained by following mechanism:

a. Intracellular cholesterol activate acyl CoA-cholesterol-acetyltransferase (ACAT) enzyme in the cell which converts cholesterol to cholesterol ester. Cholester ester is the storage form of cholesterol.

b. Increased intracellular cholesterol represses the gene for LDL receptor synthesis which further reduces uptake of cholesterol by the cell.

When the total cholesterol (sum total of dietary as well as synthesized) exceeds the cholesterol required for synthesis of membrane, bile salt and steroids, excess cholesterol gets accumulated in blood vessels and lead to atherosclerosis.

Steroid Hormone Synthesis from Cholesterol

Free cholesterol is the precursor of various steroid hormones (*see* Fig. 17.3).

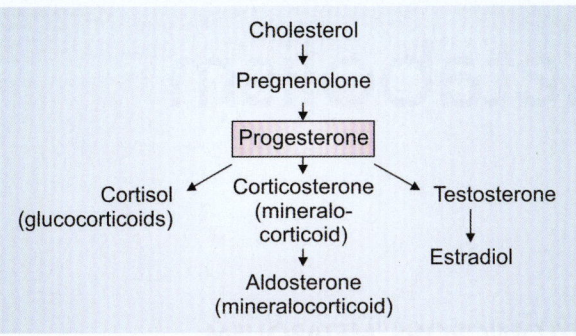

Fig. 17.3: Fate of cholesterol

Alternate Fate of Cholesterol Intermediates

Δ3-isopentenyl pyrophosphate is capable of forming huge array of biomolecules with diverse role (as exemplified in Fig. 17.4):

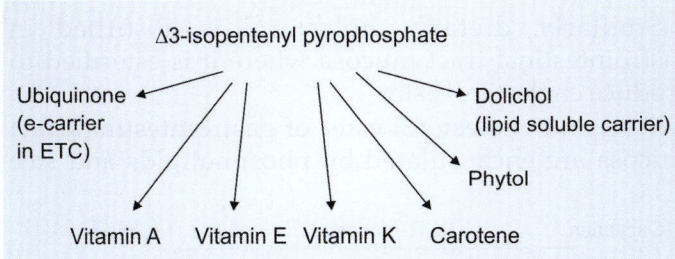

Fig. 17.4: Various fate of Δ3-isopentenyl pyrophosphate

Conversion of Cholesterol to Bile Acid

Excess cholesterol is converted to bile acid and gets excreted. Bile acids are broadly of two types (Fig. 17.5):

1. Primary bile acids
2. Secondary bile acids

Primary bile acids are synthesized in liver and secondary bile acids are produced in gastrointestinal lumen after chemical action of bacteria on primary bile acids.

Primary bile acids are:

1. Cholic acid
2. Chenodeoxy cholic acid

Secondary bile acids are:

1. Deoxycholic acid
2. Lithocholic acid

Steps of Synthesis of Bile Acid

1. 7α-hydroxylation of cholesterol is the first committed step in the biosynthesis of bile acid and it also acts as rate-limiting step for synthesis of bile acid.
   7α-hydroxylase is the microsomal enzyme which requires following coenzymes:
   - NADPH
   - Cytochrome P450
   - Vitamin C
   Vitamin C deficiency thus interfers with bile acid synthesis.
2. Primary bile acids enter the bile as glycine or taurine conjugates. Since bile contains significant amount of sodium and potassium and pH is alkaline here, bile acids and their conjugates are in bile salt form.
3. On consumption of fatty meal, bile salts enters the duodenum along with other components of bile, where bile salts help in digestion and absorption of dietary lipids.
4. On reaching terminal ileum, some of the primary bile acids are acted upon by bacterial enzyme which converts primary bile acids to secondary bile acids.
5. Following two chemical changes modify primary bile acid to secondary bile acid:
   - Deconjugation
   - 7α-dehydroxylation
6. Above two modifications convert cholic acid to deoxycholic acid and chenodeoxycholic acid to lithocholic acid (Fig. 17.5).

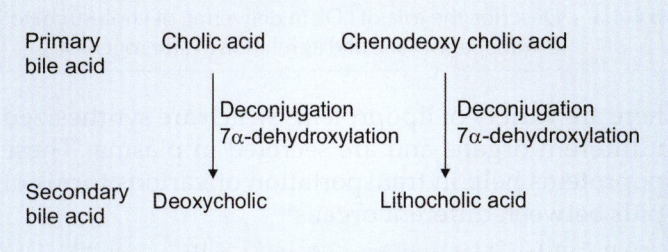

Fig. 17.5: Primary and secondary bile acids

7. 98–99% of bile acids present in the intestine is absorbed in the portal circulation and reaches the liver, and again is resecreted in the gastrointestinal tract lumen (enterohepatic circulation).
8. A small fraction of bile salt (of about 400 mg per day) escapes enterohepatic circulation and is eliminated via feces.

Section 4 ■ Metabolism of Lipids

17

18
Lipoprotein Metabolism

COMPETENCY BI 4.4

At the end of this chapter learner should be able to describe the structure and functions of lipoproteins, their functions, interrelations and relations with atherosclerosis.

COMPETENCY BI 4.3

At the end of this chapter learner should be able to explain the regulation of lipoprotein metabolism and associated disorders.

Specific Learning Objectives	
BI 4.3.1	Define lipoprotein and its various types.
BI 4.3.2	Describe metabolism of different lipoproteins.
BI 4.3.3	Discuss various dyslipoproteinemias.
BI 4.4.1	Describe the structure of a typical lipoprotein.
BI 4.4.2	Enlist diverse roles of various lipoproteins in lipid metabolism.
BI 4.4.3	Describe the role of LDL in delivering of cholesterol to extrahepatic tissue and its relation to atherogenesis.

There are variety of lipoproteins which are synthesized in different organs and are secreted in plasma. These lipoproteins help in transportation of various forms of lipids between different organs.

Following are the names of various lipoproteins:

1. Chylomicron (CM)
2. Very low density lipoprotein (VLDL)
3. Low-density lipoprotein (LDL)
4. High-density lipoprotein (HDL)
5. Remnant particles (CM remnant and VLDL remnants)

VLDL remnant is also called intermediate density lipoprotein (IDL).

CHYLOMICRONS' METABOLISM

Chylomicrons (CM) are organised in intestinal mucosa. Formation of chylomicron is an attempt to absorb dietary lipids to the blood circulation. Fatty acids which are produced in gastrointestinal tract lumen by action of lipase is absorbed in gastrointestinal tract mucosa, where it is re-esterified to produce triacylglycerol (TAG) (Fig. 18.1).

Similarly, dietary cholesterol is absorbed in gastrointestinal tract mucosa where it is esterified to produce cholesterol ester.

TAG and cholesterol ester of gastrointestinal tract mucosa are encapsulated by phospholipids and free

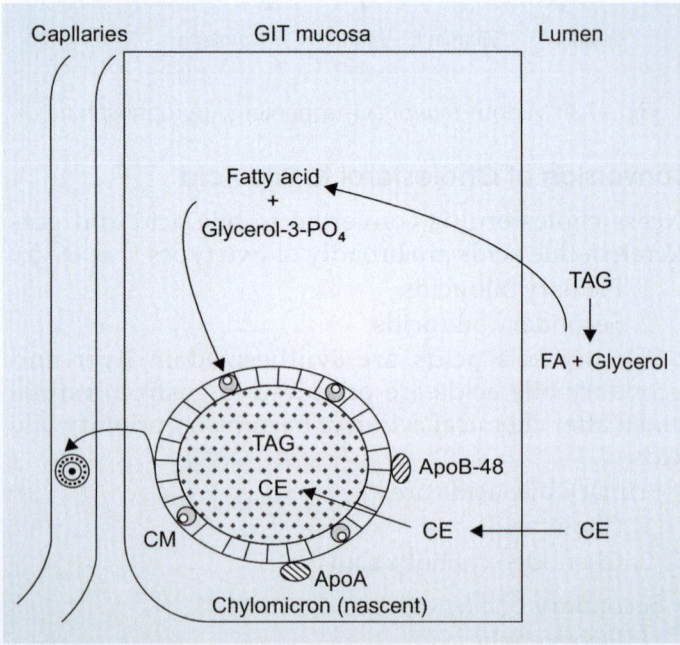

Fig. 18.1: Nascent chylomicron

cholesterol (amphipathic lipids) as to produce a shell around this nonpolar core of TAG and CE.

Later apoB-48 and apoA are incorporated in the shell of chylomicron. This chylomicron which is thus produced in the gastrointestinal tract mucosa is known as nascent chylomicron which gets absorbed in lacteals around gastrointestinal tract wall. *Finally, these lacteals join to form thoracic duct which opens in systemic circulation.*

Lipaemia of plasma, seen soon after consumption of fatty meal is due to presence of these chylomicron particles.

These chylomicrons are subjected to maturation by HDL, which donates apoC and apoE in systemic circulation (Fig. 18.2).

Once matured, chylomicron reaches capillary lumen of various tissues. Wall of capillary endothelium of certain tissues like adipose tissue and skeletal muscle and heart muscle are specially rich in lipoprotein lipase.

ApoC-II present in CM acts as an activator of lipoprotein lipase enzyme. Once activated this enzyme (LPL) acts on TAG of chylomicron core, which is hydrolyzed to fatty acid and glycerol (Fig. 18.3).

Fatty acids are taken up by adipose cell, where they are primarily meant to be stored and also by skeletal and heart muscles where they are primarily oxidized to generate energy.

Glycerol is shed to plasma, and is transported it to liver where it is utilized (either in glycolytic or gluconeogenic pathway).

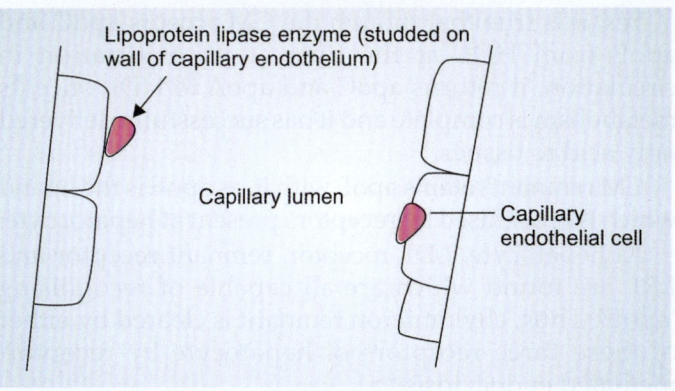

Fig. 18.3: Lipoprotein lipase enzyme

Successive removal of lots of triacyl glycerol from the core of chylomicron, reduces the size of chylomicron, which is now known as chylomicron remnant.

This chylomicron remnant which is still having all the dietary cholesterol in its core in form of cholesterol ester moves to liver.

During this journey of chylomicron remnant to its final destination (liver), apoA and apoC are returned to HDL.

This results in presence of only apoB-48 and apoE on the CM shell, by the times it represents at hepatocyte (Fig. 18.4).

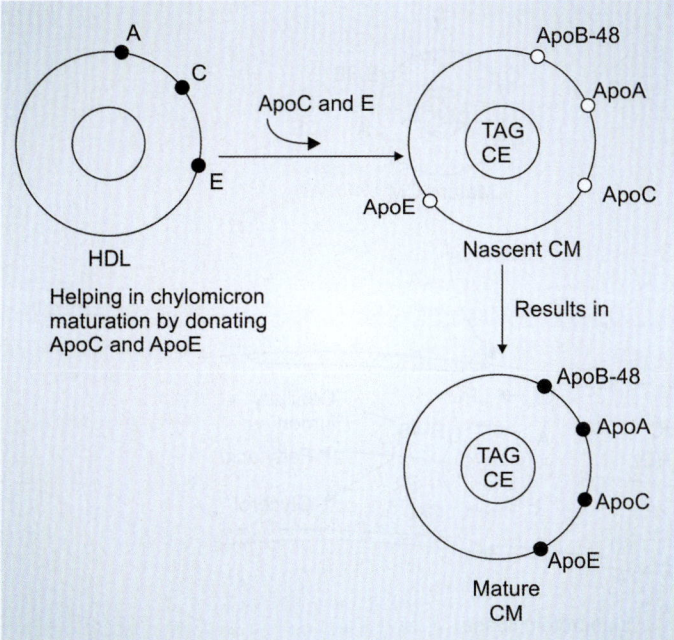

Fig. 18.2: Maturation of nascent chylomicron by HDL

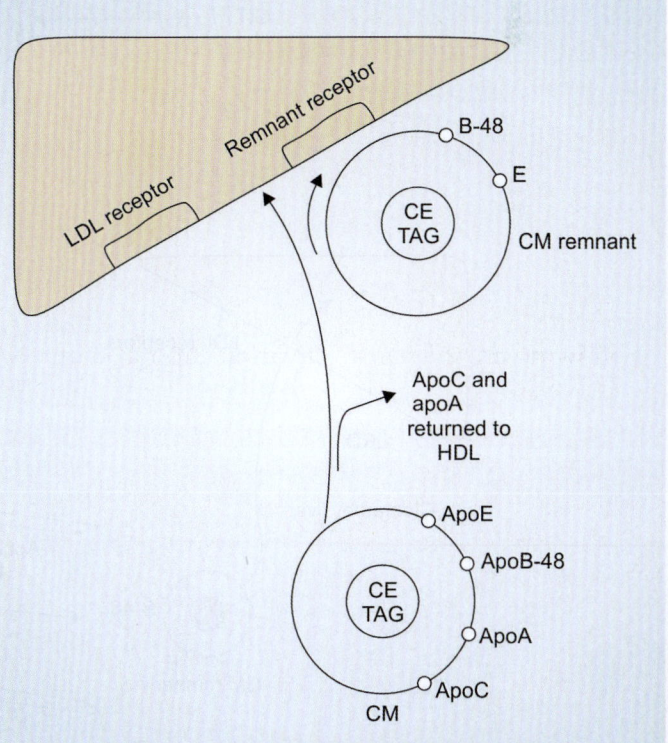

Fig. 18.4: Clearance of CM remnant by liver

Section 4 ■ Metabolism of Lipids

18

Yes, it is true that though the CM accepts apoC and apoE from HDL at the time of its maturation in circulation, it returns apoC and apoA to HDL once its metabolism is complete and it has successfully delivered fatty acid to tissues.

CM remnant retains apoE with it, as apoE is the ligand which is recognised by receptors present at hepatocoyte.

At hepatocyte, LDL receptor, remnant receptor and LRP are found which are all capable of recognising 'apoE'. Thus, chylomicron remnant is cleared by either of these three receptors of hepatocyte by receptor-mediated endocytosis.

Remaining TAG and all the cholesterol ester which the remnant particle has brought to liver are hydrolyzed and metabolized.

Complete CM metabolism is shown in Fig. 18.5.

VLDL Metabolism

Liver synthesizes VLDL particle, the core of which contains endogenous TAG and exogenous as well as endogenous cholesterol ester.

The cholesterol ester which is brought to liver by chylomicron remnant particle is dietary (exogenous) and the cholesterol ester which is synthesized by liver cell itself is endogenous.

Synthesis of VLDL in hepatocyte follows the same principle as we have seen during CM synthesis in gastrointestinal tract mucosa.

An amphipathic shell made up of free cholesterol and phospholipids encapsulates CE and TAG, giving VLDL a spherical shape.

Live encodes apoB-100, apoE and apoC.

Nascent VLDL enters the systemic circulation, where it is matured by accepting apoC and apoE from HDL. Once matured, VLDL enters the capillary lumen, where the enzyme lipoprotein lipase is adherent on endothelial wall.

In similar fashion as we have seen during CM metabolism, apoC-II activates lipoprotein lipase enzyme. Upon activation, lipoprotein lipase acts on TAG of VLDL core which is hydrolyzed to fatty acid and glycerol.

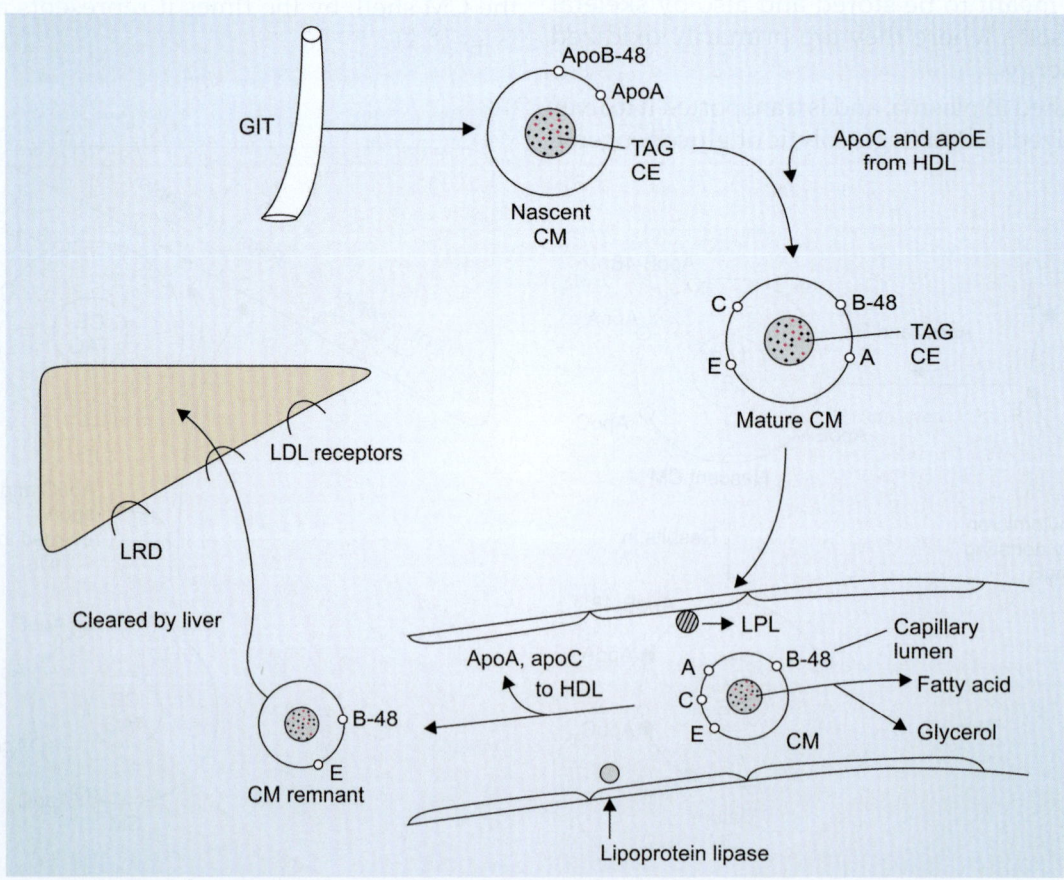

Fig. 18.5: Chylomicron metabolism (summary)

Fatty acids are supplied to cells along with other nutrients by the capillaries. During hydrolysis, apoC is returned to HDL (Figs 18.6–18.8).

Action of Lipoprotein Lipase Enzyme on VLDL

Glycerol is shed to blood and reaches the liver, where it either enters the glycolytic pathway or gluconeogenesis.

Size of VLDL shrinks due to removal of TAG from core section and it is now called VLDL remnant lipoprotein or intermediate density lipoprotein (IDL).

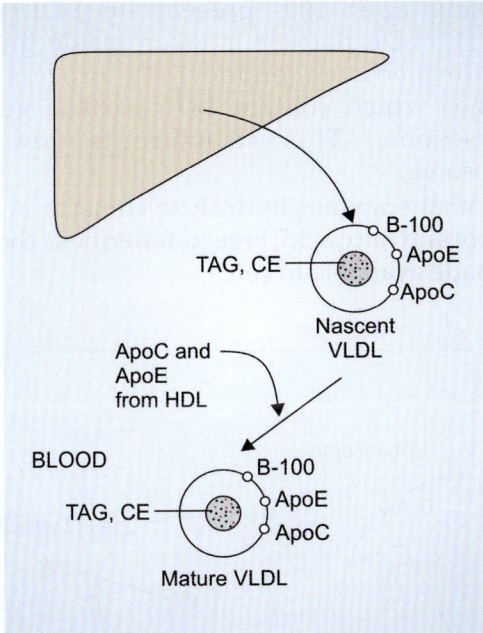

Fig. 18.6: VLDL secretion and its maturation

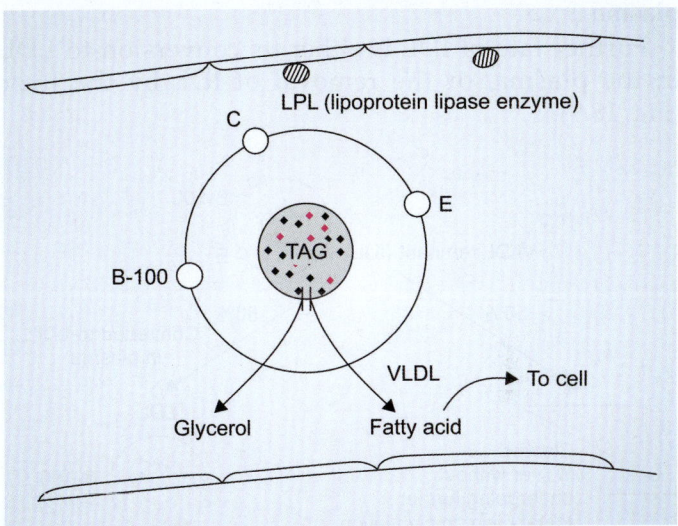

Fig. 18.7: Action of lipoprotein lipase on VLDL

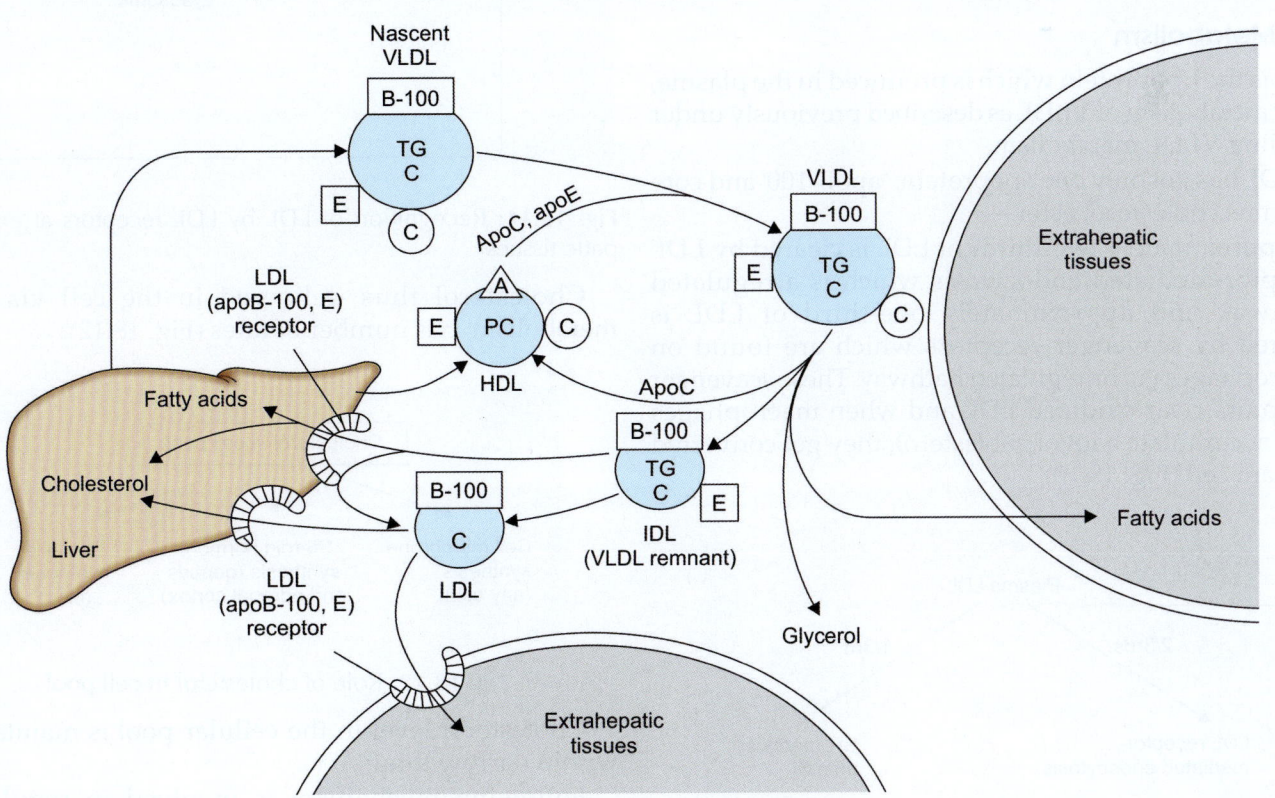

Fig. 18.8: Outline of VLDL metabolism

We find remarkable similarity in VLDL metabolism and CM metabolism till this point. After this, the metabolism of VLDL remnants is not always same as that of CM remnant. This is clearly explained in the next paragraph.

VLDL remnant is also known as intermediate density lipoprotein (IDL). IDL is transiently formed in the plasma.

Further fate of IDL is either its conversion to LDL in the plasma, or the removal of IDL by the liver (Fig. 18.9).

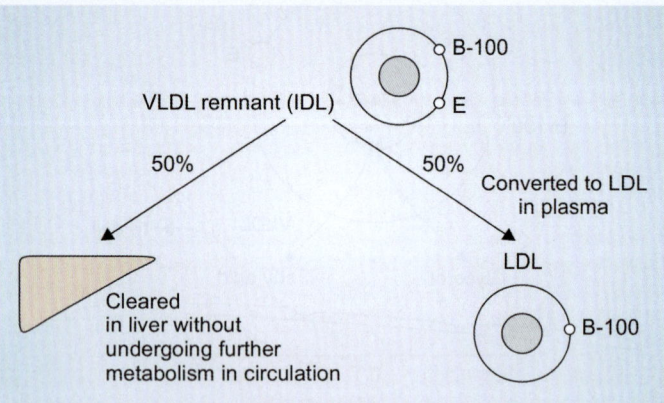

Fig. 18.9: Fate of IDL in the plasma

LDL Metabolism

LDL is the lipoprotein which is produced in the plasma, after metabolism of VLDL as described previously under heading VLDL metabolism.

LDL has got only one apoprotein, 'apoB-100' and core contains cholesterol ester.

Approximately two-thirds of LDL is cleared by LDL receptor-mediated endocytosis which is a regulated pathway and approximately one-third of LDL is cleared by scavenger receptors which are found on macrophages via unregulated pathway. These scavenger receptors clear oxidized LDL and when macrophages thus accumulate a lot of cholesterol, they get converted to foam cell (Fig. 18.10) .

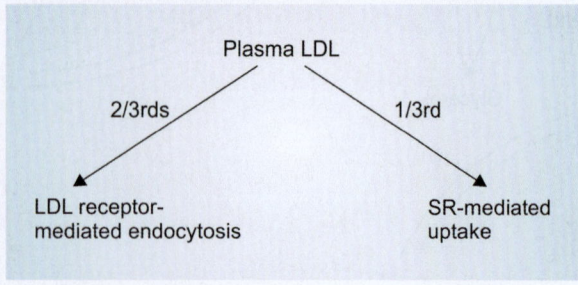

Fig. 18.10: Fate of LDL in circulation

Recognition of LDL by LDL Receptors at Extrahepatic Tissues

LDL receptor of extrahepatic tissues is capable of recognizing apoB-100, present on LDL particle (Fig. 18.11). LDL particle is taken inside the cell in a receptor-mediated endocytosis process. These endosomes which contain LDL particle get fused with lysosome. This structure is now called endolysosome.

Lysosomal enzymes hydrolyze cholesterol ester to cholesterol and fatty acid. Free (unesterified) cholesterol is thus made available to cell.

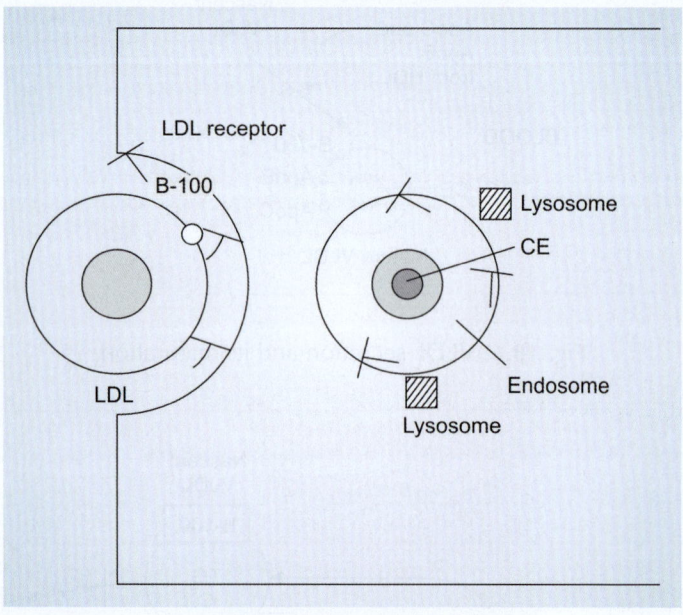

Fig. 18.11: Recognition of LDL by LDL receptors at extrahepatic tissues

Cholesterol thus delivered in the cell via LDL metabolism, has number of fates (Fig. 18.12).

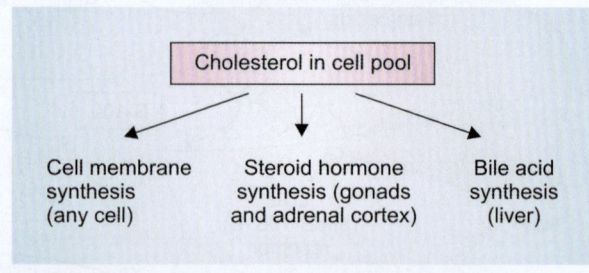

Fig. 18.12: Role of cholesterol in cell pool

Cholesterol level in the cellular pool is maintained within narrow limits.

Following mechanism is involved in regulating the level of cholesterol in cell cholesterol pool (Fig. 18.13).

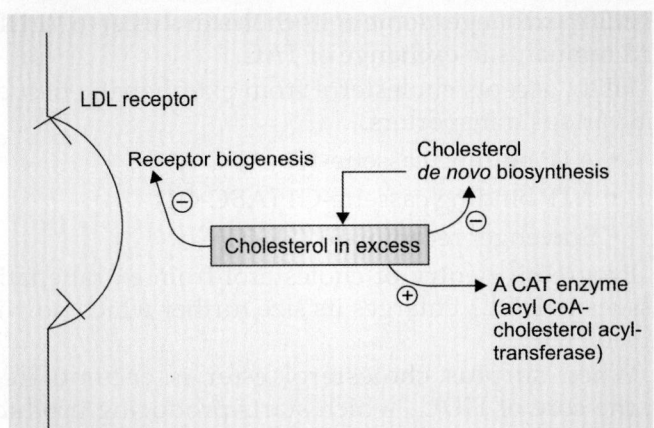

Fig. 18.13: Regulation of cholesterol in cell cholesterol pool

When the level of cholesterol in cholesterol pool increases following mechanism occurs:

1. Down regulation of *de novo* cholesterol synthesis
2. Down regulation of LDL receptor synthesis
3. Activation of ACAT enzyme.

1. **Down regulation of *de novo* cholesterol synthesis:** Cell itself synthesizes cholesterol by *de novo* pathyway. Its enzyme HMG CoA reductase activity may be inhibited by excess cholesterol of cell pool (Fig. 18.13a).

2. **Down regulation of LDL receptor synthesis:** Excess cholesterol of cell pool inhibits transcript of gene of LDL receptor protein (Fig. 18.3b).

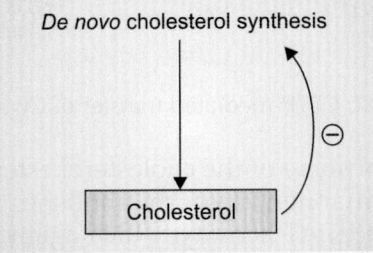

Fig. 18.13a: Down regulation of *de novo* cholesterol synthesis by pool cholesterol

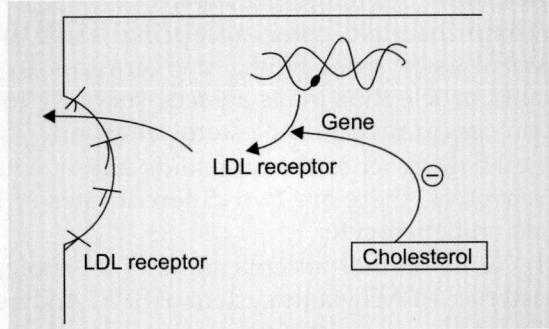

Fig. 18.13b: Down regulation of LDL receptor synthesis by free cholesterol

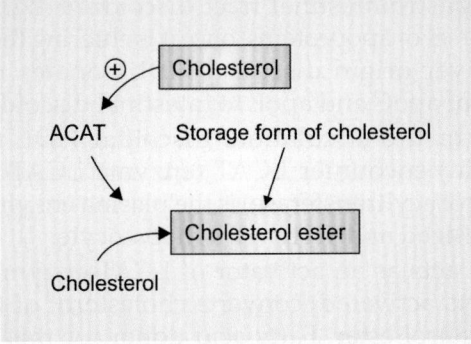

Fig. 18.13c: Conversion of cholesterol to cholesterol ester by ACAT

Less formation of LDL receptor thus reduces further uptake of LDL particle, thereby maintaining the level of cholesterol in cell pool.

3. **Activation of ACAT enzyme:** ACAT (acyl CoA-cholesterol acyltransferase) is intracellular enzyme which converts free (unesterified) cholesterol to cholesterol ester. Cholesterol ester is the storage form of cholesterol in the cell (Fig. 18.13c).

$$\text{Cholesterol} + \text{Acyl CoA} \xrightarrow{\text{ACAT}} \text{Cholesterol ester} + \text{CoA}$$

HDL Metabolism

Liver and intestine synthesize and secrete disk shaped nascent HDL particle, which is known as discoidal HDL.

Discoidal HDL is a flattened structure having shell of phospholipid and free cholesterol. Most abundant type of phospholipid is lecithin (Fig. 18.14).

Core is discoidal HDL, is almost empty except few particles of cholesterol ester which may reside there.

ApoA, apoC, and apoE are apoproteins which are found in the shell.

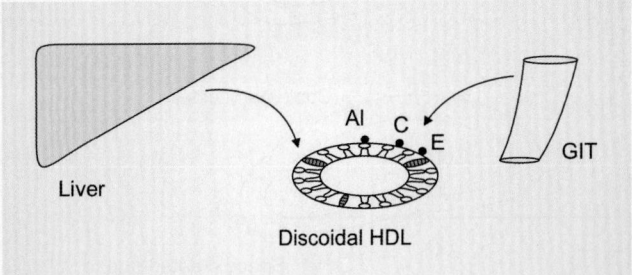

Fig. 18.14: Discoidal HDL secreted from liver and GIT

HDL secreted by liver is considered better than HDL secreted by gastrointestinal tract, because set of apoproteins (A, C, E) is more complete on HDL secreted by liver.

Section 4 ■ Metabolism of Lipids

18

Even gastrointestinal tract discoidal HDL gets the complete set of apoproteins, once it is entering the plasma where liver origin discoidal HDL donates required amount of apoC and apoE to intestinal discoidal HDL.

Once in the circulation, discoidal HDL (of both the origin) encounter LCAT (enzyme LCAT lecithin: cholesterol acyltransferase) is the plasma enzyme which is synthesized and secreted by hepatocyte.

ApoA acts as an activator of LCAT enzyme. LCAT when gets activated, converts cholesterol of the shell to cholesterol ester. Fatty acid donor for this reaction is phospholipid which donates second carbon fatty acid to cholesterol (Fig. 18.15) converting it to cholesterol ester.

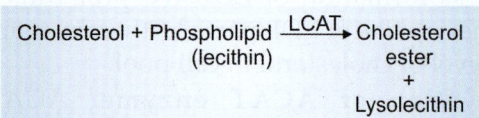

Fig. 18.15: Conversion of cholesterol to cholesterol ester by LCAT enzyme

Cholesterol ester thus produced enters the central hydrophobic core of HDL, leaving a gap/space in the shell of discoidal HDL.

This nascent HDL now accepts the cholesterol from cells and after action of LCAT enzyme, packs them in the interior core in the form of cholesterol ester (Fig. 18.16).

Filling of core with cholesterol ester changes the shape of HDL from nascent discoidal to spherical. This spherical particle is now called HDL_3.

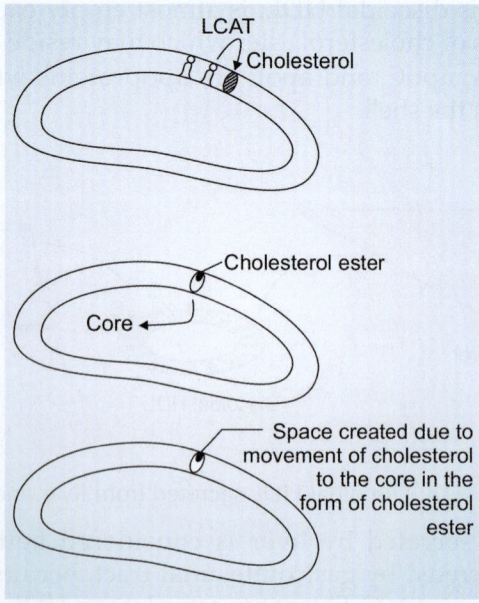

Fig. 18.16: Action of LCAT on HDL shell

HDL_3 exchanges some of its cholesterol ester to VLDL, CM ramnants in exchange of TAG.

HDL_3 accepts cholesterol from extrahepatic tissues via various transporters.

- ATP binding cassette-A1 (ABC-A1)
- ATP binding cassette-G1 (ABC-G1)
- Scavenger receptor-B1 (SR-B1)

Progressive entry of cholesterol from extrahepatic tissues to HDL_3, enlarges its size further which now is called HDL_2.

When surplus cholesterol ester is accumulated in the core of HDL_2, which starts producing product inhibition on LCAT activity, further accommodation of cholesterol in the shell is halted, as lacunae under these circumstances are sealed by last incoming cholesterol.

This type of saturated HDL_2 now moves towards liver and is encountered by CM and VLDL remnant particles on the way. Some of the HDL_2 core cholesterol is exchanged by TAG of the remnant particle. This exchange is mediated by cholesterol ester transfer protein (CETP) (Fig. 18.17).

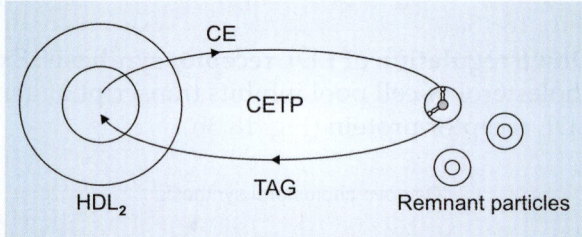

Fig. 18.17: CETP-mediated transfer of CE and TAG

Removal of some of the cholesterol ester from HDL_2 core in this manner, abruptly abolishes the product inhibition on LCAT activity, which again starts acting on this HDL_2 particle and lacunae are recreated.

These lacunae accommodate cholesterol again from extrahepatic tissue. Thus, exchange mediated by CETP increases, HDL_2 scavengering capacity.

Remnant particle after accepting some of the cholesterol ester from HDL_2, delivers this to liver. Remnant particle thus plays an accessory role to HDL in the process of reverse cholesterol transport.

If the HDL_2 reaches the sinusoids and encounters HDL receptors, there are two different fates of HDL_2 destined on hepatocyte:

1. Liver cell either accepts some of its cholesterol ester and TAG via its system of SRB1 and hepatic lipase.

   Rest of the HDL_2 is send to the circulation in the form of HDL_3, which again activates LCAT activity because of its apoA, and HDL$_3$ gets involved in the process of reverse cholesterol transport as discussed previously.

or

2. Second fate of HDL$_2$ is that it is more intensively disintegrated by hepatocyte, which removes all the phospholipid, TAG by action of hepatic lipase, cholesterol and cholesterol ester by Scavenger receptor-B (SRB). Apoproteins of HDL (apoC and apoE) also get cleared by hepatocyte. It is apoA-1 which escape to circulation where it gets incorporated in pre-β HDL.

Pre-β HDL is very much active form of HDL which starts accepting cholesterol from extrahepatic tissues; and in due course gets converted to discoidal HDL.

Discoidal HDL starts the reverse cholesterol transport once again as explained above.

It is an important observation that there is conservation of HDL during its metabolism, where the biochemical system is trying to conserve HDL in the circulation. This type of conservation of lipoprotein is not observed in metabolism of any other lipoprotein.

19

Lipoprotein Disorders

Derangement in plasma level of various lipoproteins is known as dyslipoproteinemia.

Under this heading two groups of disorders are covered:
1. Hyperlipoproteinemia
2. Hypolipoproteinemia

HYPERLIPOPROTEINEMIA

This include various conditions where specific lipoproteins are accumulated either due to lack of enzymes needed for their metabolism or due to defect in their receptors.

Most widely accepted classification for hyperlipidemia is 'Friedrickson's classification' which is described below in Table 19.1.

HYPOLIPOPROTEINEMIA

Under this heading two major groups of conditions are included:

1. **Conditions associated with low levels of apoB containing lipoproteins:**

   a. *Abetalipoproteinemia:* It is a rare autosomal recessive disorder where there is loss of function mutation of gene encoding microsomal TG transfer protein (MTP, gene: MTT).

   'Microsomal TG transfer protein' is responsible for transfer of lipid to nascent chylomicron and VLDL in the intestine and liver respectively.

   Plasma level of chylomicron, VLDL and LDL are undetectable in plasma.

TABLE 19.1	Friedrickson's classification of hyperlipoproteinemia				
Type	Metabolic defect	Elevated lipoprotein	TAG level	Cholesterol level	Inheritance
I (F. hypertriacyl glyceredemia)	Lipoprotein lipase	↑CM	↑↑	Ⓝ	AR
II A (F. hypercholesterolemia)	LDL receptor mutation or ApoB gene mutation	↑LDL	Ⓝ	↑↑	AD
II B	Defect as in IIA, additionally increased VLDL secretion	↑LDL ↑VLDL	↑	↑↑	AD
III (Remnant removal disease)	Abnormal ApoE (E$_2$)	↑Remnants (CM® and IDL)	↑	↑↑	AR
IV (F-combined hyperlipidemia)	Overproduction of VLDL	↑VLDL	↑↑	↑	Polygenic combined hyperlipidemia
V	Deficiency of apoC-II	↑VLDL ↑CM	↑↑	N	AR

Following is the presentation of a child suffering with abetalipoproteineuia:

(i) Diarrhoea due to fat malabsorption

(ii) Loss of deep tendon reflex

(iii) Blindness

(iv) Deficiency of vitamin E, A, K.

b. *Familial hypobetalipoproteinemia:* In this disorder there is mutation of apoB gene. Due to mutation of apoB gene, truncated apoB proteins are synthesised which impair VLDL and chylomicron assembly and secretion. Additionally VLDLs having truncated apoB are cleared from circulation at accelerated rate. This results in low level of LDL-C in plasma.

2. **Conditions associated with low level of HDL-C**

a. *Familial LCAT deficiency:* It is an autosomal recessive disorder. LCAT enzyme is synthesized in liver and is secreted in plasma, where it circulates after getting associated with lipoproteins.

In LCAT deficiency, free cholesterol content of circulating lipoprotein is greatly increased as it is not converted to cholesterol ester. There are two genetic variants of LCAT deficiency.

• Complete deficiency (classic LCAT deficiency)

• Partial deficiency (Fish-eye disease)

Clinical factors are:

• Corneal opacification

• Very low plasma HDL-C (<10 mg/dl)

• Variable hypertriglyceredemia

• Hemolytic anemia

• ESRD (End stage renal disease)

b. *Tangier's disease (ABC-A1 deficiency):* ABC-A1 is ATP binding cassette-A1, a transporter protein which is responsible for facilitating efflux of cellular unesterified cholesterol and phospholipid to apoA-1.

Patients with Tangier's disease have extremely low level of circulating HDL (<5 mg/dl).

Clinical features are:

• Hepatosplenomegaly

• Yellow/orange tonsil

• Intermittent peripheral neuropathy (mononeuritis multiplex)

c. *Primary hypoalphalipoproteinemia (isolated low HDL):* In this disorder, no clinical sign of low LCAT or Tangier's disease is found.

This disease is AD inheritance and here enhanced catabolism of HDL and its apoproteins are found.

EXERCISE

LONG QUESTIONS (10 MARKS EACH)

Q 1. Describe the various classes of circulating lipoproteins. Discuss their roles in health and disease.
Q 2. Discuss the metabolism of low density plasma lipoproteins.
Q 3. Discuss various steps of cholesterol synthesis. What is the rate-limiting enzyme of cholesterol biogenesis? Discuss its regulation and therapeutic measures to lower cholesterol level in the blood.
Q 4. Discuss the synthesis of palmitic acid in the cytosol.
Q 5. Which is the enzymatic pathway involved in the biosynthesis of prostaglandins ? Name one inhibitor that can block this pathway.

SHORT NOTES (5 MARKS EACH)

Q 1. Phospholipids and their function
Q 2. Fatty acid synthase complex
Q 3. Carnitine shuttle
Q 4. Hyperlipoproteinemia
Q 5. Abetalipoproteinemia
Q 6. Synthesis and utilization of ketone bodies
Q 7. Source of bile acids and its role in fat absorption and digestion
Q 8. Role of chylomicron in metabolism of exogenous fatty acid
Q 9. Lipoproteins and their classification with their composition and functions
Q 10. Liposomes and their uses in biology and medicine

SHORT NOTES (2.5 MARKS EACH)

Q 1. Role of low dose of aspirin in coronary heart diseases
Q 2. Role of polyunsaturated fatty acid in the human body
Q 3. LDL receptors
Q 4. Elongation of fatty acids
Q 5. Lipid classification
Q 6. Phospholipids
Q 7. Essential fatty acids and their biomedical importance
Q 8. Fatty acids, their nomenclature and classification with examples
Q 9. Functions and therapeutic uses of prostaglandins

MULTIPLE CHOICE QUESTIONS

19.1 Which of the following is an activator of LCAT?
a. ApoB-100
b. ApoB-48
c. ApoE
d. ApoA-l

19.2 α-linolenic acid is considered to be nutritionally essential in humans, because:
a. It is an ω3 fatty acid.
b. In humans double bonds cannot be introduced into fatty acids beyond the Δ9 position.
c. In humans double bonds cannot be introduced into fatty acids beyond the Δ12 position.
d. Human tissues are unable to introduce a double bond in the Δ9 position of fatty acid.

19.3 Which of the following regulates lipolysis in adipocytes?
a. Activation of fatty acid synthesis mediated by cyclic AMP
b. Activation of triglyceride lipase as a result of hormone-stimulated increases in cyclic AMP levels
c. Glycerol phosphorylation to prevent futile esterification of fatty acids
d. Activation of cyclic AMP production by insulin

19.4 Which one of the following is not a phospholipid?
a. Sphingomyelin
b. Plasmalogen
c. Cardiolipin
d. Galactosylceramide

19.5 Which type of lipase is controlled by glucagon?
a. Hormone sensitive lipase
b. Lipoprotein lipase
c. Gastric lipase
d. Pancreatic lipase

19.6 Which of the following will be elevated on the bloodstream about 4 hours after eating a high-fat meal?
a. Chylomicrons
b. High-density lipoprotein
c. Ketone bodies
d. Very low density lipoprotein

19.7 Ketone bodies are synthesized in liver in the fasting state, and the amount synthesized increases as fasting extends into starvation. Which one of the following statements about the fed and fasting metabolic states is correct?
a. In the fed state muscle can take up glucose for use as a metabolic fuel because glucose transport in muscle is stimulated in response to glucagon.
b. In the fed state there is decreased secretion of glucagon in response to increase glucose in the portal blood.
c. In the fed state, glucagon acts to increase the synthesis of glycogen from glucose.
d. Plasma glucose is maintained in starvation and prolonged fasting by gluconeogesis from ketone bodies.

19.8 Which one of the following statements about the fed and fasting metabolic states is correct?
a. Fatty acids and triacylglycerol are the synthesized in the liver in the fasting state.
b. In the fasting state, the main fuel for the central nervous system is fatty acid released from adipose tissue.
c. In the fasting state, the main metabolic fuel for most tissue comes from fatty acids released from adipose tissue.
d. In the fed state, muscle cannot take up glucose for use as a metabolic fuel because glucose transport in muscle is stimulated in response to glucagon.

19.9 Hormone sensitive lipase, the enzymes which mobilize fatty acid from triacylglycerol store in adipose tissue is inhibited by:
a. Glucagon
b. ACTH
c. Epinephrine
d. Prostaglandin E1

Section 4 ■ Metabolism of Lipids

19

19.10 **Regarding synthesis of triacyl glycerol in adipose tissue, all of the following are true, except:**
   a. Synthesis from dihydroxyacetone phosphate.
   b. Enzyme glycerol kinase plays an important role.
   c. Enzyme glycerol-3-phosphate dehydrogenase plays an important role.
   d. Phosphatidate is hydrolysed.

19.11 **Lipotrophic factors are all, except:**
   a. Choline
   b. Lecithine
   c. Arginine
   d. Methionine

19.12 **True about fatty acid synthesis:**
   a. Fatty acid synthase is a steroid hormone.
   b. Liver is major site.
   c. Most acetyl CoA is formed from pyruvate by pyruvate dehydrogenase in the cytosol.
   d. Oxaloacetate is reduced to malate in mitochondria.

19.13 **Arachidonic acid is synthesized from:**
   a. Linolenic acid
   b. Linoleic acid
   c. Prostaglandins
   d. Oleic acid

19.14 **A deficiency of carnitine might be expected to interfere with:**
   a. β-oxidation
   b. Ketone body formation from acetyl CoA
   c. Palmitate synthesis
   d. Mobilization of stored triacylglycerols from adipose tissue.

19.15 **In tissues affected by the predominant form of Niemann-Pick disease, which one of the following is found at abnormally high levels?**
   a. Sphingomyelin
   b. Sphingomyelinase
   c. Kerasin
   d. Acetyl coenzyme A

19.16 **Insulin causes lipogenesis by all, except:**
   a. Increasing acetyl CoA carboxylase activity
   b. Increases the transport of glucose into the cell

   c. Inhibits PDH complex
   d. Decreases intracellular cAMP level

19.17 **The metabolic adaptation in alcoholic is all of the following, except:**
   a. Lactic acidosis
   b. High NAD$^+$ level
   c. Accumulation of fat in the liver
   d. Decreased uric acid excretion

19.18 **If in a person total cholesterol = 300 mg/dl, HDL = 25 mg/dl and triglycerides = 150 mg/dl, what will be the LDL level?**
   a. 245
   b. 125
   c. 95
   d. 55

19.19 **In the well-fed state, the carnitine palmitate acyltransferase on the outer mitochondrial membrane is most potently inhibited by:**
   a. Glucose
   b. Palmitoyl CoA
   c. Malonyl CoA
   d. Acetyl CoA

19.20 **After overnight fast, level of glucose transporter is reduced in the:**
   a. Brain cell
   b. Hepatocyte
   c. Adipocyte
   d. RBC

19.21 **Phospholipid includes all, except:**
   a. Plasmalogen
   b. Dipalmityl lecithin
   c. Ceramide
   d. Cardiolipin

19.22 **Ganglioside is compose of all, except:**
   a. Galactose
   b. Phosphate
   c. Ceramide
   d. Sialic acid

19.23 **Lack of α-oxidation of fatty acid leads to:**
   a. Accumulation of phytanic acid
   b. Formation of dicarboxylic acid
   c. Formation of propionic acid
   d. Oxidation of branched chain fatty acid

19.24 The reaction: Succinyl CoA + acetoacetate and acetoacetyl CoA + succinate, occurs in all of the following, except:
a. Brain
b. Striated muscle
c. Liver
d. Cardiac muscle

19.25 Cholesterol presents in LDL:
a. Binds to a cell receptor and diffuses across the cell membrane
b. When it enters the cell, it suppresses the activity of ACAT
c. Once in the cell, it is converted to cholesteryl ester by LCAT
d. Once it has accumulated in the cell, inhibits replenishment of LDL receptor

19.26 Hypolipidemic agents act on:
a. HMG-CoA synthetase
b. HMG-CoA reductase
c. HMG-CoA mutase
d. HMG-CoA lyase

19.27 Acetyl CoA acts as a substrate for all the enzymes, except:
a. HMG-CoA synthetase
b. Malic enzyme
c. Malonyl CoA synthetase
d. Fatty acid synthetase

19.28 Which ketone body is maximum in diabetic ketoacidosis?
a. Acetone
b. Pyruvate
c. Acetoacetic acid
d. β-(OH) butyrate

19.29 Immediate precursor in the production of acetoacetate is:
a. Acetoacetyl CoA
b. Hydroxymethylglutaryl-CoA

c. Malonyl CoA
d. Isovaleric acid

19.30 All are true about LDL receptor, except:
a. They are present on clathrin coated pits on cell membrane.
b. Taken by endocytosis
c. They are present only at extrahepatic site.
d. Increased cellular cholesterol downregulates the receptors.

19.31 Ligand for LDL particle is:
a. ApoB-100
b. ApoE
c. ApoB-48
d. ApoA-11

19.32 A compound that facilitates transfer of fatty acid from cytosol into the mitochondria is:
a. TPP
b. Carnitine
c. Citrate
d. Tetrahydrofolic acid
e. Acetyl CoA

19.33 To be defined as a ganglioside, a lipid substance isolated from nervous tissue must contain in its structure:
a. N-acetylneuraminic acid (NANA), hexoses sphingosine, long-chain fatty acid
b. NANA, a hexose a fatty acid, sphigosine phosphorylcholine
c. NANA, phingosine, ethanolamine
d. NANA, sphexoses, fatty acid, glycerol

19.34 Ketone bodies cannot be utilized by which of the following?
a. Brain
b. Skeletal muscle
c. RBCs
d. Ketone bodies

Section 4 ■ Metabolism of Lipids

19

ANSWERS

19.1 (d) ApoA-I

a. **ApoA-I—synthesized in liver and intestine:**
   i. Most common protein of HDL (70–80% protein of HDL)
   ii. Is a LCAT activator.
   iii. Inversely related to risk for CHD
b. **ApoB-48**—major constituents of chylomicron synthesized in intestine
c. **ApoB-100**—major constituent of LDL—(90% protein of LDL, 60% proteins of IDL and 30% proteins of VLDL
d. **ApoE**—synthesized mainly in liver, but also in macrophages, neuron cells and glial cells; found in chylomicron VLDL, IDL, HDL
e. **ApoC-II**—activator of lipoprotein lipase
f. **ApoC-III**—inhibitor of lipoprotein lipase (Harrison 16th—inhibit lipoprotein binding to receptors)
g. **ApoA-II**—HDL, chylomicrons—inhibitor of LCAT and ApoA-I
h. **ApoB-100** is one of the longest single polypeptide chains known, having 4536 amino acid; ApoB-48 is formed from the same mRNA as ApoB-100, but in the intestine, as stop codon that is not present in genomic DNA is introduced by an RNA Editing mechanism that stops translation at amino acid residue 2153 to liberate ApoB-48.

19.2 (b) In humans double bonds cannot be introduced into fatty acids beyond the Δ9 position.

In human cell, double bond cannot be introduced beyond delta 9 position in fatty acid. This makes linoleic acid and alpha linolenic acid as essential fatty acids.

19.3 (b) Activation of triglyceride lipase as a result of hormone-stimulated increases in cyclic AMP levels

Lipolysis is directly regulated by hormones in adipocytes. Epinephrine stimulates adenylate cyclase to produce cyclic AMP, which in turn stimulates a protein kinase. The kinase activates triglyceride lipase by phosphorylating it. Lipolysis then proceeds.

19.4 (d) galactosylceramide

Galactosylceramide is a glycolipid and not the phospholipid.
List of phospholipids:
• Lecithin

• Cephalin
• Phosphatidyl serine
• Phosphatidyl inositol
• Cardiolipin
• Plasmalogens
List of glycolipids:
• Galactosylceramide
• Glucosylceramide
• Ceramide oligohexoside
• Ganglioside

19.5 (a) Hormone sensitive lipase

As the name implies, this lipase is regulated by insulin and contra-insulin hormones.

19.6 (d) Very low density lipoprotein

Very low density lipoprotein is synthesized in liver and is secreted in the plasma to distribute dietary fatty acid to peripheral tissues with the help of lipoprotein lipase enzyme.

19.7 (b) In the fed state there is decreased secretion of glucagon in response to increase glucose in the portal blood.

• Muscle glucose uptake is depended upon level of insulin as insulin increases activity of GLUT 4.
• Ketone body can never form glucose during starvation.

19.8 (c) In the fasting state, the main metabolic fuel for most tissue comes from fatty acids released from adipose tissue.

In the fasting state the main metabolic fuel for most tissues comes from fatty acids released from adipose tissue.

During fasting state, level of glucagon is high which will activate hormone sensitive lipase enzyme in adipose cell and will mobilize fatty acid from triacylglycerol.

19.9 (d) Prostaglandin E1

19.10 (b) Enzyme glycerol kinase plays an important role.

Adipose tissue does not have glycerol kinase enzyme. So, the source of glycerol-3-phosphate for the synthesis of triacylglycerol is the dihydroxyacetone phosphate which needs glycerol-3-phosphate dehydrogenase enzyme.

19.11 (c) Arginine

- Lipotrophic factors are those factors which mobilizes triacylglyserol from the hepatocytes. Following are the examples:
  - ◇ Choline
  - ◇ Folic acid
  - ◇ Betaine
  - ◇ Vitamin B$_{12}$
  - ◇ Methionine
  - ◇ Glycine
  - ◇ Inositol
  - ◇ Serine
  - ◇ Lecithin
- Lecithin is a phospholipid (phosphatidylcholine) which is important for VLDL formation and its secretion from the liver.

19.12 (b) Liver is major site.

- Fatty acid synthase (FAS) is a multienzyme. It plays a key role in fatty acid synthesis. It is not a single enzyme but a whole enzymatic system composed of 272 kDa multifunctional polypeptide.
- Liver is the major site and to lesser extent mammary glands and adipose tissue.
- Most acetyl CoA is formed from pyruvate by pyruvate dehydrogenase in the mitochondria. Acetyl CoA produced in the mitochondria is condensed with oxaloacetate by citrate synthase to form citrate, which is then transported into the cytosol and broken down to yield acetyl CoA and oxaloacetate by ATP citrate lyase.
- Oxaloacetate in the cytosol is reduced to malate by cytoplasmic malate dehydrogenase and malate is transported back into the mitochondria to participate in the citric acid cycle.

19.13 (b) Linoleic acid

- Linoleic acid produce arachidonic acid by following pathway.

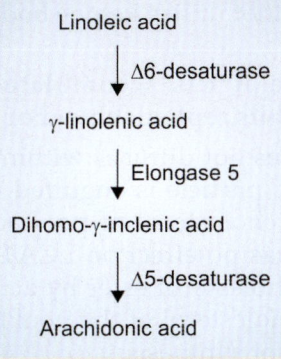

Linoleic acid
↓ Δ6-desaturase
γ-linolenic acid
↓ Elongase 5
Dihomo-γ-inclenic acid
↓ Δ5-desaturase
Arachidonic acid

19.14 (a) β-oxidation

- Carnitine functions in transport of fatty acyl CoA esters formed in cytosol into the mitochondria.
- Acetyl CoA for ketone bodies comes from sources in addition to fatty acids.
- Fatty acid synthesis is a cytosolic process.
- Mobilization is under hormonal control.

19.15 (a) Sphingomyelin

- Sphingomyelin is a lipid composed of phosphocholine and a ceramide, is characteristically found in abnormally high concentrations throughout the body tissues of patients who have any one of the forms of Niemann-Pick disease.
- Division of this disease into five categories is generally accepted: Type A, the acute neuronopathic form, is the one that has the highest incidence. The lack of sphingomyelinase in type A is the metabolic defect that prevents the hydrolytic cleavage of sphingomyelin, which then accumulates in the brain.
- Patients who have the type A form usually show hepatosplenomegaly at 6 months of age, progressively lose motor functions and mental capabilities, and die during the third year of life.

19.16 (c) Inhibits PDH complex

- Insulin rather increases the activity of PDH.
- Insulin increases the activity of acetyl CoA carboxylase activity and thus has stimulatory effect on lipogenesis.
- Insulin increases the recruitment of GLUT to the surface of various cells and thus increases the uptake of insulin via various cells.
- Insulin has inhibitory effect on adenylyl cyclase activity and so causes dephosphorylation.

19.17 (b) High NAD$^+$ level

- Oxidation of ethanol by alcohol dehydrogenase leads to excess production of NADH.
- The increased NADH/NAD$^+$ ratio, also causes increased lactate/pyruvate, resulting in hyper lactic acidemia, which decreases excretion of uric acid, aggravating gout.

19.18 (a) 245

According to Friedwald formula
LDL = Total cholesterol– HDL – VLDL
(VLDL = TG/5)
VLDL =150/5 = 30 mg/dl
LDL = 300 – 25 – 30
= 245 mg/dl

19.19 (c) Malonyl CoA

This is a question regarding regulation of ketogenesis. Ketogenesis is regulated at three crucial steps:

i. **Free fatty acids are the precursors of ketone bodies in the liver.** The liver, both in fed and in fasting conditions, extracts about 30% of the free fatty acids passing through it, so that at high concentrations the flux passing into the liver is substantial. **Therefore, the factors regulating mobilization of free fatty acids from adipose tissue are important in controlling ketogenesis.**

ii. After uptake by the liver, free fatty acids are either beta-oxidized to CO_2, ketone bodies, or **esterified** to triacylglycerol and phospholipid. There is regulation of entry of fatty acids into the oxidative pathway by **carnitine palmitoyltransferase-I** (CPT-I). CPT-I activity is low in the fed state, leading to decreased fatty acid oxidation, and high in starvation, allowing fatty acid oxidation to increase.

iii. **Malonyl CoA, the initial intermediate in fatty acid biosynthesis formed by acetyl CoA carboxylase in the fed state, is a potent inhibitor of CPT-I.**

In turn, the acetyl CoA formed in beta-oxidation is oxidized in the citric acid cycle, or it enters the pathway of ketogenesis to form ketone bodies. As the level of serum free fatty acid is raised, proportionately more free fatty acid is converted to ketone bodies and less is oxidized via the citric acid cycle to CO_2.

- The partition of acetyl CoA between the ketogenic pathway and the pathway of oxidation to CO_2 is regulated, so that the total free energy captured in ATP which results from the oxidation of free fatty acids remains constant as their concentration in the serum changes.
- Thus, ketogenesis may be regarded as a mechanism that allows the liver to oxidize increasing quantities of fatty acids within the constraints of a tightly coupled system of oxidative phosphorylation.

19.20 (c) Adipocyte

GLUT-4 is insulin dependent glucose transporter. It is found on
- Adipocyte
- Skeletal muscle
- Heart muscle

19.21 (c) Ceramide

Ceramide is sphingosine and fatty acid. It is not a phospholipid. Dipalmityl lecithin and cardiolipin are phospholipids.

Plasmalogens: Plasmalogens are also a special type of phospholipid. These compounds constitute as much as 10% of the phospholipids of brain and muscle. Structurally, the plasmalogens resemble phosphatidylethanolamine but possess an **ether link on the S_N1 carbon instead of the ester link** found in acylglycerols. Typically, the **alkyl radical is an unsaturated alcohol**. In some instances, choline, serine, or inositol may be substituted for ethanolamine.

19.22 (b) Phosphate

Ganglioside is the example of glycolipid.

Following is the structure of a ganglioside:

$$Cer—Glc—Gal—GalNAc—Gal$$
$$|$$
$$NeuAc \text{ (sialic acid)}$$

19.23 (a) Accumulation of phytanic acid

Phytanic acid is the branched chain fatty acid. This fatty acid has methyl group at the alpha carbon atom. This methyl group should be removed by alpha oxidation, then only beta oxidation can proceed.

Refsum's disease is an autosomal recessive disease. In this, there is **deficiency of enzyme phytanic α-hydroxylase** which prevents alpha oxidation. This methyl group which thus is spared from alpha oxidation, prevents beta oxidation to take place, thus leading to phytanic acid accumulation in the plasma and tissue.

Source of phytanic acid is the dairy products, ruminant fat and meat.

19.24 (c) Liver

Thiophorase (acetoacetatesuccinyl CoA, CoA transferase) is the enzyme responsible for transfer of CoA to acetoacetate converting it into acetoacetyl CoA which is responsible for utilization of ketone bodies. Liver cells do not have enzyme thiophorase and so they cannot utilize ketone bodies.

19.25 (d) Once it has accumulated in the cell, inhibits replenishment of LDL receptor

Cholesterol does not diffuses within the cell rather the whole LDL particle is engulfed via cholesterol receptor. This cholesterol of pool activates ACAT function and has no effect on LCAT function. It is converted to cholesterol ester by activity of ACAT (not LCAT). Cholesterol of the pool has got inverse effect on receptor synthesis.

19.26 (b) HMG-CoA reductase

Hypolipidemic drugs (statin) when given to reduce cholesterol content in the circulation, do so via inhibiting endogenous synthesis of cholesterol by acting on HMG-CoA reductase enzyme.

19.27 (b) Malic enzyme

HMG-CoA synthetase requires acetyl CoA as a precursor molecule. HMG-CoA in turn, is responsible for cholesterol synthesis and ketone body synthesis.

Malonyl CoA synthetase acts on acetyl CoA and carboxylates it to form malonyl CoA.

Fatty acid synthase complex use acetyl CoA and malonyl CoA as precursor molecule for fatty acid synthesis.

Malic enzyme does not require acetyl CoA as the precursor molecule.

Malic enzyme is $NADP^+$ dependent malate dehydrogenase which converts malate to pyruvate.

19.28 (d) β-(OH) butyrate

Acetoacetic acid is the precursor ketone body and β-(OH) butyrate which is formed from acetoacetate is most abundant ketone body in the circulation. Conversion of acetoacetate to β-(OH) butyrate requires presence of β-(OH) butyrate dehydrogenase which requires NAD as a coenzyme.

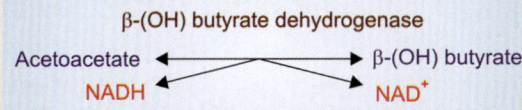

19.29 (b) Hydroxymethylglutaryl-CoA

HMG-CoA is the immediate precursor of acetoacetate which is the 1st ketone body formed.

β-(OH) butyrate is formed once β-(OH) butyrate dehydrogenase acts on acetoacetate.

β-(OH) butyrate is most abundant (predominant) ketone body formed.

19.30 (c) They are present only at extrahepatic site.

LDL receptor is present on liver as well as on extrahepatic tissue.
- LDL (ApoB-100, E) receptors occur on the cell surface in pits that are coated on the cytosolic side of the cell membrane with a protein called clathrin.

The glycoprotein receptor spans the membrane, the B-100 binding region being at the exposed amino terminal end.
- After binding, LDL is taken up intact by endocytosis. The apoprotein and cholesteryl ester are then hydrolyzed in the lysosomes, and cholesterol is translocated into the cell. The receptors are recycled to the cell surface.

This influx of cholesterol inhibits the transcription of the genes encoding HMG-CoA synthase, HMG-CoA reductase and other enzymes involved in cholesterol synthesis, as well as the LDL receptor itself, via the SREBP pathway, and thus coordinately suppresses cholesterol synthesis and uptake.

In addition, ACAT activity is stimulated, promoting cholesterol esterification. In this way, LDL receptor activity on the cell surface is regulated by the cholesterol requirement for membranes, steroid hormones, or bile acid synthesis.
- The liver and many extrahepatic tissues express the LDL (ApoB-100, E) receptor. It is so designated because it is specific for ApoB-100 but not B-48, which lacks the carboxyl terminal domain of B-100 containing the LDL receptor ligand, and it also takes up lipoproteins rich in ApoE.
- Approximately 30% of LDL is degraded in extrahepatic tissues and 70% in the liver.
- The LDL (ApoB-100, E) receptor is defective in familial hypercholesterolemia, a genetic condition which increases blood LDL cholesterol levels and causes premature atherosclerosis.

19.31 (a) ApoB-100

LDL has got only one apolipoprotein on it and it is ApoB-100. It acts as ligand as it is being recognized by LDL receptor.

19.32 (b) Carnitine

Fatty acid is transported across mitochondrial membrane via carnitine shuttle.

19.33 (a) N-acetylneuraminic acid (NANA), hexoses sphingosine, long-chain fatty acid

19.34 (c) RBCs

RBCs and liver cannot utilize ketone body.

Section 4 ■ Metabolism of Lipids

19

Metabolism of Amino Acids

Amino Acid Metabolism I: Overview and Urea Cycle

BIOSYNTHESIS AND CATABOLISM OF AMINO ACIDS (AN OVERVIEW)

Unlike plants and microorganisms, mammals can not synthesize all 20 amino acids and require some of them in their diet. The amino acids required in the diet are called essential and that which can be synthesized in the cells are called as nonessential amino acids.

Biosynthesis

Though there are diverse pathways synthesizing various amino acids, they all have an important feature in common—the source of carbon skeleton in these amino acid is the key intermediate of central metabolic pathways like glycolysis, TCA cycle, HMP shunt pathway. Amino group usually comes via transamination of the glutamate.

Catabolism

Amino acids are constantly degraded. They undergo transamination first by which the amino group is transferred to the alpha-ketoglutarate to form glutamic acid and resulting carbon skeleton is converted to one or more metabolic intermediates and are used as metabolic fuels.

It is point to note that carbon skeleton of 20 amino acids is funneled to only 7 molecules like pyruvate, acetyl CoA, acetoacetyl CoA, α-ketoglutarate, fumarate, succinyl CoA and oxaloacetate.

Transamination

Transfer of amino group from an amino acid to a keto acid is known as transamination (Fig. 20.1).

This process involves the interconversion of a pair of amino acids and a pair of keto acids, catalysed by a group of enzymes called transaminase (aminotransferases). Major acceptor α-keto acid which accepts the amino group during transamination process and produces glutamate is α-ketoglutarate. Important features of transamination are:

1. All transaminases require pyridoxal phosphate **(PLP) as cofactor**, which resides at the catalytic site.
2. Specific transaminase exists for each pair of amino and keto acids. These are specific for only one pair, but nonspecific for the other pair.
3. No free ammonia is liberated. Only the transfer of amino group occurs.
4. This reaction is reversible.
5. It is not restricted to α-amino groups.

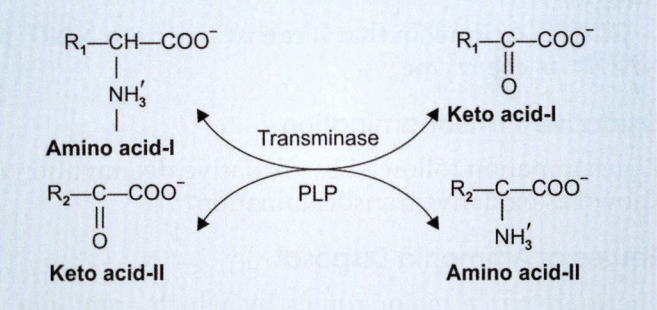

Fig. 20.1: Transamination

All amino acids undergo transamination reaction except lysine, threonine, proline and hydroxyproline (these amino acids undergo deamination).

Deamination

The removal of amino group from the amino acid as ammonia is called deamination. Liberation of free ammonia from the amino group of amino acids coupled with oxidation is known as **oxidative deamination** (Fig. 20.2).

This reaction is catalysed by **glutamate dehydrogenase** (GDH) enzyme found in the liver and kidney in mitochondrial matrix. Reaction is as follows:

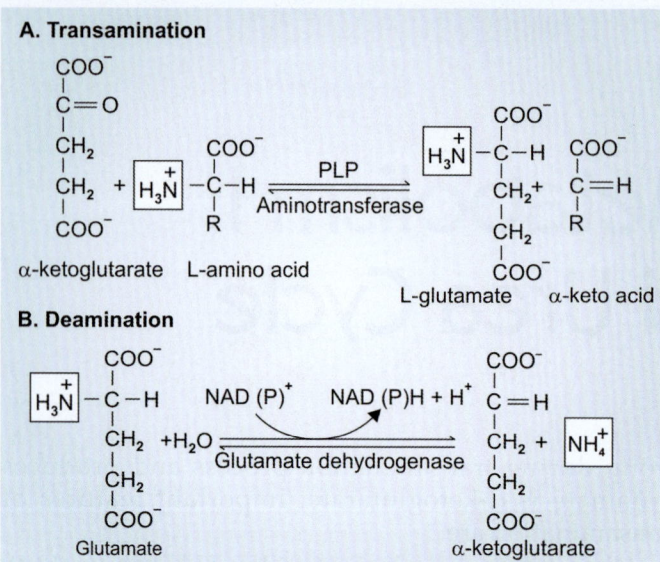

Fig. 20.2: Transamination and deamination

GDH is an important allosteric enzyme contains six subunits. GDP and ADP are important allosteric activators and GTP and ATP are important allosteric inhibitors. Low energy state of the cell (signaled by GDP and ADP) activates the GDH enzyme and accelerates the catabolism of the glutamate to α-ketoglutarate.

α-ketoglutarate is utilized in the TCA cycle to provide energy.

GDH is unique, in that it can utilize both NAD⁺ or NADP⁺ as coenzyme.

Oxidative Transdeamination

Transamination followed by oxidative deamination is known as oxidative transdeamination.

Routes of Ammonia Disposal

There are three major routes by which ammonia is detoxified:

1. Via formation of glutamate in transamination reaction
2. Via formation of glutamine in glutamine synthetase reaction
3. Via formation of urea by Krebs-Henseleit cycle.

UREA CYCLE
(Krebs-Henseleit Cycle or Ornithine cycle)

Urea cycle is the first metabolic pathway to be elucidated in 1932, by Hans Krebs and Kurt Henseleit. Hence, this cycle is known as Krebs-Henseleit cycle (also known as ornithine cycle as ornithine is the first member of this cycle).

During degradation of amino acids, α-ketoglutarate collects amino group and forms glutamate. This glutamate as well as glutamine (brain, GIT) and alanine (muscle) reach the liver.

At the liver amino group of the glutamate is oxidatively deaminated by an enzyme called glutamate dehydrogenase which is found in the liver mitochondrial matrix (see above).

This ammonia is now readily available to start the urea cycle (source of second ammonia for the urea synthesis is the aspartic acid. This aspartic acid is formed by transamination catalysed by AST enzyme where glutamate donates amino group to oxaloacetate to form aspartate.

Reactions of the Urea Cycle

Reactions of urea cycle are partly mitochondrial and partly cytosolic. Total five reactions are needed in the urea cycle. The first two reactions occur in the mitochondria, and other three reactions take place in the cytoplasm (Fig. 20.3).

Step 1: Formation of Carbamoyl Phosphate

Carbamoyl phosphate synthetase-I (CPS-I) catalyzes the formation of carbamoyl phosphate from ammonia and carbon dioxide. It is a rate-limiting enzyme and is allosterically controlled.

  i. *Energy requirement:* Two molecules of ATP are required for this reaction.
 ii. N-acetylglutamate is a positive allosteric effector of CPS 1.

Step 2: Formation of Citrulline

Ornithine transcarbamoylase (OTC) catalyzes the formation of citrulline from carbamoyl phosphate and ornithine. Citrulline is transported out in the cytosol where it is incorporated in the next metabolic step catalyzed by arginosuccinate synthetase enzyme.

Step 3: Formation of Argininosuccinate

Argininosuccinate synthetase catalyzes the formation of argininosuccinate from citrulline and aspartate. Aspartate is the source of second nitrogen atom of the urea. One molecule of ATP is required which is cleaved to AMP (equivalent to 2 ATP).

Step 4: Formation of Arginine and Fumarate

Argininosuccinate lyase (also called as arginosuccinase) removes carbon skeleton of aspartate in the form of fumarate, leaving nitrogen in the arginine.

Step 5: Formation of Urea and Ornithine

Arginase acts on arginine to convert it to urea and ornithine.

Ornithine is transported back to mitochondria where it combines with the another molecule of carbamoyl phosphate.

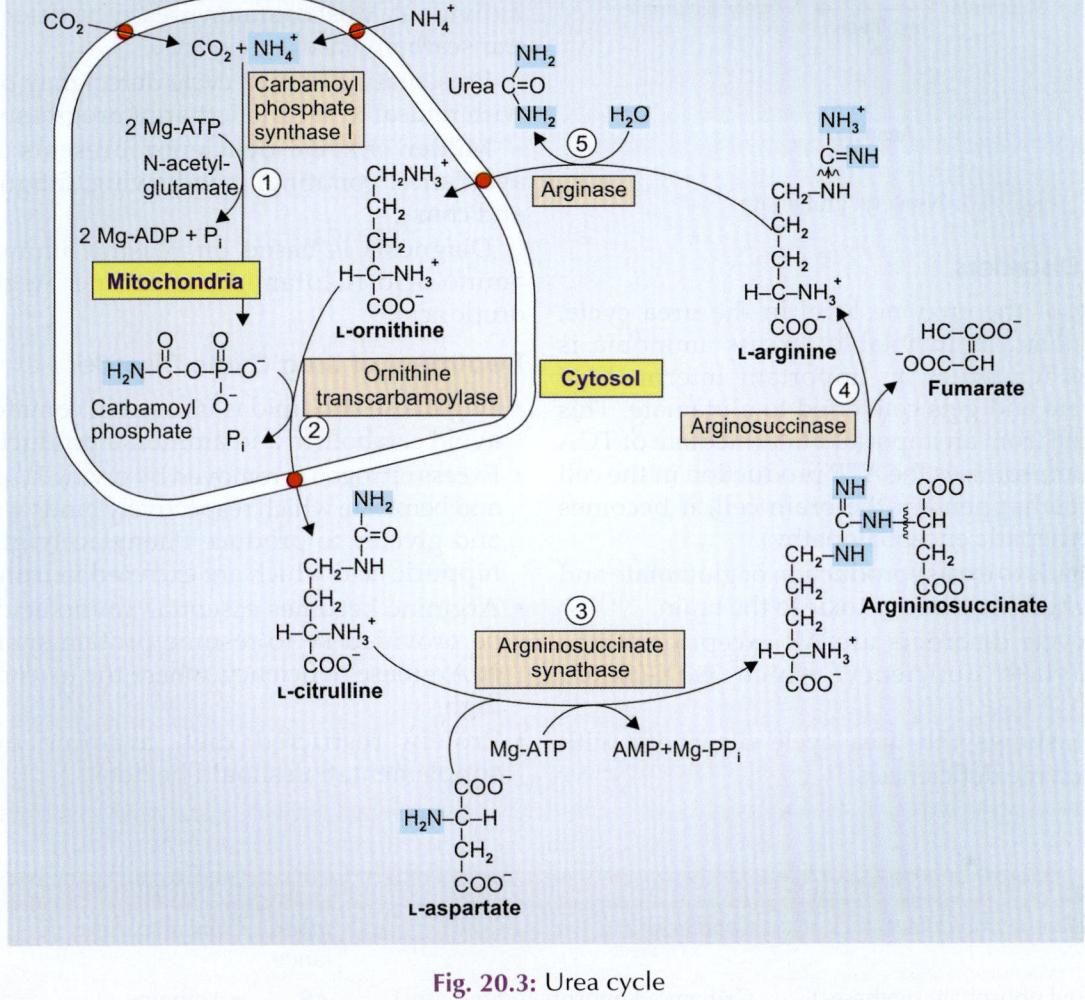

Fig. 20.3: Urea cycle

NOTE:

▶ Urea is highly soluble and nontoxic. It enters the blood and is excreted in the urine.

▶ Ornithine continues to act as an intermediate in the urea cycle. Ornithine is considered as catalyst in urea cycle.

▶ Fumarate released at the arginosuccinase step enters the TCA cycle where it is converted to malate and oxaloacetate. This oxaloacetate accepts the amino group from amino acid and is converted to aspartate.

Thus, fumarate is the link between urea cycle and the TCA cycle (sometimes called urea bicycle) (Fig. 20.4).

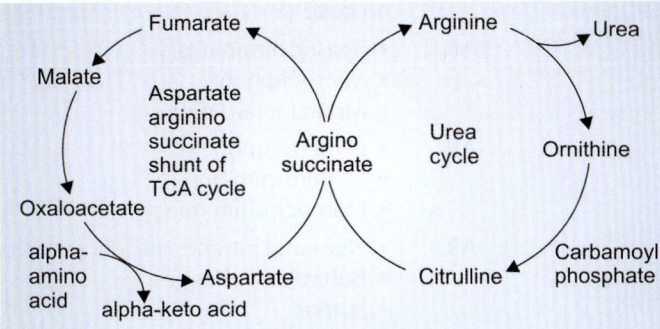

Fig. 20.4: Fumarate as a link of TCA cycle

Regulation of the Urea Cycle

• CPS I is the rate-limiting enzyme of the urea cycle which is an allosteric enzyme having 6 subunits.

• N-acetylglutamate is a positive allosteric effector for carbamoyl phosphate synthetase I. It is the rate-limiting step in the urea cycle.

• N-acetylglutamate is synthesized from acetyl CoA and glutamate with the help of NAG synthase enzyme in a recation for which arginine is needed (Fig. 20.5).

• So excess protein intake increases the concentration of arginine and thus of N-acetyl glutamate, leading to increased urea formation.

• During starvation activity of urea cycle enzyme is elevated to meet the increased rate of protein catabolism.

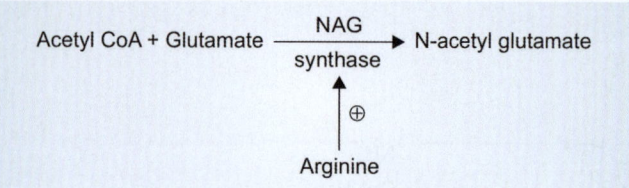

Fig. 20.5: N-acetyl glutamate

Urea Cycle Disorders

Block at any of the enzyme level in the urea cycle, hyperammonemia is inevitable. Excess ammonia is very toxic as it utilizes an important intermediate α-ketoglutarate and gets converted to glutamate. This deprive the cell from an important intermediate of TCA cycle. This compromises the ATP production in the cell and when this happens in the brain cell, it becomes pathological (hepatic encephalopathy).

This also leads to excess production of glutamate and glutamine, which are directly toxic to the brain.

All urea cycle disorders are AR except ornithine transcarbamylase deficiency, which is X-linked recessive.

Table 20.1 shows the urea cycle disorders with respective enzyme deficiencies.

Overall incidence of urea cycle defect is 1:35,000 individual. Most common urea cycle defect is 'ornithine transcarbamylase deficiency'.

Presentation of urea cycle defect may be early in life with refusal to eat and lethargy progressing to coma.

Milder enzyme deficiency presents with protein avoidance, vomiting, mood swing, fatigue, irritability and coma.

Diagnosis is based on plasma ammonia, plasma amino acid (Glutamine, citrulline, Arginine), urine orotic acid.

Treatment of Urea Cycle Disorder

- IV glucose and lipid is infused in comatose patient to avoid catabolism and ammonia production.
- Excess nitrogen is removed by giving IV phenylacetate and benzoate which respectively binds with glutamine and glycine to produce Phenylacetylglutamine and hippuric acid which are excreted in urine.
- Arginine becomes essential amino acid and should be provided IV to resume protein synthesis except in Arginase deficiency, where the level of Arginine is high.
- Protein restricted diet, arginine or citrulline supplementation should be done.

TABLE 20.1 Urea cycle disorders with respective enzyme deficiencies and clinical presentation

S. No.	Urea cycle enzyme defect	Condition	Inheritance	Clinical features
1.	Carbamoyl phosphate synthase-1	Carbamoyl phosphate synthase-1 deficiency	AR	• Lethargy • Coma • Aversion to protein • Intellectual disability • Hyperammonemia
2.	N-acetyl glutamate synthase	N-acetyl glutamate synthase deficiency	AR	-do-
3.	Ornithine Transcarbamylase (OTC)	OTC deficiency	XL	-do-
4.	Arginosuccinate synthase	Citrullinemia type 1	AR	-do-
5.	Arginosuccinate lyase	Arginosuccinic acidemia	AR	-do- and trichorhexis no dose
6.	Arginase	Arginase deficiency	AR	• Spastic tetraparesis • Microcephaly • Mental retardation
7.	Mitochondrial ornithine carrier— ORNT1	HHH syndrome	AR	• Hyperammonemia • Hyperornithema • Homocitullinemia
8.	Mitochondrial aspartate/glutamate carrier—CTLN2 (citrin deficiency)	Citrullinemia type 2	AR	• Neonatal intrahepatic cholestasis • Behavioral change • Stupor • Coma • Avoidance of carbohydrate

21

Amino Acid Metabolism II: Metabolism of Aliphatic Amino Acids

In the metabolism of various amino acids, students will be learning about diverse fate of individual amino acid in human body. In addition, the catabolism of these amino acids which may give rise to glucogenic/ketogenic or both kinds of substrates will also be discussed. For nonessential amino acids, the various routes which synthesize them, will also be described in this chapter.

▌GLYCINE

• A nonessential glucogenic acid.
• It is the only amino acid which is optically inactive as it is not having any asymmetric carbon atom.

a. Synthesis of Glycine

It can be synthesized in mammalian tissues by:
• **Serine:** Serine hydroxymethyltransferase (Fig. 21.1)

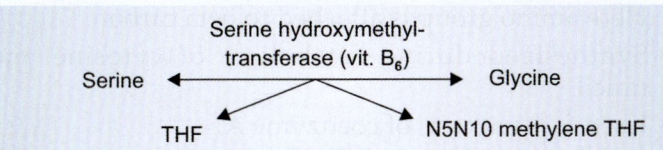

Fig. 21.1: Glycine synthesis from serine

• **Threonine:** Threonine aldolase (Fig. 21.2)
• CO_2, NH_3, one carbon moiety N5N10 methylene THFA by enzyme glycine synthase (Fig. 21.3).

b. Catabolism of Glycine

Glycine is catabolized in following ways:
• Converted to CO_2, NH_4^+ and N5N10 methylene THF (Fig. 21.3)
• Oxidative deamination by glycine oxidase (Fig. 21.4).

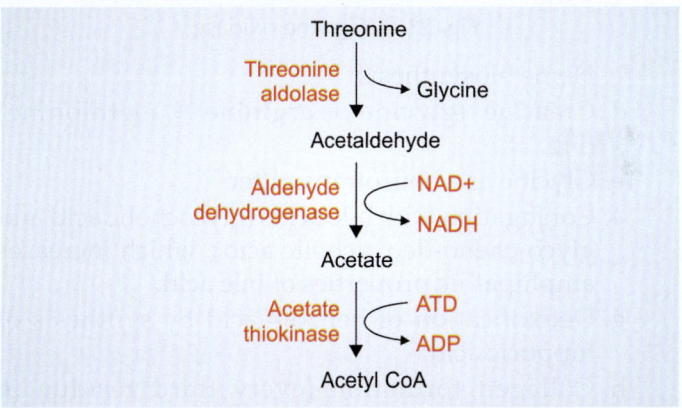

Fig. 21.2: Threonine aldolase

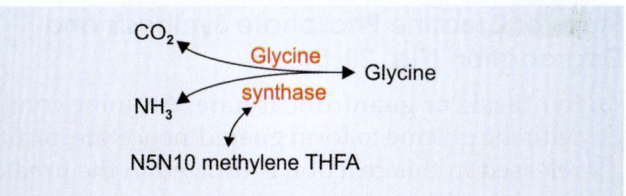

Fig. 21.3: Glycine synthase

c. Uses of Glycine

1. Glycine is utilized in the glucogenic pathway via getting converted to first serine and then pyruvate.
2. In addition, glycine is responsible for synthesis of many biological compounds and also for many important biochemical reactions like:
   a. Purine *de novo* biosynthesis (C4, C5, N7 atoms of purine ring comes from glycine)
   b. Glutathione synthesis (γ-glutamyl cysteinyl glycine)

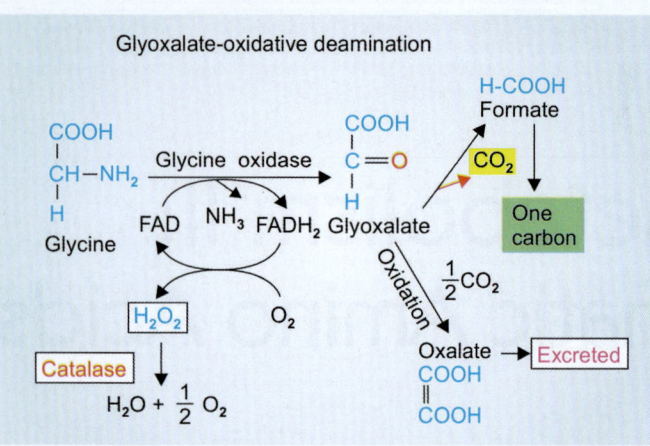

Fig. 21.4: Glycine oxidase

c. Heme biosynthesis

d. Creatine (glycine + arginine + methionine) (Fig. 21.5)

e. Glycine as a neurotransmitter

f. Conjugation with bile acids (glycocholic acid and glyco-cheno-deoxycholic acid), which increases amphipathic properties of bile acid.

g. Detoxification of benzoic acid by synthesis of hippuric acid

h. Collagen formation (every third residue in collagen polypeptide is glycine)

i. Synthesis of creatine (Fig. 21.5)

Steps of Creatine Phosphate Synthesis and Degradation (Fig. 21.5)

a. **Synthesis of guanidinoacetate:** Arginine combines with the glycine to form guanidinoacetate, ornithine released in this reaction is utilized in the urea cycle reaction.

b. **Guanidinoacetate** gets methylated to form creatine. Source of methyl group is the S-adenosyl methionine (SAM) in this reaction.

c. **Creatine** is phosphorylated to form creatine phosphate. Enzyme needed is creatine phosphokinase (CPK).

d. **Creatine phosphate** gets converted to creatinine in a spontaneous reaction which is irreversible. Excretion of creatinine per day is constant and depends on muscle mass.

Metabolic Errors in Glycine

1. Nonketotic hyperglycinemia
2. Primary hyperoxaluria

█ ALANINE

- A nonessential glucogenic amino acid.
- May be synthesized by pyruvte.
- Alanine is quantitatively most important amino acid taken up by liver from peripheral tissues specially skeletal muscles.
- **Glucose-alanine** cycle is of special significance specially in starvation. It is also called Cahill cycle (Fig. 21.6).
- Alanine coming out of the skeletal muscle during fasting reaches liver, where it undergoes transamination to produce glutamate and pyruvate.
- Pyruvate produces glucose by gluconeogenesis and glutamate provides ammonia for urea synthesis.

Beta Alanine

- Here amino group is attached to beta carbon.
- Synthesized during catabolism of cytosine and uracil.
- Used for synthesis of coenzyme A.
- Carnosine is a dipeptide made up of beta alanine and histidine.

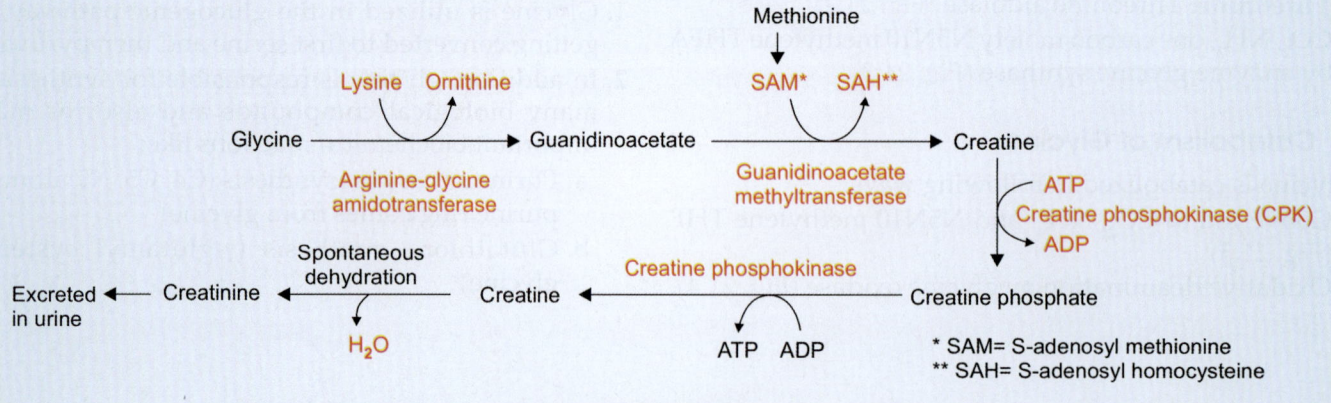

Fig. 21.5: Synthesis of creatine from glycine, arginine and methionine and its role as energy reserve

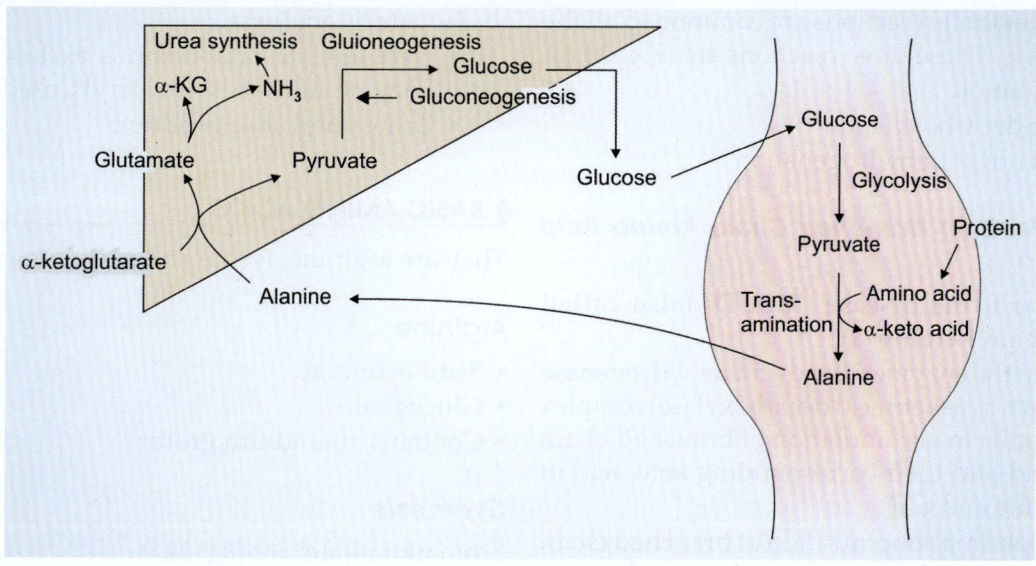

Fig. 21.6: Glucose-alanine cycle

SERINE

A nonessential glucogenic amino acid.

Synthesis

a. 3-phosphoglycerate (an intermediate of the glycolysis) is a major source of serine.
b. **From glycine:** *See* Fig. 21.1

Catabolism

Serine is deaminated to give pyruvate by serine dehydratase enzyme, but in human the main pathway of serine catabolism is conversion of serine to glycine by serine hydroxymethyltransferase (refer Fig. 21.1). Further catabolism of glycine is same as described earlier under section of glycine.

Serine contributes in the formation of following compounds:

• Glycine
• Cystein
• Alanine
• Phosphatidylserine
• Phosphatidylethanolamine
• Selenocysteine (described next)

Selenocysteine (SeCys)

Selenocysteine is considered as 21st amino acid.

Hydroxyl group of serine when replaced by selenium becomes selenocysteine. Selenocysteine is incorporated in the protein during translation .

One of the codon of mRNA UGA is read as selenocysteine incorporation codon, for which a selenocysteine insertion element, a loop structure is needed at the 3' region of the mRNA.

Selenocysteine is found at the active site of the following enzymes:

• Thioredoxine reductase
• Glutathione peroxidase
• De-iodinase
• Glycine reductase
• Selenoprotein P

THREONINE

An essential glucogenic amino acid.

No synthetic pathway as it is an essential amino acid.

Catabolism

a. By threonine aldolase: *See* Fig. 21.2
b. By threonine dehydratase: *See* Fig. 21.7

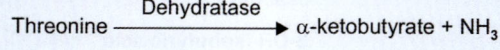

Threonine $\xrightarrow{\text{Dehydratase}}$ α-ketobutyrate + NH$_3$

Fig. 21.7: Threonine dehydratase

Branched Chain Amino Acids

There are three amino acids which has branching in the side chain.

• Valine—essential, glucogenic
• Leucine—essential, ketogenic
• Isoleucine—essential, glucogenic + ketogenic

During degradation of the branched chain amino acid,

the first three metabolic reactions are common to all the three amino acids. These three reactions are (Fig. 21.8):

1. Transamination
2. Oxidative decarboxylation
3. FAD dependent dehydrogenation

Metabolic Defects in Branched Chain Amino Acid Degradation

a. **Maple syrup urine disease (MSUD) (also called branched chain ketonuria)**
  - Defect is in the enzyme α-keto acid dehydrogenase (also known as α-keto acid decarboxylase) complex which results in accumulation of branched chain amino acid and their corresponding keto acid in blood, urine and CSF.
  - Elevated plasma concentration of branched chain amino acids and their respective keto acids.
  - Urine of patients have maple syrup or burnt sugar smell due to presence of high amount of aliphatic keto acids.

b. **Isovaleric aciduria**
  - Here leucine catabolism is exclusively affected. Enzyme affected is isovaleryl CoA dehydrogenase.
  - Urine gives cheesy odour.

■ BASIC AMINO ACIDS

They are arginine, lysine and histidine.

Arginine

- Semi-essential
- Glucogenic
- Contains guanidium group

Synthesis

From glutamate: *See* Fig. 21.9.

Catabolism

See Fig. 21.10

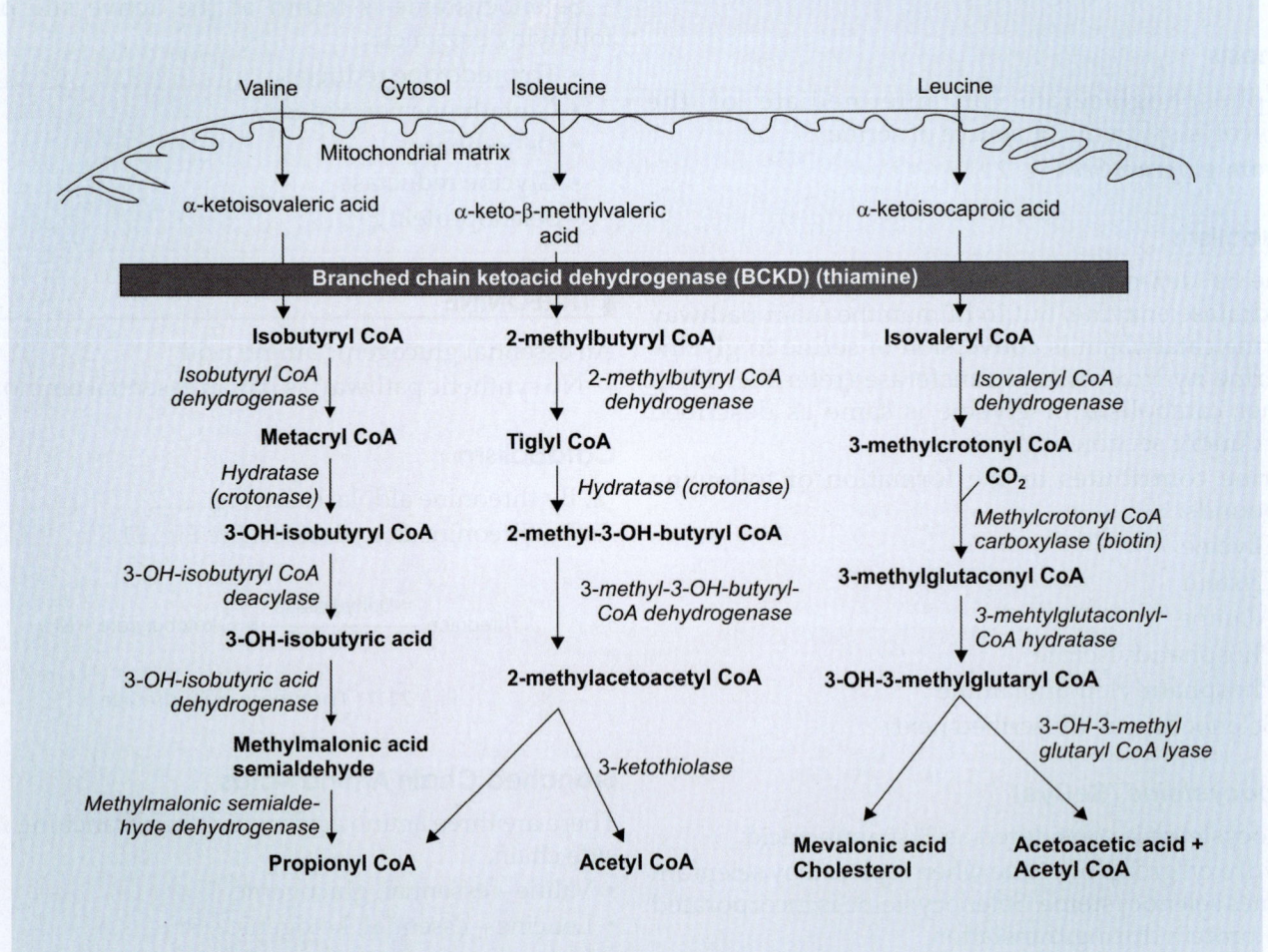

Fig. 21.8: Branched chain amino acid metabolism

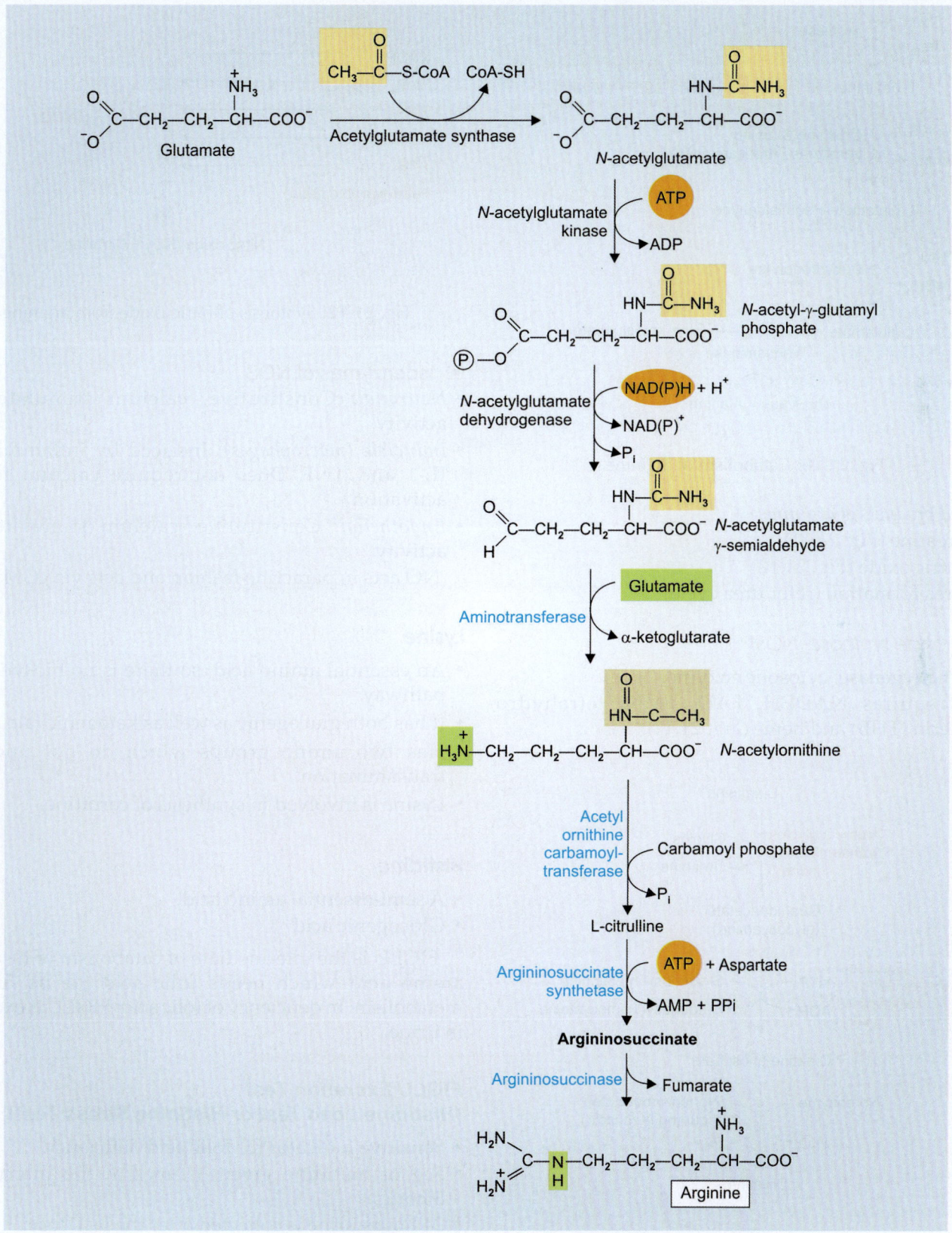

Fig. 21.9: Arginine synthesis from glutamate

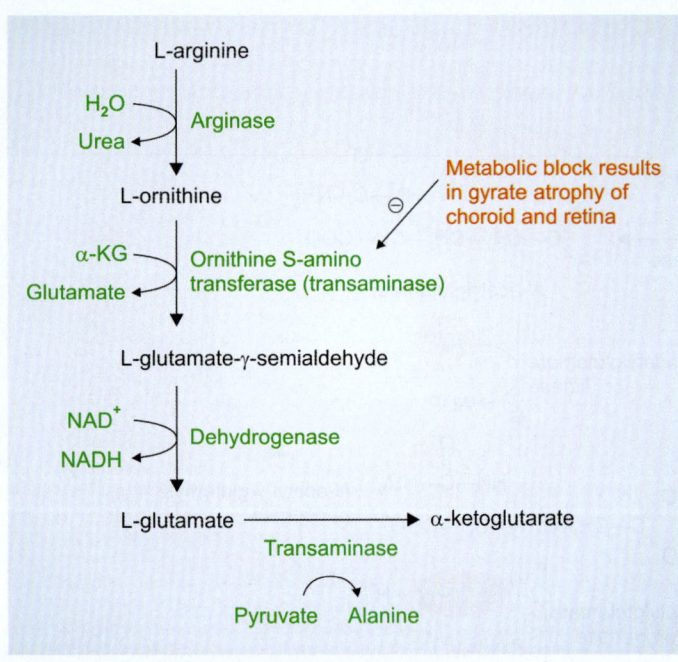

Fig. 21.10: Catabolism of arginine

Special products of arginine:
1. Creatine (Fig. 21.11)
2. Nitric oxide (Fig. 21.12)
3. Urea formation (refer urea cycle)

Nitric oxide synthase (NOS)

Mono-oxygenase, cytosolic enzyme.

It requires NADPH, FAD, FMN, tetrahydro-biopterin (THB) and heme (Fig. 21.12).

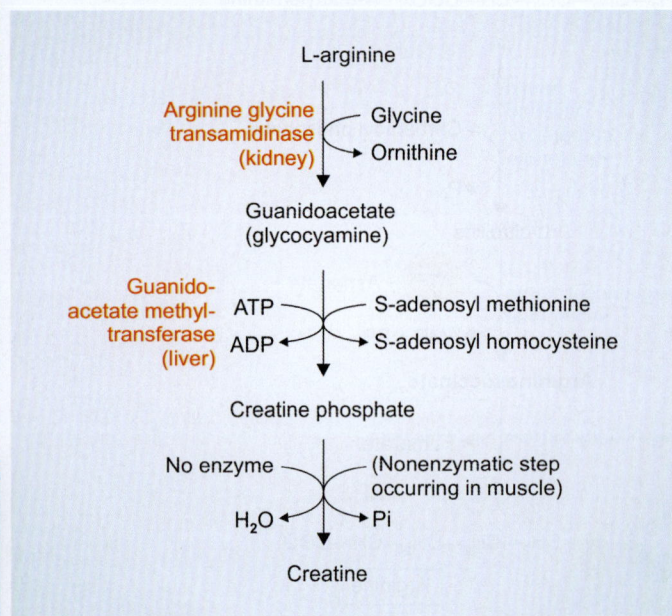

Fig. 21.11: Creatine synthesis from arginine

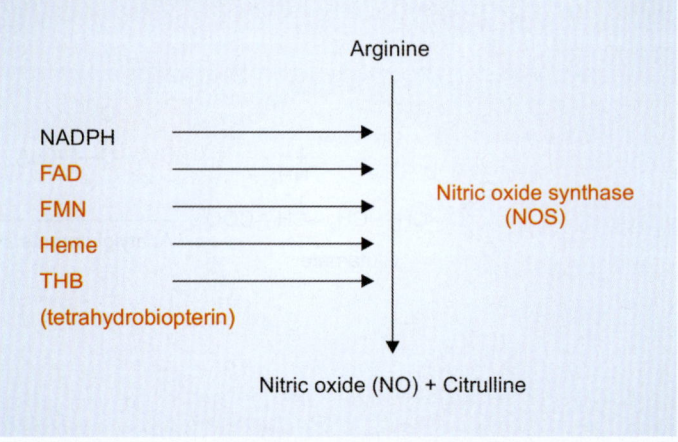

Fig. 21.12: Synthesis of nitric oxide from arginine

▣ **Isoenzymes of NOS**
- *Neuronal:* Constitutive, calcium stimulates its activity
- *Inducible (macrophages):* Induced by inflammation, IL-1 and TNF. Does not require calcium for its activation.
- *Endothelial:* Constitutive, calcium stimulates its activity.
  NO acts in paracrine fashion and acts via cGMP.

Lysine
- An essential amino acid, so there is no biosynthetic pathway.
- It has both glucogenic as well as ketogenic fate.
- Has two amino groups which do not undergo transamination.
- Lysine is involved in synthesis of carnitine.

Histidine
- A semi-essential amino acid.
- Glucogenic acid

FIGLU is the intermediate of catabolism of histidine amino acid which needs folic acid for its further metabolism. In deficiency of folic acid, FIGLU is excreted in urine.

FIGLU Excretion Test
(Histidine Load Test or Histidine Stress Test)
- Sensitive indicator for folic acid deficiency.
- 5 g of histidine given 3 times at the interval of 8 hours.
- 24 hours urine is collected after the last dose.
- Normally <30 mg of FIGLU is excreted in the urine.

- Excretion of ≥30 mg of FIGLU in the urine indicates folic acid deficiency.

SULPHUR CONTAINING AMINO ACIDS

They are methionine and cysteine.

Methionine

- An essential amino acid.
- Serves as a precursor for the synthesis of cysteine and cystine.

Metabolism of Methionine

Methionine forms S-adenosyl methionine (SAM) which acts as a methyl donor and after donation of the methyl group SAM is converted back to S-adenosyl homocysteine (SAH).

   SAH is hydrolysed into homocysteine and adenosine. Homocysteine has got two fates:

1. Converted into methionine
2. Synthesis of cysteine

1. *Conversion of homocysteine to methionine:* N5-methyl–THF acts as a methyl donor for conversion of homocysteine to methionine enzyme needed here is methionine synthase/homocysteine methyltransferase. Vitamin B_{12} is required as a cofactor.
2. *Synthesis of cysteine: See* Fig. 21.13

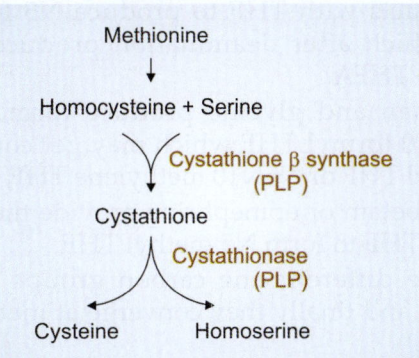

Fig. 21.13: Cysteine synthesis from methionine

Metabolic Disorders

Homocystinuria

- Heritable defects of methionine metabolism.
- Up to 300 mg of homocystine (disulphide form) is excreted in the urine.
- Cyanide nitroprusside test is done in the urine.

☐ Types of homocystinuria:
1. Type I—deficiency of cystathionine beta synthase
2. Type II—defect in homocysteine methyltransferase.

3. Type III—unavailability of N5–methyl tetrahydrofolic acid, due to defect in N5N10–methylene tetrahydro folate reductase.

Cystathioninuria

Due to cystathionase deficiency.

1. **Cystinuria (Cystine–lysinuria):**
   - Inherited metabolic disease, characterized by urinary excretion of cystine up to 30 times than normal.
   - Excretion of ornithine, lysine and arginine also rises, suggesting a defect in the renal reabsorption mechanisms for these four amino acids (COLA).
   - Since cystine is relatively insoluble, cystine calculi form in the renal tubules of these patients.
2. **Cystinosis (cystine storage disease)**
   - Rare lysosomal disorder characterized by defective carrier-mediated transport of cystine.
   - Cystine crystals are deposited in tissues and organs, particularly the reticulo-endothelial system.

Cysteine

Cysteine is synthesized from methionine (Fig. 21.13).

Special Products of Cysteine

- Cystine
- Glutathione (gamma glutamyl cysteinyl glycine)
- PAPS (3'-**p**hospho**a**denosine 5'-**p**hospho**s**ulphate)
- Taurine
- Coenzyme A

ACIDIC AMINO ACIDS

They are glutamic acid and aspartic acid.

Glutamic Acid

- Nonessential
- A glucogenic amino acid.

Synthesis of Glutamic Acid

1. Transamination reaction (Fig. 21.14)

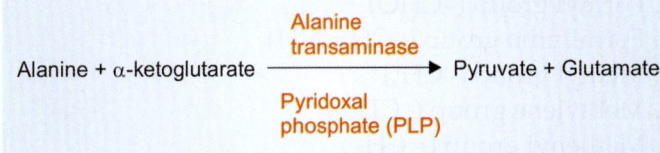

Fig. 21.14: Transamination of alanine

2. Reductive amination of α-ketoglutarate by NH_4^+ (Fig. 21.15)

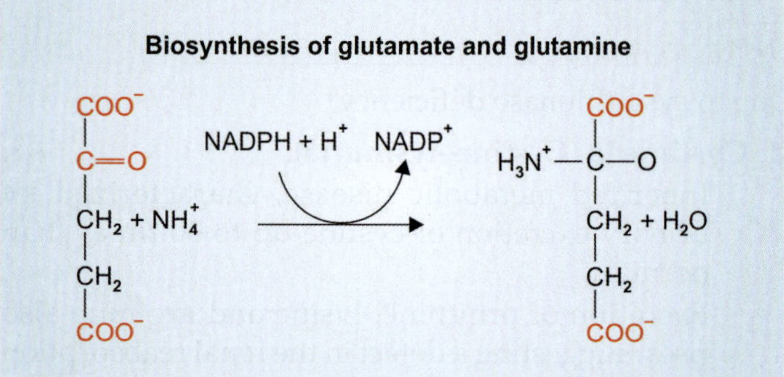

Fig. 21.15: Reductive amination

These one carbon groups are carried by tetra-hydrofolic acid (THFA) either attached to its N5 or N10 atoms. CO_2 is transferred via biotin.

Diagram of THFA : *See* Fig. 21.16.

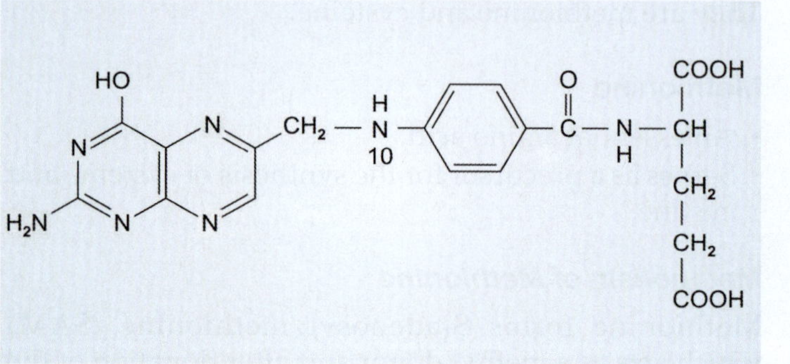

Fig. 21.16: Structure of folic acid

Importance of Glutamic Acid

- Glutamic acid is the excitatory neurotransmitter and its alpha decarboxylation gives rise to gamma amino butyric acid (GABA) which is an inhibitory neurotransmitter.
- Glutamate fixes NH_3 in brain and intestine with the help of glutamine synthetase enzyme. Glutaminase enzyme found in renal tubular cell releases NH_3 from glutamine which helps in maintaining acid-base balance via accepting H^+ from the urine and forming NH_4^+.
- Glutamine provides nitrogen for the formation of arginine, carbamoyl phosphate and purine nucleotide.

Aspartic Acid

- Nonessential
- A glucogenic amino acid.

Uses of Aspartic Acid

- Urea cycle
- Aspartate reacts with IMP to form an intermediate which is cleaved to AMP and fumarate during purine nucleotide biosynthesis.

▌ONE CARBON POOL

One carbon group plays a vital role in metabolism. Different groups containing one carbon are collectively known as one carbon group. They are:

1. Formyl group (–CHO)
2. Formimino group (–CH = NH)
3. Methyl group (–CH$_3$)
4. Methylene group (–CH$_2$–)
5. Methenyl group (= CH–)
6. Hydroxymethyl group (–CH$_2$OH)
7. Carbon dioxide (CO_2)

Source of One Carbon in One Carbon Pool

One carbon groups are contributed in one carbon pool by following amino acids:

1. **Serine (major contributor):** N5N10 methylene THFA
2. **Glycine:** N5N10 methylene THFA
3. **Histidine:** N5 formimino THFA
4. **Tryptophan:** N10 formyl THFA
5. **Choline:** N5 hydroxyl methyl THFA

- Serine is the major contributor of one carbon group
- Histidine during its catabolism produces FIGLU which reacts with THF to produce N5 formimino THFA which after deamination produces N5N10 methenyl THFA.
- Tryptophan and glycine produce formate which forms N10 formyl THF which may get converted to N5 formyl THF or N5N10 methylene THF.
- Choline, betain or epinephrine provide their methyl group to THF to form N5 methyl THF.

All these different one carbon groups are inter-convertible and finally they converge at methyl THFA (Fig. 21.17).

Utilization of One Carbon Group

One carbon units are used for the synthesis of following compounds:

1. C2 and C8 of purine
2. Synthesis of thymine base
3. Formylation of methionyl tRNA
4. Synthesis of serine from glycine
5. Synthesis of methionine from homocysteine by homocysteine methyltransferase enzyme
6. *Transmethylation reaction:* During synthesis of creatine, choline, epinephrine

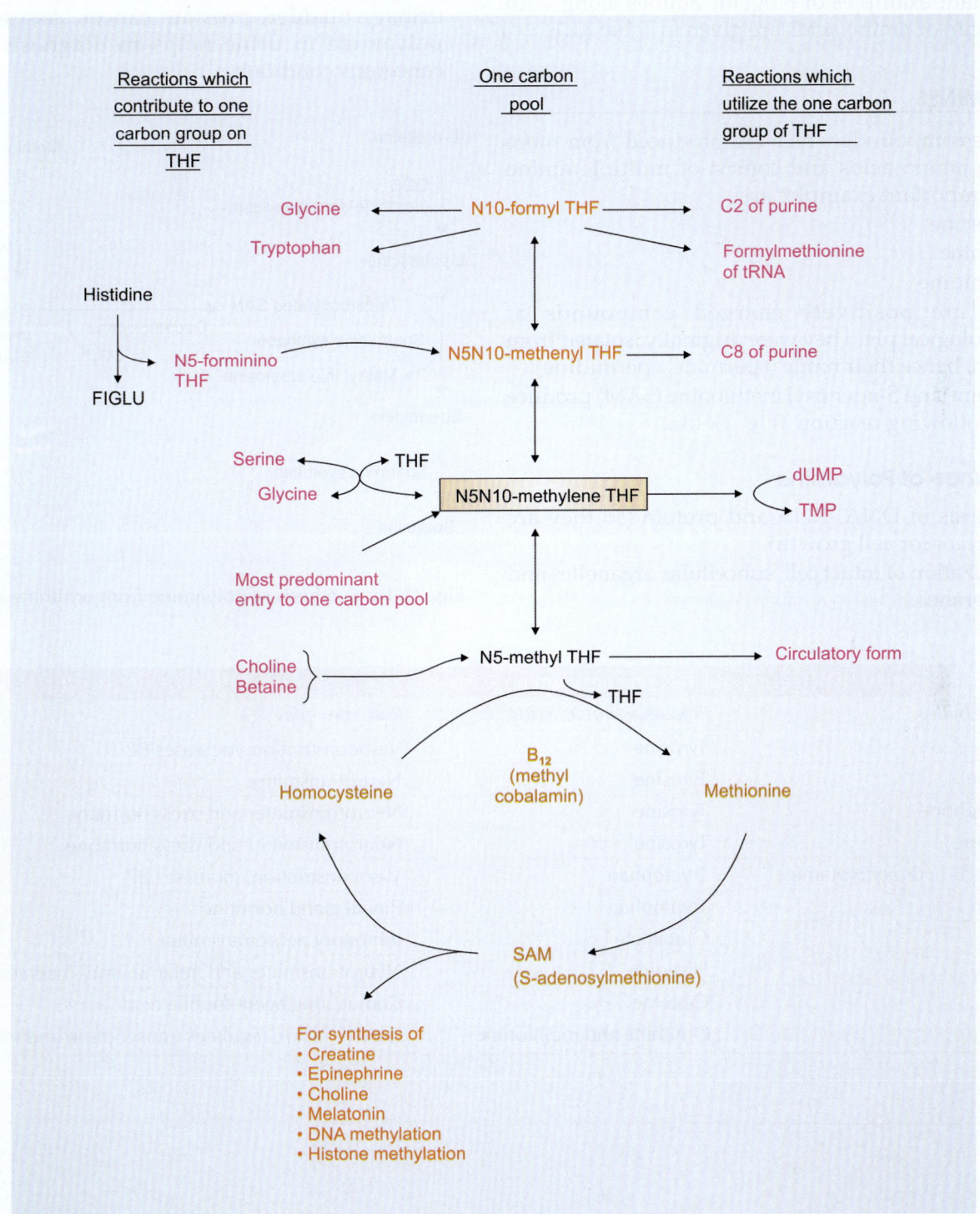

Fig. 21.17: One carbon metabolism

BIOGENIC AMINES

Biogenic amines are compounds of various significances which are produced by decarboxylation of amino acids.

Important examples of biogenic amines along with their precursor amino acids are given in Table 21.1.

POLYAMINES

These are compounds which are produced from more than one amino acids and consist of multiple amine groups. Important examples are:

1. Putrescine
2. Spermine
3. Spermidine
4. They are positively charged compounds at physiological pH. They were originally isolated from semen, hence their name (spermine, spermidine).

Ornithine and S-adenosyl methionine (SAM) produce them in following reaction (Fig. 21.18).

Significance of Polyamine

1. Synthesis of DNA, RNA and protein (so they are important for cell growth).
2. Stabilization of intact cell, subcellular organelles and membranes.

3. Clinical dose of polyamine have hypothermic and hypotensive effect.
4. Urinary excretion of polyamine increases many fold in various cancerous conditions like lung, kidney, urinary bladder, prostate cancer. Assessment of polyamine in urine helps in diagnosis of such cancerous condition.

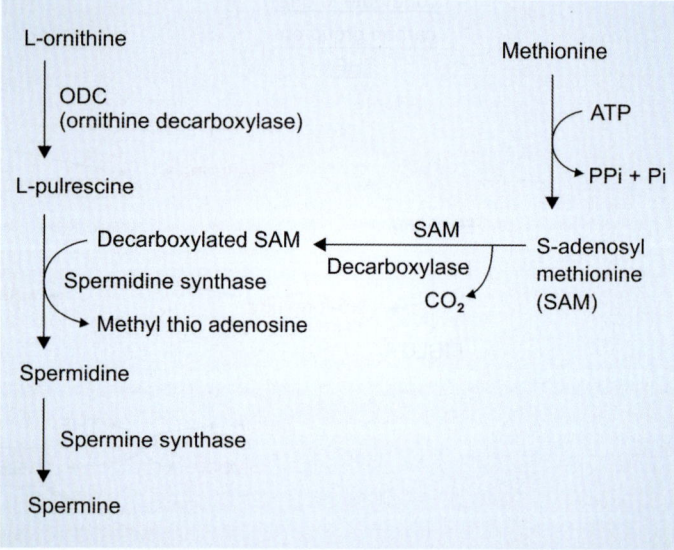

Fig. 21.18: Synthesis of polyamine from ornithine and SAM

TABLE 21.1	Biogenic amino acids and their precursor amino acids	
Biogenic amines	Precursor amino acids	Role they play
Tyramine	Tyrosine	Vasoconstriction, increases BP
Dopamine	Tyrosine	Neurotransmitter
Norepinephrine	Tyrosine	Neurotransmitter and stress hormone
Epinephrine	Tyrosine	Neurotransmitter and stress hormone
Serotonin (5-hydroxytryptamine)	Tryptophan	Vasoconstriction, increases BP
Melatonin	Tryptophan	Pineal gland hormone
GABA	Glutamate	Inhibitory neurotransmitter
Histamine	Histidine	Neurotransmitter and inflammatory mediator
Taurine	Cysteine	Conjugating agent for bile acid
Spermine	Ornithine and methionine	Growth factor, regulates transcription and translation

22

Aromatic Amino Acids

AROMATIC AMINO ACIDS

- Phenylalanine, tyrosine and tryptophan are aromatic amino acids. Out of these three amino acids, phenylalanine and tryptophan are essential and tyrosine is nonessential amino acid.
- All above three amino acids are both glucogenic and ketogenic.
- Derangement of metabolic pathways of these amino acids due to deficiency of certain enzymes results in important 'inborn error or metabolism' of clinical significance, highlighting the importance of learning of metabolic pathways of these amino acids.

PHENYLALANINE

Phenylalanine is an essential amino acid. Most of dietary phenylalanine is converted to tyrosine in human system in a biochemical reaction, where hydroxyl group is added the side chain benzene ring of phenylalanine, converting it to phenol (Fig. 22.1).

Reaction is catalyzed by phenylalanine hydroxylase which uses molecular oxygen and a source of hydrogen, 'tetrahydrobiopterin (THB)'.

THB is converted to dihydrobioptenin (DHB) which need to be reduced back to THB reducing equivalent of NADPH in presence of enzyme DHB reductase.

Phenylketonuria (PKU)

PKU is most common inborn error or metabolism (IEM) related to amino acid metabolism. It is an AR (autosomal recessive) disorder with incidence of 1 in 10,000 live births.

This diesease results due to defect of enzymes which are responsible for conversion of phenylalanine to tyrosine.

Most common type of PKU (PKU I, II, III) results due to deficiency of phenylalanine hydroxylase enzyme.

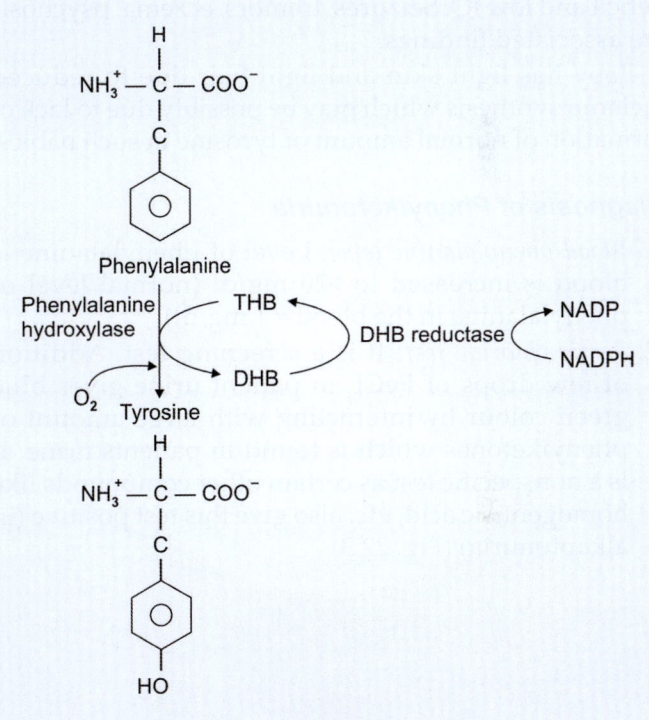

Fig. 22.1: Synthesis of tyrosine from phenylalanine

Less common type of PKU results due to deficiency of enzyme which affects the supply of THB, DHB reductase, and the deficiency of DHB synthase PKU V which reduces supply of DHB.

In case of deficiency of any of these enzymes, phenylalanine is nonconverted to tyrosine and adopts alternate route of its metabolism.

In alternate route of phenylalanine metabolism phenylalanine is converted to phenylpyruvate which may get converted to phenyllactate or phenylacetate (Fig. 22.2).

All these abnormal metabolites are phenylpyruvate, phenyllactate and phenylacetate which are excreted in the urine. Urine has characterisitic 'Mousy/Musty odour'. This odour is due to presence of phenylacetate.

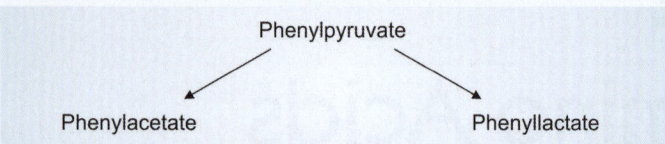

Fig. 22.2: Phenylketones

Clinical Presentation of PKU

Growth and mental retardation are seen. Increased phenylalanine and its metabolite result in neurological deficit and low IQ. Seizures, tremors, eczema, psychosis are associated findings.

Baby has light skin and light hair due to reduced melanin synthesis which may be possibly due to lack of formation of normal amount of tyrosine in such babies.

Diagnosis of Phenylketonuria

1. *Blood phenylalanine level:* Level of phenylalanine is blood is increased to >20 mg/dl (normal level of phenylalanine in the blood = 1 mg/dl)
2. *Ferric chloride test:* It is a screening test. Addition of few drops of FeCl₃ in patient urine gives blue green colour by interacting with large amount of phenylketones which is found in patients urine. It is a nonspecific test as certain other compounds like homogentisic acid, etc. also give this test positive (in alkaptonuria) (Fig. 22.3).

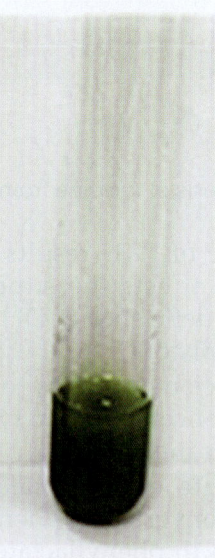

Fig. 22.3: FeCl₃ test

3. *Guthrie test:* This is a specific test to diagnose PKU.

Certain strain of *Bacillus subtilis* require phynylalanine for its growth. Addition of patient blood on media containing *Bacillus subtilis* spores, develop colonies of *Bacillus subtilis*, as the excess phenylalanine in patient blood help colonies to grow. Colonies are not formed if the blood does not contain excess phenylalanine (Fig. 22.4).

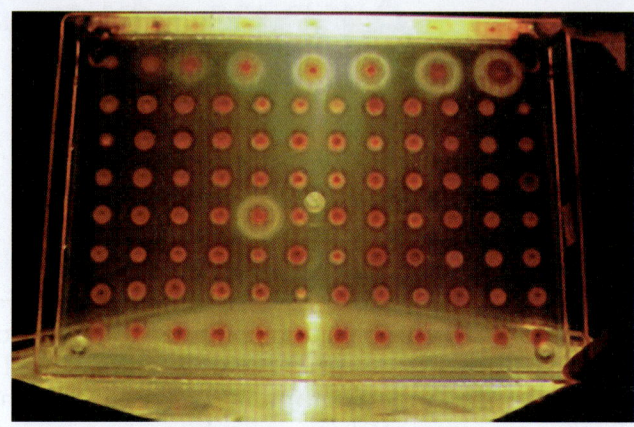

Fig. 22.4: Guthrie test

Treatment of PKU

Dietary treatment of PKU is started very early in life (within 10 days of birth) with restriction of phenylalanine in diet. Delay in starting the treatment results in irreversible loss of IQ. Dietary restriction of phenylalanine should be continued lifelong.

■ TYROSINE

Tyrosine is a nonessential amino acid, as it is synthesized from phenylalanine in above mentioned pathway (Fig. 22.1)

Tyrosine is the amino acid which produces number of biologically important compounds like:

1. Melanin
2. Catecholamines
3. Thyroid hormone

Synthesis of Melanin from Tyrosine

Melanin is a pigment which provides black colour to skin and hair. Melanin is synthesized in multistep process as described in Fig. 22.5.

As seen in Fig. 22.5, the only enzyme needed in melanin synthesis from tyrosine is 'tyrosinase'. Tyrosinase is a copper containing enzyme.

Clinical Correlation

Albinism: In this autosomal recessive disorder, there is mutation of tyrosinase gene resulting in absolute lack of synthesis of melanin. Melanin is totally absent from skin

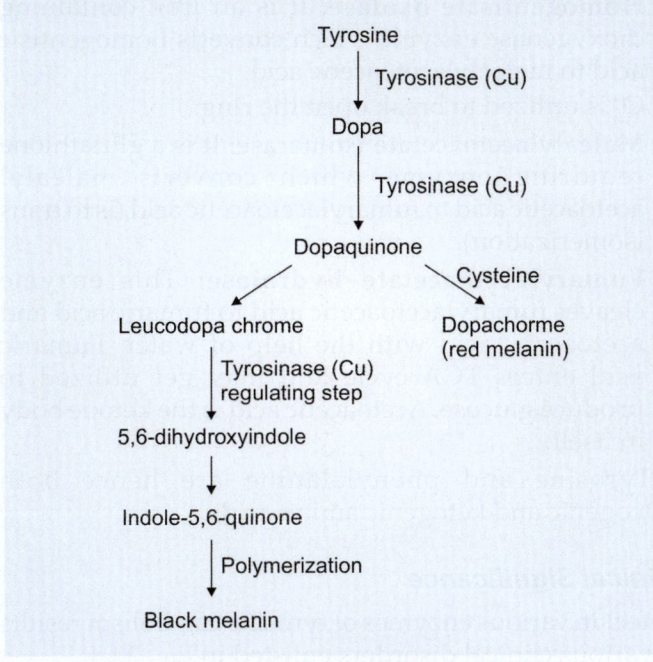

Fig. 22.5: Synthesis of melanin from tyrosine

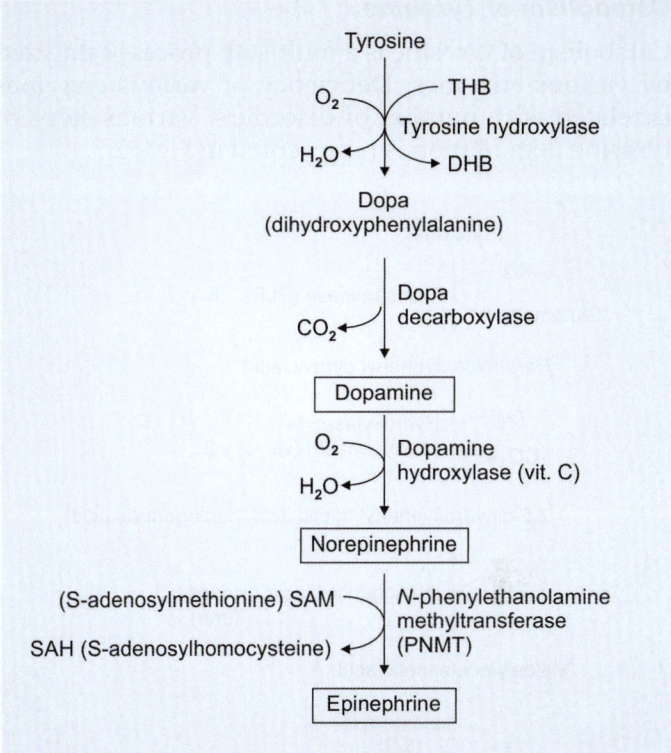

Fig. 22.6: Catecholamine synthesis from tyrosine

and hair which are characteristically white. Incidence is 1:20,000.

Leucoderma (vitiligo): It is an autoimmune disorder where autoantibodies are developed against melanoblast destroying them. So, that area of skin does not have melanin synthesis.

Copper deficiency: Cu is the cofactor for tyrosinase enzyme. In deficiency of Cu, either because of dietary deficiency or because of defect in Cu absorption from gastrointestinal tract (GIT) (Menke Kinky steely hair syndrome), melanin synthesis gets affected, resulting in graying of hair (flagging of hair in malnutrition and steely hair in Menke Kinky hair syndrome can be explained this fashion).

Synthesis of Catecholamine from Tyrosine

Important catecholamines are dopamine, epinephrine and norepinephrine. They all are synthesized from tyrosine. Pathway for synthesis of catecholamine is described below (Fig. 22.6).

Rate-limiting step during catecholamine synthesis is 'tyrosine hydroxylase'.

Pathway of catecholamine synthesis shows 'organ specific termination'.

In brain, the pathway stops at the level of dopamine synthesis and in adrenal medulla the pathway continues to produce norepinephrine and epinephrines.

Clinical Correlation

Parkinsonism

A neurological problem when patient shows symptoms like tremors, muscular rigidity, difficulty in initiating motor response is due to lack of dopamine synthesis in brain.

L-Dopa is administered, which upon entering the brain is converted to dopamine by Dopa decarboxylase enzyme and ameliorates and symptoms.

Phaeochromocytoma

In this adrenal gland tumor, there is excessive formation of catecholamine-epinephrine and norepinephrine.

Degradation of epinephrine and norepinephrine results in formation of vanillyl mandelic acid (VMA) which is excreted in urine and can be assessed.

VMA estimation in 24-hour collection urine helps in diagnosis of pheochrome cytoma.

2–6 mg of VMA in total 24 hours. Collection of urine is considered normal and amount exceeding 500 mg in 24-hour urine collection is seen in phaeochromocytoma.

Synthesis of Thyroid Hormone from Tyrosine

Thyroid hormone T_3 and T_4 are synthesized in thyroid globule.

Section 5 ■ Metabolism of Amino Acids

22

Catabolism of Tyrosine

Catabolism of tyrosine is a multistep process catalyzed by various enzymes. Deficiency of various enzymes is related with number of disorders. Various steps of tyrosine degradation is represented in Fig. 22.7.

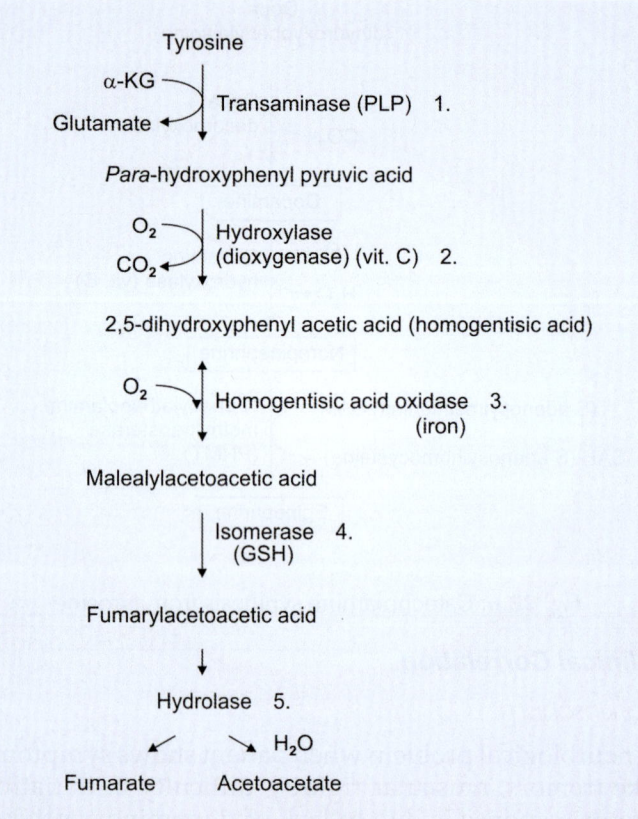

Fig. 22.7: Degradation of tyrosine

Steps of Tyrosine Degradation

1. *Tyrosine transaminase:* Tyrosine is transminated to produce *p*-hydroxyphenyl pyruvic acid. Tyrosine transaminase enzyme needs PLP (vit. B₆) (step 1).
2. *p-hydroxyphenyl pyruvic acid hydroxylase:* It is a Cu containing dioxygenase enzyme which catalyzes next reaction of tyrosine degradation (step 2). This step is a complex reaction involving number of biochemical changes like:
   * Oxidation
   * Decarboxylation
   * Migration of existing hydroxyl group from *para* to *meta* position (C2 position).
   * Incorporation of new hydroxyl group (C5 position)
     Vitamin C is required for above activities. This enzyme is dioxygenase as both the oxygen atoms are incorporated into product. One oxygen atom is incorporated in the hydroxyl group attached at C5 of ring. Another oxygen atom is incorporated in CO₂.

3. **Homogentisate oxidase:** It is an iron containing dioxygenase enzyme which converts homogentisic acid to malealylacetoacetic acid.
   O₂ is utilized to break open the ring.
4. **Malealylacetoacetate isomerase:** It is a glutathione requiring enzyme which converts malealyl acetoacetic acid to fumarylacetoacetic acid (is to trans isomerization).
5. **Fumarylacetoacetate hydrolase:** This enzyme cleaves fumarylacetoacetic acid to fumaric acid and acetoacetic acid with the help of water. Fumaric acid enters TCA cycle and may get utilized to produce glucose. Acetoacetic acid is the ketone body in itself.

   Tyrosine and phenylalanine are hence both glucogenic and ketogenic amino acids.

Clinical Significance

Defect in various enzymes of tyrosine catabolism results in various clinical disorders enlisted in Fig. 22.8.

Tyrosinemia Type II

* An autosomal recessive disorder
* An oculocutaneous disorder

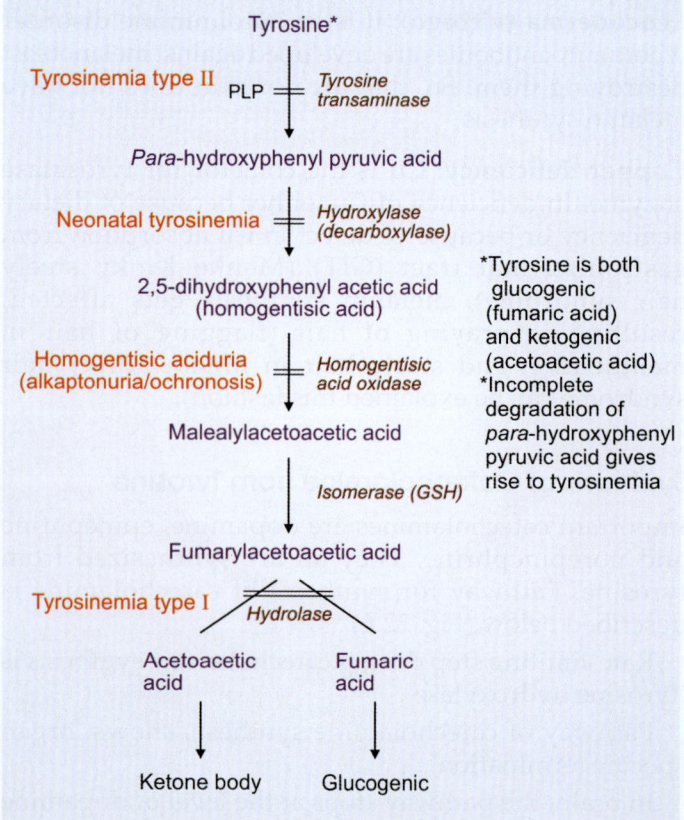

Fig. 22.8: Clinical disorders associated with tyrosine catabolism

Tyrosinemia Type I

* An autosomal recessive disorder
* A hepatorenal disorder

Tyrosinemia Type III

Also called neonatal tyrosinemia.

Alkaptonuria

* Due to deficiency of homogentisic acid oxidase enzyme.
* Urine shows characteristic black discolouration on exposure to atmospheric oxygen. Addition of alkali in the urine fasten the process of black discolouration of urine (Fig. 22.9).
* $FeCl_3$ test is positive (greenish blue colour)
* Disease characterized by back pain, arthritis, etc.

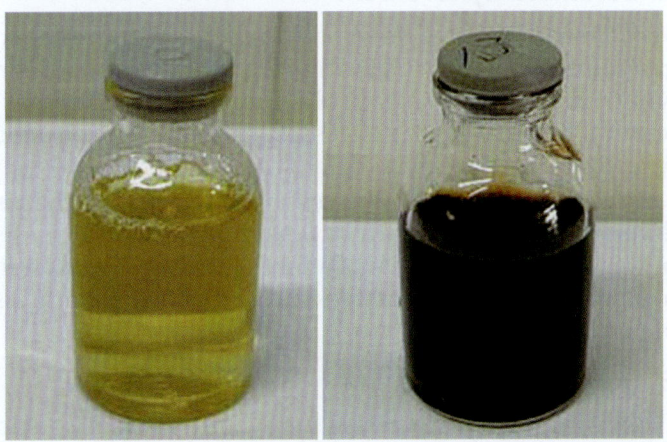

Fig. 22.9: Alkaptonuria

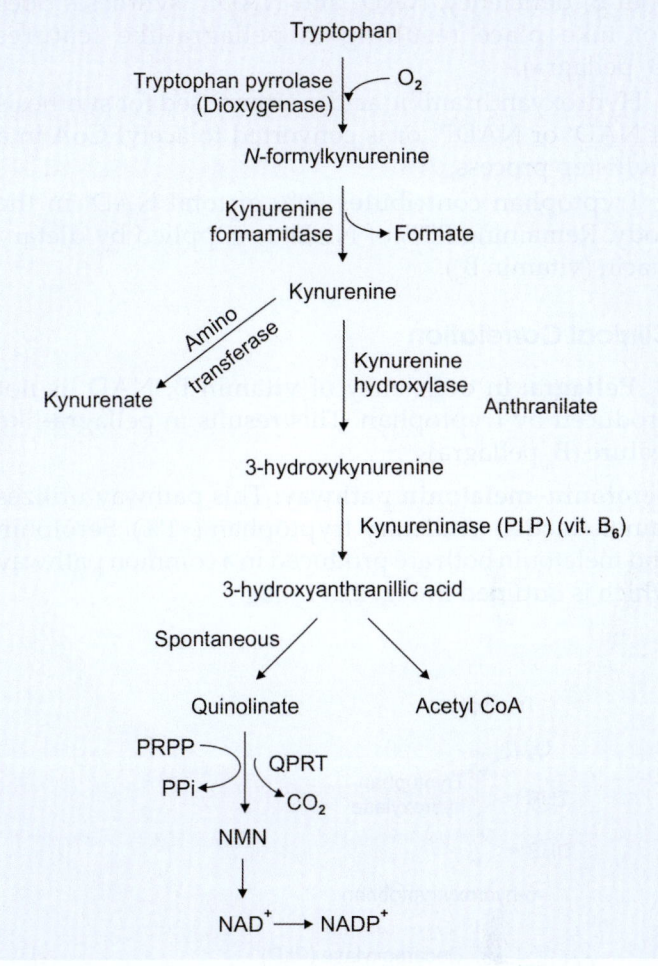

Fig. 22.10: Kynurenine pathway or NAD^+ pathway of tryptophan

■ TRYPTOPHAN

Tryptophan is an essential aromatic amino acid. Its side chain has an indole ring. Tryptophan is both glucogenic and ketogenic.

Important compounds which are produced from tryptophan are:

$$\left.\begin{array}{l} NAD^+ \\ NADP^+ \end{array}\right\} \text{In kynurenine–nicotinate pathway}$$

$$\left.\begin{array}{l} \text{Serotonin} \\ \text{Melatonin} \end{array}\right\} \text{In serotonin–melatonin pathway}$$

Major amount of dietary tryptophan is utilized in NAD^+ or $NADP^+$ formation. The pathway is called NAD^+ pathway or Kynurenine pathway or Major metabolic pathway of tryptophan.

Kynurenine–nicotinate pathway: Outline of this pathway is given in Fig. 22.10.

■ DESCRIPTION OF NAD⁺/KYNURENINE PATHWAY

Tryptophan pyrrolase is a dioxygenase which opens the indole ring and converts tryptophan to N-formyl kynurenine. Glucagon and cortisol induce tryptophan pyrrolase enzyme favouring catabolism of tryptophan.

Formamidase removes formate from formyl kynurenine to produce kynurenine. Kynureinine thus produced is predominantly hydroxylated to produce hydroxykynurenine.

Hydroxykynurenine is converted to hydroxy anthranilic acid by enzyme kynureninase (PLP dependent). Alanine is produced in this reaction which is glucogenic.

In deficiency of PLP, kynureninase enzyme does not work, resulting in excess hydroxykynurenine which is diverted to alternate route to produce xantheurenic acid.

Xantheurenic acid is a nontoxic metabolite which gets excreted in urine in patients having B_6 deficiency.

Section 5 ■ Metabolism of Amino Acids

22

In B_6 deficiency, NAD$^+$ and NADP$^+$ synthesis does not take place resulting in pellagra-like features (B_6 pellagra).

Hydroxyanthranillic acid is either used for synthesis of NAD$^+$ or NADP$^+$ or is converted to acetyl CoA in a multistep process.

Tryptophan contributes 50% of total NAD$^+$ in the body. Remaining 50% of NAD$^+$ is supplied by dietary niacin (vitamin B_3).

Clinical Correlation

B_6 Pellagra: In deficiency of vitamin B, NAD$^+$ is not produced by tryptophan. This results in pellagra-like feature (B_6 pellagra).

Serotonin–melatonin pathway: This pathway utilizes minor fraction of dietary tryptophan (~1%). Serotonin and melatonin both are produced in a common pathway which is outlined in Fig. 22.11.

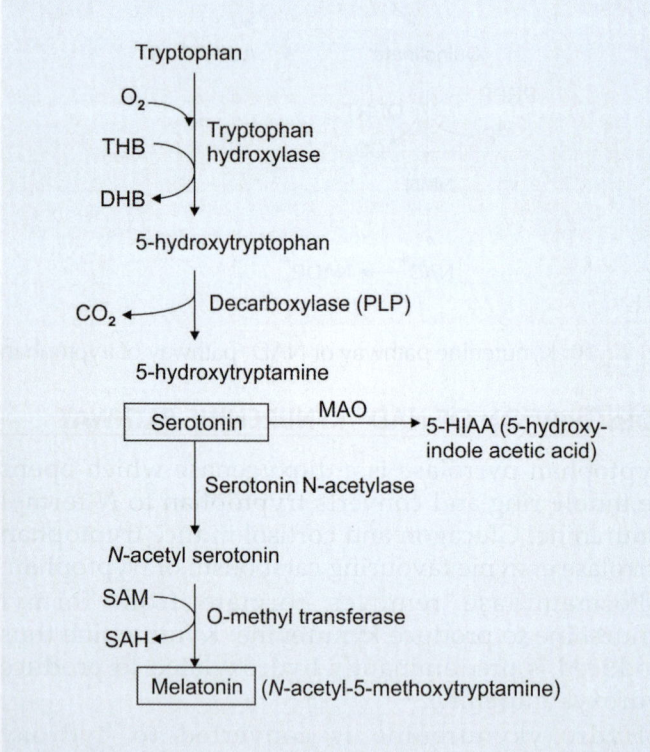

Fig. 22.11: Serotonin/melatonin pathway of tryptophan

DESCRIPTION OF SEROTONIN/MELATONIN PATHWAY

Serotonin is a neurotransmitter distributed in platelet, GIT, retina and brain.

Tryptophan is hydroxylated by tryptophan hydroxylase enzyme with the requirement of tetrahydrobiopterin (THB). Resulting 5-hydroxy-tryptophan is undergoing decarboxylation to produce 5-hydroxytryptamine (serotonin).

Mono amino oxidase (MAO) enzyme acts on scrotonin and converts it to 5-hydroxy indole acetic acid (5HIAA) which is excreted in urine.

Melatonin is a pineal gland hormone which is produced from serotonin by N-acetylation and then methylation by S-adenosylmethionine.

Clinical Correlation

A. Carcinoid Syndrome

Serotonin is produced by argentaffin cells in gastrointestinal tract (GIT). In a rare malignant condition where argentaffin cells proliferate (argentaffinomas) (carcinoid syndrome) excess serotonin is produced resulting in excess level of 5HIAA.

In carcinoid syndrome excess of dietary tryptophan is diverted to serotonin pathway resulting in less synthesis of NAD$^+$ from tryptophan. Patient with this condition so has pellagra-like manifestation due to lack of synthesis of NAD$^+$ from tryptophan.

B. Hartrup's Disease

This is an AR disorder, where neutral amino acid transporter is mutated in gastrointestinal tract (GIT) and kidney tubules.

This results in loss of neutral amino acid from gastro-intestinal tract (GIT) and kidney tubules.

Due to decreased level of tryptophan, patient has pellagra-like features as tryptophan is not available for synthesis of NAD$^+$.

Unabsorbed tryptophan in intestinal lumen is acted upon by intestinal bacteria which convert tryptophan to indole compounds. Indole compounds are absorbed in blood and are filtered in urine. Baby diaper turns blue due to presence of these indole compounds. These indole compounds in urine can be detected by 'Obermeyer test'.

EXERCISE

LONG QUESTIONS (10 MARKS EACH)

Q 1. How is melanin synthesized from tyrosine? Name the disease and the biochemical defect associated with their formation.

Q 2. Describe the steps involved in synthesis of various catecholamines from tyrosine.

Q 3. Discuss the various mechanisms of ammonia transport and outline the reactions of urea cycle.

Q 4. Name the inborn errors of metabolism in phenylalanine pathway and mention the enzyme which is missing in each case.

Q 5. How is ammonia detoxified in brain ? How is it different from the detoxication of ammonia in liver?

SHORT NOTES (5 MARKS EACH)

Q 1. Urea cycle disorder

Q 2. Homocysteinuria

Q 3. Specilized products of tyrosine

Q 4. Inborn errors of sulphur containing amino acids

Q 5. Various specialized products synthesized from tryptophan

Q 6. A typical transamination reaction

Q 7. Ammonia transportation

Q 8. Oxidative transdeamination

SHORT NOTES (2.5 MARKS EACH)

Q 1. Phenylketonuria

Q 2. Essential amino acids

Q 3. Semi-essential amino acids

Q 4. Alkaptonuria

Q 5. Vanillyl mandelic acid (VMA)

Q 6. Cysteine as nonessential amino acid

Q 7. Important product from glycine

Q 8. Tyrosinosis

Q 9. Zwitter ion

Q 10. Glycine

Q 11. Polyamines

Section 5 ■ Metabolism of Amino Acids

22

MULTIPLE CHOICE QUESTIONS

22.1 A 2 years old male child is brought with pellagra-like symptoms and dermatitis. Elder sister has similar symptoms. Two siblings are normal. Most likely diagnosis is:
a. Tyrosinemia
b. Alkaptonuria
c. PKU
d. Hartnup's disorder

22.2 Tryptophan load test helps in the evaluation of deficiency of which vitamin?
a. Folic acid
b. Niacinamide
c. Pyriodoxine
d. Cyanocobolamine

22.3 Amino acid producing ammonia in kidney is:
a. Glutamine
b. Alanine
c. Methionine
d. Glycine

22.4 S-adenosylmethionine (SAM) serves as the methylating agent for each of the following, except:
a. The conversion of norepinephrine to epinephrine
b. The synthesis of creatine from guanidinoacetate
c. The synthesis of phosphatidylcholine from phosphatidylethanolamine
d. The conversion of dUMP to dTMP

22.5 Which of these amino acids does not enter the Krebs' cycle by forming acetyl CoA via pyruvate?
a. Tyrosine
b. Hydroxyproline
c. Glycine
d. Alanine

22.6 For metabolic disorder of urea cycle, which statement is not correct?
a. Ammonia intoxication is most severe when the metabolic block in the urea cycle occurs prior to the reaction catalyzed by arginosuccinate synthase.
b. Clinical symptoms include mental retardation and the avoidance of protein rich foods.
c. Clinical signs can include acidosis.
d. Aspartate provides the second nitrogen of arginine succinate.

22.7 Hyperammonemia blocks which phase of Krebs' cycle?
a. Malate dehydrogenase
b. Isocitrate dehydrogenase
c. α-ketoglutarate dehydrogenase
d. Succinate dehydrogenase

22.8 Precipitation of proteins is done by all these, except:
a. Salts of heavy metals
b. Adding trichloroacetic acid
c. Adding acetyl alcohol and acetone
d. Adjusting pH to other than the isoelectric point

22.9 In the synthesis of collagen, the hydroxylation of proline and lysine occurs in which of the following?
a. Golgi apparatus
b. Secretory vesicles
c. Rough endoplasmic reticulum
d. Smooth endoplasmic reticulum

22.10 Transmembrane region of a protein is likely to have:
a. A stretch of hydrophilic amino acids
b. A stretch of hydrophobic amino acids
c. A disulphide loop
d. Alternating hydrophilic and hydrophobic amino acids

22.11 In collagen synthesis, hydroxyproline is formed from:
a. Proline
b. Lysine
c. Hydroxylysine
d. None of the above

22.12 Chaperones are:
a. Mediators of the post-translational protein complexes
b. Antigen presenting cells
c. Purine metabolism mediators
d. None of the above

22.13 Sickling in HbS disease is primarily caused by:
a. Decreased solubility
b. Decreased stability
c. Altered function
d. Altered O_2 binding capacity

22.14 Which of the following is not used for protein estimation?
a. Biuret method
b. Barfoed method
c. Lowry's method
d. Bromocresol green method

22.15 Glycoproteins may have protein linked to the carbohydrate moiety through any of the following bonds:
a. O-glycosidic linkage
b. N-glycosidic linkage
c. GPI linkage
d. Either O- or N-glycosidic linkage

22.16 Myoglobin:
a. Contains four heme per molecule
b. Shows the Bohr effect
c. Has an O_2 dissociation curve that is unaffected by wide range of pH
d. None of the above

22.17 Quaternary structure of protein is:
a. The arrangement sequence of amino acids in the polypeptide chain
b. Interrelation between amino acids in a single polypeptide chain
c. Interrelation and arrangement of polypeptides in a protein with more than 2 polypeptide chain
d. None of the above

22.18 Alpha-helix and beta-pleated sheet are examples of:
a. Primary structure
b. Tertiary structure
c. Secondary structure
d. Quaternary structure

22.19 Which among the following amino acids absorbs UV light?
a. Leucine
b. Lysine
c. Tyrosine
d. Valine

22.20 All are true about glutathione, except:
a. It is a tripeptide.
b. It converts hemoglobin to methemoglobin .
c. It conjugates xenobiotics.
d. It is a cofactor of various enzymes.

22.21 Amino acid residue having imino side chain is:
a. Lysine
b. Histidine
c. Tyrosine
d. Proline

22.22 Catecholamines:
a. Production terminates with dopamine in the brain but epinephrine in the adrenal gland
b. Production begins with the action of tyrosinase on tyrosine
c. Are metabolized to both glucogenic and ketogenic fragments
d. All contain methyl group donated by S-adenosylmethionine

22.23 In Hartnup's disease .... is excreted in the urine.
a. Ornithine
b. Glycine
c. Tryptophan
d. Phenylalanine

22.24 The rationale for feeding benzoic acids to subjects with an urea cycle enzyme defect is:
a. It provides an alternative route for N_2 excretion through glycine conjugate, hippuric acid.
b. It provides an alternative route for N_2 excretion through the N-acetyl glucuronic acid conjugate kynurenine.
c. It inhibits adenylate deaminase.
d. It inhibits glutamate dehydrogenase.
e. It neutralizes NH_3 in both blood as well as urine.

22.25 Tyrosinemia type II is due to deficiency of:
a. Tyrosine transaminase
b. Fumarylacetoacetyl hydrolase
c. Tyrosine hydroxylase
d. Tyrosinase

Section 5 ■ Metabolism of Amino Acids

22

ANSWERS

22.1 (d) Hartnup's disorder

Neutral amino acids absorption from kidney tubules and GIT is effected in Harnup's disease. This results in decreased availability of tryptophan for niacin synthesis. This manifests as pellagra-like symptoms.

22.2 (c) Pyriodoxine

Kynureninase enzyme requires PLP for its action. To detect the latent deficiency of vitamin B$_6$ tryptophan load test is done.

22.3 (a) Glutamine

Kidney is involved in buffering. Ammonia is important in buffering action of the kidney. Source of this ammonia is the glutamine. Glutaminase is the enzyme which removes ammonia from the glutamine and this ammonia is used in buffering action.

22.4 (d) The conversion of dUMP to dTMP

Tetrahydrofolate is involved in the conversion of dUMP to dTMP.

Rest all the reactions given in options a, b and c need methyl group, the donor of which is the S-adenosyl-methionine (SAM).

22.5 (a) Tyrosine

Following amino acids enter TCA cycle via giving acetyl CoA:

- Tryptophan
- Alanine
- Hydroxyproline
- Serine
- Cysteine
- Threonine
- Glycine

22.6 (d) Aspartate provides the second nitrogen of arginine succinate.

In urea cycle disorder there is respiratory alkalosis. True statements regarding urea cycle disorder are :
- Ammonia intoxication is most severe when the metabolic block in the urea cycle occurs prior to the reaction catalyzed by arginosuccinate synthase.
- Clinical symptoms include mental retardation and the avoidance of protein rich foods.
- Aspartate provides the second nitrogen of arginine succinate.

22.7 (c) α-ketoglutarate dehydrogenase

Ammonia binds with α-ketoglutarate dehydrogenase of TCA cycle and converts it to glutamate. This removes α-ketoglutarate dehydrogenase from the TCA cycle and inhibits this pathway. This is the biochemical explanation for the hepatic encephalopathy.

22.8 (d) Adjusting pH to other than the isoelectric point.

At pH other than isoelectric pH, proteins are either positively or negatively charged which makes it soluble.

Methods to precipitate the proteins are as follows:
- Neutralization of charge of protein (isoelectric pH)
- Removal of shell of hydration (alcohol or acetone)

22.9 (c) Rough endoplasmic reticulum

- Prolyl and lysyl hydroxylase are the two enzymes that carry out hydroxylation of proline and lysine.
- The process is both co- and post-translational and, therefore, occurs during, or more often after, the amino acids are inserted into nascent collagen polypeptide chains in the RER.
- Hydroxyproline, which constitutes 10% of collagen, is often used to determine the collagen content of various tissues.
- Hydroxylation of proline stabilizes the triple helix through interchain hydrogen bonds, and hydroxylation of lysine is critical for the cross-linking stage of collagen assembly.

22.10 (b) A stretch of hydrophobic amino acids

22.11 (a) Proline

During collagen formation, proline is hydroxylated in position 4 (when situated at the amino-side of the glycine) or in position 3 (when situated at the carboxy-side of the glycine). Lysine is hydroxylated in position 5.

22.12 (a) Mediators of the post-translational protein complexes

- Chaperones are proteins that assist the noncovalent folding/unfolding and the assembly/disassembly of other macromolecular structures.
- Molecular chaperone' was invented by Ron Laskey to describe the ability of a nuclear protein called nucleoplasmin to prevent the aggregation of folded

histone proteins with DNA during the assembly of nucleosomes.

- The term was later extended by John Ellis in 1987 to describe proteins that mediated the post-translational assembly of protein complexes.
- Many chaperones are heat shock proteins, that is, proteins expressed in response to elevated temperatures of other cellular stresses.

22.13 (a) Decreased solubility

Replacement of a polar amino acid (glutamic acid) with a nonpolar amino acid (valine) results in decreased solubility of HbS.

HbC and HbD are other hemoglobins which show decreased solubility.

22.14 (b) Barfoed method

Barfoed test is done to differentiate monosaccharide from disaccharide and thus it is a carbohydrate test. Monosaccharide gives red precipitate with this test.

Biuret, Lowry's, BCG (bromocresol green) are methods to estimate (quantitate) the protein.

22.15 (d) Either O- or N-glycosidic linkage

O-glycosylation occurs between OH group of the amino acid and oligosaccharide, while N-glycosylation occurs between amino group of the amino acid and an oligosaccharide chain.

Serine, threonine and hydroxylysine are OH group containing amino acids which get attached with the oligosaccharide chain with the help of O-glycosidic linkage.

Asparagine is an amide group containing amino acid which gets attached with the oligosaccharide chain with the help of N-glycosidic linkage.

22.16 (c) Has an O_2 dissociation curve that is unaffected by wide range of pH

22.17 (c) Interrelation and arrangement of polypeptides in a protein with more than 2-polypeptide chain

22.18 (c) Secondary structure

22.19 (c) Tyrosine

Amino acids which absorb 250–290 nm UV light are:
- Tryptophan
- Tyrosine
- Phenylalanine

(In decreasing order of extent of absorbtion of UV light).

22.20 (b) It converts hemoglobin to methemoglobin

- Glutathione is a tripeptide (γ-glutamyl-cysteinyl-glycine)
- It helps in conjugation reaction
- It is a cofactor of various enzymes

Its reduced form is necessary for converting methemoglobin to hemoglobin.

(Not the hemoglobin to methemoglobin)

22.21 (d) Proline

The side chain of the proline makes **pyrrolidine ring** structure with the imino group.

22.22 (a) Production terminates with dopamine in the brain but epinephrine in the adrenal gland

- Synthesis of catecholamine is organ specific, so option a is correct.
- Production of catecholamine begins once tyrosine hydroxylase enzyme acts on tyrosine and forms dopa, so option b is wrong. (Tyrosinase action on tyrosine which forms dopa synthesizes melanin.)
- All catecholamines are metabolized to vanillylmandelic acid (VMA) which gets excreted in urine unchanged. VMA has neither glucogenic nor ketogenic fate. So, option c is also wrong.
- Out of various catecholamines, only epinephrine has one methyl group. Dopamine and norepinephrine do not contain any methyl group. So, option d is also wrong.

22.23 (c) Tryptophan

22.24 (a) It provides an alternative route for N_2 excretion through glycine conjugate, hippuric acid

22.25 (a) Tyrosine transaminase

Section 5 ■ Metabolism of Amino Acids

22

Integrated Pathways

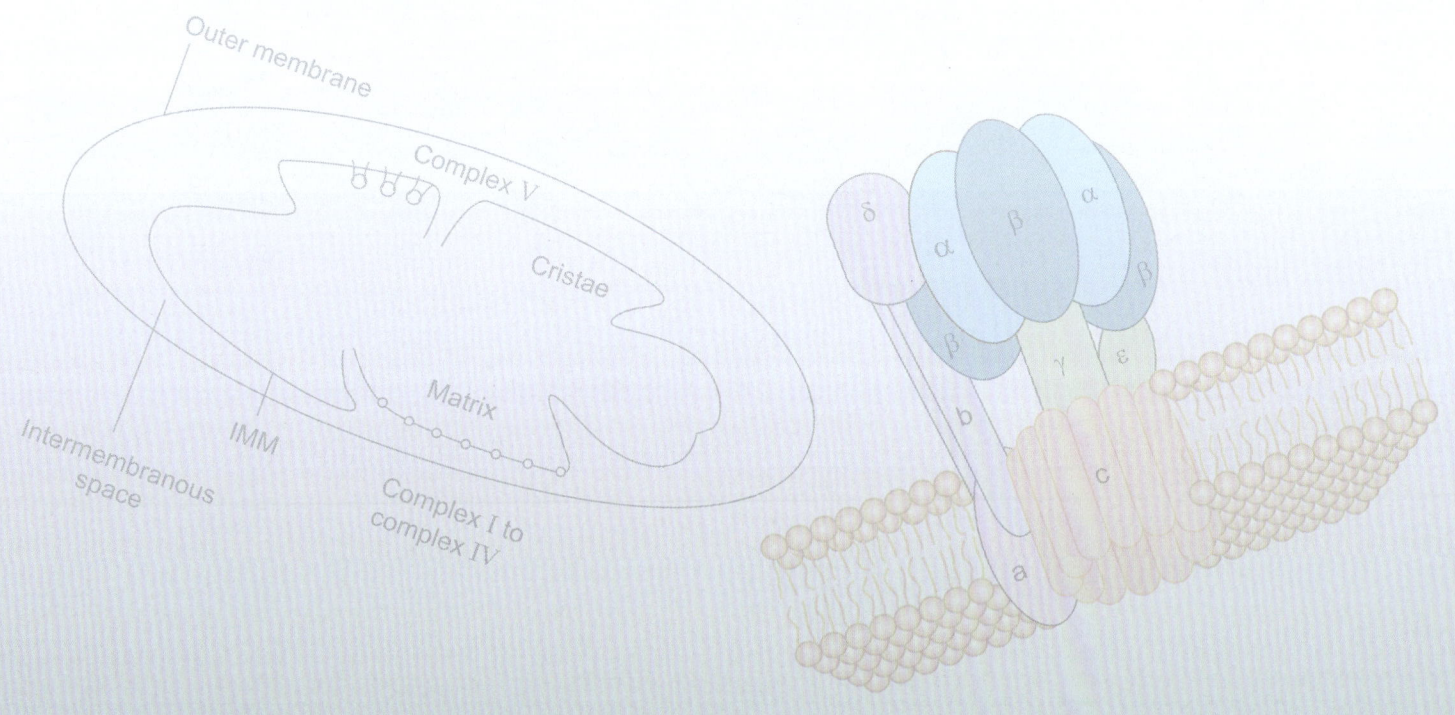

5

Integrated Pathways

23

TCA Cycle

COMPETENCY BI 3.6

Specific Learning Objectives

BI 3.6.1 Discuss the steps of TCA cycle with special emphasis on rate limiting step.

BI 3.6.2 Explain the amphibolic role of TCA cycle.

CITRIC ACID CYCLE/KREBS' CYCLE OR TCA (TRICARBOXYLIC ACID) CYCLE

Definition: It is a series of enzyme catalyzed reactions that form a common pathway for final oxidation of all metabolic fuels (carbohydrate, free fatty acids, ketone bodies and amino acids).

Location: Mitochondrial matrix.

Reactions of TCA cycle: *See* Fig. 23.1

TCA cycle is an aerobic pathway as the reduced coenzyme NADH and $FADH_2$ generated during this cycle needs O_2 molecule in ETC for their oxidation, which generates ATP and converts them to NAD^+ and FAD respectively which continue the TCA cycle.

Bioenergetics: One molecule of acetyl CoA produces 10 ATP in a complete turn of citric acid cycle. One glucose molecule which produces 2 pyruvate and thus 2 acetyl CoA produces 20 ATP in the TCA cycle (Table 23.1).

Anaplerotic reactions: Reactions providing the intermediates of the TCA cycle are known as anaplerotic reactions. As these reactions supply the intermediate of TCA cycle, they are also known as filling up reactions. Important examples are (Fig. 23.2):

TABLE 23.1	ATP calculation in TCA cycle (one acetyl CoA produces 10 ATP in TCA cycle)	
Step catalysed by	*Gain from 1 acetyl CoA*	*ATP*
Isocitrate dehydrogenase (ICD)	1 NADH	2.5 ATP
α-ketoglutarate dehydrogenase (α-KGD)	1 NADH	2.5 ATP
Succinate thiokinase	1 ATP	1 ATP
Succinate dehydrogenase (SCD)	1 $FADH_2$	1.5 ATP
Malate dehydrogenase	1 NADH	2.5 ATP
Total	–	**10 ATP**

1. Formation of oxalo acetate (OAA) from pyruvate.

$$Pyruvate \xrightarrow[carboxylase]{Pyruvate} OAA \rightarrow TCA\ cycle$$

2. Propionyl CoA $\rightarrow\rightarrow\rightarrow$ Succinyl CoA

3. Phenylalanine
   Tyrosine $\longrightarrow$ Fumarate

Out of above list, the most important anaplerotic reaction is pyruvate carboxylase reaction which converts pyruvate to oxaloacetate.

Cataplerotic reactions: Reactions which utilize TCA intermediate to non-TCA reactions and divert them, are known as cataplerotic reactions.

These reactions are also known as emptying reactions as they vacate TCA of its intermediate.

Important examples are:

1. Diversion of succinyl CoA to heme synthesis:

$$Succinyl\ CoA + Glycine \xrightarrow{ALA\ synthase}$$
$$Amino\ levullinic\ acid \rightarrow Heme$$

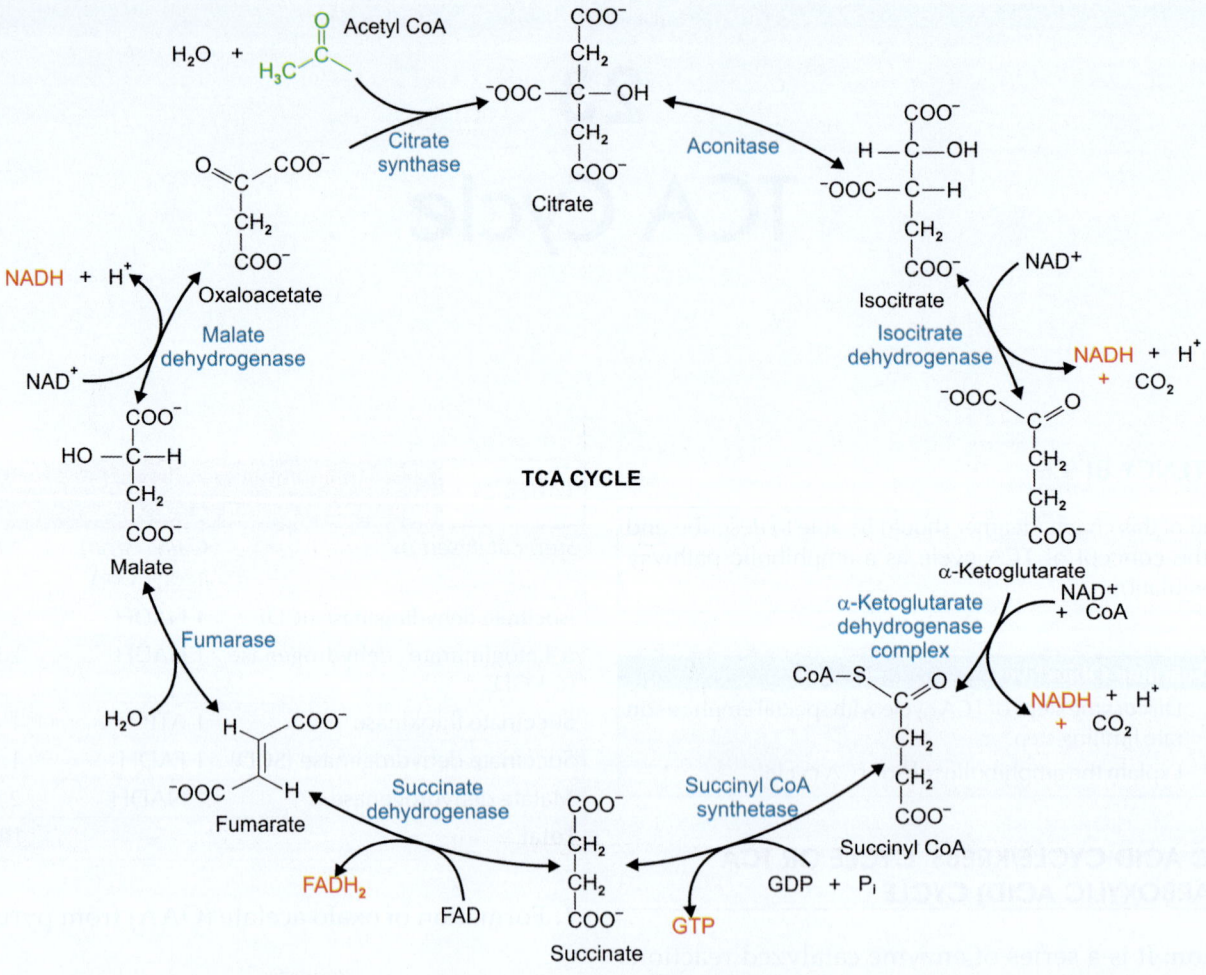

Fig. 23.1: TCA cycle/Krebs' cycle

2. Diversion of citrate to fatty acid:

$$\text{Citrate} \xrightarrow[\text{Lyase}]{\text{ATP citrate}} \text{OAA + Acetyl CoA}$$

$$\downarrow$$

$$\text{Fatty acid}$$

3. Diversion of citrate to cholesterol synthesis:

$$\text{Citrate} \xrightarrow[\text{Lyase}]{\text{ATP citrate}} \text{OAA + Acetyl CoA}$$

$$\downarrow$$

$$\text{Cholesterol}$$

4. Diversion of α-ketoglutarate in transamination reactions.

α-ketoglutarate + Amino acid →

Glutamate + α- keto acid

TCA cycle is an amphibolic pathway, as its reactions are involved both in catabolic and anabolic reactions.

Regulation of TCA Cycle (Table 23.2)

Enzymes which are regulatory in TCA cycle are:
1. Citrate synthase
2. Isocitrate dehydrogenase (ICD)
3. α-ketoglutarate dehydrogenase

Following are the positive and negative allosteric modifiers for these enzymes.

TABLE 23.2	TCA cycle regulators	
Enzyme	Positive allosteric modifier	Negative allosteric modifier
Citrate synthase	ADP	ATP NADH Succinyl CoA Acyl CoA (LCFA)
Isocitrate dehydrogenase	Ca++ ADP	ATP NADH
α-ketoglutarate dehydrogenase	Ca++	ATP NADH Succinyl CoA

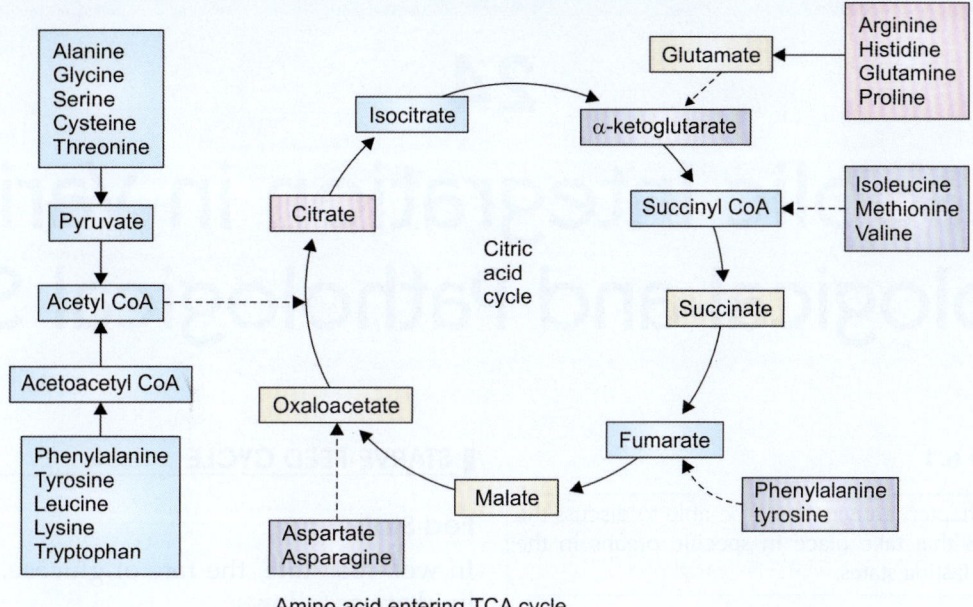

Fig. 23.2: Amino acid entering TCA cycle by providing various intermediates of TCA cycle

Kindly note that energy abundant state in the cell (NADH, ATP) has negative allosteric effect and energy deficient state in the cell (ADP) has positive allosteric effect on TCA cycle regulatory enzymes.

Inhibitors of TCA cycle

1. Fluoroacetate inhibits aconitase enzyme.
2. Arsenite inhibits α-ketoglutarate dehydrogenase.
3. Malonate inhibits succinate dehydrogenase enzyme.

Metabolic Integration in Various Physiological and Pathological States

COMPETENCY BI 6.1

At the end of this chapter learner should be able to discuss the metabolic processes that take place in specific organs in the body in the fed and fasting states.

Specific Learning Objectives	
BI 6.1.1	Discuss the metabolism of adipose cell in fed and fasting state.
BI 6.1.2	Discuss the metabolism of liver in fed and fasting state.
BI 6.1.3	Discuss the metabolism of heart in fed and fasting state.
BI 6.1.4	Discuss the metabolism of brain in fed and fasting state.

There are number of metabolic pathways in a biochemical system. For example:
- Glycolysis
- Fatty acid synthesis
- Glycogenesis
- Glycogenolysis
- Fatty acid oxidation
- Ketogenesis/ketolysis
- TCA cycle
- Protein synthesis
- Proteolysis
- Urea synthesis, etc.

It is important to have a clear idea of following:
1. In which tissues these pathways occur predominantly?
2. When are these pathways most active?
3. How are these pathways regulated in different metabolic states and diseased condition?

It is important to learn starve-feed cycle to understand the interrelation of various organs.

STARVE-FEED CYCLE

Fed State

In well-fed state, the fate of glucose, amino acid and lipid are as follows:

Glucose

Glucose gets absorbed from gastrointestinal tract lumen to portal blood and reaches liver (Fig. 24.1).

Liver: In liver glucose is either converted to glycogen for later use, or is undergoing glycolysis to generate ATP.

Some amount of glucose in liver is used in pentose phosphate pathway for NADPH production, which is required for reductive biosynthesis like fatty acid synthesis, etc.

Much amount of glucose passes through the liver to reach other organs where it is utilized for various purpose. For example in:

Brain: Glycolysis

Muscle: Glycogenesis, glycolysis

RBC: For glycolysis

Renal medulla: Glycolysis

Adipose cells: Glucose is primarily converted to glycerol which is required for triacylglycerol synthesis.

In well-fed state Cori cycle (glucose → lactate in peripheral tissue and lactate → glucose in liver) is interrupted as during well-fed state, liver is involved in glycolysis rather than gluconeogenesis.

Amino Acid

Fate of dietary amino acid is that some of it is utilized by gastrointestinal tract cells, but majority of it is send to portal blood by which it reaches the liver. Liver utilizes some of these amino acid, but majority of it is passed to

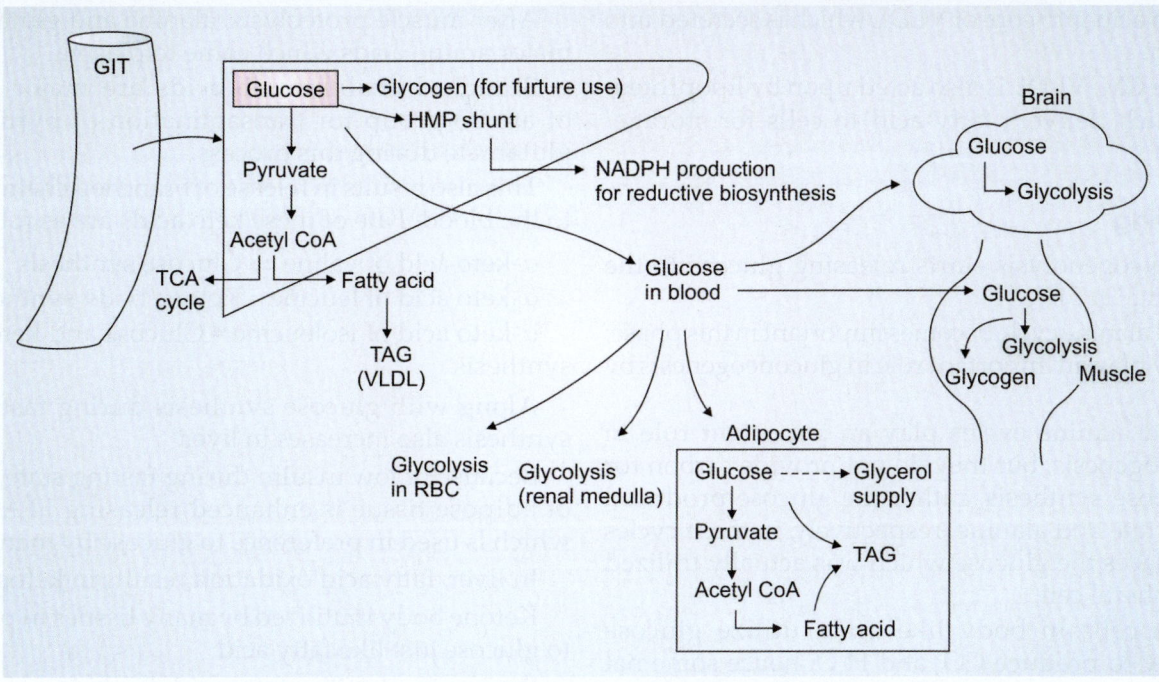

Fig. 24.1: Fate of dietary glucose in well-fed state

other tissues. It is specially true for essential amino acids as they are very much required to be supplied to tissues for protein synthesis (Fig. 24.2).

Liver: Though the liver catabolise the amino acid, the K_m of enzyme needed for such catabolism is quite high which means that excess of amino acid is required for their liver catabolism.

Liver uses excess amino acid to convert them to CO_2, urea, H_2O or intermediate for lipogenesis.

Other tissues: Amino acid which escapes liver and reaches other tissues is utilized either for protein synthesis or is utilized for energy production (Fig. 24.2).

Lipid

Dietary triacylglycerol reaches the blood stream directly from gastrointestinal tract via lymphatics in the form of chylomicron.

Lipoprotein lipase present on the wall of capillary endothelium acts upon chylomicron to release free fatty acid from its core TAG. Fatty acid is delivered to respective tissue and leftover chylomicron which is now known as 'CM remnant' remains in circulation.

Adipose tissue capillary is specially having rich amount of lipoprotein lipase, hence major amount of dietary fatty acid and is given here.

This fatty acid is re-esterified with glycerol-3-phosphate to produce TAG, which is stored as lipid droplet within the adipocyte.

Liver clears chylomicron remnant particles from circulation. In liver, lysosomal lipase hydrolyzes TAG of chylomicron remnant and utilises its fatty acid for re-esterification with glycerol-3-phoshate to form triacylglycerol.

Liver pack this TAG and also smaller amount of TAG produced by *de novo* fatty acid synthesis from glucose

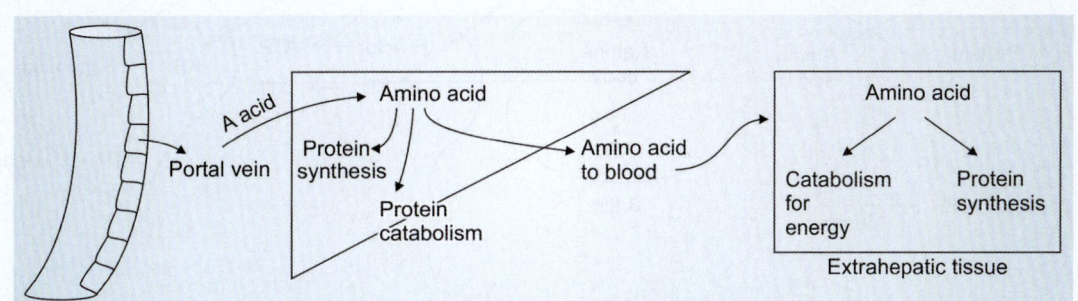

Fig. 24.2: Fate of dietary amino acid in well-fed state

Section 6 ■ Integrated Pathways

24

and amino acid into core of VLDL which is secreted into circulation.

Just like CM, VLDL is also acted upon by lipoprotein lipase which delivers fatty acid to cells for storage/utilization.

Early Fasting

- Liver glycogenolysis starts releasing glucose to the blood (Fig. 24.3).
- Cori and alanine cycle becomes important in this phase; and they play an important role in gluconeogenesis by liver.
- Cori and alanine cycles play an important role in gluconeogenesis, but they do not provide carbon for net glucose synthesis, rather the glucose produced from lactate and alanine, respectively, in these cycles just replaces the glucose which was actually utilized by peripheral cell.

Certain cells in body like brain utilize glucose completely to produce CO_2 and H_2O, hence some net glucose synthesis is mandatory during fasting state.

This role is fulfilled by protein of skeletal muscle and 'glycerol' a byproduct of lipolysis in adipose cell.

Most of the carbon for net glucose synthesis comes from protein of skeletal muscle.

After muscle proteolysis, alanine and glutamine are major amino acids which come to plasma.

Branched chain amino acids are major provider of amino group for transamination of pyruvate and glutamate during this process.

This also results in release of branched chain keto acid to the blood. Fate of these keto acids are as follows:

α-keto acid of valine ⇒ Glucose synthesis
α-keto acid of leucine = Ketone body synthesis
α-keto acid of isoleucine = Glucose and ketone body synthesis

Along with glucose synthesis during fasting, urea synthesis also increases in liver.

Because of low insulin during fasting state, lipolysis of adipose tissue is enhanced releasing FFA in blood which is used in preference to glucose by many tissues.

In liver, fatty acid oxidation results in ketogenesis.

Ketone body is utilized by many tissues in preference to glucose just like fatty acid.

Brain cannot utilize fatty acid due to impermeability of blood brain barrier to fatty acid.

It is capable of utilizing ketone body for its ATP need during fasting, once the level of ketone bodies is high enough in plasma for its utilization.

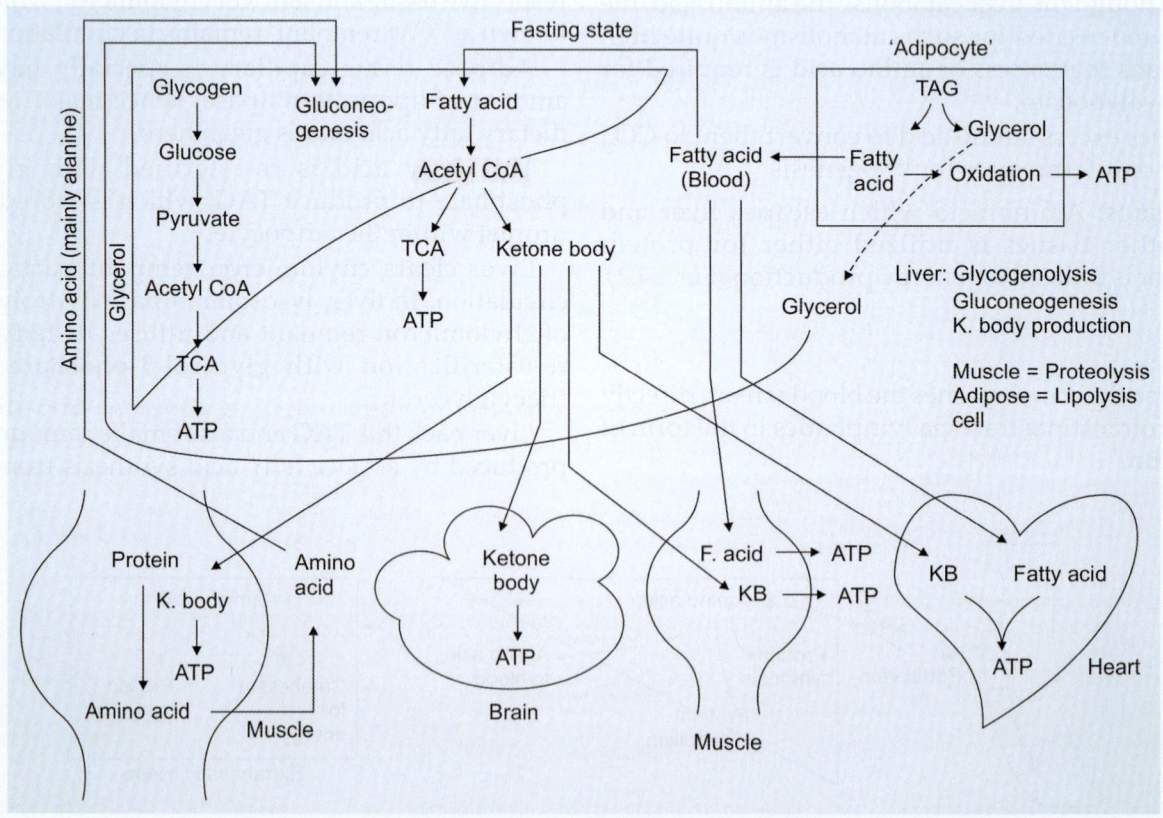

Fig. 24.3: Interaction of various organs during fasting and starvation

Ketone body may also suppress proteolysis and branched chain amino acid oxidation in muscle and decreases alanine release.

This decreases muscle wasting and also reduces gluconeogenesis by liver.

Liver, adipose cell and muscle play important role to provide glucose to brain.

Liver: Site of gluconeogenesis

Muscle and ENT: Supply substrate for gluconeogenesis, i.e. alanine.

Adipose cell: Supply fatty acid which is oxidised in the liver to produce ATP.

Reye's syndrome (Aspirin used by children with varicella): Brain dysfunction and oedema (characterized by irritability, lethargy and coma) and liver dysfunction (plasma FFA, fatty liver; hypoglycemia, hyperammonemia, accumulation of short chain organic acid).

- Liver mitochondria are damaged.
- Fatty acid oxidation is impaired.
- CPS-I, PDH, pyruvate carboxylase, adenine nucleotide transporter are all inhibited by CoA ester of organic acid.
- Liver mitochondrial damage
- Hypoglycemia
- Lactic acidosis
- Fatty liver
- Liver failure

Energy Reserve of Human

Fuel	Tissue	Fuel (g)	Reserve (kcal)
Glycogen	Liver	70	280
Glycogen	Muscle	120	480
Fat	Adipose	15,000	135,000
Protein	Muscle	6,000	24,000

MECHANISM RESPONSIBLE FOR METABOLIC CONTROL IN WELL-FED AND STARVED STATE IN LIVER

Factors controlling the switch mechanism in the liver between fed state and starvation are:

1. Substrate supply
2. Allosteric regulation of key enzymes
3. Covalent modification of key enzymes
4. Induction-repression of enzymes

1. Substrate Supply

a. Fatty acid supply to liver → determines ketogenesis.
b. Gluconeogenic substrate entry in liver → determines gluconeogenesis.

2. Allosteric Regulation of Key Enzymes

Example of important allosteric regulators (in liver):

a. Glucose $\xrightarrow{\oplus}$ Glucokinase (GK) (by translocating GK from nucleus to cytosol)

b. Glucose $\xrightarrow{\ominus}$ Glycogen phosphorylase

c. Glucose $\xrightarrow{\oplus}$ Glycogen synthase

d. Fructose-2,6-bisphosphate $\xrightarrow{\oplus}$ PFK-1

e. Fructose-2,6-bisphosphate $\xrightarrow{\ominus}$
$$\text{F-1,6-bisphosphatase}$$

f. Fructose-1,6-bisphosphate $\xrightarrow{\oplus}$ Pyruvate kinase

g. Pyruvate $\xrightarrow{\oplus}$ PDH complex

h. Citrate $\xrightarrow{\oplus}$ Acetyl CoA carboxylase

i. Malonyl CoA $\xrightarrow{\ominus}$
$$\text{CPT-I (carnitine palmitoyltransferase-I)}$$

j. Acetyl CoA $\xrightarrow{\oplus}$ Pyruvate carboxylase

k. Acetyl CoA $\xrightarrow{\ominus}$ PDH complex

l. Long chain acyl CoA $\xrightarrow{\ominus}$ Acetyl CoA carboxylase

m. Fructose-6-phosphate $\xrightarrow{\ominus}$ Glucokinase (translocating it to nucleus from cytosol)

n. Citrate $\xrightarrow{\ominus}$ PFK-1

o. NADH $\xrightarrow{\ominus}$ TCA cycle

cAMP is an important allosteric regulator which is greatly increased in starvation, it is important for covalent modification of enzymes.

AMP $\xrightarrow{\oplus}$ Glycogen phosphorylase
AMP $\xrightarrow{\oplus}$ PPK-1
AMP $\xrightarrow{\oplus}$ F-1,6-bisphosphatase

3. Covalent Modification of Key Enzymes

Covalent modification of key enzyme of pathway also controls switch mechanism in liver between fed and starved state.

Phosphorylation and dephosphorylation of enzyme are the most important covalent modifications.

Mostly, it is serine residue which undergoes phosphorylation but it may be threonine residue also.

Two enzymes are involved (Fig. 24.4):
   a. Protein kinase A (cAMP dependent)
   b. AMP activated protein kinase (AMPK)

In well-fed state, almost all the enzymes in liver are in dephosphorylated form. This is due to high insulin–glucagon ratio which results in low cAMP level in liver (Fig. 24.5).

Section 6 ■ Integrated Pathways

24

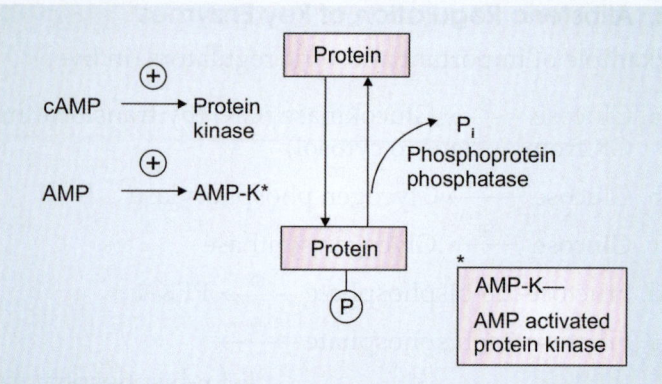

Fig. 24.4: Protein kinase

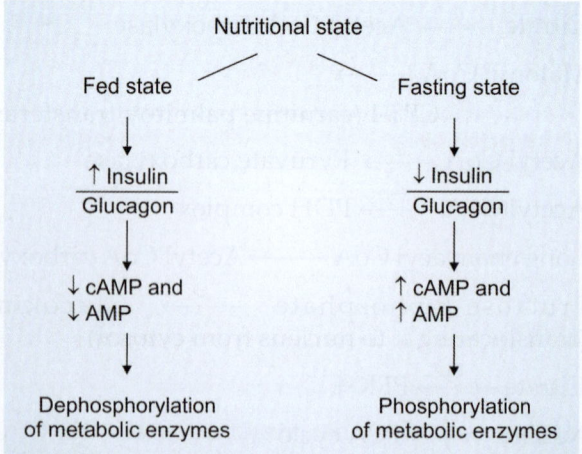

Fig. 24.5: Covalent modification of enzymes based on nutritional state

In this condition, there is low protein kinase activity and high phosphoprotein phosphatase activity resulting in dephosphorylation of enzymes.

Following enzymes in liver are in dephosphorylated state in well-fed condition:
- Glycogen synthase
- Glycogen phosphorylase
- Phosphorylase kinase
- PFK-2/F-2,6-bisphosphatase
- Pyruvate kinase
- Acetyl CoA carboxylase

Pathways favoured in well-fed state:
- Glycogenesis
- Glycolysis
- Lipogenesis

Pathways inhibited in well-fed state
- Glycogenolysis
- Gluconeogenesis
- Ketogenesis

During fasting state, the liver enzymes are in phosphorylated state. Insulin is low and glucagon is high resulting in high cAMP level which activates protein kinase A and inactivates protein phosphatase (Fig. 24.6).

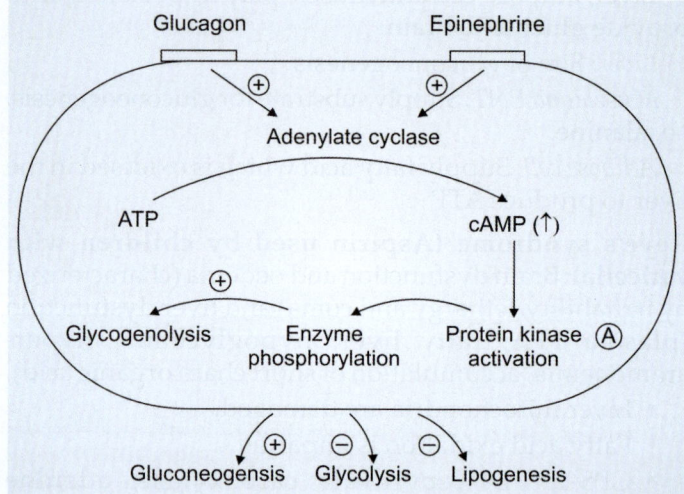

Fig. 24.6: Effect on cAMP production by glucogon and α-adrenergic agonist (epinephrine) and metabolic consequences

Enzymes active in phosphorylated state are:
- Glycogen phosphorylase
- Phosphorylase kinase
- F-2,6-bisphosphatase

This results in glycogenolysis, gluconeogenesis and ketogenesis to dominate in fasting state.

In addition to the 'hormones' insulin and glucagon, regulating cAMP level and thus having affect on metabolic pathways as described in above paragraph, the 'energy status' of the cell also determines the activity of key enzymes of metabolic pathways.

Under condition of high energy demand when the level of ATP is low, and level of AMP is high, a kinase termed AMP-K (AMP activated protein kinase) gets activated and phosphorylates enzymes (Fig. 24.4).

AMPK in-turn turns off the anabolic pathways which utilize ATP and turn on the catabolic pathways which generate ATP (Fig. 24.7).

Following enzymes are phosphorylated by AMPK:
- Glycogen synthase → gets inactivated
- Glycerol-3-phosphate acyltransferase → gets inactivated
- Acetyl CoA carboxylase → gets inactivated
- Malonyl CoA decarboxylase (MDC) →
                                    gets activated
- HMG-CoA reductase → get inactivated

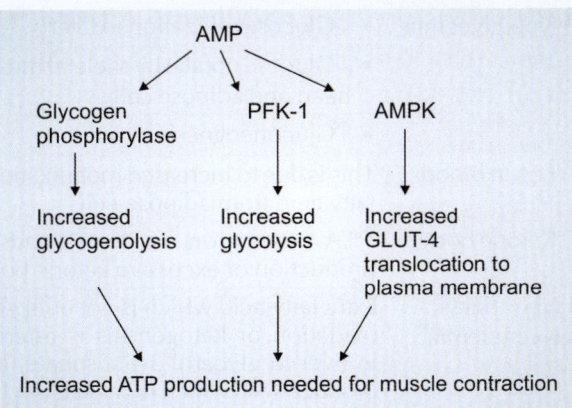

Fig. 24.7: AMP and AMP activated protein kinase and their effect on ATP production

All the above enzymes except MDC are inactive in phosphorylated state and hence following metabolic pathways are turned off:

- Glycogenesis
- TAG synthesis
- Fatty acid synthesis
- Cholesterol synthesis

MDC is active in phosphorylated state hence level of malonyl CoA is reduced. Malanyl CoA is a blocker of CPT-I, so lowering of malonyl CoA removes block of CPT-I and increases fatty acid oxidation.

Above three mechanisms described, i.e. substrate supply, allosteric regulation of key enzymes and covalent modification of key enzymes are only short-term regulation operating on a minute-to-minute basis.

Long-term regulation of enzyme activity is via controlling the amount of concentration of enzyme via effect on transcription.

This is described below.

4. Induction-Repression of Enzyme

Induction of enzyme	Repression of enzyme
Glucokinase	PEP carboxy kinase
PFK-1	PDH kinase
Pyruvate kinase	Pyruvate carboxylase
G6PD	F-1,6-bisphosphatase
6-PG dehydrogenase	Glucose-6-phosphatase
Malic enzyme	Aminotransferase
ATP citrate lyase	
Acetyl CoA carboxylase	
Fatty acid synthase	
Δ9 desaturase	
HMG-CoA reductase	
Glycerol-3-phosphate acyltransferase	

Fasting state: Lipogenic enzymes are decreased and gluconeogenic enzymes are induced.

▌ADIPOSE TISSUE IN STARVE-FEED CYCLE

Fed state: Following enzymes in adipose cell are dephosphorylated:

1. Pyruvate kinase (active in dephosphorylated form)
2. PDH complex (active in dephosphorylated form)
3. Acetyl CoA carboxylase (active in dephosphorylated form)
4. Hormone sensitive lipase (active in phosphorylated form)

Above states of enzymes favor lipogenesis.

Fasting state: All the above enzymes undergo phosphorylation which inhibits lipogenesis and increases lipolysis (mobilization of fatty acid from adipose cell).

Skeletal Muscle in Starve-feed Cycle

Fed state: Following enzymes are in dephosphorylated state:

1. Glucogen synthase (active)
2. Glycogen phosphorylase (inactive)
3. PDH complex
4. Acetyl CoA carboxylase
5. Malonyl CoA decarboxylase

GLUT-4 also is recruited to plasma membrane by insulin.

This results in increased glucose uptake, glycogenesis and fatty acid synthesis.

Fatty acid oxidation is inhibited due to block of CPT-I by malonyl CoA.

Fasting state: Glucose, alanine, lactate and pyruate are spared and fatty acid is oxidized.

▌OBESITY

It is a common problem in developed countries.

Obesity is due to excessive deposit of fat in adipocyte which is mainly due to excess consumption of food.

Main source of body fat is diet, only small amount is synthesized by the liver and is transported to adipose cell or is synthesized *de novo* in adipose cell.

Obesity is often associated with insulin resistance, with increased level of insulin.

Section 6 ■ Integrated Pathways

24

TYPE 2 DIABETES MELLITUS

β cell failure and insulin resistance are two components of this type of diabetes mellitus (DM). To overcome the insulin resistance, insulin is secreted, though this does not overcome the problem.

Hyperglycemia occurs due to lack of inhibition of gluconeogenesis in liver and also due to reduced glucose uptake in cells having GLUT-4.

GLUT-4 is insulin dependent glucose transporter which is distributed on heart, skeletal muscles and adipose cells.

Ketogenesis is rare in this disease, as enough insulin is present which prevents excessive mobilization of fatty acid from TAG of adipose cell.

Fatty acid reaching the liver or synthesized *de novo* is preferably used for triacylglycerol synthesis.

Hence, diabetic patients show hypertriacylglyce-reclemia along with increased VLDL, without hyper-chylomicronemia.

Normally gluconeogenesis and lipogenesis do not occur together, but in type 2 DM both these processes take place simultaneously.

Diet, exercise and weight control are first choice for treating type 2 DM.

Medications (oral hypoglycemia agents or insulin) may be given in advanced form of the disease.

POLYOL PATHWAY

Enzymes which constitute polyol pathway are:
1. Aldose reductase
2. Sorbitol dehydrogenase

These enzymes are distributed in:
- Lens
- Peripheral nerves
- Renal papillae
- Schwann cell
- Glomerulus
- Retinal capillaries

TYPE I DIABETES MELLITUS

In this disease, pancreas fail to produce insulin, so there is complete lack of insulin.

In this disease liver is in gluconeogenic and ketogenic modes, as there is no insulin to prevent these pathways.

GLUT-4 remains in cytosolic vesicles in adipose cell and muscle, which prevent glucose uptake by these cells.

In addition, VLDL and chylomicron (CM) are not metabolized properly by lipoprotein lipase, as insulin is required for synthesis of lipoprotein lipase enzyme.

a. Hyperglycemia	• ↓Glucose utilization in liver
	• ↓Glucose uptake by skeletal muscle, heart and adipose cell
	• ↑Gluconeognesis by liver
b. ↑FFA in blood	This is due to increased mobilization of fatty acid from adipose cell
c. ↑Ketone body	↑F.A. oxidation in liver leads to production of excessive ketone body.
d. Hypertriacyl glyceredemia	Extra fatty acid which is not utilized for oxidation or ketogenesis is esterified in liver to glycerol-3-phosphate, as to produce TAG which is packed in VLDL, which comes to plasma.

CANCER

Cancer cells differ from normal cells in that they do not adapt to starve-feed cycle as many normal cells in body do.

Cancer cell always demands glucose for their energy purpose irrespective of metabolic state of the body.

Even hormonal changes do not effect tumor cell, unlike many other normal tissues.

Cancer cell utilizes very large amount of glucose for ATP production. This can be explained by the fact that cancer cells are comparatively hypoxic and hypoxia increases HIF-α (hypoxia inducible factor-α). HIF-α is a potent transcription factor which increases transcription of gene producing glucose transporter and glycolytic enzymes.

Cancer Cachexia

Unexplained weight loss in cancer is known as cancer cachexia which is due to loss of remarkable protein from skeletal tissues and adipose tissues.

Various interleukins (IL-1, IL-6) and tumor necrosis factor α (TNF-α) play an important role in this condition.

AEROBIC AND ANAEROBIC EXERCISES

'Long distance running' is an example of aerobic exercise and weight lifting and sprinting are examples of 'anaerobic exercises'.

Anaerobic Exercise

- Little or no interorgan cooperation
- Phosphocreatine is the immediate source of ATP followed by glycolysis and glycogenolysis.

Aerobic Exercise

- Muscle glycogenolysis
- Activation of AMPK (AMP activated protein kinase)

ATP is decreased and AMP is increased.

AMP is an allosteric activator of:

- Glycogen phosphorylase
- PFK-1
- AMPK

Increases ATP production needed for muscle contraction.

Fatty acid oxidation soon follows glycogenolysis during a race. Just like fasting, in exercise also muscle uses fatty acid in preference to glucose.

AMPK not only promotes fatty acid oxidation in muscle, but also directs fatty acid into oxidation in liver and away from esterification into triacylglycerol.

ALCOHOL

Liver is the main organ for alcohol oxidation.

Alcohol consumption increases NADH production.

Alcohol inhibits gluconeogenesis, fatty acid oxidation, resulting in fasting hypoglycemia and fatty liver.

TCA cycle is inhibited due to excess NADH, so acetate is not oxidized. So much of the acetate escapes the liver to reach the blood and form adducts with various biological compounds (Fig. 24.8).

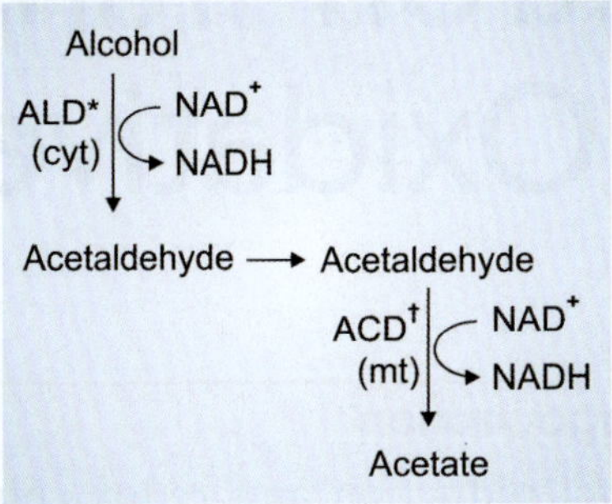

* ALD = Alcohol dehydrogenase † ACD = Acetaldehyde dehydrogenase

Fig. 24.8: Alcohol metabolism

25

Electron Transport Chain (ETC) and Oxidative Phosphorylation

Chapter Organization

1. Oxidation, reduction and redox couple (pair), redox potential.
2. Substrate level phosphorylation and oxidative phosphorylation.
3. High energy compounds
4. Mitochondria and shuttle transportation.
5. ETC and oxidative phosphorylation
   a. ETC arrangement
   b. Chemiosmotic model
   c. ATP synthase
6. ETC inhibitors
7. Uncouplers

Oxidation: Defined as the loss of e⁻.

Reduction: Defined as the gain of e⁻. Reductant is e⁻ donating molecule and oxidant is e⁻ accepting molecule.

```
Reductant    Oxidant
   A    +    B  ———→  A⁺ + B⁻
        e⁻
```

In the above example 'A' is reductant and 'B' is oxidant.

In biological system and otherwise too, oxidation–reduction is a coupled process.

A/A⁺ and B/B⁻ are redox couples.

Redox potential: It is a quantitative measure of redox pair to loose or gain electrons.

▌ELECTRON TRANSPORT CHAIN (ETC)

Electron transport chains are set of enzyme complexes where all the components (except cytochrome c) are embedded in the inner mitochondrial membrane (IMM)

(Fig. 25.1). ETC is the final common pathway where e⁻ derived from oxidation of carbohydrate, lipid and amino acid is finally channelled to oxygen molecule, which forms water (H_2O) (Fig. 25.2).

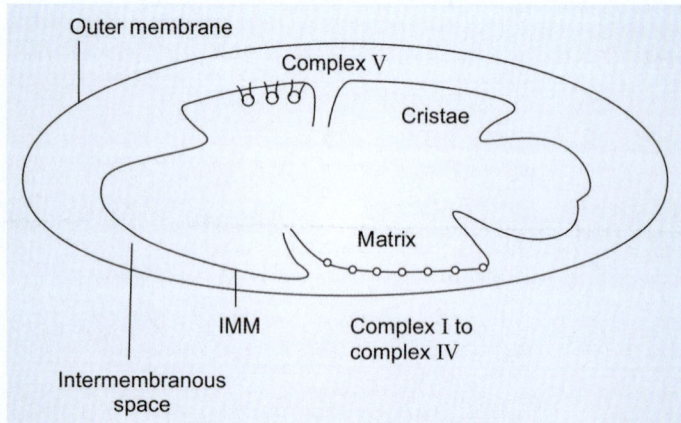

Fig. 25.1: ETC on mitochondria

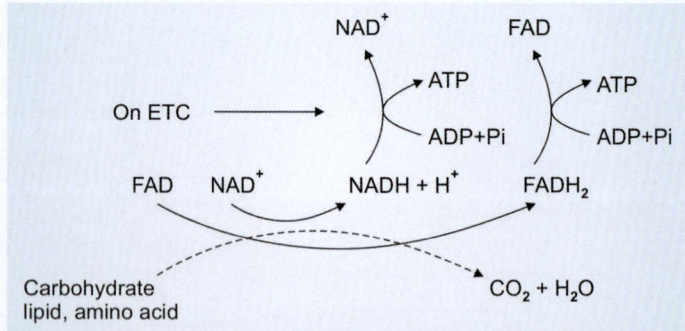

Fig. 25.2: NADH and $FADH_2$ producing ATP on ETC

Inner mitochondrial membrane is not permeable to small ions and small as well as large molecules. To move ions or molecules, specialized carriers or transport system is required.

Mitochondrial matrix is a gel-like solution which is having enzymes like PDH complex, enzymes of TCA cycle [except succinate dehydrogenase (SCD) enzyme which is on IMM], enzymes of amino acid oxiation, fatty acid oxidation, urea, heme and glucose synthesizing enzymes. NAD$^+$, FAD, ADP and Pi are also richly found here.

mt-DNA, mt-RNA and ribosomes are also found in matrix which are involved in mitochondrial protein synthesis.

ETC Components

Organization of ETC components is dependent upon their redox potential.

ETC components are organized in order of increasing redox potential (Figs 25.3 and 25.4).

Except CoQ, which is quinone, all other components of ETC are proteins in nature.

Redox Couple and Redox Potential (Reduction Potential)

Each molecule or atom which can donate or accept e$^-$ exists in two forms (a) reduced and (b) oxidised state. Together these two states constitute the redox couple.

The tendency of redox couple to donate e$^-$ is called redox potential.

Important redox couples and their redox potentials are shown in Tables 25.1a and b.

Complex I

e$^-$ flow at complex I: Dehydrogenases which use NAD$^+$ as coenzyme, remove two hydrogen atoms from their substrate. Both e$^-$ and one H$^+$ are transferred to NAD$^+$ resulting in formation of NADH and H$^+$.

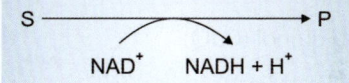

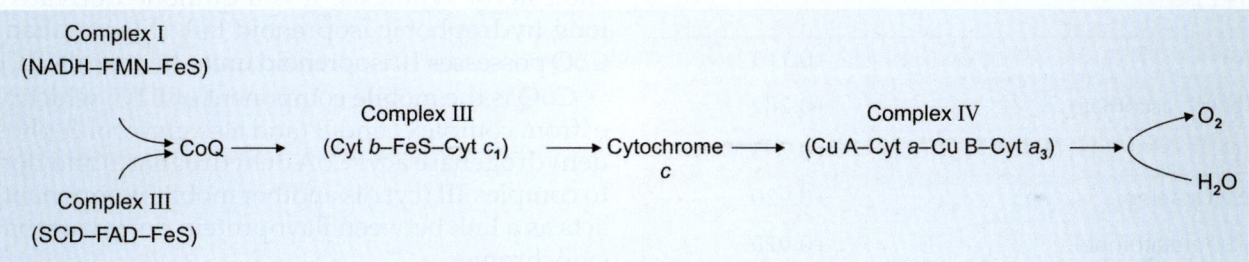

Fig. 25.3: ETC (electron transport chain)

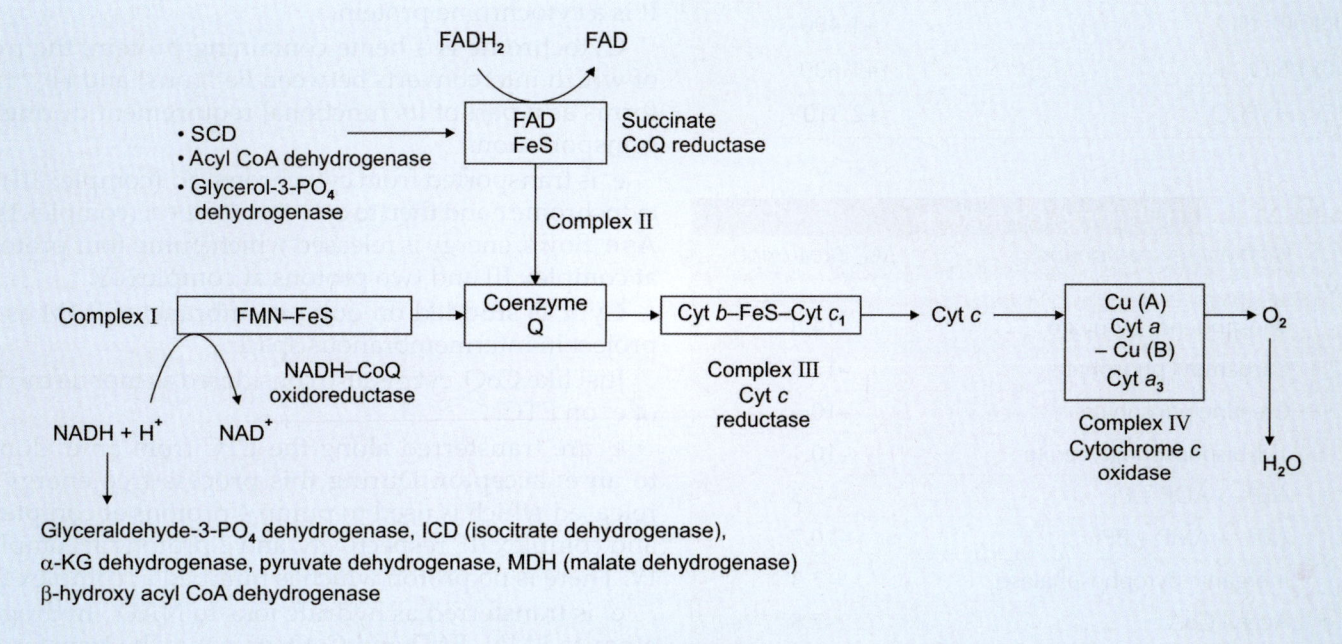

Fig. 25.4: Arrangement of various components in electron transport chain (ETC)

TABLE 25.1a	Various redox couples and their respective redox potentials
Redox couple	Reduction potential ($\Delta E°$; V)
$NAD^+/NADH$	–0.316
$NADP^+/NADPH$	–0.315
Pyruvate, H^+/lactate	–0.183
Oxaloacetate, $2H^+$/malate	–0.166
H^+/H_2	–0.42
Menaquinone/red. menaquinone	–0.074
ESSE/2ESH (ergothioneine)	–0.060
$CoQ/CoQ^{•–}$	–0.036
$FAD^+/FADH_2$	+0.00
Ubiquinone/ubiquinol (CoQ)	+0.10
Cytochrome a (Fe^{+++}/Fe^{++})	+0.29
$\frac{1}{2}O_2/H_2O$	+0.82
Fe^{3+}/Fe^{2+}	+0.110
$Ascorbate^{•–}/ascorbate^-$	+0.282
O_2/H_2O	+0.295
$RS^{•}/RS^-$ (cysteine)	+0.920
$GS^{•}/GS^-$ (glutathione)	+0.920
$NO_2^{•}/NO_2^-$	+0.990
$HO_2/H^+/H_2O_2$	+1.060
$ONOO^-/NO_2$	+1.400
NO_2^+/NO_2	+1.600
$HO^{•}, H^+/H_2O$	+2.310

TABLE 25.1b	High energy compounds	
S. No.	High energy compounds	$\Delta G°'$(kcal/mol)
1.	Phosphoenol pyruvate	–14.8
2.	Carbamoyl phosphate	–12.3
3.	Creatine phosphate	–10.5
4.	1,3-bisphosphoglycerate	–10.1
5.	ATP → ADP + Pi	–7.3
6.	ATP → AMP + PPi	–10.7
7.	Inorganic pyrophosphatase	–7.3
8.	Acetyl CoA	–7.5
9.	S-adenosylmethionine	–7.0

This NADH hydride [:H^+] and H^+ are then transferred to FMN by NADH dehydrogenase.

FMN is converted to $FMNH_2$. From $FMNH_2$ the e^- is transfered to Fe of FeS centre and then to CoQ.

NADH ⟶ FMN ⟶ Iron of FeS center

This e^- transfer from NADH to FMN, then to Fe of FeS and CoQ results in loss of energy. This energy pumps protons from the matrix of mitochondria to intermembrane space.

Complex II

e^- flow at complex II: Here e^- from $FADH_2$ is transferred to FeS protein and from it to CoQ. As there is no loss of energy at this movement, no proton is pumped out of matrix to intermembranous space in the mitochondria.

Coenzyme Q

It is made from one of the intermediate during cholesterol synthesis. It is a quinone derivative with long hydrophobic isoprenoid tail. (Mammalian tissue CoQ possesses 10 isoprenoid units, hence called CoQ10.)

CoQ is the mobile component of ETC, which accepts e^- from complex I and II (and also glycerol-3-phosphate dehydrogenase acyl CoA dehydrognase) and donates it to complex III (cyt c is another mobile component). CoQ acts as a link between flavoprotein dehydrogenase and cytochromes.

Complex III

It is a cytochrome protein.

Cytochrome is a heme containing protein, the iron of which interconverts between Fe^{++} (ous) and Fe^{+++} (ic) forms as a part of its functional requirement during e^- transportation.

e^- is transported from cytochrome bc_1 (complex III) to cytochrome c and then to cytochrome $a + a_3$ (complex IV). As e^- flows, energy is released which pump four protons at complex III and two protons at complex IV.

Cyt c is studded on outer membrane of IMM as to project in intermembranous space.

Just like CoQ, cyt c is also considered as mobile carrier of e^- on ETC.

e^- are transferred along the ETC from an e^- donor to an e^- acceptor. During this process free energy is released which is used to pump 4 protons at complex I and complex III, respectively, and 2 protons at complex IV. There is no proton which is pumped at complex II.

e^- is transferred as hydride ions to NAD^+, hydrogen atom to FMN, FAD and CoQ; or it may be transferred as electron itself to cytochromes.

Complex IV heme iron has got coordination site for 'O' atom and hence this complex reacts with 'O' atom to form water.

$2e^-$ are required to form one molecule of H_2O by one 'O' atom, $2H^+$. Cu atom is also needed for this complex reaction.

$$Cu\,A \longrightarrow Cyt\,a \longrightarrow Cu\,B \longrightarrow Cyt\,a_3 \longrightarrow 'O'$$

Leaked e^- from ETC are very toxic, as they tend to generate free radicals like superoxide ion (O_2^-), H_2O_2, hydroxyl radicals (OH^-).

Superoxide dismutase (SOD), catalase, glutathione peroxidase (GPO) are enzymes which handle these free radicals efficiently.

Following are important components of ETC:

1. Nicotinamide nucleotides = NAD^+ (not $NADP^+$)
2. Flavoproteins
   - FMN → Prosthetic group of NADH dehydrogenase
   - FAD → It is a coenzyme for succinate dehydrogenase.
3. **Iron-sulphur protein:** FeS participates in the transfer of e^- from
   - FMN to CoQ
   - Cyt b to cyt c_1.
4. **Coenzyme Q (ubiquinone):** It can accept e^- from $FMNH_2$ or $FADH_2$.
5. **Cytochromes:** Cytochromes are conjugated proteins having heme group. Heme contains iron, but unlike iron of heme of Hb and myoglobin, iron of cytochrome, heme undergoes alternate oxidation (Fe^{+++}) and reduction (Fe^{++}) which is important for its role in e^- transportation.

The order of cytochromes which are encountered during e^- flow from coenzyme Q to oxygen molecule are:

- Cytochrome b
- Cytochrome c_1
- Cytochrome c
- Cytochrome a
- Cytochrome a_3

P:O RATIO

P:O ratio refers to the number of inorganic phosphate utilized for ATP generation when one atom of oxygen is consumed.

P:O ratio for NADH is 2.5 and for $FADH_2$ it is 1.5.

$2e^-$ flow from NADH and H^+ through complexes I, III and IV, accumulate 10 protons $(4 + 4 + 2)$ and $2e^-$ flow from $FADH_2$ through complexes II, III and IV result in accumulation of 6 protons $(4 + 2)$.

As 4 protons return back to matrix to produce 1ATP, total 10 protons produce 2.5 ATP and 6 protons produce 1.5 ATP in the matrix of mitochondria.

When one molecule of NADH is oxidized, about 35% of energy is trapped in the form of 2.5 ATP, rest is lost as heat.

ATP synthesis in a cell may occur via two mechanisms:

1. Substrate level phosphorylation
2. Oxidative phosphorylation

Substrate Level Phosphorylation (SLP)

Here ATP production occurs at the reaction level itself without the need of O_2, ETC, mitochondria, NADH or $FADH_2$. ATP production via this mechanism is a rare phenomenon, and only three reactions in biochemical system produce ATP by substrate level phosphorytation (SLP) (Fig. 25.5).

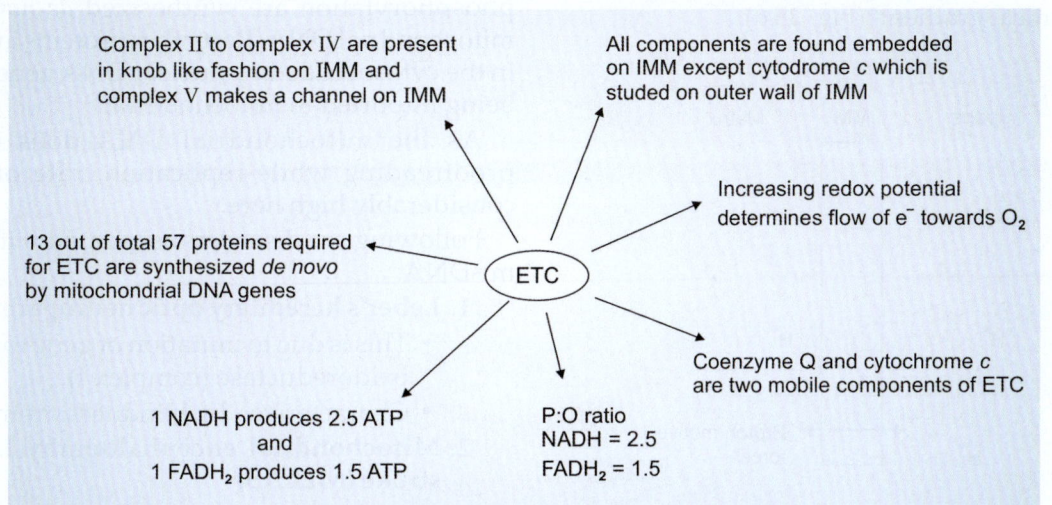

Fig. 25.5: Important points regarding ETC

Content of figure:
- Complex II to complex IV are present in knob like fashion on IMM and complex V makes a channel on IMM
- All components are found embedded on IMM except cytodrome c which is studed on outer wall of IMM
- 13 out of total 57 proteins required for ETC are synthesized *de novo* by mitochondrial DNA genes
- Increasing redox potential determines flow of e^- towards O_2
- ETC
- Coenzyme Q and cytochrome c are two mobile components of ETC
- 1 NADH produces 2.5 ATP and 1 $FADH_2$ produces 1.5 ATP
- P:O ratio NADH = 2.5 $FADH_2$ = 1.5

Two reactions belong to glycolysis and one reaction belongs to TCA cycle. These reactions are:

1. Phosphoglycerate kinase
2. Pyruvate kinase
3. Succinate thiokinase

Major advantage of SLP to a cell is that this takes place even in anaerobic condition, so cell lacking mitochondria (like RBC), SLP is the only mechanism by which ATP production takes place in these cells.

Oxidative Phosphorylation

In this mechanism of ATP production, ATP is produced by ETC for which O_2 is a must component as a final acceptor of e^-. The donors of e^- are NADH and $FADH_2$ in this route.

Hence, ATP production via oxidative phosphorylation occurs in aerobic condition alone.

The major route of ATP production in a cell (except those cell where mitochondria is absent, e.g. RBC) is oxidative phosphorylation only.

The mechanism of oxidative phosphorylation and factor contributing into this is described in detail in this chapter.

e^- transport from complex I to complex IV at ETC is linked with ATP production at complex V. In other words, oxidation at ETC is coupled with phosphorylation (ATP production) at complex V, this coupling is known as oxidative phosphorylation.

To explain oxidative phosphorylation, chemiosmotic hypothesis was put forward by Peter Mitchell in 1961.

According to this model, protons are translocated in the intermembraneous space from the matrix during e^- transportation on ETC. This accumulation of proton in the intermembranous space, generates 'proton gradient' or 'electrochemical gradient' (Fig. 25.6).

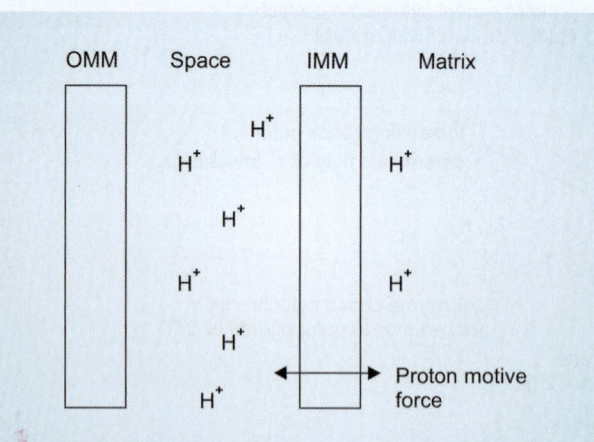

Fig. 25.6: Proton motive force across IMM

OMM   Space   IMM   Matrix

Proton motive force

This elecrtochemical gradient force proton to move back to matrix via F_0 channel of complex V.

Complex V is ATP synthase, which is also called ATPase, as it is a reversible enzyme. This enzyme is multisubunit complex. Broadly, it can be divided into two subunits—F_0 and F_1 (Fig. 25.7).

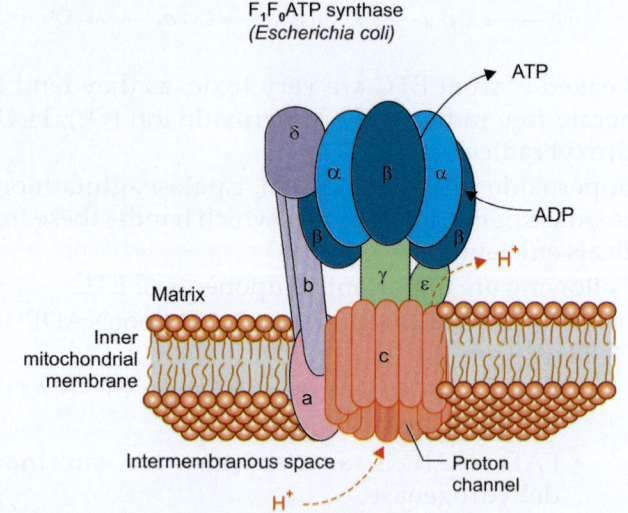

F_1F_0ATP synthase
(*Escherichia coli*)

Fig. 25.7: ATP synthase/complex V

BINDING CHANGE MODEL/ROTARY MOTOR/ ENGINE DRIVING MODEL

- Proposed by Paul Boyer in 1964.
- Rotation of γ subunit induces conformational change in β subunit.

Inherited Disorder Related to Mitochondrial DNA Mutation

13 out of total 67 proteins required for oxidative phosphorylation are synthesized *de novo* by gene of mitochondrial DNA. Rest other proteins are synthesized in the cytosol coded by nuclear DNA gene; and are then being imported to mitochondria.

As the mitochondrial DNA does not undergo proofreading while replication, rate of mutation is considerably high here.

Following are disorders associated with mutation of mt-DNA:

1. **Leber's hereditary optic neuropathy (LHON)**
   - This is due to mutation of gene for NADH-CoQ oxidoreductase (complex I)
   - Characterized by blindness, tremor and ataxia
2. **Mitochondrial encephalopathy lactic acidoss, stroke (MELAS)**
   - Mutation of gene encoding tRNA for leucine.

- Characterized by deafness, diabetes mellitus, dementia, lactic acidosis and stroke.
3. **Myoclonic epilepsy and ragged red fiber (MERRF)**
   - Unidentified mutation of mt-DNA gene
   - Abnormal eye movement, deafness, lactic acidosis, ragged red muscle fiber.

FACTORS ADVERSLY AFFECTING THE PROCESS OF BIOLOGICAL OXIDATION

ETC Inhibitors

Number of chemicals block the e⁻ transmission at various sites on ETC (Fig. 25.8).

1. **Examples of inhibitors which block e⁻ transmission from complex I to CoQ:**
   a. Rotenone (fish poison)
   b. Piericidin A (antibiotic)
   c. Amytal (barbiturates)
   d. Chlopromazine (tranquilizer)
   e. Guanethide (hypotensive agent)
2. **Inhibitors which block e⁻ transmission from complex II to coenzyme Q:**
   a. Carboxin
   b. Tritheonyl fluoroacetate (TTFA)
3. **Inhibitors which block the e⁻ transmission within complex III:**
   a. British anti-Lewisite: antidote to war gas (BAL)
   b. Antimycin A

4. **Inhibitors which block e⁻ transmission within complex IV:**
   a. Cyanide
   b. H_2S
   c. Carbon monoxide (CO)
   d. Sodium azide

Inhibitors of Oxidative Phosphorylation

1. Atractyloside → Inhibits ATP-ADP translocase
2. Oligomycin → Blocks inflow of protons through F_0
3. Valinomycin: Ionophore which dissipates proton gradient and prevents ATP formation via complex V.

Uncouplers

Uncouplers may be chemical or physiological (natural).
A. **Chemical**
   1. 2,4-dinitrophenol (2,4-DNP)
   2. 2,4-dinitrocresol (2,4-DNC)
   3. Chloro-carbonyl cyanophenyl hydrazone (CCCP)
B. **Physiological (natural)**
   1. Thermogenin
   2. Thyroxine
   3. Bilirubin
   4. Free fatty acid

Inhibitors which either stop entry of e⁻ from complex I to CoQ or from complex II to CoQ prevent the oxidation of respective channel.

Blockers of common channel, i.e. channel III and IV are most toxic as they prevent the transport of e⁻ to oxygen from both complex I and complex II.

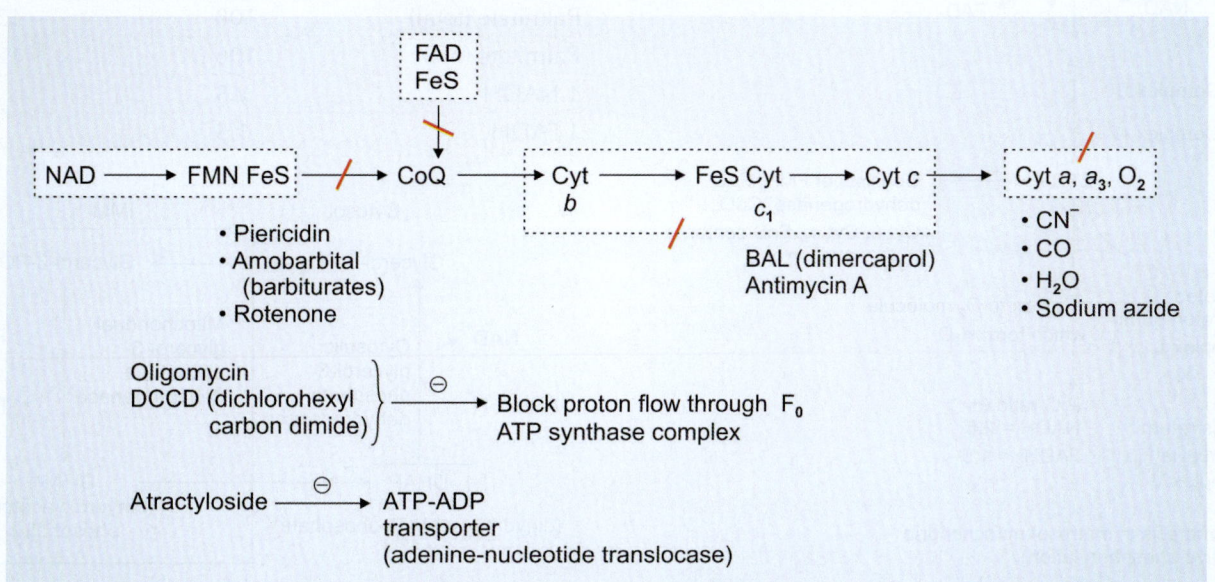

Fig. 25.8: ETC blockers at various levels

ATRACTYLOSIDE

Atractyloside blocks ATP-ADP translocase (antiport) on IMM. This results in reduced or no supply of ADP in the mitochondrial matrix (Fig. 25.9).

ATP synthesis thus stops in the matrix of mitochondria due to lack of substrate (ADP) in spite of normal oxidation going on.

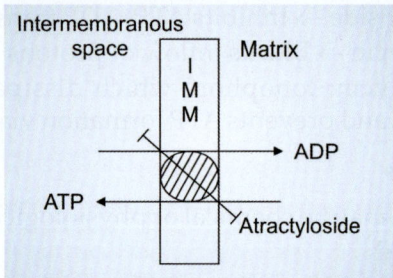

Fig. 25.9: Action of atractyloside on ATP-ADP antiport

Oligomycin

Oligomycin blocks F_0 channel and prevents proton entry back to mitochondria. This prevents ATP synthesis in the mitochondrial matrix.

Important points regarding ETC are summarized in Figs 25.5 and 25.10.

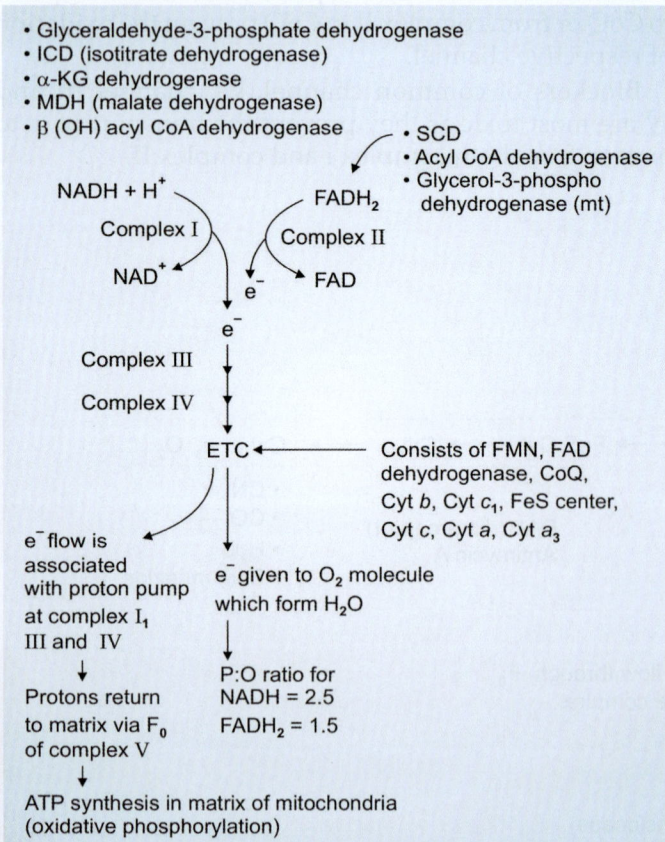

Fig. 25.10: ETC in nutshell

SHUTTLE TO TRANSPORT REDUCING EQUIVALENT OF CYTOSOLIC NADH TO THE COENZYME INSIDE THE MITOCHONDRIAL MATRIX

As NADH is not permeable to mitochondrial membrane there are two types of shuttle systems, which function to transport reducing equivalent from cytosolic NADH to matrix coenzyme (NAD^+ or FAD).

1. Malate-aspartate shuttle
2. Glycerophosphate shuttle

These shuttle have organ specific distribution.

Malate-asparate shuttle is preferably distributed to liver, kidney, heart and glycerophosphate shuttle is preferably distributed to brain and muscle.

Reactions involved in glycerophosphate shuttle are summarised in Fig. 25.11.

Reactions involved in malate-aspartate shuttle are summarized in Fig. 25.12.

Value of various ATP generators as per new and old calculation method (Table 25.3):

- 1 NADH = 2.5 ATP, as per new calculation method and 3 ATP, as per old calculation method
- 1 $FADH_2$ = 1.5 ATP as per new calculation method and 2 ATP, as per old calculation method.

TABLE 25.3	ATP generation with respective old and new values for NADH and $FADH_2$	
ATP generators	*New* *1 NADH = 2.5 ATP* *1 FADH₂ = 1.5 ATP*	*Old* *1 NADH = 3 ATP* *1 FADH₂ = 2 ATP*
Acetyl CoA	10	12
Glucose (total)	34	40
Glucose (net)	32	38
Palmitate (total)	108	131
Palmitate (net)	106	129
1 NADH	2.5	3
1 $FADH_2$	1.5	2

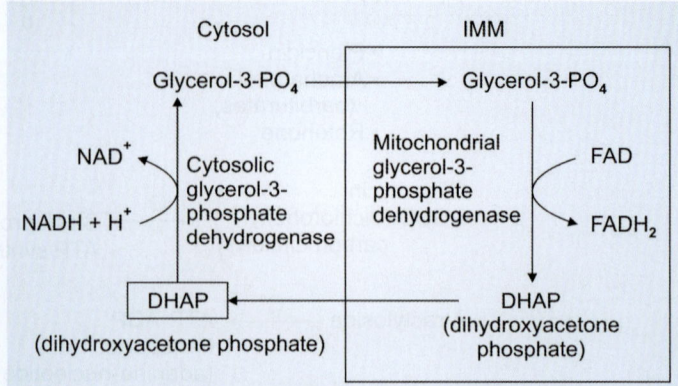

Fig. 25.11: Reactions involved in glycerophosphate shuttle

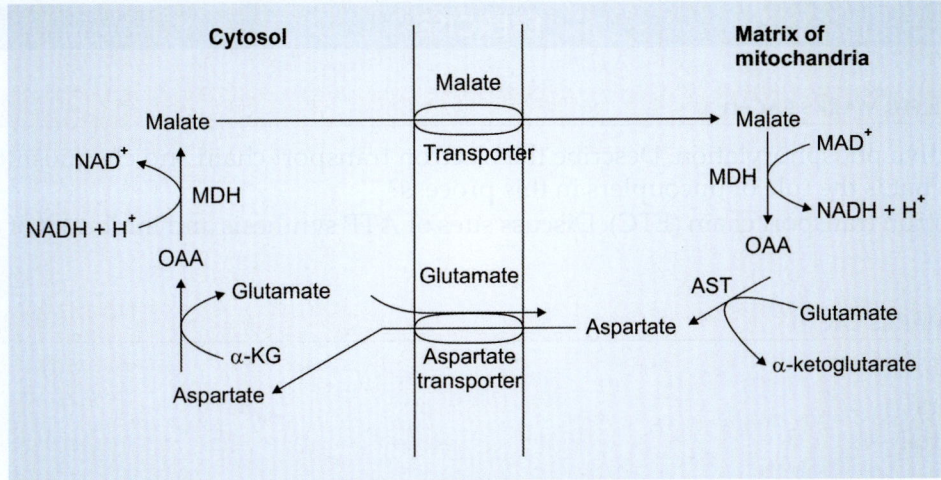

Fig. 25.12: Reactions involved in malate-aspartate shuttle

EXERCISE

LONG QUESTIONS (10 MARKS EACH)

Q 1. Define oxidative phosphorylation. Describe the electron transport chain and chemiosmotic model of ATP formation. What is the role of uncouplers in this process?

Q 2. Describe electron transport chain (ETC). Discuss sites of ATP synthesis and inhibitors of electron transport chain.

SHORT NOTES (5 MARKS EACH)

Q 1. ATP synthase
Q 2. ETC inhibitors
Q 3. Redox potential
Q 4. Uncouplers

MULTIPLE CHOICE QUESTIONS

25.1 During exercise the most rapid way of resynthesis of ATP is:
   a. Glycolysis
   b. Glycogenolysis
   c. Phosphocreatine breakdown
   d. Citric acid cycle

25.2 Dinitrophenol causes:
   a. Inhibition of ATP synthase
   b. Inhibition of ETC
   c. Uncoupling of oxidation and phosphorylation
   d. Accumulation of ATP

25.3 Cytochrome oxidase is inhibited by:
   a. Cyanide
   b. Aluminium phosphide
   c. Phenobarbitone
   d. Carbon monoxide

25.4 The specialized mammalian tissue/organ in which fuel oxidation serves not to produce ATP but to generate heat is:
   a. Adrenal gland
   b. Skeletal muscle
   c. Brown adipose tissue
   d. Heart

25.5 The effect of 2,4-dinitrophenol is to:
   a. Lower BMR
   b. Raise R, Q
   c. Lower R, Q
   d. Decrease proton gradient

25.6 Which of the following statements is true regarding 'cyanide' ?
   a. Only minimally inhibits the ETC because cytochrome oxidase is the terminal component of the chain
   b. Inhibits mitochondrial respiration, but energy production is unaffected
   c. Also binds the copper of cytochrome oxidase
   d. Bind to Fe^{+++} of cytochrome a_3

25.7 Which among the following is not an inhibitor of complex I of electron transport chain?
   a. Barbiturates
   b. Piericidin A
   c. Rotenone
   d. Antimycin

ANSWERS

25.1 (c) Phosphocreatine breakdown

During exercise existing ATP in the skeletal muscle last only for 2 seconds. In case of continued exercise rapid resynthesis of muscle ATP is required for which phosphocreatine is cleaved rapidly to resynthesize ATP. Role of glycolysis to provide the ATP comes only next followed by TCA cycle.

[Ref. Harper's Illustrated Biochemistry, 28th ed, Chapter 11, pg 95].

[Voet and Voet Biochemistry, chapter 27, pg 1092].

25.2 (c) Uncoupling of oxidation and phosphorylation.

2,4-dinitrophenol, 2,4-dinitrocresol and CCCP are chemical uncouplers which damage the inner membrane of the mitochondria. Due to formation of these noncatalytic pores in the mitochondrial membrane, H$^+$ passes from intermembranous space to the matrix of the mitochondria utilizing these noncatalytic pores, this does not lead to any ATP synthesis in contrast to the situation when protons pass through the ATP synthase channel which leads to ATP synthesis.

25.3 (a) Cyanide

25.4 (c) Brown adipose tissue

25.5 (d) Decrease proton gradient

22.6 (d) Bind to Fe^{+++} of cytochrome a_3

- That is why methhemoglobin is an effective antidote since it also has Fe^{+++}.
- Respiration and energy production is the coupled process, so inhibition of one inhibits the other as well.
- Cu is an important part of cytochrome oxidase, but cyanide does not bind it.

25.7 (d) Antimycin

Inhibitors of respiratory chain

Inhibitors of electron transport	
Via complex I	Barbiturates Piericidin A Rotenone
Via complex II	TTFA CarboxinE
Via complex III	BAL Antimycin A
Via complex IV	Cyanide CO H$_2$S Sodium azide

Nutrition, Vitamins and Minerals

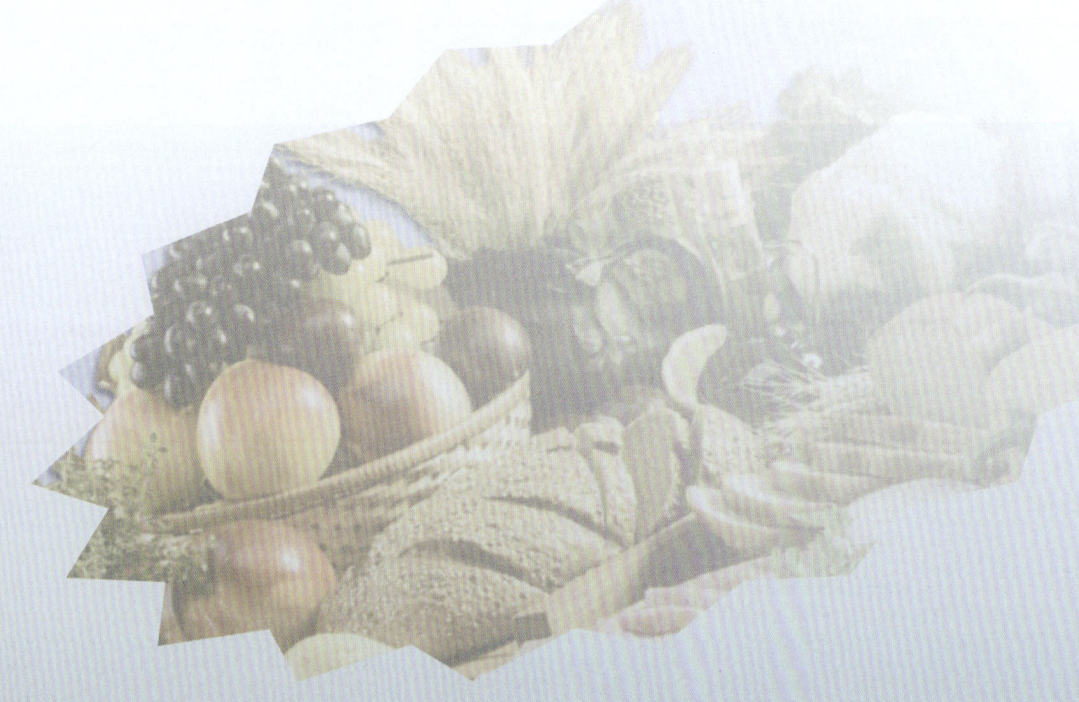

7

Nutrition,
Vitamins and Minerals

26

Nutrition

COMPETENCY BI 8.2

At the end of this chapter learner should be able to describe the types and causes of protein energy malnutrition and its effects.

COMPETENCY BI 8.3

At the end of this chapter learner should be able to provide dietary advice for optimal health in childhood and adult, in disease conditions like diabetes mellitus, coronary artery disease and in pregnancy.

COMPETENCY BI 8.5

At the end of this chapter learner should be able to summarize the nutritional importance of commonly used items of food including fruits and vegetables (macromolecules and their importance).

Specific Learning Objectives	
BI 8.2.1	Define protein energy malnutrition (PEM).
BI 8.2.2	Discuss various types of PEM.
BI 8.3.1	Discuss dietary advice for optimal health in adults.
BI 8.5.1	Describe the role of macromolecules in diet.
BI 8.5.2	Explain the importance of carbohydrates in diet (starch, sucrose and dietary fibers).
BI 8.5.3	Describe importance of dietary fats.
BI 8.5.4	Discuss benefits of essential fatty acids and atherogenic effect of trans fatty acids.
BI 8.5.5	Elaborate importance of dietary proteins (essential amino acids).

■ NUTRITION

Macronutrients

Balanced diet: A balanced diet is defined as one which contains a variety of foods in such quantity and proportion that need for energy and all nutrients are adequately met for maintaining health, vitality and general wellbeing.

Major macronutrients providing energy are the following:
• Carbohydrates • Lipids • Proteins

65–80% of total energy intake should be provided by carbohydrates, 10–30% by lipids and 7–15% by proteins.

Proximate principle of the food: Carbohydrates, lipids and proteins are called proximate principle of the food items.

Unit of energy: The unit of energy is calorie (cal).

Definition of a calorie: It is defined as the amount of heat required to raise temperature of 1.0 g of water by 1°C (specifically from 15°C to 16°C).

$$1 \text{ kcal} = 4.12 \text{ kJ}$$

Calorific value of various food items: Calorific value is defined as 'amount of heat energy obtained by burning 1.0 g of food stuff completely in the presence of oxygen.

Calorific value of different food stuffs is determined in an apparatus called bomb calorimeter. Calorific value of (Table 26.1):
• Carbohydrate—4 kcal/gram
• Protein—4 kcal/gram
• Lipid—4 kcal/gram
• Alcohol—7 kcal/gram

TABLE 26.1	Calorific value, RQ, SDA of various food items		
Nutrient	RQ	Calorific value	SDA
Carbohydrate	1.0	4 kcal/gram	5%
Protein	0.8	4.2 kcal/gram	30%
Lipid	0.7	9 kcal/gram	15%
Mixed diet	0.85	—	10%
Alcohol	—	7 kcal/gram	—

DIETARY REFERENCE INTAKE (DRI)

DRI is a quantitative estimate of the nutrient amount which should be consumed to prevent deficiencies and to maintain the optimum health.

Under DRI, following definitions are to be considered:

1. **Estimated average requirement (EAR):** Amount of nutrient estimated to meet the nutrient requirement of half (50%) of healthy individual in an age and gender group.
2. **Recommended dietary allowance (RDA):** Amount of nutrient estimated to meet the nutrient requirement of 97–98% of healthy individual population.

    Consumption of nutrient in excess and less quantity than RDA is associated with various disease states.

    RDA may be calculated as per following formula:

$$RDA = [EAR + 2 SD]$$

3. **Adequate intake (AI):** It is useful, if the experimental data is not available to calculate the EAR or SD, in that case adequate intake is defined. It is defined as the amount of nutrient estimated to meet the requirement of most of the individuals in a population.
4. **Tolerable upper intake level (UL):** It is the highest average intake of a nutrient that poses no risk for adverse health effect for almost all the individuals in a population.

BASAL METABOLIC RATE (BMR)

- It is minimal energy required by the body to sustain life and maintain vital function of the body.
- It is defined as 'energy expenditure by the body when at rest (physical, emotional and digestive) but not asleep, under thermal neutrality (at 25°C), estimated after 12 hours of fasting'.

Determination of BMR

1. Open circuit system, e.g. Tiscot and Douglas method.
2. **Closed circuit method:** BMR measured by Benedict-Roth metabolism apparatus.

Normal Value of BMR

Adult male: 35 kcal/m^2/hour

Adult female: 32 kcal/m^2/hour.

For easier calculation BMR for adult may be taken as 24 kcal/kg/day.

Factors Influencing BMR

1. **Age:** BMR of children is much higher than the adult. Maximum BMR is seen at the age of 5 years.
2. **Sex:** Women normally have lower BMR than men.
3. **Surface area:** BMR is directly proportional to surface area expressed as kcal/m^2/hour.
4. **State of nutrition:** BMR lowered in condition of malnutrition, starvation and wasting diseases.
5. **Exercise:** BMR increases during exercise.
6. **Drugs:** Drugs like caffeine, benzedrine, epinephrine, nicotine, alcohol, etc. increase the BMR.
7. **Hormones:** Thyroid hormones, adrenal medulla and anterior pituitary hormones increase BMR.
8. **Pregnancy:** BMR of pregnant mother after 6 months of gestation rises.
9. **Climate:** In cold climate BMR is increased.

Clinical Aspect (Pathological Variations in BMR)

1. **Fever:** Infections and febrile diseases elevate BMR usually in proportion to increase in temperature.
2. **Diseases:** BMR increased in diseases characterized by increased activity of cells, e.g. leukemia and polycythemia.
3. **Endocrine diseases**
    a. BMR is increased in hyperthyrodism, Cushing's disease, Cushing's syndrome also in acromegaly.
    b. BMR is reduced in hypothyroidism and Addison disease.

RESPIRATORY QUOTIENT (RQ)

RQ is 'ratio of volume of CO_2 produced by a volume of O_2 consumed during a given time by utilizing one gram of proximate principle' (Table 26.1).

RQ = volume of CO_2 produced/volume of O_2 consumed

a. RQ of the carbohydrate is 1.
b. RQ of the protein is 0.84.
c. RQ of the fat is 0.71.
d. RQ of mixed diet is about 0.85.

Clinical Aspects

1. **In acidosis:** During acidosis, CO_2 output is greater than O_2 consumption, hence RQ increased.
2. **In alkalosis:** RQ will fall, because respiration is depressed and CO_2 is retained in body and less CO_2 is produced.
3. **Febrile conditions:** Increase RQ.
4. **In diabetes mellitus:** RQ will fall initially because energy is supplied by oxidation of fats.

SPECIFIC DYNAMIC ACTION (SDA)/DIET INDUCED THERMOGENESIS

- This is the energy utilized in the processing of food like digestion, absorption, active transport, etc.
- This energy is utilized from previously available energy, so actual energy produced from the food is lesser than that of calculated value.
- SDA can be considered as activation energy needed for a chemical reaction.
- Proteins have greatest SDA, amounting to about 30% above its caloric value. Carbohydrate and lipid have SDA of 5% and 15% respectively (Table 26.1).
- For mixed diet, SDA may be calculated as 10%.

How to Calculate the Energy Requirement of a Normal Person

Factors taken into consideration for calculation of energy required by a normal person is the following:
a. Energy required for BMR
b. Physical activity based energy requirement
c. SDA of the food
d. Only additional requirement in pregnancy and lactation.

a. Energy required for BMR

For an adult, BMR is 24 kcal/kg body weight/day. So, according to the body weight, the energy required for BMR is to be calculated.

b. Physical activity based energy requirement:

Physical work may be sedentary, moderate or heavy. Energy requirement varies according to physical activity done by a person (as per his job requirement).

Sedentary worker require least energy (30% of BMR) to perform work. Moderate worker will require energy which is 40% of BMR but the heavy worker will need energy which is 50% of BMR.

c. SDA of mixed diet should be 10% of (a + b).

d. During pregnancy additional 300 kcal/day and during lactation additional 500 kcal/day energy has to be added in above calculation.

Calculate the energy required per day for a healthy adult of 60 kg doing moderate work.

Per day energy calculation for a 60-year-old male doing moderate work is shown in Fig. 26.1.

	Energy Required		
For BMR	24×60	=	1440 kcal
Moderate activity	40% of BMR	=	$\frac{40}{100} \times 1440$
		=	576 kcal
Subtotal (1)		**=**	**2,016 kcal**
Now,			
SDA @ 10% for mixed diet (2)		=	$\frac{10}{100} \times 2,016$
		=	**201.6 kcal**
Total (1) + (2)	= 2,016 + 201.6		
	= 2,217.6		
Round off (nearest of 50)	= 2,250 kcal		

Fig. 26.1: Energy calculation per day for a 60-year-old male doing moderate work

GLYCEMIC INDEX

It is defined to describe the effect of carbohydrate on blood glucose level. It is defined as effect of 50 grams of carbohydrate in a particular food on blood glucose level compared to 50 grams of glucose.

In other words,

It is a ratio of incremental area under glucose tolerance curve after 50 g of test meal to that of incremental area under glucose tolerance curve after 50 g of reference meal (glucose).

Simple carbohydrates like glucose have high glycemic index compared to complex carbohydrates such as starch (Table 26.2 and Fig. 26.2).

TABLE 26.2	Glycemic index of various food items
• Potato chips	80–90
• Bread	70–79
• White rice (polished)	70–79
• Parboiled (brown) rice	60–69
• Banana	60–69
• Beans, peas	40–49
• Legumes, peanuts	35–40
• Milk	35–40
• Ice cream	35–40

Section 7 ■ Nutrition, Vitamins and Minerals

26

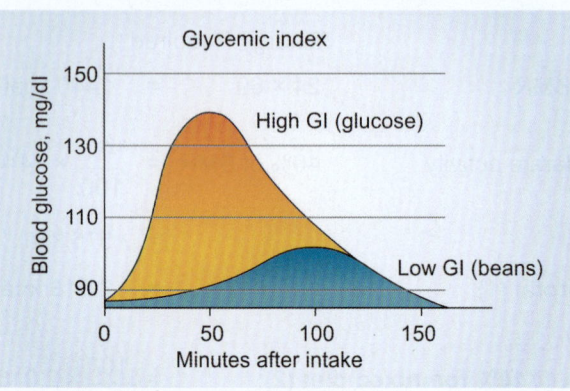

Fig. 26.2: Glycemic index

▌DIETARY FIBER

They are those components of the food that can not be broken down by human digestive enzymes. It is incorrect however to assume that fiber is indigestible since some fibers are, in fact, at least partially broken down by intestinal bacteria (Fig. 26.3).

Dietary fibers are undigestible and unavailable carbohydrates.

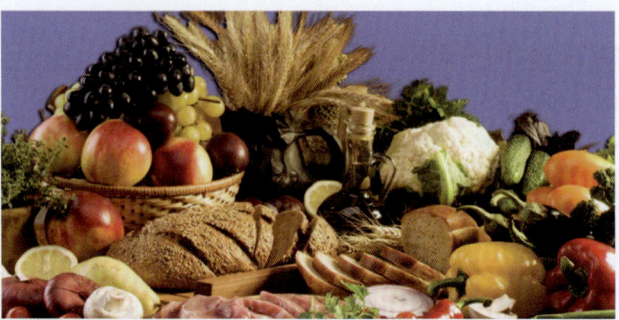

Fig. 26.3: Food rich in dietary fiber

Insoluble fiber increases stool bulk, improves gut motility and decreases transit time.

Daily requirement of dietary fiber for an healthy adult:

Male: 38 g/day
Female : 25 g/day
Examples of dietary fibers are:
1. Cellulose
2. Hemicellulose
3. Lignin
4. Pectins
5. Gums

26 Nutritional Indices of Protein

1. **Biological value (BV) of protein:** Ratio of nitrogen retained and nitrogen absorbed during a specific interval.

$BV = $ Nitrogen retained/Nitrogen absorbed $\times 100$
2. **Net protein utilization (NPU):** Ratio of nitrogen retained to that of the nitrogen intake multiplied by 100.

$NPU = $ Nitrogen retained/Nitrogen intake $\times 100$

Limiting amino acid: Amino acid deficient in a protein is known as limiting amino acid.

Methionine is the limiting amino acid in the pulses. Lysine is limiting amino acid in the cereals.

Nitrogen balance: When dietary nitrogen intake (calculated as 16% of protein intake) is equal to daily loss through urine, faeces, and sweat, it is called state of nitrogen balance.

When intake is excess of loss, it is said to be positive nitrogen balance.

When loss is excess of intake, it is said to be negative nitrogen balance.

Factors which lead to positive nitrogen balance (Fig. 25.4)
a. Period of growth
b. Pregnancy

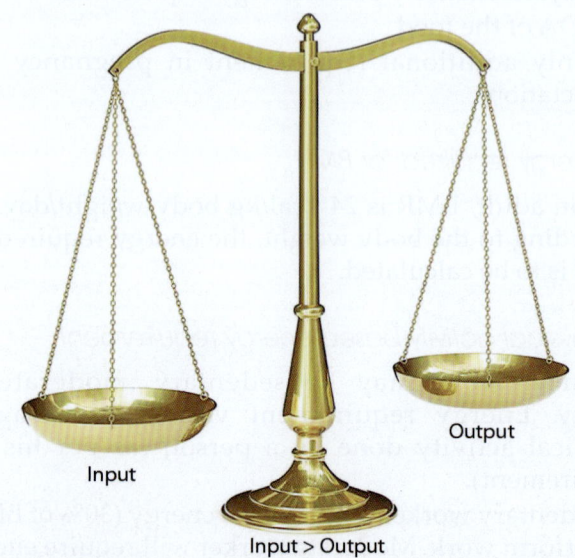

Fig. 26.4: State of positive N$_2$ balance

c. Lactation
d. Convalescence
e. Hormones like insulin, growth hormone, androgens.

Factors which lead to negative nitrogen balance (Fig. 25.5)
a. *Acute illness:* Surgery, trauma, burns
b. *Chronic illness:* Malignancy, uncontrolled diabetes mellitus
c. Protein deficiency in malnutrition
d. Starvation

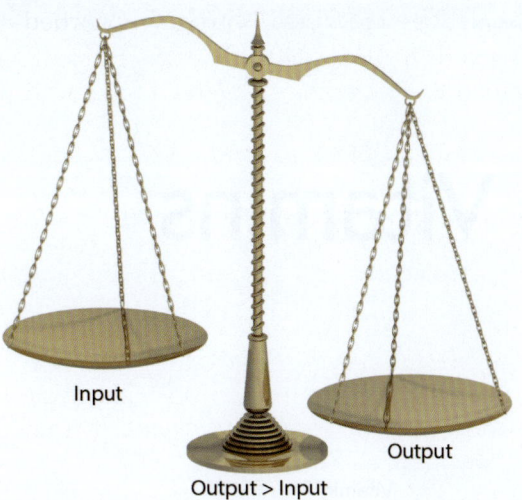

Fig. 26.5: State of negative N$_2$ balance

PROTEIN ENERGY MALNUTRITION (PEM)

Marasmus

Due to continuous deficiency of both dietary energy and protein (Fig. 26.6)

- No oedema
- Thin skin
- Frequent diarrhoea
- Weight loss of the baby
- Face shrunken
- Good appetite

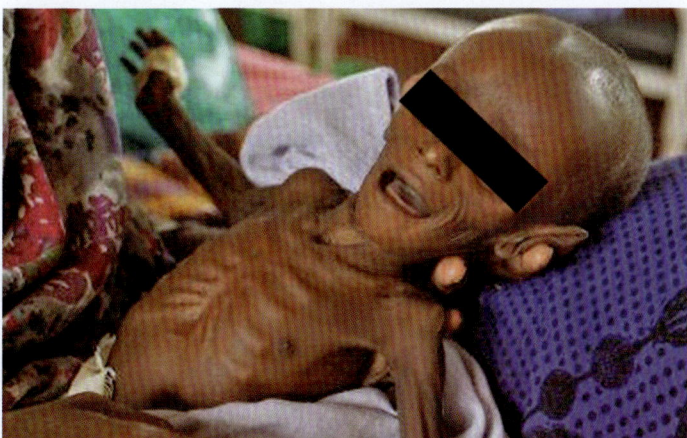

Fig. 26.6: Marasmus child

Kwashiorkor

- Due to isolated deficiency of protein alone along with adequate supply of calorie.
- Oedema is a characteristic sign (Fig. 26.7).
- Hypoalbuminemia
- Puffy face

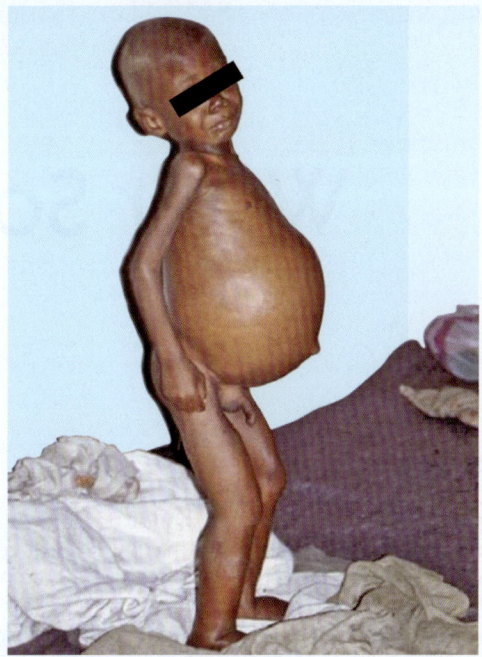

Fig. 26.7: Kwashiorkor (protuberant abdomen and puffy face to note)

- Abdomen protuberant
- Poor appetite

Biochemically such patients show altered value of serum protein, deficiency of mineral, vitamin, electrolyte imbalance due to associated infection and diarrhoea.

Fig. 26.8 shows the comparison of kwashiorkor and marasmus patients.

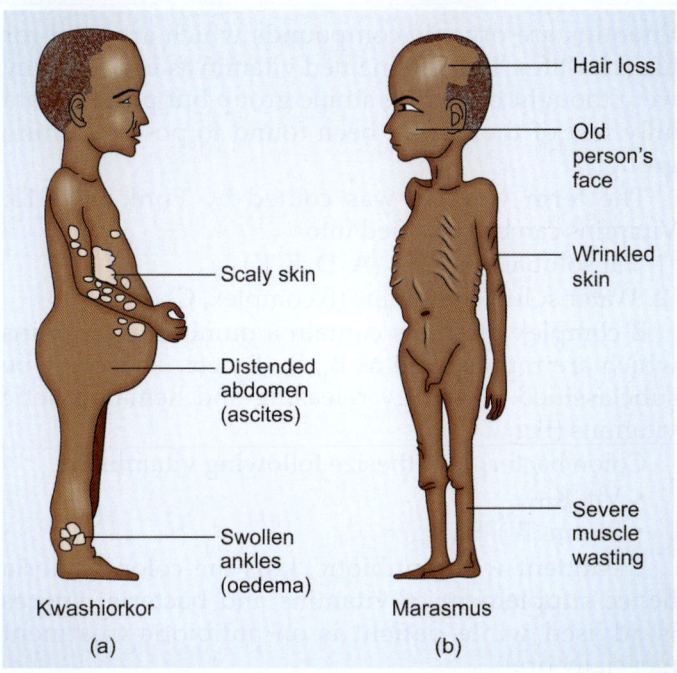

Fig. 26.8: Comparison of kwashiorkor and marasmus

Section 7 ■ Nutrition, Vitamins and Minerals

26

Water Soluble Vitamins

COMPETENCY BI 6.5

At the end of this chapter learner should be able to describe the biochemical role of vitamins in the body and explain the manifestations of their deficiency.

Specific Learning Objectives	
BI 6.5.1	Describe the biochemical role of vitamin A.
BI 6.5.2	Describe the biochemical role of vitamin C.
BI 6.5.3	Describe the biochemical role of vitamin D.
BI 6.5.4	Describe the biochemical role of vitamin K.
BI 6.5.5	Enumerate the good sources of vitamin A.
BI 6.5.6	Enumerate the good sources of vitamin D.
BI 6.5.7	Enumerate the good sources of vitamin E.
BI 6.5.8	Enumerate the good sources of vitamin K.
BI 6.5.9	Enumerate the deficiency manifestations of vitamin A.
BI 6.5.11	Enumerate the deficiency manifestations of vitamin D.
BI 6.5.12	Enumerate the deficiency manifestations of vitamin E.
BI 6.5.13	Enumerate the deficiency manifestations of vitamin K.

Vitamins are organic compounds which are vital for life (vita-life). They are named vitamin as initially they were thought of having amine group but present data only few of them have been found to possess amino group.

The term vitamin was coined by Funk in 1913. Vitamins can be classified into
1. Fat soluble vitamins (A, D, E, K)
2. Water soluble vitamins (B complex, C)

B complex vitamins contain a number of vitamins which are represented as B_1, B_2, B_3, etc. They may be subclassified as energy releasing and hematopoietic vitamins (Fig. 27.1).

Colon bacteria synthesize following vitamins:
• Vit. K
• Biotin (B_7), B_2, B_{12}

Treatment with antibiotic, kills the colon bacteria hence supplement of vitamins and bacterial spores is advised while patient is on antibiotic treatment (specially oral).

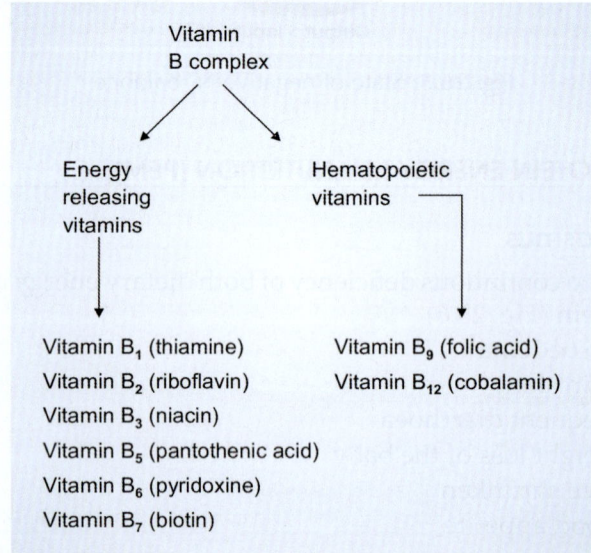

Fig. 27.1: Vitamin B complex

❚ FAT SOLUBLE

• Requires chylomicron for absorption
• Stored in liver and adipose tissue
• All fat soluble vitamins are isoprenoid compounds since they all are made up of one or more 5C isoprene units.
• They are mostly toxic in excess dose, e.g. vit. A and vit. D.

❚ WATER SOLUBLE

• Not stored in body except vitamin B_{12} which is considerably stored in liver.
• They are nontoxic in excess dose.
• Water soluble vitamins function as coenzyme for various enzymes.

Vitamin B$_1$

Vitamin B$_1$ is also known as
- Thiamine or
- Anti-beriberi factor or
- Antineuritic vitamin

Coenzyme form of thiamine is thiamine pyrophosphate (TPP).

In structure of thiamine, a pyrimidine ring is attached to thiazole ring through methylene bridge (Fig. 27.2).

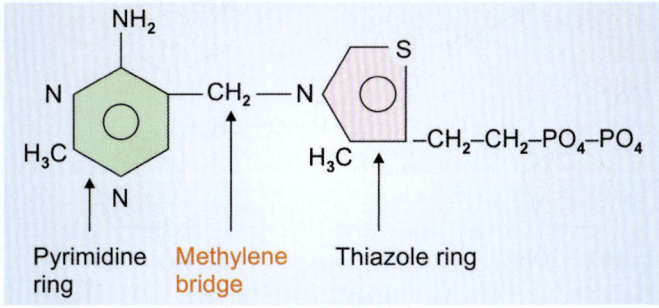

Pyrimidine ring   Methylene bridge   Thiazole ring

Fig. 27.2: Vitamin B$_1$ (thiamine)

TPP as coenzyme needed in following biochemical reactions:
  i. Branched chain α-keto acid dehydrogenase (decarboxylase) enzyme complex.
 ii. PDH complex
iii. Transketolase
 iv. α-keto glutarate dehydrogenase complex

RDA

1.0–1.5 mg/day	:	Adult
0.7–1.2 mg/day	:	Children
2.0 mg/day	:	Pregnancy, lactation, old age and alcoholism

Dietary Sources

Cereals (aleurone layer of cereals)
- Pulses
- Oil seeds
- Nuts
- Yeast
- Pork
- Liver
- Heart
- Kidney
- Milk

Deficiency Manifestation

Deficiency results in beriberi (Fig. 27.3).
1. Anorexia
2. Weakness
3. Constipation
4. Nausea
5. Depression

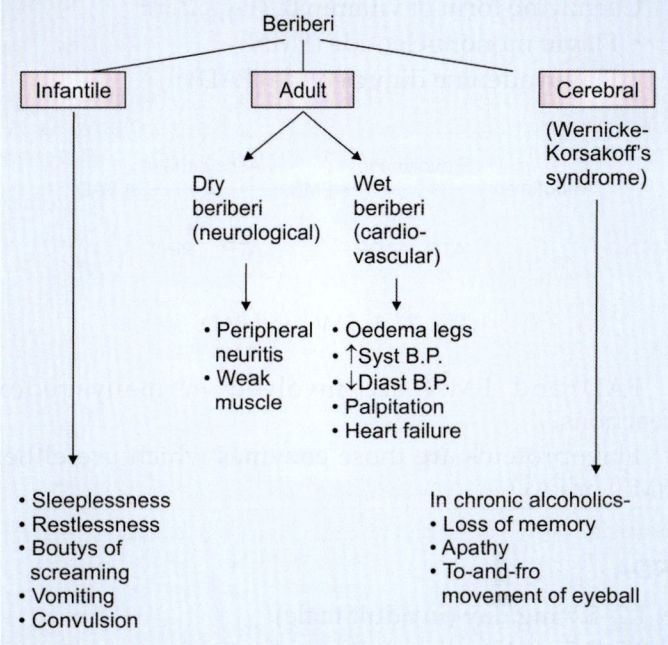

Fig. 27.3: Beriberi

6. Neuropathy
7. Pin and needle sensation in legs (numbness too).

RBC transketolase activity to be assessed to find out B$_1$ deficiency.

Sea food contain thiaminase.

Fern contains pyrithiamine.

Life-threatening lactic acidosis may be found in B$_1$ deficiency.

Vitamin B$_2$ (Riboflavin)

- It is intense yellow coloured vitamin (yellow vitamin of Warburg).
- Associated with cellular oxidation-reduction reaction.
- D-ribitol is attached to iso-alloxazine ring through 'N' atom (Fig. 27.4).
- Heat stable but photosensitive.

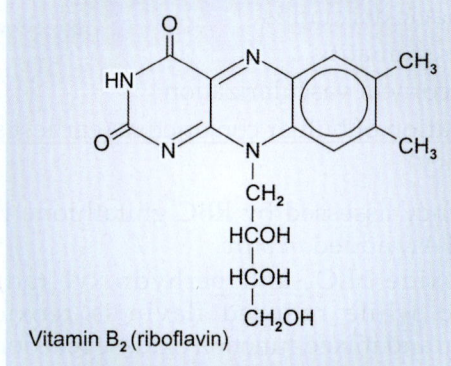

Vitamin B$_2$ (riboflavin)

Fig. 27.4: Structure of vitamin B$_2$

Section 7 ■ Nutrition, Vitamins and Minerals

27

Coenzyme form of vitamin B$_2$ (Fig. 27.5):
- Flavin mononucleotide (FMN)
- Flavin adenine dinucleotide (FAD)

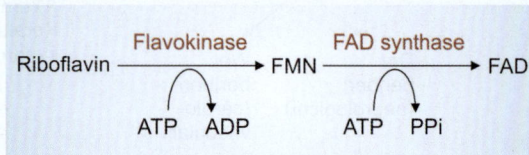

Fig. 27.5: FMN and FAD

FAD and FMN are involved in many redox reactions.

Flavoproteins are those enzymes which use either FMN or FAD.

RDA

- 1.2–1.7 mg/day (in adult male)
- 0.2–0.5 mg/day (in adult female)

Dietary Sources

- Milk
- Meat
- Egg
- Liver
- Kidney
- Cereals
- Fruits
- Vegetables
- Fish

(Galactoflavin is an antimetabolite of riboflavin.)

Deficiency Symptoms

- Cheilosis (lips)
- Glossitis (tongue)
- Seborrhocic dermatitis
- Angular stomatitis
- Circumcorneal vascularization
- Proliferation of bulbar conjunctiva (earliest sign of B$_2$ deficiency)

Deficiency assessed by RBC glutathione reductase assay by FAD added *in vitro*.

Superoxide H$_2$O$_2$ and perhydroxyl radicals are generated while reduced flavin is reoxidized in oxygenase and mixed function oxidase reactions. Flavin oxidase makes significant contribution to total oxidant stress in the body.

Vitamin B$_3$ (Niacin)

Pellagra preventing factor (PPF) of Goldberger. Active form of niacin is NAD$^+$ and NADP$^+$ (Fig. 27.6).

NAD$^+$ and NADP$^+$ can be synthesized by tryptophan 60 mg of tryptophan is equivalent to 1 mg of niacin (Fig. 27.7).

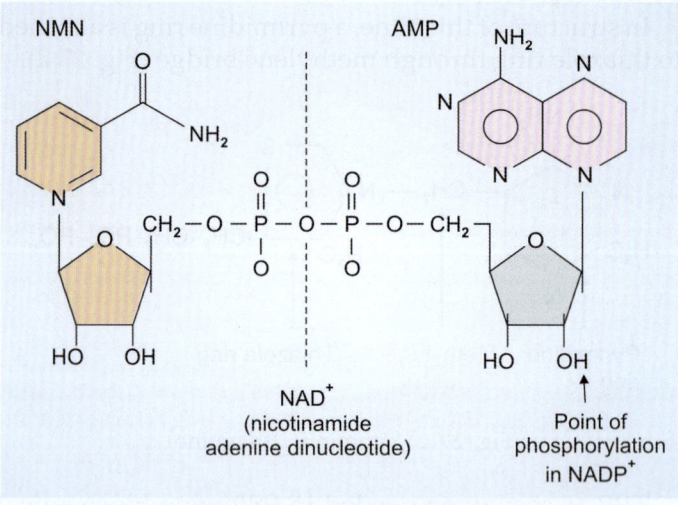

Fig. 27.6: NADP$^+$ structure
Niacin is pyridine-3-carboxylic acid

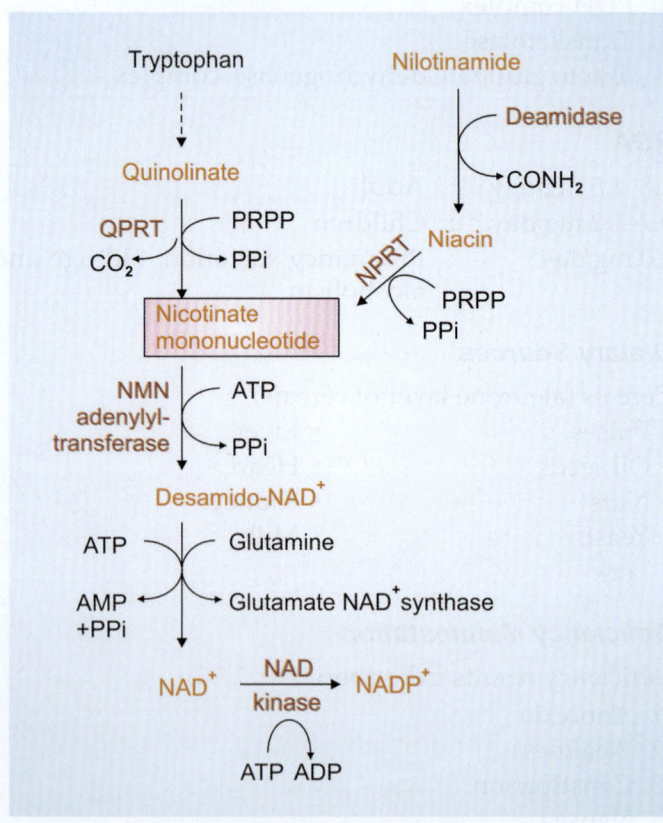

Fig. 27.7: Synthesis of NAD$^+$/NADP$^+$ from tryptophan

RDA

Adult: 15–20 mg
Child: 10–15 mg
One Niacin Equivalent [NE] = 1 mg of niacin

One Niacin Equivalent [NE] = $\dfrac{1}{60}$ mg of tryptophan

Dietary Sources

Meat, peanut, legumes, liver, yeast, whole grain, cereals, pulses (beans, peanut), milk, fish, egg, vegetable.

Deficiency Symptoms

Pellagra characterized by '4Ds':
- **Diarrhoea**
- **Dermatitis** (Fig. 27.8)
- **Dementia**
- **Death**

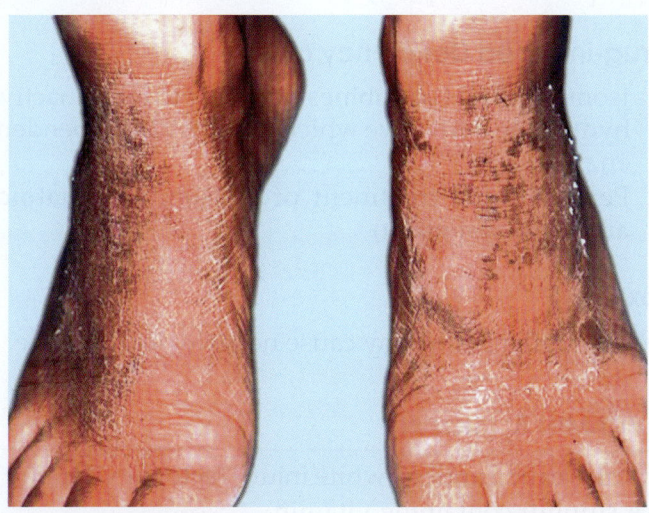

Fig. 27.8: Pellagra: Dermatitis

Deficiency of niacin is seen in corn/maize eating population who consumes it as staple diet.

Niacin in maize is in bound form, so it is not available for absorption.

Tryptophan content is low in maize.

Sorghum contains leucine in high amount.

Leucine inhibits conversion of niacin to NAD+ (leucine pellagra) by inhibiting QPRT enzyme.

Therapeutic Role of Niacin

2–4 g/day (200 times the RDA) is associated with
1. Inhibition of lipolysis in the adipose cell.
2. Decreased TAG synthesis in liver.
3. Decreased serum level of LDL, TAG, VLDL and HDL hence niacin is used in treatment of hyperlipidemia type II b.

4. In high doses niacin is found to be useful to decrease lipoprotein levels.

Niacin is not strictly a vitamin as it is synthesized in body during tryptophan metabolism.

Toxicity of B₃

- Dilatation of blood vessel
- Flushing
- Skin irritation
- Liver damage
- Hyperuricemia

VITAMIN B₅

(Pantothenic acid, *Pantos*: Everywhere)
- Chick antidermatitis factor or filtrate factor
- Panthothenic acid is important for
    a. Coenzyme A
    b. Phosphopantotheine moiety of FAS

Coenzyme A is the active form for pantothenic acid (CoA-SH).

CoA serves as a carrier of activated acetyl/acyl group (as thiol ester). It is synthesized in following steps from pantothenic acid (Fig. 27.9).

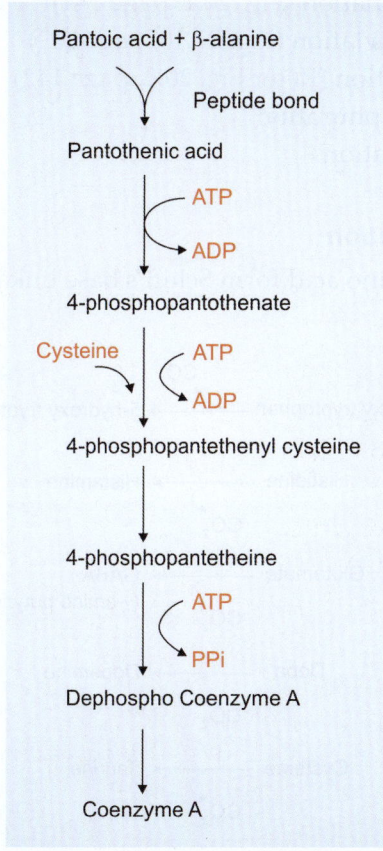

Fig. 27.9: Coenzyme A synthesis from pantothenic acid

Section 7 ■ Nutrition, Vitamins and Minerals

27

RDA

5–10 mg/day

Dietary Sources

Widely available, so deficiency is rare. Main sources are egg, liver, meat, yeast, milk.

Burning Feet Syndrome

Occurs in B_5 deficiency described by Indian scientist Gopalan.

VITAMIN B_6

Vitamins of B_6 are
- Pyridoxamine
- Pyridoxal
- Pyridoxine

Chemically similar substances that possess qualitatively similar vitamin activity.

Pyridoxal phosphate (PLP) is attached to ε-amino group of lysine of enzyme.

Vitamin B_6 (PLP) Requiring Process

1. Transamination (Fig. 20.1, page 141)
2. Decarboxylation (Fig. 27.10, page 202)
3. Deamination (Refer Fig. 20.2, page 142)
4. Trans-sulphuration
5. Condensation

Transamination

PLP and amino acid form Schiff's base linkage.

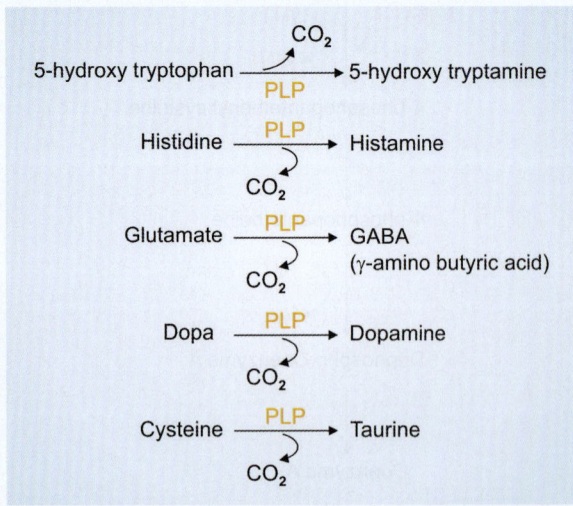

Fig. 27.10: Decarboxylation of amino acids

RDA

1.5 – 2.0 mg/day
Pregnancy
Lactation } 2.5 mg/day
Old age

Dietary Sources

Meat, vegetables, whole grain cereals and egg yolk are rich sources.

Deficiency Manifestation

- Fits in newborn
- Depression
- Irritability
- Confusion
- Convulsion (infantile fits)
- Peripheral neuropathy

Drug-induced Deficiency of B_6

1. Isoniazid (INH) combines with PLP to form inactive hydrazone derivative which inhibits PLP dependent enzymes.
2. Penicillamine treatment of Wilson, rheumatoid, arithritis, cystinuria)

Toxicity

Doses > 200 mg/day may cause neurological damage.

VITAMIN B_7 (BIOTIN)

It is also called antiegg white injury factor or vitamin H.
- A sulphur containing vitamin
- Prosthetic group for carboxylase enzyme
- Avidin is heat labile glycoprotein found in egg white and was called egg white injury factor.
- Heterocyclic, sulphur containing monocarboxylic acid
- Imidazole and thiophene ring fused with valeric acid side chain.
- Biotin is covalently bound to ε-amino group of lysine residue of carboxylase enzyme to form biocytin.
- Role of biotin in the action of pyruvate carboxylase is intensively studied. With the expenditure of ATP, CO_2 is first attached to lysine residue of enzyme to produce carboxybiotin enzyme complex.

This high energy complex then hand over the CO_2 to pyruvate to produce OAA.

Reactions where biotin is required are (Fig. 27.11):
1. Pyruvate → OAA (4C)
2. Acetyl CoA (2C) → Malonyl CoA (3C)
3. Propionyl CoA → Methyl malonyl CoA (4C)

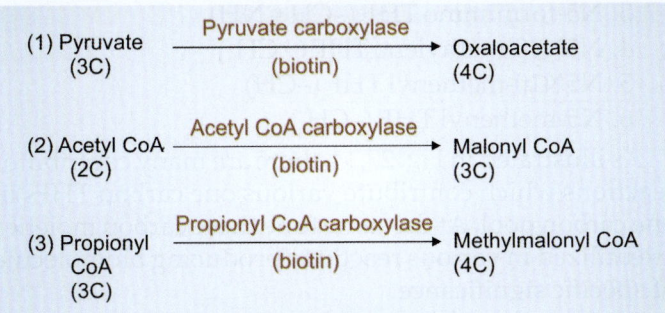

Fig. 27.11: Biotin needed as cofactor for carboxylase enzyme

4. Leucine metabolism
    β-methylcrotonyl CoA → β-methylglutaconyl CoA
5. Biotin plays role in cell cycle.

RDA

20–30 mg

Food/Dietary Sources

• Liver
• Kidney
• Egg yolk
• Milk
• Tomatoes
• Grain

Deficiency Symptoms

• Depression
• Hallucination
• Anemia
• Loss of appetite
• Nausea
• Dermatitis
• Glossitis

Dietary deficiency is rare and it may be associated with
    • Antibiotic use (kill gastrointestinal tract flora)
    • High consumption of raw egg.

VITAMIN LIKE COMPOUNDS

A. α-lipoic acid → Both fat and water soluble (Thioctic acid)
    • A sulphur containing fatty acid, it is required as coenzyme for decarboxylation in following enzyme complexes:
        a. PDH complex
        b. α-ketoglutarate dehydrogenase complex
        c. Branched chain α-ketoacid dehydrogenase enzyme complex.

• α-lipoic acid improves glucose utilization and decreases insulin resistance in metabolic syndrome and T2DM.
• 100–600 mg/day.

B. **Choline**
    • It is synthesized from serine.
    • It is included in B complex vitamin.
    • It is an important component of phospholipid lecithine.
    • Choline is lipotropic factor preventing the occurrence of fatty liver.
    • Choline is important for acetyl choline synthesis. Acetylcholine is an important neurotransmitter.

C. **Inositol**
    • Myoinositol is a constituent base of phospholipid 'Phosphatidyl inositol' (Fig. 27.12).
    • Phosphatidyl inositol diphosphate releases inositol triphosphate and diacyl glycerol by action of phospholipate C. IP_3 and DAG act as second messenger.
    • Inositol is also included in the list of lipotropic factor.

D. *Para*-amino benzoic acid (PABA)
E. **Bioflavonoids**

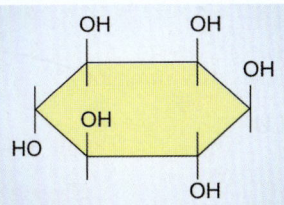

Fig. 27.12: Myoinositol

HEMATOPOIETIC VITAMINS (B₉, B₁₂)

Folic Acid (Vitamin B₉)

Folic acid consists of three components:
1. Pteridine ring
2. *Para*-aminobenzoic acid (PABA) (Fig. 27.13)
3. Glutamic acid

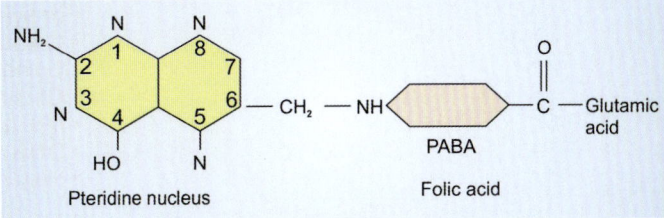

Fig. 27.13: Folic acid composition

Glutamic Acid

- Folic acid mostly has one glutamic acid residue and is called as pteroylglutamic acid (PGA)
- For absorption, monoglutamate of folic acid is required.
- For action as THF (tetrahydrofolate) polyglutamate (5–6 glutamate residues) is the most potent form.
- Stored in liver (10–12 mg) in polyglutama form. This store lasts for 2–3 months.
- N5-methyl THF is the circulatory form.

Biochemical role

THF is involved in one carbon metabolism.

THF acts as one carbon carrier. Various one carbon moieties which are transferred by THF are:

1. N5-formyl THF (–CHO)
2. N10-formyl THF (–CHO)
3. N5-formimino THF (–CH=NH)
4. N5N10-methylene THF (=CH$_2$)
5. N5N10-methenyl THF (–CH)
6. N5-methenyl THF (–CH$_3$)

As illustrated in Fig. 27.14, there are many contributor reactions which contribute various one carbon THFs in one carbon pool. At the same time these carbon moieties are utilized in various reactions producing biomolecule of specific significance.

For example, synthesis of following compounds needs one carbon THF:

1. Purine ring
2. Formyl methionine (initiator amino acid of protein synthesis in prokaryotes)
3. TMP (pyrimidine nucleotide) and hence DNA.

When one carbon folate has excess formyl THF, gets oxidized to yield CO_2.

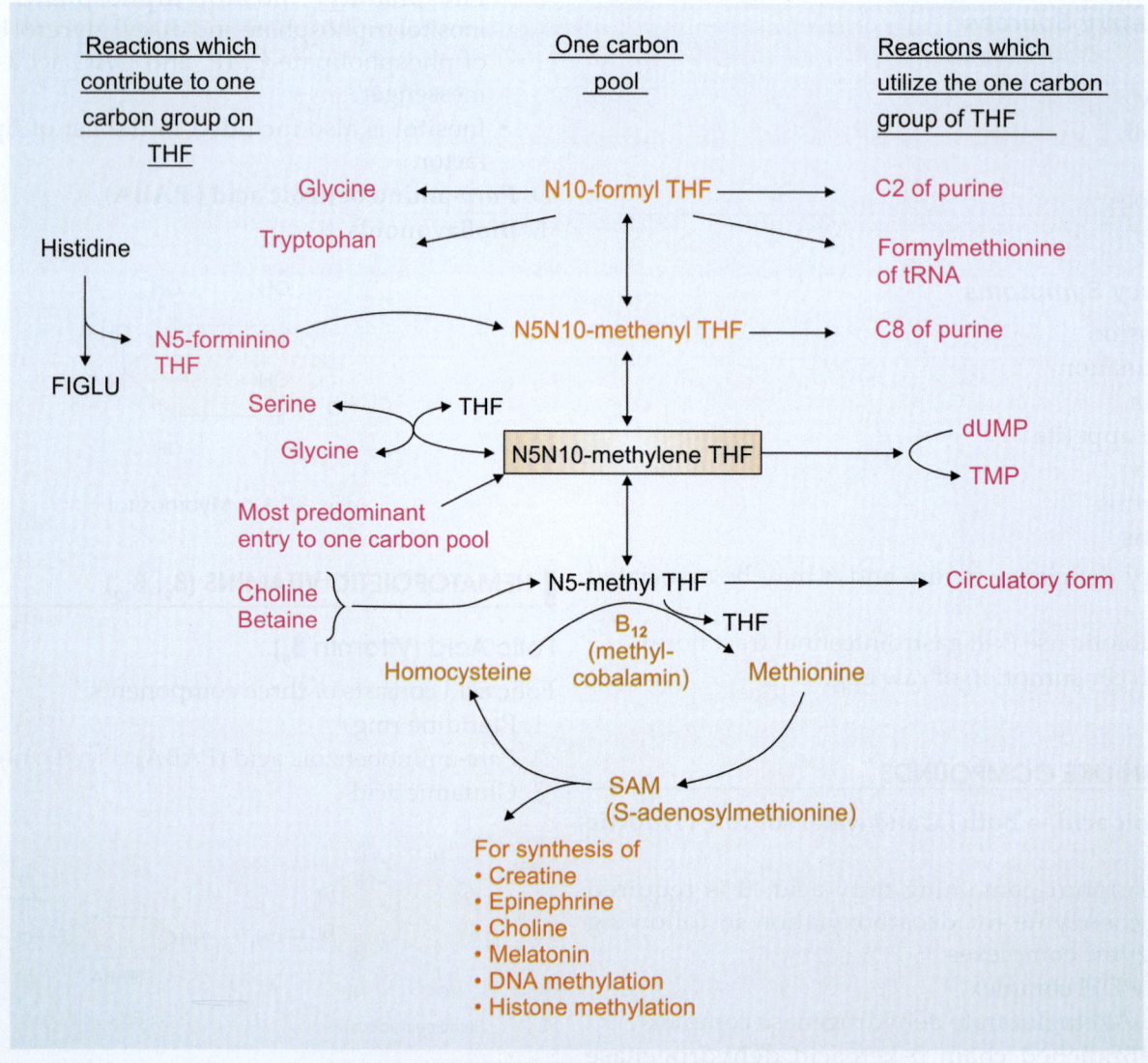

Fig. 27.14: One carbon metabolism

RDA

200 µg/day = Adult
400 µg/day = Pregnancy
300 µg/day = Lactation

Dietary Sources

- Green leafy vegetables
- Whole grains
- Cereals
- Liver
- Kidney
- Yeast
- Egg
- Milk

Deficiency Symptoms

- Most common vitamin deficiency is folic acid deficiency.
- Deficiency may be either due to inadequate intake, deficient absorption or increased demand.
- DNA synthesis is affected in folic acid deficiency due to nonavailability of purines and TMP. This leads to macrocytic RBC (cell cycle arrest at S phase).
- Folic acid deficiency in pregnant ladies is seen to be associated with neural tube defect. Early supplementation of folic acid (even before conception) is important for ladies in reproductive age group.
- In folic acid deficiency FIGLU is excreted in urine. To assess folic acid deficiency 'histidine load test' or 'FIGLU excretion test' is done.
- Macrocytic anemia with megaloblastic changes in bone marrow.

Folic Acid Antagonist

Following are competitive inhibitors of dihydrofolate reductase (DHF) reductase:

1. Aminopterin
2. Methotrexate (amethopterin)

So, above two drugs are used as anticancer agents.

In addition, antibacterial drugs like trimethoprim and pyrime-thamine antimalarial are also structural analogue of folic acid.

Sulphonamide is PABA analogue which inhibits incorporation of PABA into pteridine and hence blocks folic acid synthesis in bacteria. Bacteria thus is killed by sulphonamide therapy.

Human cell is not affected by sulphonamide as folic acid is not synthesized in human cell, rather it is needed in readymade form.

GIT enzyme removes glutamate residue and monoglutamate form of folic acid is absorbed. This absorption takes place at jejunum.

Anticonvulsants like dilantin and phenobarbitone inhibit gastrointestinal tract enzymes which remove the glutamate folate absorption, are reduced on such therapy.

Colon and cervical cancer is seen to be associated with folic acid deficiency.

VITAMIN (B₁₂)

- Also called antipernicious anemia factor, extrinsic factor of castle or cobalamin.
- Synthesized only by microorganisms.
- Corrin is tetrapyrrole ring with the central cobalt atom in it.
- Cobalt is having 6 valency, 4 valency of Co is coordinated with N atom of 4 pyrole ring and 6th valency of Co may bind either to
    i. Cyanide (cyanocobalamin)
    ii. Hydroxyl (hydroxylcobalamin)
    iii. Adenosylcobalamin (Ado-B₁₂)
    iv. Methylcobalamin

Functional coenzyme forms of B₁₂ in the body are Ado-B₁₂ and methyl B₁₂.

Vit. B₁₂ is red in color, H_2O soluble and heat stable.

Major storage forms: Ado-B₁₂.

Major form in plasma = methylcobalamin

Injectable preparation: Hydroxylcobalamin.

Absorption of B₁₂

- Intrinsic factor secreted by stomach parietal cell is required for absorption of vitamin B₁₂. It is a glycoprotein with molecular weight of 50,000 Da. One intrinsic factor binds with two molecule of vitamin B₁₂).
- Absorption of vit. B₁₂ takes place from ileum.
- In mucosal cell, B₁₂ is converted to methylcobalamin which when comes to blood binds with transcobalamins (TC I and II) (TC I > TC II)
- 4–5 mg lasting for 4–5 years in stock in liver. Vitamin B₁₂ is the only water soluble vitamin, which is stored in body.
- Excess of methylcobolamin is taken up by liver and is converted to deoxyadenosyl cobalamin and is stored.

Clinical Aspect

Pernicious anemia

Metabolic Role

Out of total 10 enzymes which are seen to be required vitamin B_{12} as cofactor, only 2 enzymes are found in mammals. They are:

1. Homocysteine methyltransferase (methionine synthase) (Fig. 27.15).

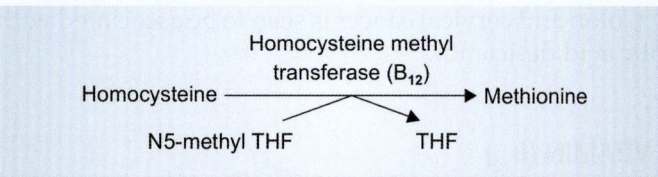

Fig. 27.15: Homocysteine methyltransferase

2. Methylmalonyl CoA mutase (Fig. 27.16)

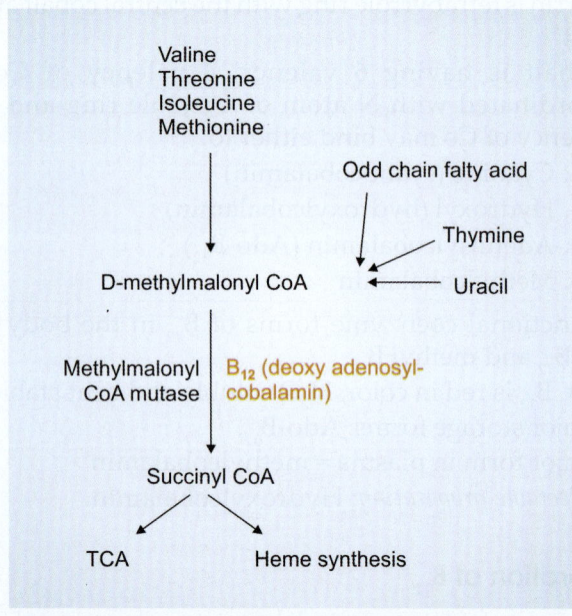

Fig. 27.16: Methylmalonyl CoA requiring vitamin B_{12}

Clinical Aspect

1. Methylmalonic aciduria
2. Folate trap
3. Megaloblastic anemia

RDA

Adult	1–2 µg/day
Children	0.5–1.5 µg/day
Pregnancy	
Lactation	3 µg/day

Dietary Sources

- Unique characteristic of vitamin B_{12} is that it is exclusively synthesized by microorganisms. So, an individual obtains vitamin B_{12} either by consuming items of animal origin or by his own gastrointestinal tract flora.
- Strict vegans who do not even consume curd or milk are prone to develop vitamin B_{12} deficiency.
- Milk, egg, curd, fish, pork, chicken are sources of vit. B_{12}.

Deficiency Manifestations

1. Megaloblastic anemia
2. Neuronal degeneration and demyelination of nervous system, [subacute combined degeneration (SACD)]
3. Hyperhomocysteinemia

Therapeutic Dose

100–1000 µg IM injection.
- Folic acid supplementation reverses the hematological abnormality observed in vitamin B_{12} deficiency, but neurological symptoms persist.
- Simultaneous administration of both vitamin B_{12} and folic acid is advised to treat megaloblastic anemia.

Folate Trap

In B_{12} deficiency plasma level of folate (N5-methyl THF) is found to be high. This is due to decreased action of homocysteine methyl transfer or methionine synthase which spares N5-methyl THF which circulates in plasma in excess quantity.

At the same time amount of free THF is reduced which affects DNA synthesis.

Factors Responsible for Vitamin B_{12} Deficiency

1. **Nutritional:** Inadequate intake which is commonly seen in vegans.
2. **Deficient absorption:** Seen in
   - Gastrectomy
   - Resection ileum
   - Malabsorption syndrome
3. **Addisonian pernicious anemia:** Uncommon in India but common in western countries. It is an autoimmune disorder where antibodies are developed against parietal cell leading to no partial absorption of vitamin B_{12}.
4. **Gastric atrophy**
5. **Pregnancy**
6. **Fish tapeworm:** *Diphillobothrium latum* infection in population eating live fish.

Assessment of B_{12} Deficiency

1. Serum B_{12} quantitation by RIA
2. Peripheral smear

VITAMIN C (ASCORBIC ACID)

- Water soluble
- Heat and alkali labile
- Vitamin C is a strong reducing agent ($Fe^{+++} \rightarrow Fe^{++}$)
- Reducing property is due to enediol carbon.
- L-ascorbic acid
- Dehydroascorbic acid
- D-ascorbic acid
- Ascorbic acid is a hexose (6 C) derivative, closely resembling the structure of monosaccharide (Fig. 27.17).

Dehydroascorbic acid is spontaneously and irreversibly, converted to inactive form 'diketogulonic acid'. Cu stimlates oxidation of ascorpic acid (Cu inactivates vitamin C) (Fig. 27.18).

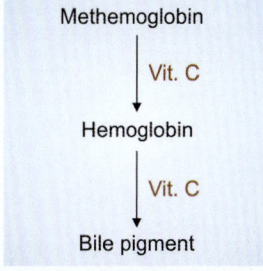

Fig. 27.17: Structure of ascorbic acid (vitamin C)

Fig. 27.18: Vitamin C (ascorbic acid)

Synthesis of Vitamin C in the Body

Many animals synthesize vitamin C via uronic acid pathway, but man, primate, guinea pig, and bat do not synthesize vitamin C in uronic acid pathway due to lack of enzyme L-gulonolactone oxidase.

Biochemical Role

a. Vitamin C is important for hydroxylation reactions. Following are important examples where vitamin C plays role in hydroxylation reactions (Fig. 27.19):

i. Proline	$\rightarrow$ Hydroxypoline
ii. Lysine	$\rightarrow$ Hydroxylysine
iii. Tryptophan	$\rightarrow$ 5-hydroxytryptophan

Hydroxylation of lysine and proline is important for cross-linking in procollagen, which converts it to collagen fibril.

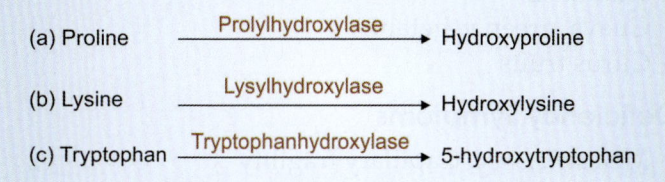

Fig. 29.19

b. Vitamin C helps in iron absorption in gastrointestinal tract lumen.

Vitamin C converts Fe^{+++} to Fe^{++} form, which is then transported across mucosal cell by DMT-1.

c. Methemoglobin is converted to Hb and then to bile pigment (Fig. 27.20).

d. Tyrosine metabolism

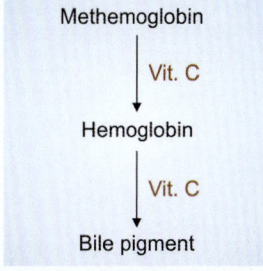

Fig. 27.20: Role of vitamin C

Vitamin C spares vitamin A, E and certain B complex vitamins by protecting them from oxidation.

f. Activation of folic acid requires vitamin C (Fig. 27.21).

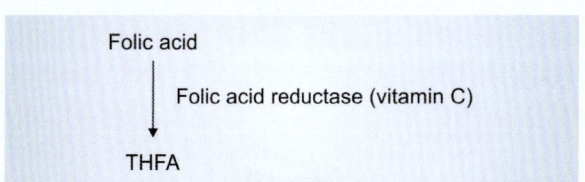

Fig. 27.21

g. Vitamin C acts as an antioxidant vitamin and helps protection against cataract, cancer, CAD.

h. Vitamin C enhances the synthesis of Ig and increases the phagocytic action of WBC.

i. Vitamin C is needed for carnitine synthesis which is important for fatty acid oxidation.

Section 7 ■ Nutrition, Vitamins and Minerals

27

RDA

75–90 mg/day for adult nonsmokers and 110–125 mg/day for smokers.

Additional 10–20 mg during pregnancy and lactation.

Dietary Sources

- Indian gooseberry (*Amla*) is the richest source of vitamin C.
- Guava, green vegetables
- Citrus fruits

Deficiency Symptoms

- *Mild deficiency:* Capillary fragility
- *Severe deficiency:*
  - Decreased wound healing
  - Osteoporosis
  - Hemorrhages
  - Anemia

Scurvy: Characterised by 'bleeding gums, loose teeth'.

Infantile Scurvy (Barlow's disease): Vitamin C is an antioxidant and is found to be useful in wound healing and common cold.

HEMATOLOGICAL AND NEUROLOGICAL CHANGES IN ALCOHOLICS IN VITAMIN DEFICIENCY

1. Megaloblastic erythropoiesis due to folate deficiency
2. Sideroblastic anemia due to B_6 (pyridoxine) deficiency
3. Peripheral neuropathy due to B_6 (pyridoxine) deficiency
4. Wernicke-Korsakoff syndrome

   Confusion, loss of memory, ataxia, uncoordinated eye movement, cogestive heart failure
5. Chronic alcoholics have redistribution of vitamin A in the body. Liver store is decreased while plasma and other tissues show normal or slightly elevated level of vitamin A.
6. Decreased bone density and increased incidence of osteoporosis
7. Zn, Ca, Mg are lowered in plasma.
8. Increased iron due to excess iron content in alcohol and iron absorption by alcohol

28

Fat Soluble Vitamins

COMPETENCY BI 6.5

At the end of this chapter learner should be able to describe the biochemical role of vitamins in the body and explain the manifestations of their deficiency.

Specific Learning Objectives	
BI 6.5.1	Describe the biochemical role of vitamin A.
BI 6.5.2	Describe the biochemical role of vitamin C.
BI 6.5.3	Describe the biochemical role of vitamin D.
BI 6.5.4	Describe the biochemical role of vitamin K.
BI 6.5.5	Enumerate the sources of vitamin A.
BI 6.5.6	Enumerate the sources of vitamin D.
BI 6.5.7	Enumerate the sources of vitamin E.
BI 6.5.8	Enumerate the sources of vitamin K.
BI 6.5.9	Enumerate the deficiency manifestations of vitamin A.
BI 6.5.11	Enumerate the deficiency manifestations of vitamin D.
BI 6.5.12	Enumerate the deficiency manifestations of vitamin E.
BI 6.5.13	Enumerate the deficiency manifestations of vitamin K.

▌VITAMIN D

It is also called sunshine vitamin, antirachitic vitamin and prohormone.

Two types of vitamin D:
  i. Vitamin D_2 (ergocalciferol)
  ii. Vitamin D_3 (cholecalciferol)

The compound which was named as vitamin D, was later proved to be not a vitamin D compound.

• Vitamin D_3 is produced from 7-dehydrocholesterol, a minor metabolite of cholesterol produced in gastrointestinal tract and is found in skin (Fig. 28.1).

  • Vitamin D_2 is produced from ergosterol found in plant via commercial photolysis (Fig. 28.2).

  • Difference of vitamin D_2 and vitamin D_3 is that vitamin D_2 has one additional methyl group and an additional double bond in its structure compared to vitamin D_3.

  • Potency of cholecalciferol (vitamin D_3) and ergocalciferol (vitamin D_2) is same.

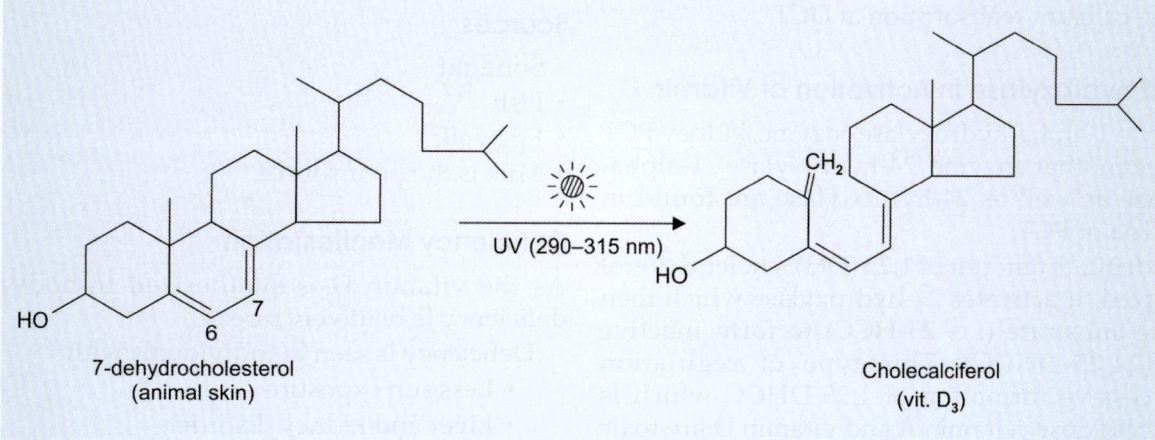

7-dehydrocholesterol
(animal skin)

UV (290–315 nm)

Cholecalciferol
(vit. D_3)

Fig. 28.1: Synthesis of vitamin D_3 (in animal skin)

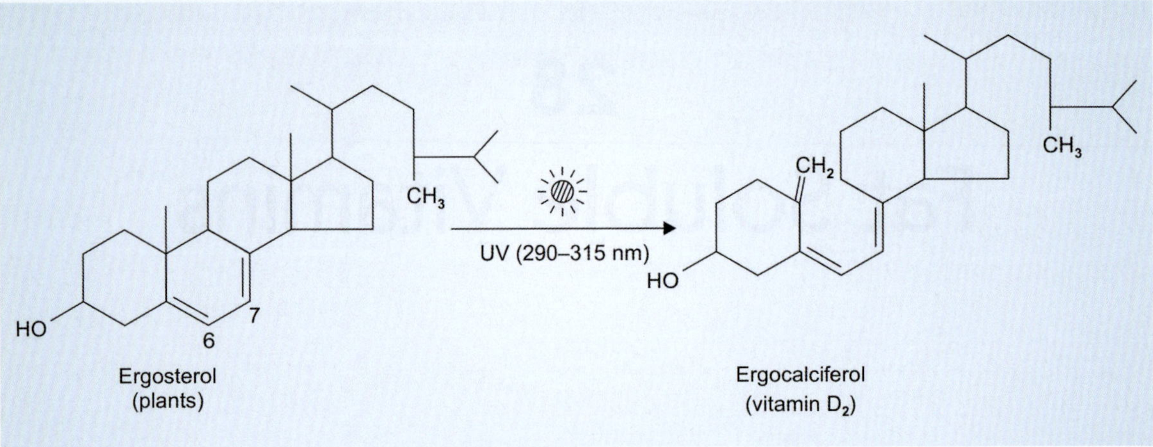

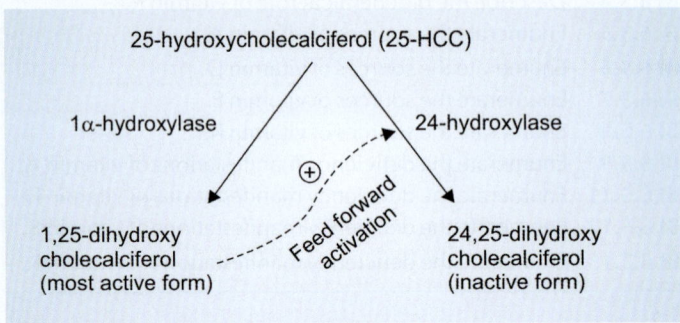

Fig. 28.2: Synthesis of vitamin D$_2$ (in plants)

Activation of Vitamin D

Activation of vitamin D occurs in proximal convoluted tubule of kidney (Figs 28.3 and 28.4).

Effect on Calcitriol on GIT, Bone and Kidney

Vitamin D maintains calcium homeostasis via following roles it play on various organs (Fig. 28.5):

On GIT: 1,25-dihydroxycholecalciferol acts as typical steroid hormone in gastrointestinal tract mucosa where it induces the synthesis of calbindin, the protein required for calcium transport from gastrointestinal tract lumen to mucosal cell.

On bone: 1,25-dihydroxycholecalciferol and PTH acts synergistically to promote bone resorption (demineralization) by stimulating osteoblast formation and activity.

On kidney (DCT): 1,25-dihydroxycholecalciferol and PTH inhibit calcium excretion via kidney by stimulating calcium reabsorption at DCT.

Role of 24-hydroxylase in Activation of Vitamin D

In addition to 1-alpha-hydroxylase enzyme, kidney PCT also has yet another enzyme '24-hydroxylase'. 1-alpha-hydroxylase as well as 24-hydroxylase are found in mitochondria of PCT.

When adequate amount of 1,25 (OH)$_2$ cholecalciferol is synthesized, it activates 24-hydroxylase which then diverts the substrate (i.e. 25-HCC) to form inactive product (24,25-DHCC). This type of regulation avoids excessive formation of 1,25-DHCC which is toxic in excess dose (vitamin A and vitamin D are toxic vitamins).

Half-life of 1,25-DHCC is only 6–8 hours and it is excreted mainly through bile.

RDA

Children   =   400 IU/day
Older   =   200 IU/day
Lactation =   400 IU/day
(1 mg of cholecalciferol or ergocalciferol = 40 IU)

Fig. 28.3: Regulated activation of vitamin D

Sources

- Sunlight
- Fish
- Egg yolk
- Milk is the poor source.

Deficiency Manifestation

As the vitamin D is synthesized in body itself, its deficiency is relatively rare.

Deficiency is seen in individuals with
- Less sun exposure
- Liver and kidney disorder
- Fat malabsorption syndrome

Deficiency of vitamin D results in rickets in children and osteomalacia in adults.

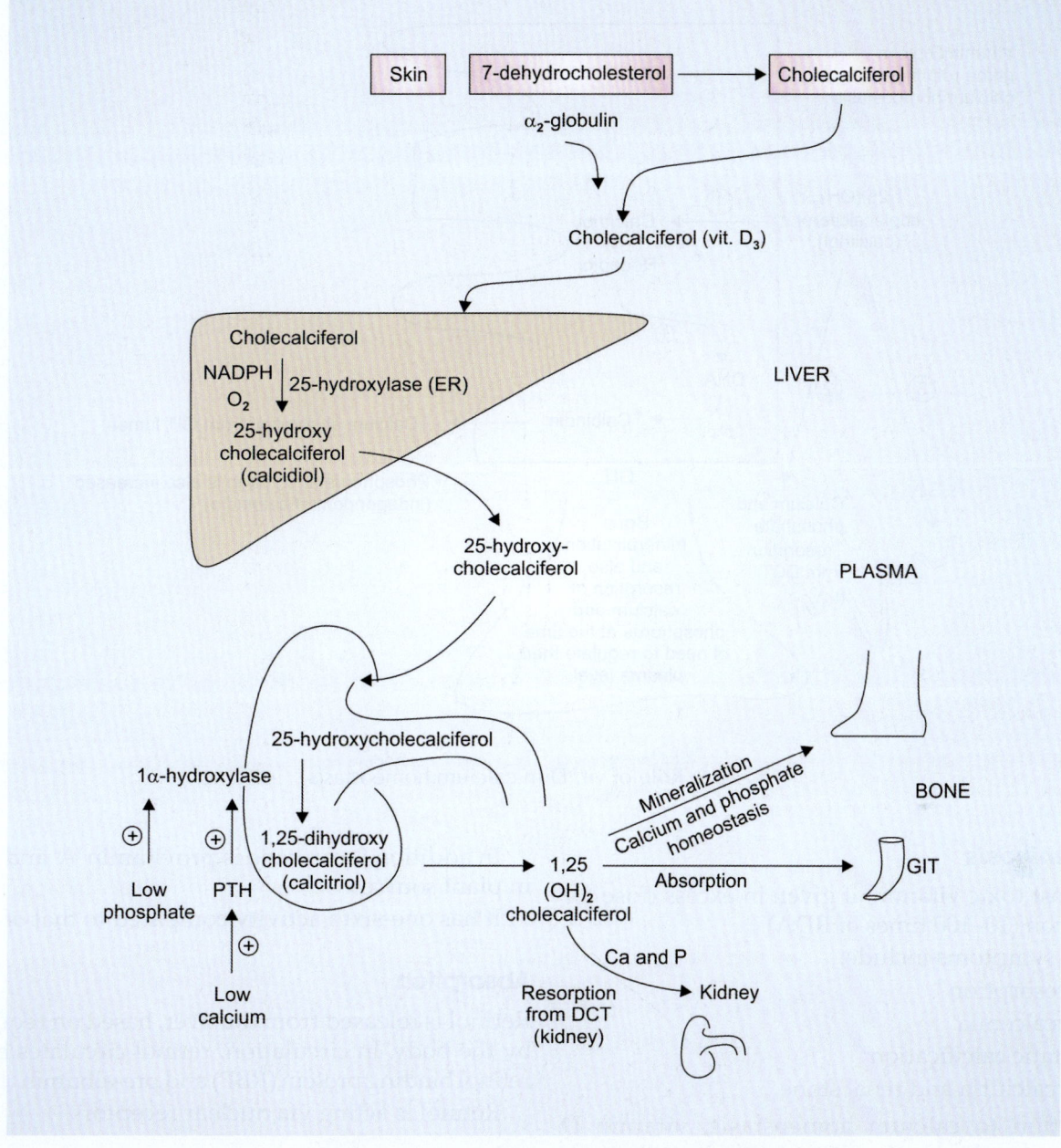

Fig. 28.4: Synthesis and activation of vitamin D

A. Rickets

Clinical presentation of rickets are:
 a. Bow legs
 b. Delayed teeth former
 c. Soft and pliable bone due to less mineralization. (Osteoid matrix is formed normally.)

Biochemical Feature

1. Decreased calcitriol level
2. Increased ALP

B. Osteomalacia

Here bones are soft and brittle. It fractures easily. It is due to demineralization of the pre-existing bone in lack of vitamin D.

Osteomalacia: Osteoid matrix is normal or intact.

Osteoporosis: Osteoid matrix is reduced.

Renal rickets (renal osteodystrophy)

In patient with chronic renal failure, calcitriol is not formed in the kidney. This results in deficiency manifestation.

Section 7 ■ Nutrition, Vitamins and Minerals

28

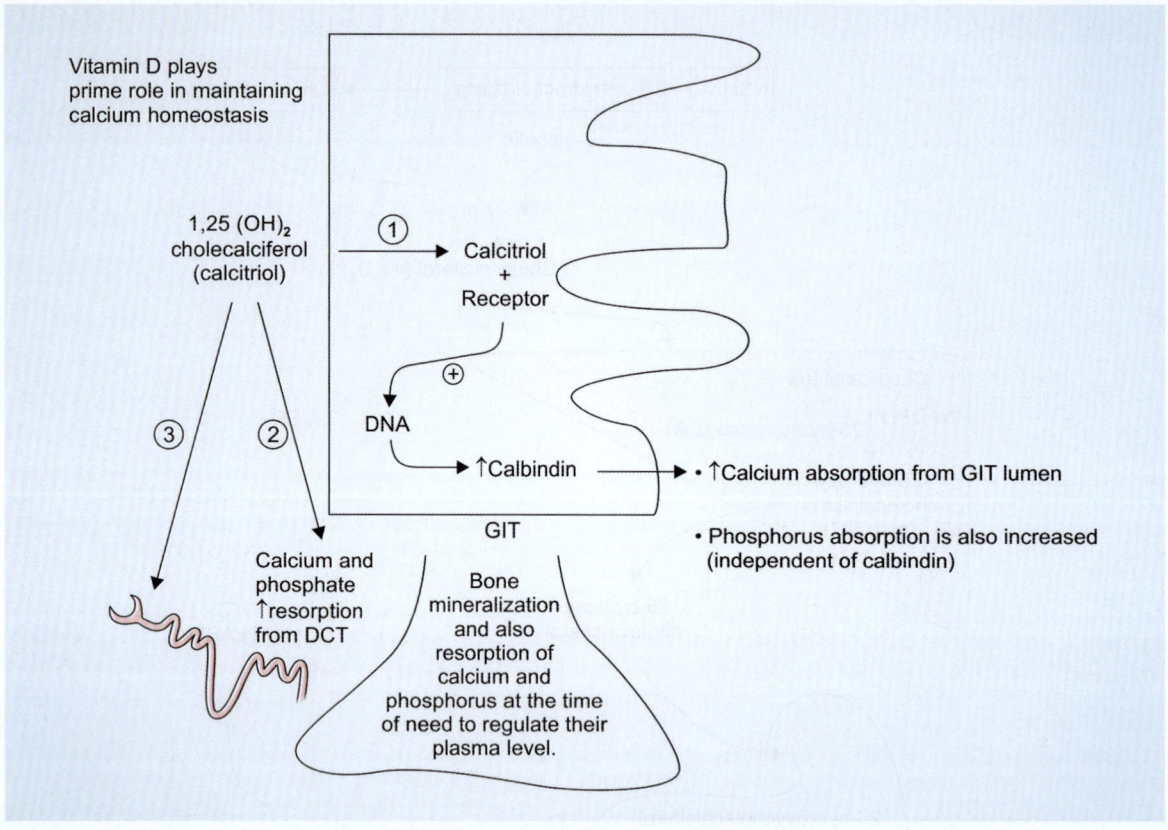

Fig. 28.5: Role of vit. D in calcium homeostasis

Hypervitaminosis

It is the most toxic vitamin, if given in excess dose for long duration (10–100 times of RDA).

Toxicity symptoms include:
- Bone resorption
- Hypercalcemia
- Metastatic calcification
- Hypercalciuria and renal stone.

In addition to calcium homeostasis, vitamin D is also seen to play an important role in cell proliferation, immune system, insulin secretion by beta cell, blood pressure control and neuromuscular functioning.

Best indicator of vitamin D sufficiency is 25-hydroxycholecalciferol level in blood.

▌ VITAMIN A

Number of compounds which all have vitamin A-like activity are included in terminology 'retinoids'.

These compounds are:
1. Retinol
2. Retinal
3. Retinoic acid

In addition β-carotene is provitamin 'A' and is found in plant sources.

It has one-sixth activity compared to that of retinol.

Absorption

Retinol is released from the liver, based on requirement by the body. In circulation, retinol circulates bound to retinol binding protein (RBP) and pre-albumin (Fig. 28.6).

Retinol is acting via nuclear receptors.

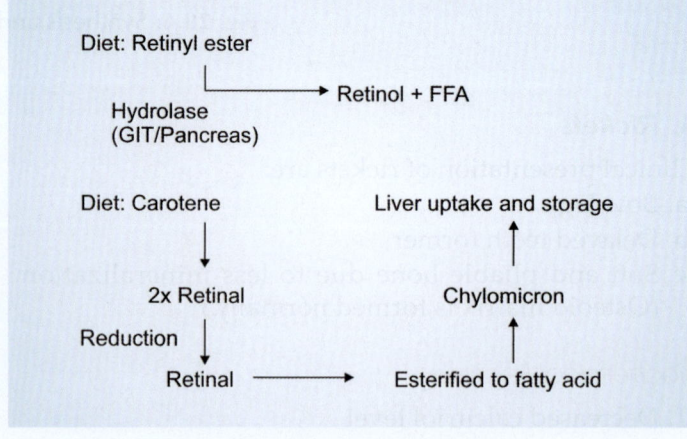

Fig. 28.6: Absorption of vitamin A

Biochemical Role of Vitamin A

Vision

Wald visual cycle (rhodopsin cycle) (Figs 28.7a and b).

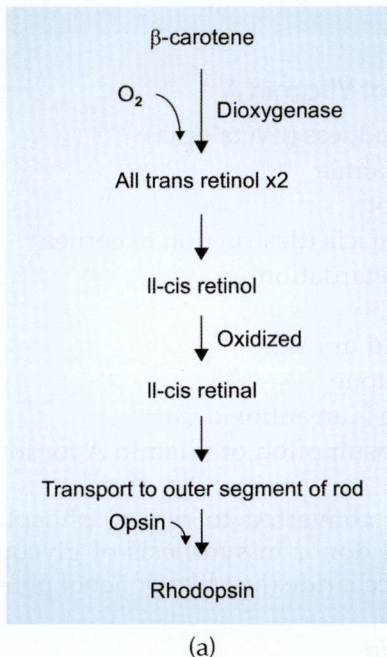

(a)

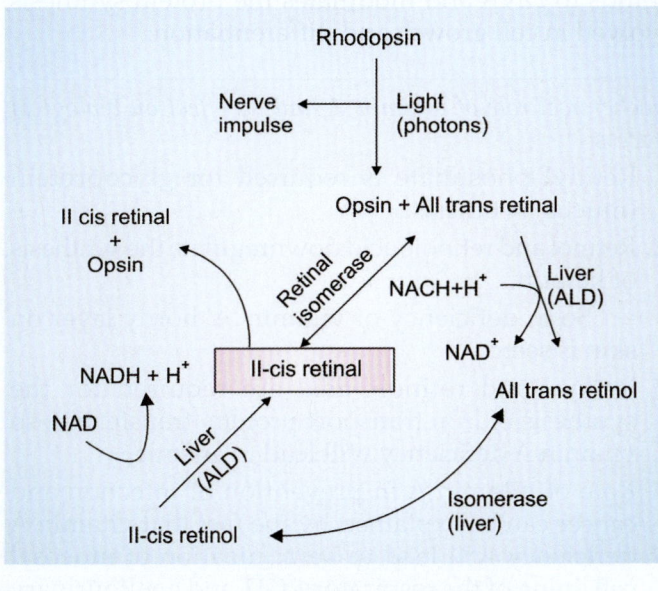

(b)

Fig. 28.7: Wald visual cycle

Rhodopsin is a conjugated protein in rods:

Opsin + II-cis retinal → Rhodopsin

Opsin is the protein, where ε-amino group of lysine is linked with –CHO of retinal.

Difference in rods and cones role in vision is summarized in Table 28.1.

TABLE 28.1 Differences between rods and cones	
Rods	*Cones*
Periphery	Center
Dim light	Bright light
Vision	Colour vision
10 millions	5 millions

Bleaching of Rhodopsin

See Fig. 28.8.

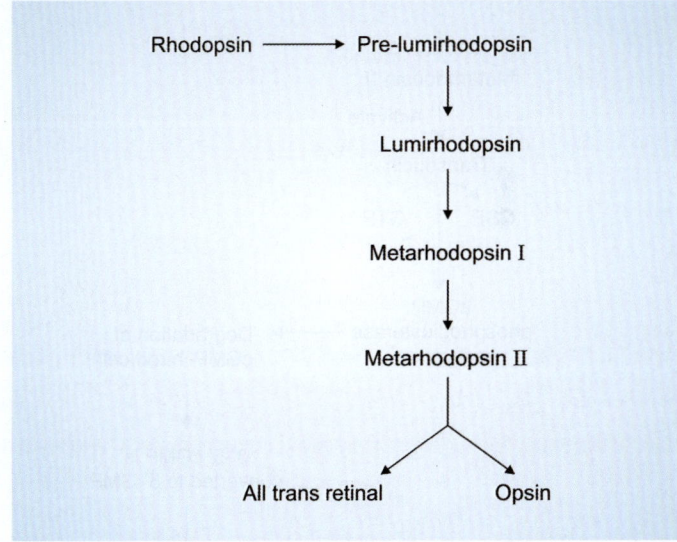

Fig. 28.8: Bleaching of rhodospin

Role of cGMP in Visual Cascade

Fall of photons on retina evokes membrane hyper-polarization which results in generation of nerve impulse (Fig. 28.9).

cGMP plays an important role in this.

Colour Vision

Cones are responsible for bright and colour vision. Colour sensitive pigments are:

Long porphyropsin → Splits to sense red

Medium iodopsin → Splits to sense green

Short cyanopsin → Splits to sense blue

All above pigments are made up of II-cis retinal and opsin.

When a particular colour light falls, the corresponding respective pigment is bleached (split). For example red colour light splits porphyropsin and green colour light splits iodopsin. This split sends signal to brain just like the phenomenon seen in rods.

Section 7 ■ Nutrition, Vitamins and Minerals

28

Other Roles of Vitamin A

1. Cell growth and differentiation
2. Prevent keratin synthesis
3. Synthesis of glycoprotein
4. Synthesis of transferrin
5. Maintaining immune system
6. Cholesterol synthesis
7. β-carotene and other carotenoids play an important role as an antioxidant.

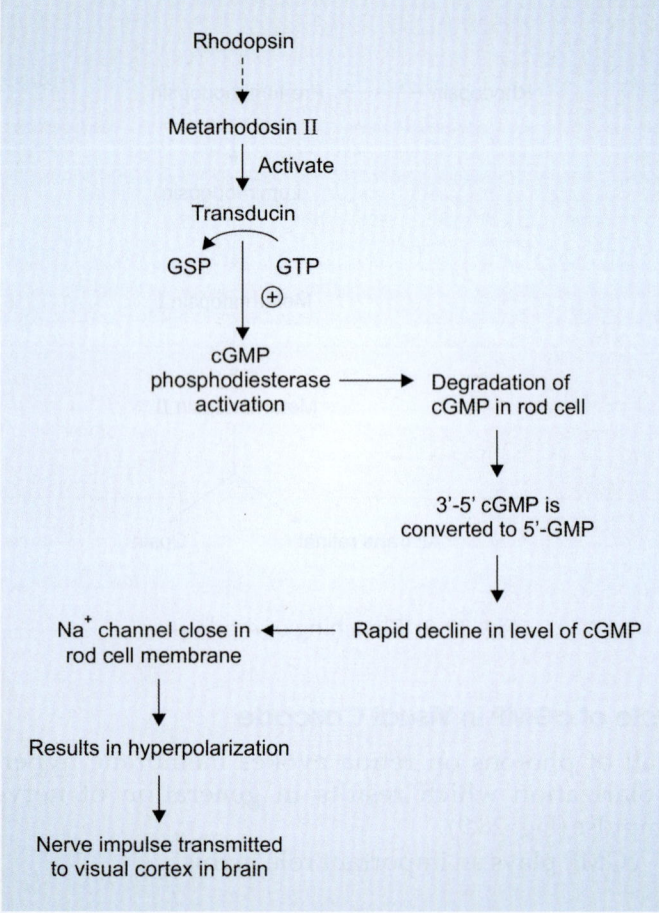

Fig. 28.9: Role of cGMP in visual cascade

RDA

Adult :   1000 RE in male
            (3000 IU/day)
            and
            800 RE in female
            (2500 IU/day)

1IU   =   0.3 mg of retinol
1 RE   =   1 μg of retinol
       =   12 μg of β-carotene
       =   24 μg of other carotenoids

Dietary Sources

Liver, kidney, egg yolk, milk, cheese, butter, fish (cod/shark) liver oil is rich source of vitamin A. Yellow and dark green vegetables and fruits contain carotene.

Deficiency of Vitamin A

1. Night blindness (nyctalopia)
2. Xerophthalmia
3. Bitot's spot
4. Keratomalacia (destruction of cornea)
5. Growth retardation
6. Male sterlity
7. Rough and dry skin
8. Urinary stone
   β-carotene is an antioxidant.

Excess consumption of vitamin A for long duration is toxic.

Retinol is converted to retinyl phosphate, which is a glycosyl donor in synthesis of glycoprotein and mucopolysaccharide (just like dolichol phosphate).

Retinoic Acid

It binds to DNA and modulates the protein synthesis, involved in cell growth and differentiation.

Biochemical role of vitamin A and its effect on biological process:

1. Retinyl phosphate is required for glycoprotein (mucus) synthesis.
2. Retinol and retinoic acid downregulate the synthesis of keratin.
   So in deficiency of vitamin 'A' horny layer on skin is seen.
3. Retinol and retinoic acid are required for the synthesis of iron transport protein 'transferrin', so vitamin A deficiency will lead to anemia.
4. Role of vitamin A in prevention of infection and cancer can be explained by the fact that vitamin A deficiency will lead to keratinization of mucosal cell lining of the respiratory, GIT and genitourinary tract, which results in fissure formation and promotes infection.

Toxicity

Excess of vitamin A consumption (25,000–50,000 IU/day) for over months or years will result in bone pain, scaly dermatitis, liver enlargement, spleen enlargement, nausea, diarrhoea, etc.

VITAMIN E (TOCOPHEROL)

Vitamin E is the most potent biological antioxidant. This is also known as antisterility or anti-infertility vitamin.

Vitamin E is constituent of group of tocopherols and tocotrienols. Eight vitamers have been identified α, β, γ, δ etc.

To scavenger reactive oxygen species (ROM), most potent is α-tocopherol while to scavenger reactive nitrogen species (RNS), most potent is γ-tocopherol.

Tocopherols are derived of 6-hydroxychromane (tocol) ring with 3 units of isoprenoids in the side chain (Fig. 28.10).

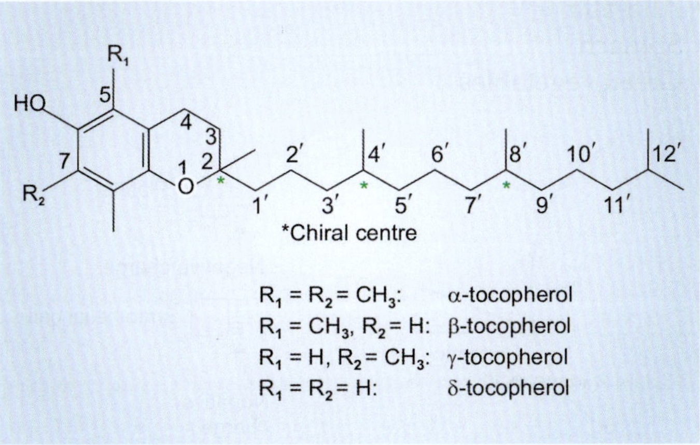

R₁ = R₂ = CH₃: α-tocopherol
R₁ = CH₃, R₂ = H: β-tocopherol
R₁ = H, R₂ = CH₃: γ-tocopherol
R₁ = R₂ = H: δ-tocopherol

Fig. 28.10: Structure of vitamin E

Absorption from GIT

Vitamin E, like many other fatsoluble vitamins, are absorbed from gastrointestinal tract lumen through chylomicron.

Liver sends it in plasma by incorporating it in VLDL and LDL core.

Plasma level of tocopherol is <1 mg/dl.

Biochemical Role of Vitamin E

Biochemical role of vitamin E can be broadly discussed under following headings:
- Antioxidant role
- Effect on enzyme
- Effect on transcription

Vitamin E as an Antioxidant

- Vitamin E is a scavenger of free radical. In that process vitamin E itself is oxidized to quinone form.
- Vitamin E protects cell membrane
  - Vitamin E protects RBC membrane

- Vitamin E is important for normal reproductive function
- Vitamin E is needed in heme synthesis (ALA synthase and ALA dehydratase).
- Vitamin E stabilizes coenzyme Q.
- Vitamin E delays onset of cataract.

Synergistic Role of Vitamin E and Selenium

Vitamin E is an antioxidant and selenium is seen component amino acid Se-Cys (selenocysteins) found in glutathione peroxidase (GPO).

GPO is an important enzyme which detoxify H_2O_2.

Selenium and vitamin E are seen to be mutually sparing requirement of each other.

RDA

Male = 10 mg of tocopherol (15 IU)
Female = 8 mg of tocpheorol (12 IU)

Vitamin E supplementation to be increased with increased consumption of PUFA.

Dietary Sources

- Wheat gram oil
- Cotton seed oil
- Peanut oil
- Corn oil
- Sunflower oil

Deficiency Symptoms

- Sterility
- Degenerative changes in muscle
- Megaloblastic anemia
- CNS changes
- Fragile RBC

Vitamin E is least toxic amongst fat soluble vitamins.

VITAMIN K

Vitamin K is the only fat soluble vitamin which has specific coenzyme function.

Three forms of vitamin K are:
1. **Vitamin K₁ (phylloquinone):** Plant sources
2. **Vitamin K₂ (menaquinone):** Animal sources
3. **Vitamin K₃ (menadione):** Synthetic analogue

Vitamin K₁, K₂ and K₃ are naphthoquinone derivatives. Vitamin K₁ and K₂ have isoprenoid side chain.

Vitamin K is heat stable but acid and alkali labile.

Section 7 ■ Nutrition, Vitamins and Minerals

28

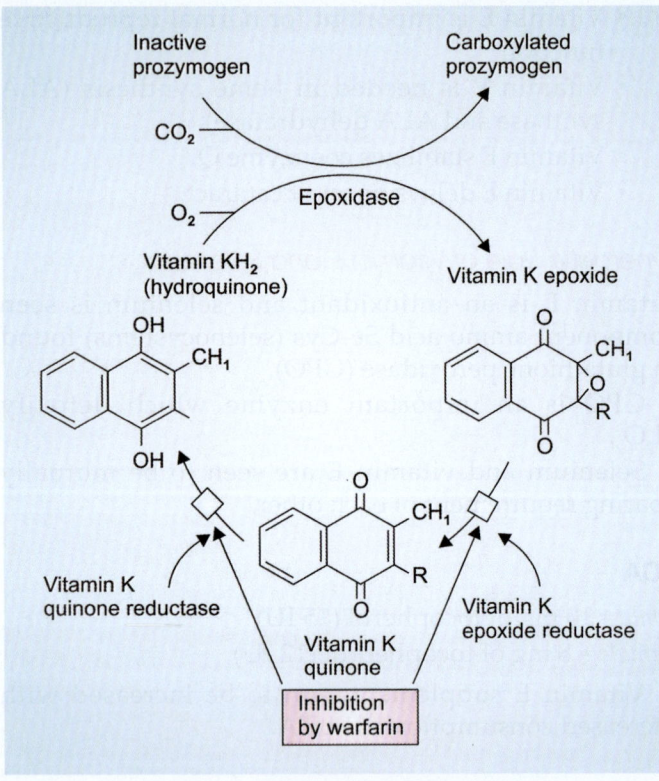

Fig. 28.11: Vit. K cycle or epoxide cycle

Biochemical Role

Vitamin K and Carboxylation

Vitamin K is involved in carboxylation of clotting factor II, VII, IX, X and also in carboxylation of bone proteins like osteocalcin, matrix Gla protein (MGP), Gas6. Vit. K cycle is important for carboxylation of these proteins (Fig. 28.11). Carboxylation of osteocalcin helps in bone mineralization and carboxylation of Gas6 and MGP are important to prevent vascular calcification. Even nephrocalcin in kidney undergoes vitamin K dependent carboxylation.

Gamma carboxyglutamic acid is a good chelator of calcium and it allows the binding of calcium to protein (Fig. 28.12).

Vitamin K_1 is stored in liver.

Vitamin K_2 is accumulated in peripheral tissues.

RDA

70–100 microgram/day in adults

Dietary Sources

• Cabbage
• Cauliflower
• Tomato
• Alfa-alfa
• Spinach
• Green vegetables

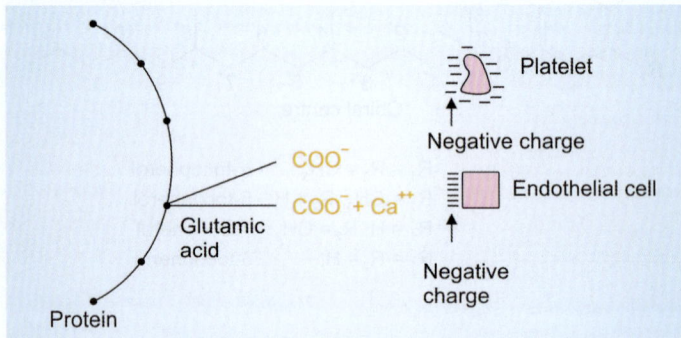

Fig. 28.12: Carboxylation of glutamic acid

Deficiency Symptoms

• Increased clotting time
• Vitamin K deficiency is common in newborn infant of mother who is on anticonvulsant therapy.
• Vitamin K deficiency is commonly associated with obstructive jaundice due to fat malabsorption.
• Vitamin K deficiency is common in patients with long term antibiotic therapy.

EXERCISE

LONG QUESTIONS (10 MARKS EACH)

Q 1. How is vitamin D synthesized in human body? Describe its activation. How does vitamin D help maintain serum calcium level? Name two disorders which are related with vitamin D deficiency.

Q 2. Write in detail about chemistry, absorption, metabolism and biological functions of vitamin A. How does vitamin A help in growth and tissue differentiation?

Q 3. Describe various biochemical roles of vitamin C. How is the deficiency of vitamin C responsible for bleeding gums seen in scurvy?

SHORT NOTES (5 MARKS EACH)

Q 1. Biochemical role of cobalamin and vitamin B_{12} deficiency

Q 2. Biochemical role of vitamin A

Q 3. Physiological roles of thiamine and folic acid

Q 4. Folate trap and its affect on the metabolism of one carbon moiety

Q 5. Biological role of vitamin K and mechanism of its function

Q 6. Role of vitamin C in connective tissue formation

Q 7. Role of folic acid in one carbon metabolism

Q 8. Beri-beri

Q 9. Vitamin K cycle

Q 10. Antioxidant vitamins

Q 11. Vitamins as coenzymes

Q 12. Role of vitamin E and selenium as antioxidants

Q 13. Rickets

Q 14. One carbon metabolism

MULTIPLE CHOICE QUESTIONS

28.1 Respiratory quotient after heavy carbohydrate meal is:
a. 1.2
b. 0.8
c. 1.0
d. 0.7

28.2 Calcium absorption is increased in the GUT by:
a. 1,25-dihydroxycholecalciferol
b. Intrinsic factor
c. Calcitonin
d. PTH

28.3 For single carbon transfer, which coenzyme is responsible?
a. Acetyl CoA
b. Biotin
c. THFA
d. Pyridoxine

28.4 A person ingests 100 g of proteins/day and excretes 25 g of nitrogen. What is he/she?
a. Normal healthy individual
b. Pregnant lady
c. Clinically ill
d. Nephrotic syndrome

28.5 Anion gap means:
a. Gap in anion molecule
b. Difference between high and normal anion gap acidosis
c. Unmeasured ions
d. Primary deficit of anions

28.6 Thermogenic food is present in which of the following?
a. High protein diet
b. High carbohydrate diet
c. High fat diet
d. It does not depend on the macronutrients

28.7 Vitamin B$_{12}$ acts as a coenzyme to which of the following enzymes?
a. Isocitrate dehydrogenase
b. Homocysteine methyltransferase
c. Glycogen synthase
d. Glucose-6-phosphate dehydrogenase

28.8 Which among the following reactions requires pyridoxal phosphate as a coenzyme?
a. Carboxylation
b. Glycogen synthesis
c. One carbon transfer
d. PDH complex

28.9 Thiamine pyrophosphate is a coenzyme required for:
a. Branched chain amino acid dehydrogenase complex
b. 2-hydroxyphytanoyl-CoA lyase
c. Transketolase
d. All of the above

28.10 Which of the following conditions most rapidly produces a functional deficiency of vitamin K?
a. Coumadin therapy to prevent thrombosis in patients prone to clot formation.
b. Broad spectrum antibiotic therapy
c. Lack of red meat in the diet
d. Lack of citrus fruits in the diet

28.11 Neural tube effects such as anencephaly and spina bifida have higher frequencies in certain population. Deficiency of which of the following vitamins is associated with the occurrence of neural tube defects ?
a. Thiamine (vit. B$_1$)
b. Riboflavin (vit. B$_2$)
c. Biotin
d. Folic acid

28.12 Vitamin K is involved in the post-translational modification of:
a. Glutamate
b. Aspartate
c. Lysine
d. Proline

28.13 Active form of vitamin D is:
a. Cholecalciferol
b. 1,25 (OH)$_2$ cholecalciferol
c. 24,25 (OH)$_2$ cholecalciferol
d. 25 (OH) cholecalciferol

28.14 Which is true about BMR?
a. Is not influenced by energy intake.
b. Increases in response to starvation.

c. May decrease up to 50% during period of starvation.
d. Not responsive to change in the hormonal level.

28.15 Vitamin B$_{12}$ is:
a. Extrinsic factor of Castle
b. Intrinsic factor of Castle
c. Cyanocobalamin
d. Decrease Ca^{2+} and decrease PO$_4$

28.16 Which vitamin is also acting as hormone?
a. Vitamin D
b. Vitamin A
c. Vitamin B$_1$
d. Vitamin C

28.17 Vitamin B$_{12}$ is absorbed in the:
a. Stomach
b. Duodenum
c. Lower jejunum
d. Proximal ilium
e. Terminal ilium

28.18 Glutathione peroxidase contains:
a. Selenium
b. Iron

c. Zinc
d. Copper

28.19 Amount of proteins excreted in urine/24 hour is:
a. Less than 150 mg
b. 200 mg
c. 450 mg
d. 800 mg

28.20 Thiamine is not used in which of the following reactions?
a. Lactate to pyruvate
b. Alpha-ketoglutarate to succinyl CoA
c. Glucose to pentose
d. Oxidative decarboxylation of alpha-keto acid of branched chain amino acid

28.21 Which is not pyridoxine dependent?
a. Oxaluria
b. Homocystinuria
c. Maple syrup urine disease
d. Xanthurenic aciduria

28.22 Specific dynamic action (SDA) is greatest of:
a. Protein
b. Carbohydrates
c. Fat
d. Vitamins

ANSWERS

28.1 (c) 1.0

Respiratory quotient: It is the ratio of CO_2 produced and O_2 consumed to completely combust 1 g of proximate principles.

RQ of various food iteams:

Food item	RQ
Carbohydrate	1.00
Protein	0.80
Fat	0.70
Mixed food	0.85

28.2 (a) 1,25-dihydroxycholecalciferol

- In liver, vitamin D is hydroxylated at the 25th position, and in kidney further hydroxylation is affected at the 1st position to produce dihydroxycholecalciferol or calcitriol.
- The calcitriol induces a carrier protein in the intestinal mucosa, which increases the absorption of calcium. Hence, blood calcium level tends to be elevated.
- Vitamin D is acting independently on bone. Vitamin D increases the number and activity of osteoblasts, the bone forming cells.
- Secretion of alkaline phosphatase by osteoblasts is increased by vitamin D.

28.3 (c) THFA

Folic Acid

- Coenzyme from tetrahydrofolic acid (THFA).

Function: Transporter for single carbon units ($-CH_3$, $-CH_2$, $COOH$) for purine, thymidylate synthesis and methionine synthesis from homocysteine—requires B_{12}.

Deficiency

- Most common vitamin deficiency in humans
- Hematopoietic tissue—anemia
- Epithelial cells—nutrient absorption impaired.

28.4 (c) Clinically ill

Nitrogen Balance

- Nitrogen balance can be actually measured by calculating the dietary intake of protein nitrogen (16% of the weight of the ingested proteins) and comparing it with the daily nitrogen excretion.
- A normal healthy adult is said to be in nitrogen balance if the dietary intake of nitrogen (I) = daily loss in urine (U) + feces (F) + skin (S).

$$I = U + F + S$$

- In the above question, the person ingests 100 g (which amounts in 16 g of ingested nitrogen) of proteins/day and excretes 25 g of nitrogen/day.
- Hence, the rate of nitrogen excretion is more than that of ingestion. Hence, the person is in a state of negative nitrogen balance which is common in illness.

28.5 (c) Unmeasured ions

Anion Gap

- A clear concept of the anion gap (AG) is essential. The sum of cations and anions in ECF is always equal, so as to maintain the electrical neutrality.
- Sodium and potassium together account for 95% of the cations whereas chloride and bicarbonate account for only 86% of the anions.
- Only these electrolytes are commonly measured. Hence, there is always a difference between the measured cations and the anions. The unmeasured anions constitute the anion gap which is due to the presence of protein anions, sulphate, phosphate and organic acids. The anion gap is calculated as the difference between ($Na^+ + K^+$) and ($HCO_3 + Cl^-$).

  Anion Gap = $[Na^+ + K^+] - [HCO_3^- + Cl^-]$
- Normally this is about 12 ± 5 mmol/liter. The alternation in anion gap is extremely useful in the clinical assessment of patients with acid–base disorders.

28.6 (a) High protein diet

- Thermogenic foods may help increase metabolism and calorie burning by enhancing thermogenesis
- The main determinant of DIT (diet-induced thermogenesis) is the energy content of the food, followed by the protein fraction of the food.
- The intestinal absorption of nutrients, the initial steps of their metabolism and the storage of the absorbed nutrient but not immediately oxidized nutrient.

28.7 (b) Homocysteine methyltransferase

- This enzyme is needed for conversion of homocysteine to the methionine.
- This is B_{12} dependent enzyme, which requires methyl THF as a methyl donor. Deficiency of vitamin B_{12} leads to accumulation of methyl THF (folate trap).
- As free form of THF is required for the synthesis of N5N10-methylene THF, which is required for the synthesis of dTMP from dUMP by the enzyme

thymidylate synthase, the deficiency of B_{12} leads to defective synthesis of the dTMP and thus that of the DNA and thus megaloblastic anemia.

28.8 (b) Glycogen synthesis

Pyridoxal phosphate is the coenzyme required for following reactions:

- Transaminases
- Decarboxylation of amino acid
- ALA synthase
- Kynureninase
- Glycogen phosphorylase
- Cystathionine beta-synthase

28.9 (d) All of the above

Thiamine pyrophosphate (TPP) or thiamine diphosphate (TDP) is a thiamine derivative which is cleaved by thiamine pyrophosphatase.

Thiamine pyrophosphate is a coenzyme to many enzymes, such as:

- Pyruvate dehydrogenase complex
- Alpha-ketoglutarate dehydrogenase complex
- Branched chain amino acid dehydrogenase complex
- 2-hydroxyphytanoyl CoA lyase
- Transketolase.

28.10 (a) Coumadin therapy to prevent thrombosis in patients prone to clot formation

- Coumadin is an analogue of vitamin K and acts as anticoagulant via competing with vitamin K.
- Even broad spectrum antibiotics do not sterilise intestine completely.
- Red meat and citrus fruit are not the source of vitamin K. Vitamin K is richly found in green and leafy vegetables.

28.11 (d) Folic acid

B_1 deficiency in chronic alcoholics is associated with Wernicke-Korsakoff psychosis (loss of memory, rhythmic eyeball movement). Thiamine deficiency from excess consumption of polished rice leads to beri-beri.

Riboflavin (vit. B_2) deficiency leads to mouth ulcer (stomatitis), glossitis, cheilosis (dry and scaly lips), scaly skin (seborrhoea) and photophobia.

Biotin deficiency leads to dermatitis, lethargy and dehydration. Lactic acidosis may be an important finding in biotin deficiency. This is due to lack of functional pyruvate carboxylase enzyme in biotin deficiency.

28.12 (a) Glutamate

- Vitamin K is responsible for post-translational modification of glutamate residue of clotting factors II, VII, IX, X.
- It facilitates γ-carboxylation of this residue in these clotting factors which facilitate clotting process.
- Vitamin K also carboxylates the bone protein osteocalcin which is synthesized by osteoblast and thus helps in mineralization of bone. (Osteocalcin also contains hydroxyproline, so it is dependent on both vitamins C and K.)

28.13 (b) 1,25 (OH)$_2$ cholecalciferol

Vitamin D is derived either from 7-dehydrocholesterol (Malpighian layer of the epidermis) or ergosterol (fungus derived) by the action of ultraviolet radiation.

7-dehydrocholesterol of the skin cell is isomerised to form cholecalciferol which is a prohormone. It is first transported to liver where it is hydroxylated by microsomal enzyme 25-hydroxylase.

25-hydroxycholecalciferol is the major transportable form and it is bound to vitamin D binding protein '$α_2$ globulin'.

In the kidney it is further hydroxylated at 1st position to form 1,25 (OH)$_2$ cholecalciferol which is also known as calcitriol. This is most active form of the vitamin D.

Rate-limiting enzyme of vitamin D synthesis is 25α-hydroxylase.

28.14 (c) May decrease up to 50% during period of starvation

This is a part of survival mechanism in starvation.

Reduced energy intake reduces BMR and increased energy intake increases BMR.

BMR changes in response to hormone level. Thyroid hormone, cortisol, etc. increase the BMR.

28.15 (a) Extrinsic factor of Castle

Vitamin B_{12} needs intrinsic factor (a small glycoprotein secreted from parietal cell of stomach) for its absorption from terminal ilium.

Hence, vitamin B_{12} is also known as extrinsic factor of Castle.

28.16 (a) Stomach and (b) Duodenum

28.17 (e) Terminal ilium

28.18 (a) Selenium

28.19 (a) Less than 150 mg

Section 7 ■ Nutrition, Vitamins and Minerals

28

28.20 (a) Lactate to pyruvate

Option b: By action of alpha-ketoglutarate dehydrogenase complex.

Option c: By action of transketolase (in HMP shunt pathway).

Option d: By action of branched chain alpha-keto acid dehydrogenase/decarboxylase complex.

28.21 (c) Maple syrup urine disease

28.22 (a) Protein

Specific Dynamic Action (SDA)

This refers to the increased heat production following the intake of food.

This **energy is trapped in the food from previously available energy, so that the actual energy produced from the food** is lesser than that of calculated value.

SDA can be considered as activation energy needed for a chemical reaction.

1. **Proteins have greatest SDA, amounting to about 30% above its caloric value.**
2. *Fats:* SDA value is 15%.
3. *Carbohydrates:* SDA value is 5%.

Nutrient	RQ	SDA
Carbohydrate	1.00	5%
Lipid	0.70	15%
Protein	0.85	30%

29

Minerals and their Metabolism

COMPETENCY BI 6.9

At the end of this chapter learner should be able to describe the functions of various minerals in the body, their metabolism and homeostasis.

COMPETENCY BI 6.10

At the end of this chapter learner should be able to enumerate and describe the disorders associated with mineral metabolism.

Specific Learning Objectives	
BI 6.9.1	Describe calcium absorption from intestine and influences.
BI 6.9.2	Discuss function of calcium.
BI 6.9.3	Discuss function of iron.
BI 6.9.4	Discuss role of iron containing proteins.
BI 6.9.5	Discuss normal level of sodium in blood.
BI 6.9.6	Describe iron deficiency manifestations.
BI 6.9.7	Discuss the enzymes containing zinc.
BI 6.9.8	Describe the role of selenium containing enzymes.
BI 6.10	Enumerate and describe the disorders associated with mineral metabolism.
BI 6.10.1	Discuss influence of serum calcium level.
BI 6.10.2	Describe the factors which will retard iron absorption.
BI 6.10.3	Describe mucosal block.
BI 6.10.4	Discuss hepcidin.
BI 6.10.5	Describe carrier protein in iron in blood.
BI 6.10.6	Describe hemopexin.
BI 6.10.7	Describe major cause for hemosiderosis.
BI 6.10.8	Describe ceruloplasmin.

Minerals play diverse role in biochemical system. They are substances which are required in small quantities by the body.

Minerals are not only important to play a role as a cofactor for enzymes but also are needed for bone formation.

Minerals may be classified into macromineral and micromineral category depending upon their daily requirements by an adult human.

1. **Macrominerals:** Those minerals whose daily requirement exceeds 100 mg (>100 mg/day) belong to this category. Examples are:
   a. Calcium (Ca)
   b. Phosphorus (P)
   c. Magnesium (Mg)
   d. Sodium (Na)
   e. Chloride (Cl^-)
   f. Potassium (K)
2. **Microminerals:** Those minerals whose daily requirement is either 100 mg or lesser (<100 mg) belong to this category. They are further subclassified into:
   i. Trace element (daily requirement 1–100 mg)
   ii. Ultratrace element (daily requirement <1 mg)
   i. *Trace element (daily dose needed is 1 to 100 mg):* Examples are:
      a. Copper (Cu)
      b. Zinc (Zn)
      c. Iron (Fe)
      d. Fluorine (as fluoride F^-)
      e. Chromium (Cr)
      f. Manganese (Mn)
   ii. *Ultratrace element (daily dose needed is <1 mg):* Examples are:
      a. Iodine (I)
      b. Selenium (Se)
      c. Molybdenum (Mo)

The characteristic features of all these minerals will be described in sequential order.

MACROMINERALS

▌CALCIUM (Ca)

Total calcium content in an adult human body is 1.0–1.5 kg. Its distribution in various forms is shown in Fig. 29.1

RDA

Adult	:	500 mg/day
Children	:	1200 mg/day
Pregnancy	:	1500 mg/day
Lactation	:	1500 mg/day

Normal plasma level of total calcium is 9–11 mg/dl.
- Hypocalcemia is the state when plasma total calcium level is below 8.8 mg/dl.
- Mild tremor is seen when plasma total calcium level is below 8.5 mg/dl.
- Tetany is seen when plasma total calcium level is below 7.5 mg/dl.

Absorption of dietary calcium through gastrointestinal tract: Calcium is absorbed in first and second parts of duodenum. It is an energy requiring process.

Absorption increased by:
- Calcitriol
- PTH
- Acidity

Absorption decreased by:
- Phytic acid
- Oxalates
- Phosphates
- Malabsorption

Calmodulin is a calcium binding protein, which changes its conformation after binding with the calcium. One calmodulin is capable of binding 4 ions of calcium.

There are multiple enzymes which are regulated by calmodulin. These are:
- i. Ca^{++}-Mg^{++} ATPase
- ii. Protein kinase
- iii. Adenylyl cyclase
- iv. Glycogen synthase
- v. Phospholipase C
- vi. Phosphorylase kinase
- vii. PDH
- viii. Pyruvate carboxylase
- ix. Glycerol-3-phosphate dehydrogenase
- x. Pyruvate kinase

Dietary Sources

Milk, cheese, sunlight, fish, liver, nuts.

Role of Calcitriol (Vitamin D), PTH and Calcitonin in Regulation of Blood Calcium Level

A. Role of Calcitriol on Calcium Homeostasis

Vitamin D has its effect on gastrointestinal tract, bone and distal convoluted tube of nephron. These effects are now discussed one by one (Table 29.1).

1. **Vitamin D enhances absorption of calcium from GIT:** Vitamin D enters the gastrointestinal tract cell and after binding with its receptor. It increases transcription of gene for calbindin. Calbindin is a calcium-binding protein which increases calcium absorption from GIT.
2. **Vitamin D helps in bone mineralization:** Vitamin D enhances the number of osteoblasts in the cell. These osteoblasts secrete alkaline phosphatase (ALP) which increases local concentration of calcium and phosphorous. This leads to bone mineralization and remodelling.
3. **Vitamin D helps in calcium and phosphorus reabsorption from DCT of kidney:** PTH conserves only calcium.

B. Role of PTH on Calcium Homeostasis

PTH increases level of calcium in blood by following mechanism:

1. **PTH and bone:** PTH increases number of osteoclasts in the bone. This results in resorption of bone which in turn increases level of calcium in the blood.
2. **PTH and kidney:** PTH decreases calcium excretion through kidney and increases level of the calcium in the blood. On the other hand PTH increases phosphorus excretion thus lowering its level.

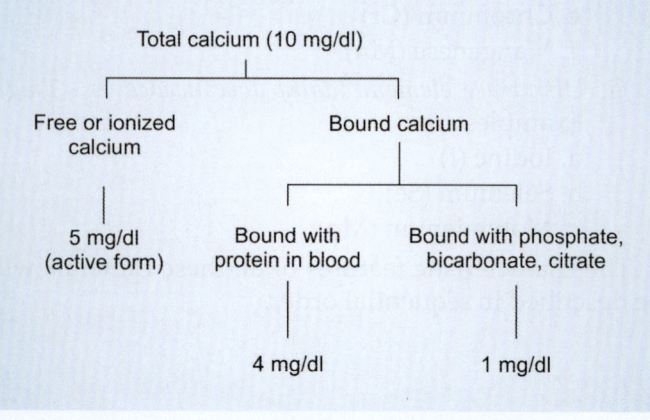

Fig. 29.1: Total calcium and its various forms

TABLE 29.1	Impact of vit. D, PTH and calcitonin on metabolism					
Role of vitamin D	Blood calcium level	Predominant action	GIT calcium absorption	Bone resorption	Deficiency
Vit. D	Increased	Calium absorption from of GIT	↑	↓	Rickets
PTH	Drastically increased	Bone resorption (demineralization)	↑	↑	Tetany
Calcitonin	Decreased	Opposes demineralization	Nil	↓	Nil

3. **PTH and intestine:** PTH stimulates activity of 1α-hydroxylase which acts on 25-hydroxycholesterol to convert it to 1,25-dihydroxycholecalciferol (calcitriol). Calcitriol then increases calcium absorption from gastrointestinal tract by increasing transcription of calbindin gene. Calbindin in turn increases calcium absorption from gastrointestinal tract.

C. Role of Calcitonin in Calcium Homeostasis

Calcitonin plays a role to decrease serum calcium level.

Calcitonin decreases the activity of osteoclast and increases the activity of osteoblast.

Calcitonin and PTH are antagonist in term of their effect on plasma calcium level (Table 29.1).

Tetany is manifested by (a) Trousseau's sign and (b) Chvostek's sign.

▌PHOSPHORUS (P)

- Total body content of phosphorus is 1 kg.
- Phosphorus is needed by the body in many forms.
- Majority of body phosphorus in the body is found in inorganic hydroxyl appetite (85% of total).
- Remaining phosphorus (15%) is distributed in phospholipid, ATP and other nucleotides, creatine phosphate.
- Phosphorus is required in (Pi) in organic form for action of phosphorylase enzyme.

RDA

RDA of phosphorous is 500 mg/day.

Dietary Sources

Milk is a good source of phosphorus (100 mg/100 ml). Other sources are:
- Cereals
- Nuts
- Meat

Serum Level

Total phosphorous in the serum is 3–4 mg/dl.

Multiple factors may lead to derangement of phosphorus level in the blood. They have been enumerated in Table 29.2.

TABLE 29.2	Derangement of phosphate in blood
Hyperphosphatemia	Hypophosphatemia
• Increased GIT absorption (excess vitamin D)	• Decreased GIT absorption → Malabsorption
• Cell lysis	→ Malnutrition
→ Cancer chemotherapy	→ Diarrhoea
→ Bone secondaries	→ Deficiency of vitamin D
• Reduced renal excretion	• Respiratory alkalosis
→ Renal impairment	• Insulin therapy
→ Decreased PTH (hypoparathyroidism)	• Hyperparathyroidism
(PTH reabsorbs calcium from kidney tubules, but enhances excretion of phosphate)	• Chronic alcoholic
• Hypocalcemia	• Drugs
• Massive blood transfusion (Whole blood phosphate is 40 mg/dl)	• Antacids • Diuretics • Salicylates

▌MAGNESIUM (Mg)

- Total body content of Mg is 25 grams.
- 60% of total body content of magnesium is lying in the bone.

Important enzymes which require Mg are as follows:
- Kinases
- DNA polymerase
- RNA polymerase
- Alkaline phosphatase (ALP)
- Adenylyl cyclase

Magnesium therapy lowers blood pressure. Magnesium sulphate is used in the treatment of pre-eclampsia, a hypertensive disorder of pregnancy.

RDA

Male   = 400 mg/day
Female = 300 mg/day

Section 7 ■ Nutrition, Vitamins and Minerals

29

Dietary Sources

- Cereals
- Beans
- Leafy vegetables
- Fish

Serum Level

1.8–2.2 mg/dl

Deranged magnesium level in the plasma may be because of following reasons (Table 29.3):

TABLE 29.3	Reasons for deranged Mg level in plasma
Hypomagnesemia	*Hypermagnesemia*
i. Hyperaldosteronism	i. Excessive oral or parentral administration
ii. Urinary loss in tubular necrosis	ii. ↑PTH
iii. Familial hypomagnesemia	iii. Renal failure
iv. Diarrhoea	iv. Multiple myeloma
v. Laxatine abuse	
vi. Nasogastric tube aspiration, vomiting	
vii. ↓PTH	
viii. Malnutrition	
ix. Thiazide diuretics	

▌ SODIUM (Na) AND CHLORIDE (Cl⁻)

- These two macrominerals are described together as they play important role in many physiological processes in collaboration of each other.
- They are important to maintain water balance, osmotic equilibrium and membrane potential.
- Na^+ and Cl^- are mainly extracellular electrolytes.
- NaCl (common salt) is important source of Na^+ and Cl^-.
- Na^+ is important for renal and gastrointestinal absorption of glucose, galactose and amino acids.

▌ POTASSIUM

- Potassium is mainly intracellular electrolyte.
- Normal serum level of potassium is 3.5–5.0 mEq/L (mmol/L)
- Hypokalemia and hyperkalemia are associated with cardiac arrhythmias.

MICROMINERALS

Microminerals are further subclassified in trace elements and ultratrace elements.

▌ TRACE ELEMENTS: DAILY REQUIREMENT (1–100 mg/day)

Under this heading following elements will be described:

Copper (Cu), zinc (Zn), iron (Fe), fluorine (F), chromium (Cr), manganese (Mn).

Copper

Multiple number of enzymes require Cu for their functioning:

- Cytochrome *c* oxidase
- Ferroxidase (ceruloplasmin, hephaestin)
- Lysyl hydroxylase
- Dopamine β-hydroxylase
- Tyrosinase
- Cytosolic and extracellular superoxide dismutase (SOD)
- ALA synthase
- Monoamino oxidase (MAO)
- Phenol oxidase

RDA

1.5–3.0 mg/day

Dietary Sources

- Meat
- Shellfish
- Nuts
- Whole grains
- Green leafy vegetables

In plasma, ceruloplasmin is the major copper containing protein. 90% of plasma Cu is tightly bound with ceruloplasmin.

Plasma ceruloplasmin level is 25–50 mg/dl.

10% of plasma Cu is bound to albumin, which constitutes transport form of Cu.

Functional Aspect of Cu

1. *Role of Cu in heme metabolism:* Cu is not only important for iron absorption, but also it helps in incorporation of iron into the heme.
2. Role in hydroxylations (norepinephrine synthesis)
3. Role in melanin synthesis (via its role in tyrosinase activity)
4. Role in collagen cross-linking (via lysyl oxidase activity)

Diseases Associated with Derangement in Cu Metabolism

1. **Menkes' kinky hair syndrome (Table 29.4):** It is an X-linked disorder which results due to defect in Cu transportation across the basolateral wall of gastrointestinal mucosal cell. It is due to mutation of gene 'ATP7A'.

   'ATP7A' is the transporter protein which helps in transportation of Cu from gastrointestinal tract mucosal cell to blood vessels (Fig. 29.2).

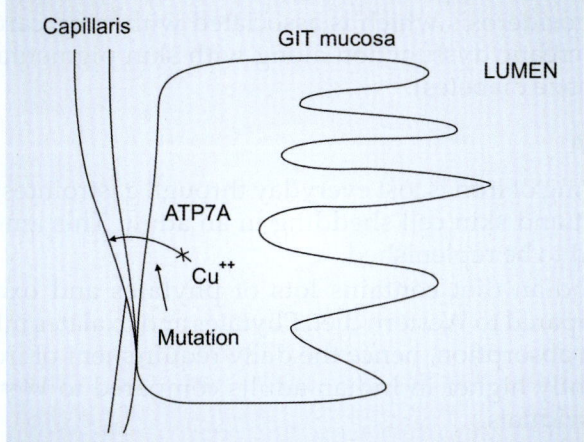

Fig. 29.2: Absorption of copper via ATP7A transporter

Clinical manifestation of Menkes disease:
- Poor growth
- Mental retardation
- Loose skin and joints
- Hypothermia
- Hypopigmentation
- Kinky hair
- Symptoms appear early in life (2–3 months) and death occurs by 3 years of age.
- Injection of copper-histidine complex is used in therapy which is only moderately successful.
- ATP7A and ATP7B are Cu transporting ATPase, whose main role is Cu efflux from the cells when copper is in excess amount.

- ATP7B is abundantly found in liver and brain while ATP7A is abundantly found in gastrointestinal tract cells.

2. **Wilson disease (Table 29.4):** It is an autosomal recessive disorder characterized by excessive copper deposition in certain organs specially liver and brain.

   Liver and neurological tissues release excess of their copper through ATP7B copper transporter.

   In Wilson disease, there is mutation of ATP7B which results in abnormal accumulation of excess Cu in liver, substantia, nigra, descement membrane of cornea which respectively results in liver cirrhosis, chronic hepatitis and liver failure, Parkinsonians symptom, seizure and psychiatric manifestation, Kayser-Fleischer ring (golden-brown ring around cornea).

   Treatment of Wilson disease is Zn supplementation. Zn is a copper chelating agent which reduces copper absorption from GIT.

3. **Copper deficiency and cardiovascular disorder:** Cu deficiency results in weakening of arterial wall, aneurysm and fatal rapture of aortic wall.

4. **Anemia:** Copper deficiency results in microcytic normochromic anemia.

5. **Hypopigmentation and flagging of hair:** Melanin is synthesized from amino acid tyrosine for which tyrosinase enzyme is required. Tyrosinase is a copper containing enzyme which does not function in Cu deficiency. This results in lack of melanin synthesis and graying of hair grown during the period of copper deficiency.

   Deficiency of Cu is rare except in circumstances when excessive Zn is consumed (Zn impairs Cu absorption from gastrointestinal tract lumen) and also in Menke disease (Cu transporter ATP7A is mutated). Deficiency of copper results in:
   - Anemia
   - Bone demineralization
   - Blood vessel fragility
   - Demyelination of neuronal tissues

TABLE 29.4	Comparison of Menkes and Wilson disease	
Parameters	Menkes disease	Wilson disease
Whole body Cu	Low	High
Plasma Cu	Low	High
Urinary Cu	Low	High
Liver Cu	Low	High
Inheritance	X-linked	AR
Cu transporting	ATP7A	ATP7B
ATPase affected	—	—

Zinc (Zn)

Total Zn content in an adult human is approximately 2 grams.

Zn is important for storage of insulin in β cell pancreas.

Dietary Sources

- Grains
- Beans
- Nuts
- Cheese
- Meat

Section 7 ■ Nutrition, Vitamins and Minerals

29

Role of Zn in Body

Zn as a cofactor for enzymes. Important enzymes where Zn acts as a cofactor are enumerated below:

    a. Carbonic anhydrase
    b. Alkaline phosphatase (ALP)
    c. Carboxypeptidase
    d. Lactate dehydrogenase (LDH)
    e. Superoxide dismutase (SOD)
    f. DNA polymerase
    g. RNA polymerase
    h. PBG synthase (ALA dehydratase)

Zn is also found in center of **Zn finger motifs** seen in certain proteins which are DNA binding regulatory proteins.

RDA

Adults and children	:	10 mg/day
Pregnancy and lactation	:	15–20 mg/day

Zn Toxicity

Zinc toxicity is seen in welders which is due to inhalation of zinc oxide fumes while welding.

Deficiency Manifestation

- Poor growth in children
- Poor wound healing
- Skin lesion
- Hyperkeratosis
- Dermatitis
- Alopecia
- Decreased taste activity
- Immune dysfunction
- *Acrodermatitis enteropathica:* Due to malabsorption of Zn during diarrhoea, oral lesions are found.

Iron (Fe)

Iron is an important trace element which is needed for many biological functions like oxygen transport, energy metabolism, cell proliferation, etc. Total amount of iron in adult human body is 3–4 grams which is distributed in various compartments. Major fraction of this iron is incorporated in the heme of hemoglobin.

Free iron is toxic as it generates free radical through Fenton's reaction and also supports the growth of microbial pathogens increasing the risk of systemic infection. Hence, iron is always in sequestered form in body, sequestered with ferritin in mucosal cell and sequestered with transferring in the blood stream.

Ferritin: Apoferritin is a multisubunit protein having capacity to bind 4500 atoms of iron (in the ferric form).

Transferrin: It is a monomer having two binding sites, hence one transferrin binds two iron atoms (in the ferric form).

Hemosiderosis: Once the amount of cellular iron exceeds which could bind the apoferritin, excess iron starts depositing in the form of amorphous mixture of iron hydroxide, iron phosphate and protein called hemosiderin. Such deposits are seen in liver, heart, pancreas and pituitary gland. This condition is called hemosiderosis which is associated with liver, cardiac, pancreatic dysfunction along with skin pigmentation (bronze diabetes).

RDA

1–2 mg of iron is lost everyday through gastrointestinal tract and skin cell shedding in an adult. This amount need to be replenished.

Indian diet contains lots of phytates and oxalate compared to Western diet. Phytates and oxalates inhibit iron absorption, hence the daily requirement of iron is slightly higher in Indian adults compared to Western individuals.

Efficiency of iron absorption from gastrointestinal tract varies from 10–15% in Indians while efficiency of iron absorption varies from 15–20% in Western individual.

Keeping these facts in mind, following are the RDA of iron:

Indian adults	=	20 mg/day
Western adults	=	15 mg/day
Children	=	30 mg/day
Pregnancy	=	40 mg/day

Mother transfers iron and calcium to the foetus only in last trimester of pregnancy. Preterm babies are thus very much prone to develop deficiency of iron.

Dietary Sources

- Green leafy vegetables
- Jaggery
- Meat
- Dry fruits
- Enriched cereals

It is important to note that iron is poor in breast as well as in cow's milk, so newborn should be supplemented with this essential element.

Absorption of Iron from Gastrointestinal Lumen

Regulation of iron homeostasis occurs almost entirely at the level of iron uptake and delivery to the bloodstream by the intestine.

Iron is absorbed by upper part of duodenum.

Both heme and nonheme iron is absorbed from gastrointestinal tract lumen. Mechanism of heme iron uptake is not clear at present, but the mechanism of nonheme iron is well explained by the scientists.

Digestion of nonheme iron protein in gastrointestinal tract lumen produce Fe^{+++} (+3 state); but it is important to note that iron is transported across the membrane only in Fe^{++} (ous/+2 state) form. Additionally, it is important to notice that storage of iron with the ferritin or the transportation of iron with transferrin warrants ferric form of iron.

Keeping these facts in mind, the absorption, storage and transportation of iron can be easily understood (Fig. 29.3).

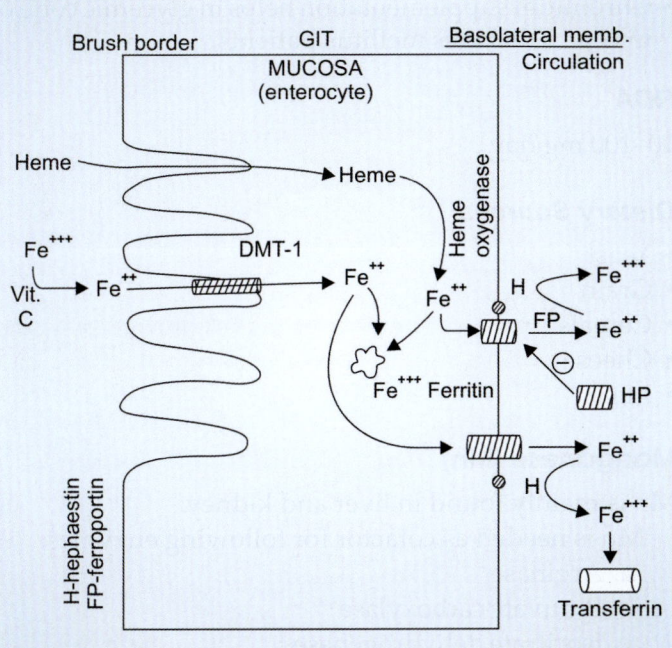

Fig. 29.3: Absorption of dietary iron from GIT mucosa

A. Steps of iron absorption, storage and transport

- Heme is taken up by gastrointestinal tract cell by heme carrier protein, there heme is acted upon by heme oxygenase to release Fe^{++}.
- Nonheme ferric is converted to ferrous form in gastrointestinal tract lumen by duodenal cytochrome *b* enzyme which needs vitamin C as a coenzyme (it is a known fact that vitamin C enhances iron absorption).
- Ferrous is transported from gastrointestinal tract lumen to mucosal cell by divalent metal transporter-1 (DMT-1).
- Ferrous in the gastrointestinal tract cell is either stored by intracellular protein ferritin (4500 iron atoms in the ferric forms per apoferritin) or is directly transported

to blood via ferroportin (FP), at basolateral membrane. During its transportation by FP, Fe^{++} is oxidized to Fe^{+++} form by a copper containing protein 'hephaestin'.

- This Fe^{+++} is binding to apotransferrin to form transferring (one apoferritin binds two Fe^{+++}).
- Hepcidin is a polypeptide which is secreted by the liver, is involved in internalization and lysosomal degradation of FP, thus reducing iron export in the blood by cell.
- Level of hepcidin goes hand-in-hand with iron status in the circulation. If iron is excess, more hepcidin is transcribed, which reduces further iron expert in the blood. On the other hand, when the level of iron is low in circulation, less of hepcidin is synthesized, favouring iron transport to blood vessels by ferroportin, thus balancing the level of iron in the blood.

Mucosal block theory: Absorption of iron depends upon body requirement. If body store of iron is less, more is absorbed and vice versa. This is called mucosal block theory.

B. Recycling of Iron

Macrophages ingest old and damaged RBC. Iron of the heme is then freed which is transported to blood via ferroportin. Ceruloplasmin converts Fe^{++} to Fe^{+++} in the circulation. This Fe^{+++} is then reutilized for erythropoiesis (Fig. 29.4).

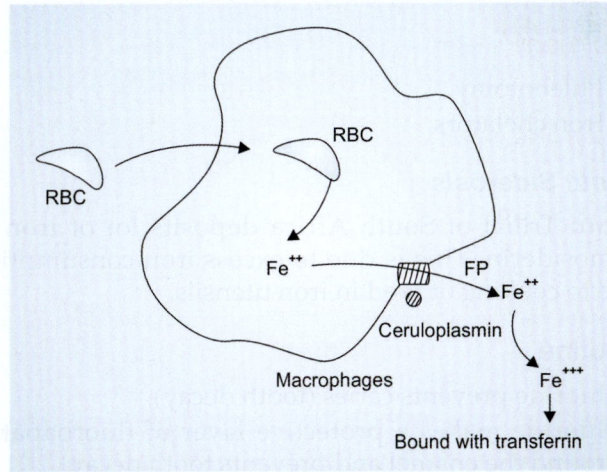

Fig. 29.4: Recycling of iron

C. Uptake of Iron by Erythroblast and Other Cells

Erythroblast and other cells have transferring receptor (TfR), which binds transferrin-Fe^{+++} complex and internalize them (Fig. 29.5).

The iron is freed from transferrin and is either stored as ferritin or is utilized for erythropoiesis etc.

TfR- Tf is recycled to the surface.

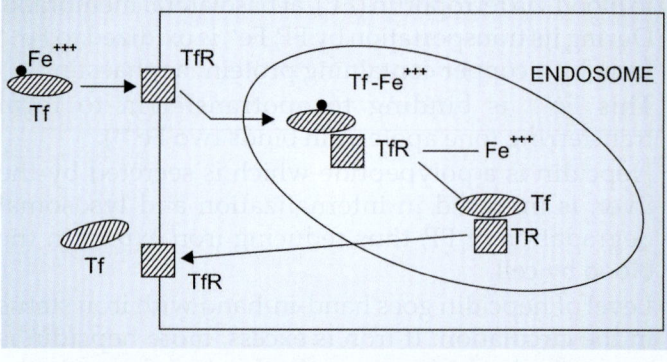

Fig. 29.5: Transferrin receptor and iron intake

> **NOTE:** Both ceruloplasmin and hephaestin are copper containing proteins, thus Cu deficiency may lead to iron deficiency anemia.

Iron Deficiency

It is very common in India as well as in Western countries.

Iron deficiency leads to microcytic, hypochromic anemia characterized by pale and small sized RBC on peripheral blood smear.

Iron Excess

Hemochromatosis: An autosomal recessive (AR) disorder where excess iron deposition is seen in liver, heart, pancreas, skin and pituitary gland.

Treatment

a. Phlebotomy
b. Iron chelators

Bantu Siderosis

Bantu Tribal of South Africa deposits lot of iron in hemosiderin. This is due to excess iron consumption due to cooking of food in iron utensils.

Flourine

- Fluoride prevents caries (tooth decay).
- Fluoride makes a protective layer of fluoroapatite around the enamel and prevents tooth decay.
- The safe limit of fluorine is about 1 ppm in water
- Fluoride is a two-edge word in the sense that its deficiency results in caries and excess consumption is also toxic known as fluorosis.
  1. **Dental caries:** Drinking water having <0.5 ppm of fluoride is associated with dental caries in children.
  2. **Fluorosis:** Excess consumption (>5 ppm) leads to mottling of enamel and discolouration of teeth. Yellow and brown patches are seen on teeth (dental fluorosis).

- If consumption of fluoride is >20 ppm, it is toxic to the bones, characterized by excessive calcification of vertebra and long bones leading to stiffness. It is called skeletal fluorosis.
- Genuvalgum is seen due to deformity of lower limbs.

Chromium (Cr)

- Chromium is an important mineral which is also called 'glucose homeostatis factor' due to its favorable role on insulin action.
- Chromium binds with chromodulin, which facilitates insulin binding to insulin receptor and thus potentiates the effect of insulin.
- Chromium decreases level of LDL and increases level of HDL in the plasma.
- Chromium supplementation helps in glycemic control in type 2 diabetes mellitus patients.

RDA

10–100 mg/day

Dietary Sources

- Yeast
- Grain
- Cereals
- Cheese
- Meat

Manganese (Mn)

Mn is mainly found in liver and kidney.

Mn is needed as cofactor for following enzymes:
  a. Arginase
  b. Pyruvate carboxylase
  c. Isocitrate dehydrogenase
  d. Superoxide dismutase (mitochondrial)
  e. Peptidase
  f. Hexokinase
  g. Phosphoglucomutase
  h. Glutamine synthetase
  i. Glucosyltransferase
  j. RNA polymerase
  k. Phosphoenol pyruvate carboxykinase (decarboxylase)

RDA: 5 mg/day

Dietary Sources

- Nut
- Tea leaves
- Leafy vegetables
- Fruits

Mn is involved in synthesis of mucopolysaccharide, glycoprotein, hemoglobin and cholesterol synthesis.

Mn Deficiency

- Growth retardation
- Bone deformity
- Sterility

ULTRA-TRACE ELEMENTS

Iodine (I)

Majority of body iodine is found in thyroid gland.

Iodine is needed for synthesis of thyroid hormone namely T_3 and T_4.

Thyroid hormone regulates BMR in adults and growth and development in children.

RDA

Adult   : 100–150 μg/day
Pregnancy : 200 μg/day

Dietary Sources

- Seafood
- Drinking water
- Vegetables
- Fruits

Iodine Deficiency

Iodine deficiency is common in India.

Goiter: Enlargement of thyroid gland in an attempt to increase the thyroid hormone in hypothyroidism.

Cretinism: Characterized by mental retardation, growth retardation.

Selenium (Se)

RDA: 50–100 mg/day

Dietary Sources

- Liver
- Kidney
- Sea food

'Selenium' and 'Vitamin E' Play Synergistic Role as Antioxidants.

Glutathione peroxidase (GPO) destroys peroxide in cytosol which complements the effect of vitamin E, since vitamin E is limited primarily to the membrane.

Selenium is an important component of selenocysteine (Se-Cys).

Se-Cys is derived from serine when its oxygen is replaced by selenium during its transportation on seryl tRNA.

This modification of serine to Se-Cys requires ATP, selenide and enzyme selenocysteine synthetase; seryl-tRNA.

More than two dozen human proteins are now found to have Se-Cys in them.

The UGA codon which otherwise is a stop codon, incorporates Se-Cys in the elongating polypeptide.

The mRNA, whose UGA codes for Se-Cys and does not acts as stop codon, has Se-Cys insertional sequence (SECIS) at 3′ UTR end of mRNA.

Se-Cys is seen in following enzymes:

- Glutathione peroxidase
- Phospholipid-hydroperoxide
- Thioredoxin reductase (purine nucleotide metabolism)
- Iodothyronine deiodinase responsible for conversion of T_4 to T_3.
- Selenoprotein P (extracellular protein)
- Sperm capsule selenoprotein GP × 4 (involved in sperm motility)
- Muscle selenoprotein W (muscle metabolism)

Research have shown that supplementation with Se may reduce the risk of lung, breast and bladder cancer.

Keshan disease: Deficiency of Se in China is associated with endemic cardiomyopathy.

Toxicity of Se: Selenosis occurs due to excess consumption of selenium. Following features are seen:

- Diarrhoea
- Hair loss
- Garlic odor
- Breath (dimethyl selentide)
- Weight loss
- Emotional disturbance

Molybdenum (Mo)

Molybdenum is a cofactor for certain enzymes enumerated below.

1. Xanthine oxidase
2. Aldehyde oxidase
3. Sulphite oxidase

Molybdenosis: Excessive consumption of molybdenum leads to molybdenosis. This is characterized by:

- Diarrhoea
- Anemia
- Growth impairment

Section 7 ■ Nutrition, Vitamins and Minerals

29

Miscellaneous Topics

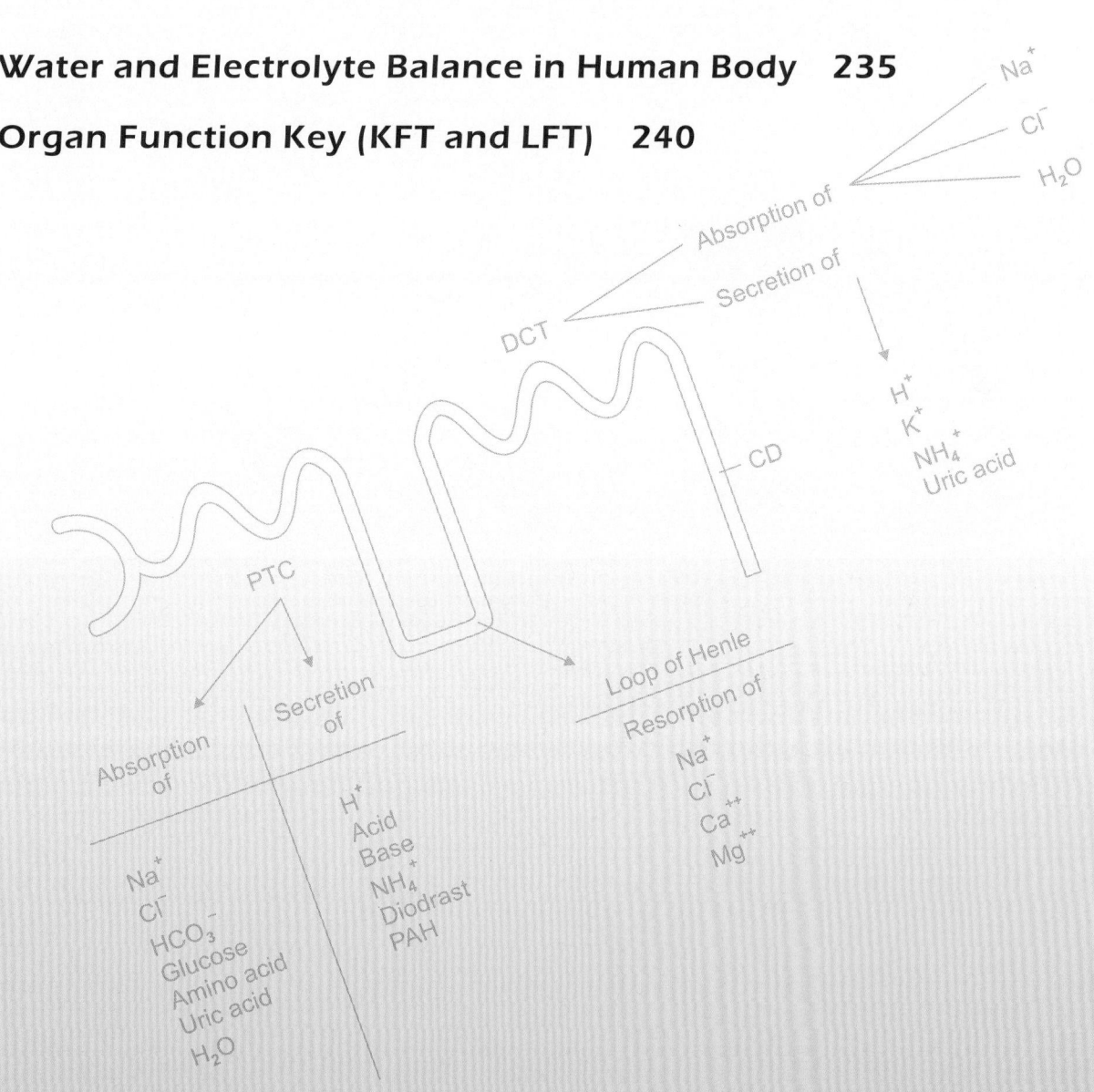

8

Miscellaneous Topics

Chapter

30

Water and Electrolyte Balance in Human Body

Total body water in a healthy adult is 42 liters (60% of total body weight). This water is distributed in intracellular and extracellular compartments (Fig. 30.1).

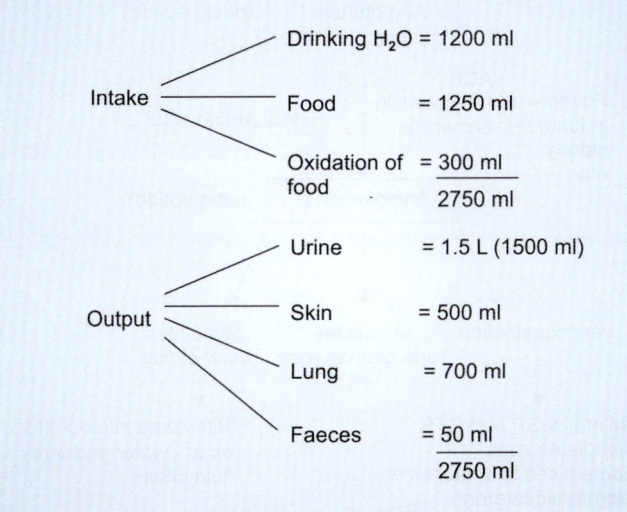

Fig. 30.1: Distribution of water in human system

Osmolarity = Osmotic pressure exerted by number of moles per liter of solution

Osmolality = Osmotic pressure exerted by number of moles per kg of solvent.

(Osmolality of plasma = 285–295 mOsm/kg)

Albumin is the main protein which maintains osmotic balance.

▌OSMOLALITY

a. **Hypertonic:** When osmolality is increased.
b. **Hypotonic:** When osmolality is decreased.

Osmolality affects hydration status of cell. when osmolality is increased, it leads to dehydration of cell and on the other hand when osmolality is decreased, it leads to swelling of cell manifesting headache, vomiting and brain medullary herniation.

Various components contributing to osmolality of plasma are enumerated in Table 30.1.

▌WATER AND SODIUM BALANCE (Figs 30.2–30.5)

Water is an important constituent of all living organisms including human.

Homeostasis of water ensures that:

1. Total water content of the body is maintained within narrow limits.
2. The distribution of water among various compartments like intracellular, intravascular and interstitial (extravascular) is well maintained.

Osmotic and hydrostatic force determines the water distribution in various compartments.

Sodium is the most abundant extracellular cation, which along with its associated anions plays as a chief factor to determine osmotic force.

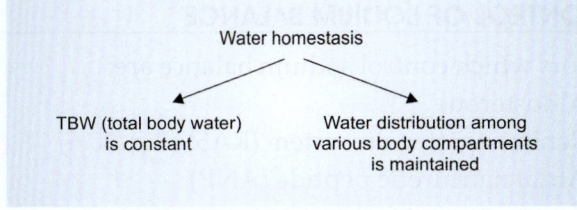

Fig. 30.2: Water homeostasis

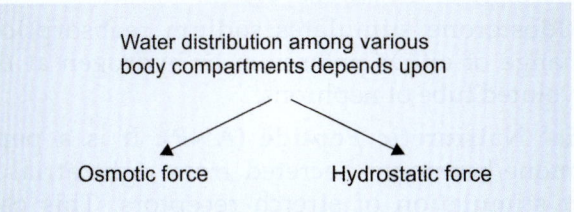

Fig. 30.3: Water distribution

235

Osmotic activity depends upon relative amount of sodium and water, rather than on absolute quantity of either.

Everyday approximately 200 L of water and 30,000 mmol of sodium pass through kidney, out of which 99% is reabsorbed resulting in loss of only 1.5–2 L of water and 100 mmol of sodium in the urine.

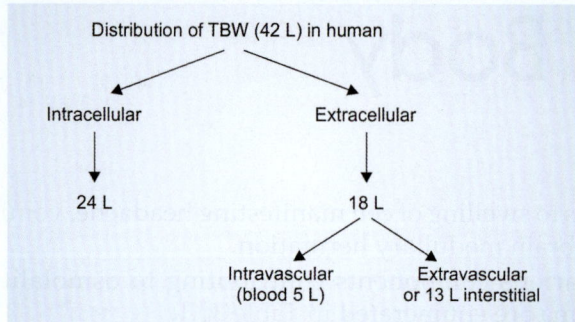

Fig. 30.4: Water distribution in different body compartments

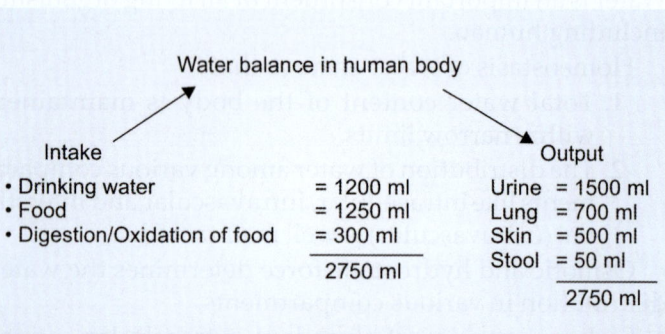

Fig. 30.5: Water distribution

CONTROL OF SODIUM BALANCE

Factors which control sodium balance are:
1. Aldosterone
2. Renin-angiotensin system (RAS) (Fig. 30.6)
3. Atrial natriuretic peptide (ANP)

Most important factor out of above list is aldosterone, a mineralocorticoid hormone secreted by the zona glomerulosa of the adrenal cortex.

Aldosterone stimulates sodium reabsorption in exchange of either potassium or hydrogen at distal convoluted tube of nephrons.

Atrial Natriuretic Peptide (ANP): It is a peptide hormone/hormones secreted from right atrial wall after stimulation of stretch receptors. This causes high sodium excretion (natriuresis) by increasing GFR and by inhibiting renin and aldosterone secretion.

CONTROL OF WATER BALANCE

Antidiuretic Hormone (ADH)
- Increase in plasma osmolality stimulates osmoreceptors of hypothalamus, which results in ADH secretion.
- ADH is synthesized in hypothalamus and is secreted from posterior pituitary gland.
- ADH enhances H_2O reabsorption from the collecting duct of nephrons.

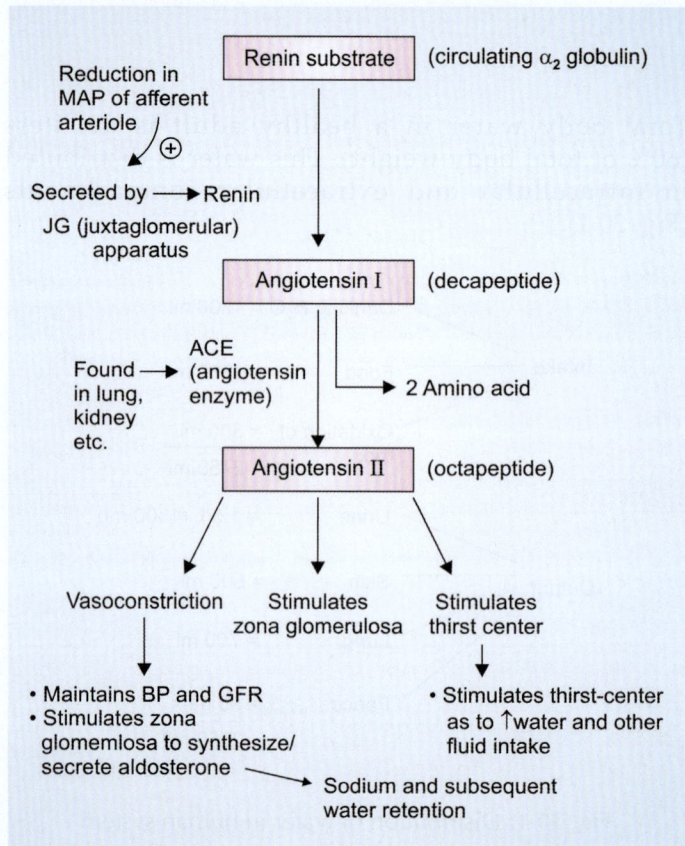

Fig. 30.6: Renin angiotensin system (RAS)

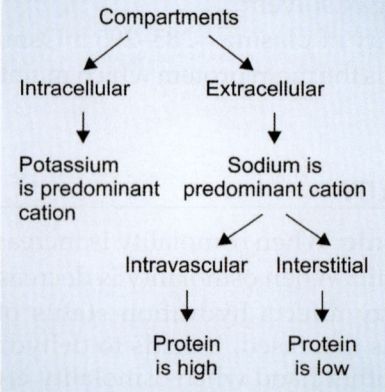

Fig. 30.7: Distribution of ions

Sodium is predominantly extracellular and potassium is predominantly intracellular ion (Fig. 30.7).

This differential concentration of sodium and potassium in intracellular and extracellular space is maintained by Na^+ - K^+ ATPase/pumps.

Osmotic Gradient

'It is the concentration gradient of particles (either ion or molecules) across the membrane which is not permeable to such particles'.

Crystalloids and water can diffuse across the membrane and do not provide osmotic gradient.

Units of Measurement of Osmotic Pressure

Osmolarity: mmol/L of solution
Osmolality: mmol/kg of solvent

TABLE 30.1	Contribution of various components in determining osmolality of plasma	
Sodium and anion	270 mmol/kg	92%
Potassium, Ca, Mg and their anions	11 mmol/kg	4%
Urea, glucose, protein	11 mmol/kg	4%
Total	292 mmol/kg	100%

Hypernatremia

This is the condition when concentration of sodium in body is increased (Fig. 30.8).

Clinical symptoms are:
- Excess thirst
- Restlessness
- Dry mucus membrane
  1. *Inadequate water intake:* It may be due to:
     - Unavailability of H_2O
     - Infant
     - Unconsciousness/coma
  2. *Impaired water retention*
     - Osmotic diuresis
     - Diabetes insipidus
  3. *Excess sodium intake*
     - *Drugs:* Carbenicillin, metronidazole
     - *Diet*
  4. *Excess sodium retention:*
     - *Due to excess mineralocorticoids:* Conn's syndrome, Cushing's syndrome.

Increased osmolality leads to dehydration of cell and decreased osmolality results in hydration/swelling of cell.

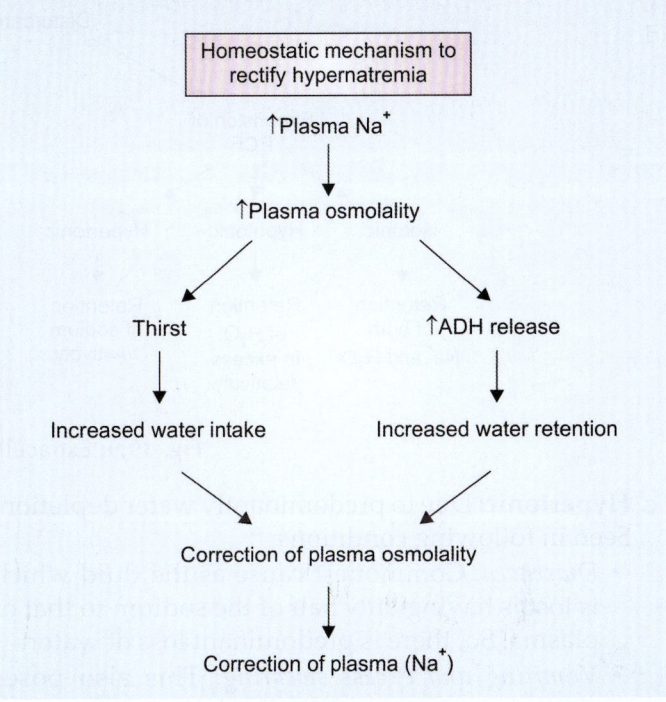

Fig. 30.8: Hypernatremia

Clinical Associations

ECF Expansion (Fig. 30.9)

a. **Isotonic:** Both Na^+ and water retention. Seen in following conditions:
   - Hypertension
   - Cardiac failure
   - Secondary hyperaldosteronism
b. **Hypotonic:** Due to retention of water alone. Seen in following conditions:
   - ADH excess
   - Glomerular dysfunction
c. **Hypertonic:** Due to retention of sodium alone. Seen in the following conditions:
   - Conn's syndrome
   - Cushing's syndrome

ECF Contraction (Fig. 30.9)

a. **Isotonic:** Both Na+ and water are lost. Seen in following conditions:
   - Loss of the gastrointestinal fluid
   - Severe cases may be associated with hypotension
b. **Hypotonic:** Due to predominant loss of sodium. Seen in following conditions:
   - Dextrose infusion

Section 8 ■ Miscellaneous Topics

30

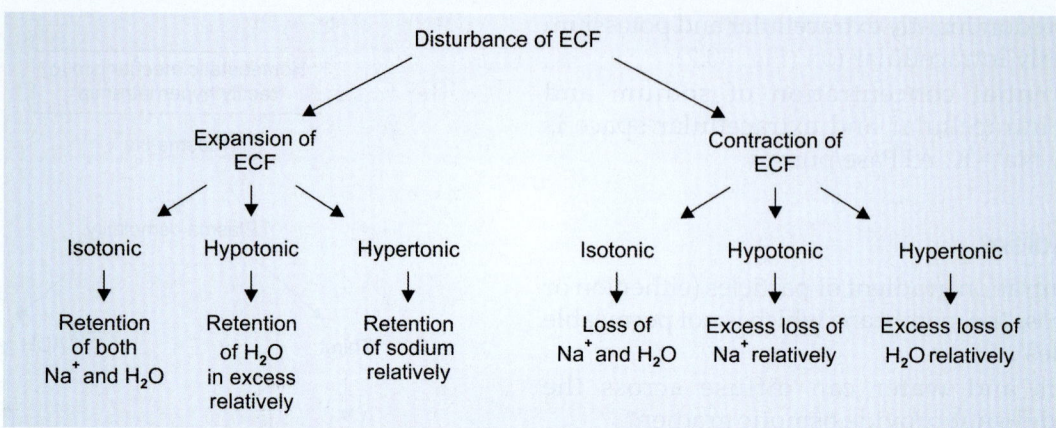

Fig. 30.9: Extracellular fluid derangement

c. **Hypertonic:** Due to predominantly water depletion. Seen in following conditions:
  - *Diarrhoea:* Commonest cause as the fluid which is lost is having only half of the sodium to that of plasma. So, there is predominant loss of water.
  - *Vomiting and excess sweating:* This also poses similar picture as seen in diarrhoea.

Hyponatremia

This is the condition when concentration of sodium in the body is decreased (Fig. 30.10).

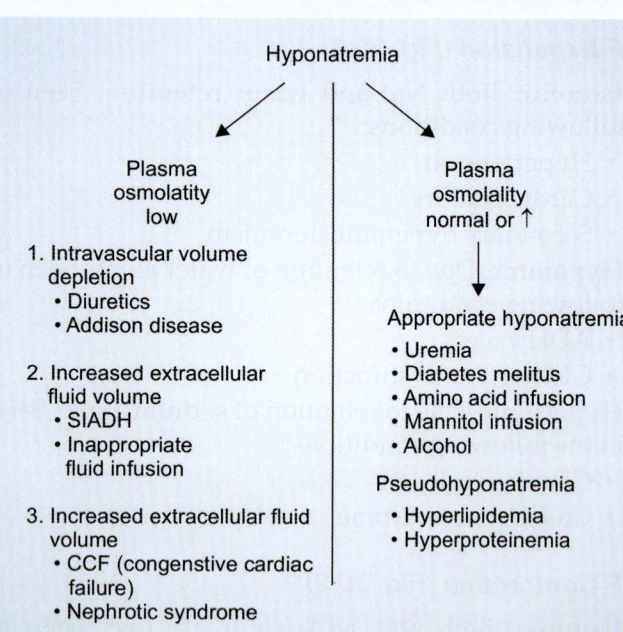

Fig. 30.10: Hyponatremia

Clinical Features

- Low BP
- Lethargy

- Confusion
- Tremors
- Cornea

Potassium and its Derangement

Potassium is the major intracellular cation.
  Intracellular concentration gradient is maintained by Na^+- K^+ ATPase.

Plasma Level

3.5–5.0 mmol/L

Intracellular Level

160 mmol/L

Sources

- Tender coconut
- Banana
- Orange
- Apple
- Pineapple
- Almond
- Dates, beans

Hypokalemia (Plasma K^+ Less Than 3 mmol/L)

Following are the clinical signs and symptoms of hypokalemia:
- Muscle weakness
- Fatigue
- Muscle cramps
- Hypotension
- Decreased reflex
- Palpitation
- Cardiac arrhythmia

- Cardiac arrest
- ECG shows inverted 'T' waves
- Lowering of ST segment

Causes of hypokalemia

- Cushing's syndrome
- Hyperaldosteronism
- Renal tubular acidosis
- Adrenogenital syndrome
- Alkalosis
- Insulin therapy
- Diarrhoea, vomiting
- Less dietary intake
- Excess saline infusion

Hyperkalemia (Plasma K⁺ More Than 5.5 mmol/L)

Following are clinical signs and symptoms of hyperkalemia:

- Ventricular arrhythmia
- Ventricular fibrillation
- Bradycardia
- Cardiac arrest
- ECG: 'T' wave elevation
- 'QRS' widening
- 'PR' lengthening

Causes of hyperkalemia

- Renal failure
- Heart failure
- Hemolysis
- Chemotherapy
- Metabolic acidosis
- Spironolactone
- Beta blockers
- ACE inhibitors

31

Organ Function Key
(KFT and LFT)

COMPETENCY BI 6.13

At the end of this chapter learner should be able to describe the functions of the kidney, liver, thyroid and adrenal glands.

COMPETENCY BI 6.14

At the end of this chapter learner should be able to describe the tests that are commonly done in clinical practice to assess the functions of these organs (kidney, liver, thyroid and adrenal glands).

Specific Learning Objectives

BI 6.13	Describe the functions of the kidney, liver, thyroid and adrenal glands.
BI 6.13.1	Describe thyroid hormones.
BI 6.13.2	Describe kidney function test.
BI 6.13.3	Describe liver function test.
BI 6.13.4	Describe thyroid function test.
BI 6.13.5	Discuss in detail the synthesis and biochemical functions of thyroid hormones.
BI 6.14.1	Describe briefly on the different laboratory investigations employed to assess liver function.
BI 6.14.2	Discuss the biochemical parameters for the different diagnosis of jaundice.
BI 6.14.3	Describe the renal function tests.
BI 6.14.4	Discuss an account of the serum enzymes derived from liver and their importance in LFT.
BI 6.14.5	Discuss hemolytic jaundice, Van den Bergh reaction.

KIDNEY FUNCTION TEST (KFT)

Major functions of kidney are:
1. Excretion of metabolic waste products like urea, uric acids, creatinine and modified drugs.
2. Role in buffering action—maintain pH
3. Role in maintaining water homeostasis
4. Proximal convoluted tubule is involved in activation and regulation of synthesis of vitamin D via enzyme 1α-hydroxylase and 24α-hydroxylase, respectively.

FORMATION OF URINE BY NEPHRONS

Nephron is the functional unit of kidney. This is made up of Bowman's capsule with the glomerulus, PCT, loop of Henle, DCT and collecting duct (Fig. 31.1).

When the blood passes through the glomerulus, it is filtered, where cell and proteins are retained in the blood and waste products like urea, creatinine, uric acid are filtered out.

Renal blood flow: 1200 ml blood/min
700 ml plasma/min

GFR = 120–125 ml/min

Total filtrate = 170–180 L/day

Final volume of formed urine = 1.5 L/day

Reabsorption and secretion of various ions and other metabolites at various segments of nephron.

Threshold Substance

These substances are those substances whose urinary excretion is dependent on their level in the plasma. These substances and their treshold levels are:

Glucose = 180 mg/dl
Lactate = 60 mg/dl
Bicarbonate = 28 mEq/L
Calcium = 10 mg/dl

Water Absorption

PCT : Obligatory resorption of water.
(movement of water along with Na^+, Cl^-, HCO_3^-)
DCT : Facultative resorption of water
(water resorption under the influence of ADH)

Urine Color

Straw colored/clear	:	Normal
Cloudy/opalescent	:	Pus
Yellow	:	Bilirubin

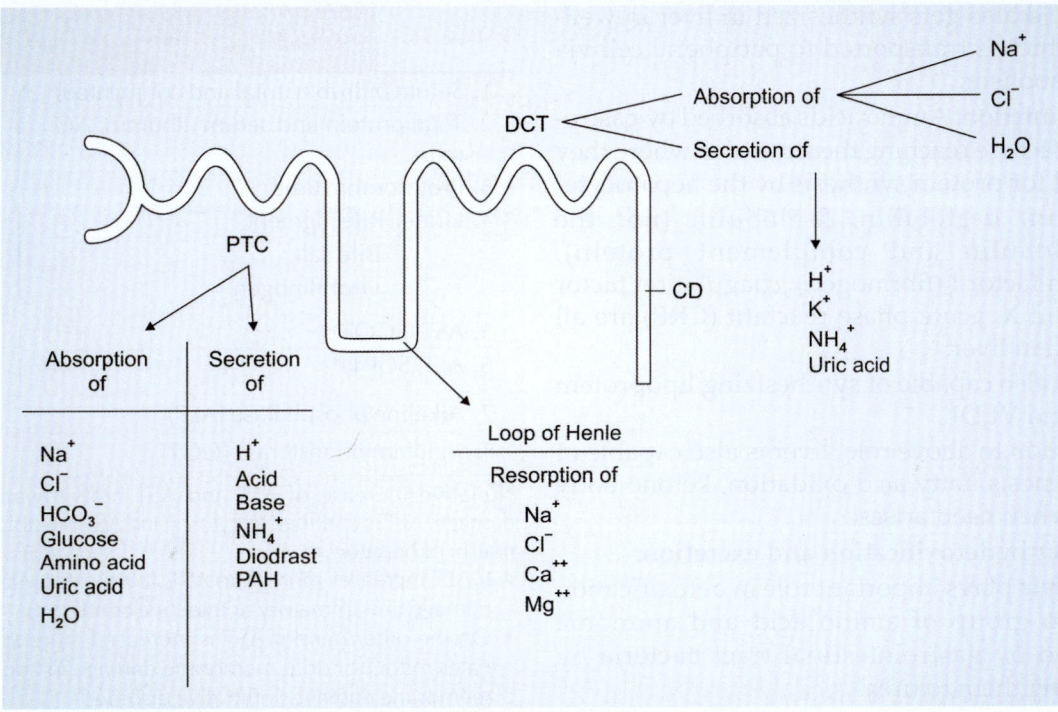

Fig. 31.1: Kidney tubule and exchange of various ions

Smoky red	:	Blood in urine
Brownish red	:	Hemoglobinuria
Orange	:	Rifampicin, bilirubin
Red	:	Porphyria
		Red beet consumption
Black	:	Alkaptonuria
		Formic acid, posion
Milky urine	:	Chyluria

Nonprotein nitrogen (NPN) substances:
1. Urea
2. Creatinine
3. Uric acid
4. Urobilinogen (UBG)
5. Indican
6. NH_3 and amino acid

▌LIVER FUNCTION TEST (LFT)

It is important to review the architecture of liver before learning this topic of LFT.

Anatomy: Liver is made up of number of hexagonal lobules of cells which are structural subunits of liver. Cords of hepatocyte radiate from central vein outwards and are separated by sinusoids.

Sinusoids: Blood from systemic circulation (hepatic artery) and (portal vein) get mixed here. Kuffer cells are found here.

Central vein: Large vessel in the center of each lobule which receives blood from sinusoids.

Portal triad: Present at border of liver lobule. It has following components.
- Hepatic artery
- Portal vein
- Bile duct
  - Portal vein brings blood from capillary bed of stomach, small intestine, large intestine, spleen and pancreas to the liver where nutrients are processed by hepatocyte before coming to systemic circulation.

Metabolic Role of Liver

Overall function of liver may be categorized in three broad headings:
1. Metabolic function
2. Synthetic function
3. Role in detoxification and excretion

1. **Metabolic function:** Many nutrients from gastrointestinal tract (except chylomicron and its constituents) reach liver via portal circulation. They all enter hepatic sinusoids where they are metabolized by hepatocyte before entering in systemic circulation. Glucose thus entering either is immediately utilized in glycolysis or any other pathway like HMP shunt or uronic acid pathway or is stored in liver in the form of glycogen for later use.

Section 8 ■ Miscellaneous Topics

31

Fatty acid also gets synthesized in liver in well-fed state which is transported to peripheral cell via VLDL metabolism.

2. **Synthetic function:** Amino acids absorbed by gastro-intestinal tract are reaching the sinusoids where they are utilized for protein synthesis by the hepatocyte.

Albumin, α-globulin, β-globulin (not the immunoglobulin and complement protein), coagulation factor I (fibrinogen), coagulation factor II, V, VII and X, acute phase reactant (CRP) are all synthesized in liver.

Liver is also capable of synthesizing lipoprotein like HDL and VLDL.

In addition to above role, liver is also capable of gluconeogenesis, fatty acid oxidation, ketone body synthesis when need arises.

3. **Role of liver in detoxification and excretion:**
   • Hepatocyte plays important role in detoxification of amino group of amino acid and ammonia produced by gastrointestinal tract bacteria by converting them to urea.
   • Excess unwanted cholesterol which are brought back to liver by HDL metabolism, is converted to bile acid in hepatocyte. Conversion of cholesterol to bile acid increases the polarity of compound which makes it easily excretable.
   • Many of the drugs are metabolized and get inactivated by enzymes of endoplasmic reticulum.
   • Toxins which are absorbed from gastrointestinal tract are tackled by Kupffer cells.

LFT

Two important points to be noticed regarding LFT are:

1. LFT is a misnomer, as all the test done under this heading do not necessarily assess the liver function. For example, enzyme assays (AST, ALT, ALP) done under LFT, rather denote the extent of damage of hepatocyte (in other words the dysfunction of hepatocyte) (Table 31.1).
2. Because of large reserve capacity of liver, test done to assess impairment of metabolic function (synthetic and excretory) of the liver, e.g. albumin level, clotting factor assessment (prothrombin test), bilirubin level assessment is relatively an insensitive indicator of liver disease.

Serum Bilirubin

Normal level of serum bilirubin:

_____
* Sulphanilic acid in HCl and sodium nitrite.

TABLE 31.1	Tests which are done under LFT to assess diverse roles of liver	
1. Serum bilirubin (total and conjugated)		
2. Total protein and serum albumin, AG ratio		To assess the liver dysfunction
3. Prothrombin time		
4. Urine: Bile pigment		
Bile salt		
Urobilinogen		
5. AST (SGOT)*		To assess cell damage
6. ALT (SGPT)*		
7. Alkaline phosphatase (ALP)		
8. γ-glutamyltransferase (GGT)		

*Relative increase of ALT and AST hints towards type of cell damage. ALT is confined to cytosol and AST is within mitochondrial matrix of hepatocyte.
• If ALT increases more than AST, it indicates plasma membrane damage (inflammatory or infective condition).
• On the other hand if AST is increased more than ALT, it indicates mitochondrial membrane damage in addition to plasma membrane damage (infiltrative disorder).

Total = 0.2–1.0 mg/dl

Unconjugated bilirubin (indirect): 0.2–0.7 mg/dl

Conjugated bilirubin (direct): 0.1–0.4 mg/dl

Level of bilirubin may be estimated by Van den Bergh reaction:

Diazotized sulphanilic acid* + Bilirubin → Azobilirubin (purple)

Direct test: Given by conjugated bilirubin. It is positive in obstructive juandice when level of conjugated bilirubin increases.

Indirect test: Given by unconjugated bilirubin. Here Van den Bergh test gives positive result only after addition of alcohol and hence it is called indirect test and unconjugated bilirubin is known as indirect bilirubin. In hemolytic anemia, unconjugated bilirubin increases, which gives indirect test +ve.

Biphasic: When serum has increased conjugated and unconjugated bilirubin (as seen in hepatic disease) the Van den Bergh reaction is biphasic which means that purple colour is produced immediately which gets intensified on adding the alcohol.

▌URINE

Bilirubin

• Fouchet's test
• Conjugated bilirubin (soluble) denotes obstructive jaundice.

Test for Bile Pigments

Fouchet's Test

Procedure: Add 5 ml of 10% BaCl$_2$ to 10 ml of urine and filter. Dry the filter paper and add a few drops of Fouchet's reagent (prepared by adding 10 mg of 10% FeCl$_3$ to 100 ml of 25% TCA). A green color is obtained due to oxidation of bilirubin to biliverdin (Fig. 31.2).

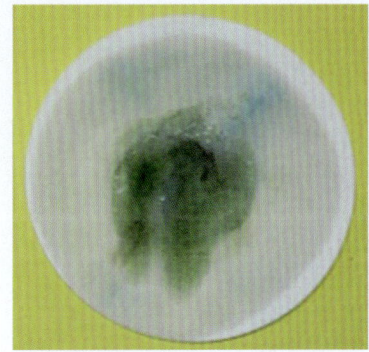

Fig. 31.2: Fouchet's test

Urobilinogen (UBG)

• UBG is produced in gastrointestinal tract lumen after action of bacteria on bilirubin.
• UBG is absent in urine in case of obstructive jaundice.
• UBG is assessed in urine by Ehrlich's test (Fig. 31.3).

Bile Salt

• Regurgitate in blood in obstructive jaundice case.
• Detected in urine by *Hay's sulphur test* (Fig. 31.4).

• Obstruction may be seen even in hepatic jaundice where cell inflamed may cause obstruction of biliary channels.

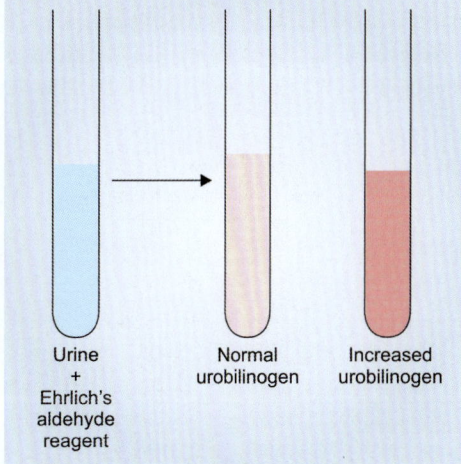

Fig. 31.3: Ehrlich's test for urobilinogen

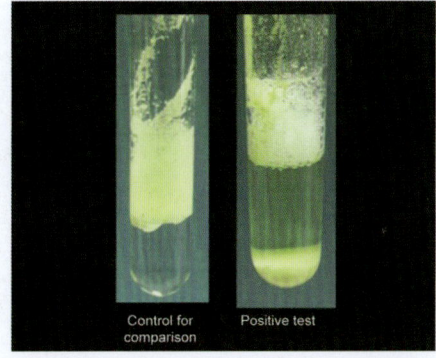

Fig. 31.4: Hay's sulphur test (for bile salt)

Nucleic Acids: Chemistry, Metabolism and Applied Aspects

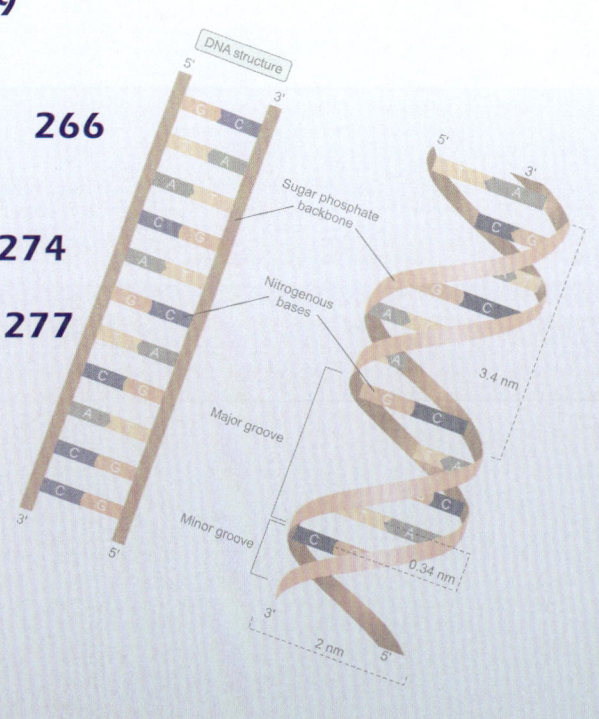

9

Nucleic Acids: Chemistry, Metabolism and Applied Aspects

32

Nucleotides: Chemistry and their Metabolism

COMPETENCY BI 6.2

At the end of this chapter learner should be able to describe and discuss the metabolic processes in which nucleotides are involved.

COMPETENCY BI 6.3

At the end of this chapter learner should be able to describe the common disorders associated with nucleotide metabolism).

Specific Learning Objectives	
BI 6.2	Describe and discuss the metabolic processes in which nucleotides are involved.
BI 6.2.1	Describe synthesis of purine nucleotides.
BI 6.2.2	Describe salvage pathway of nucleotides.
BI 6.2.3	Enumerate amino acids required for purine synthesis.
BI 6.2.4	Enumerate amino acids required for pyrimidine synthesis.
BI 6.2.5	Enumerate the molecules having regulatory effect on synthesis of purine.
BI 6.3.1	Enumerate the causes of primary hyperuricemia.
BI 6.3.2	Enumerate the causes of secondary hyperuricemia.
BI 6.3.3	Describe the sources of carbon and nitrogen atoms in purine ring.
BI 6.3.4	Discuss salvage pathway of purine synthesis.
BI 6.3.5	Describe the purine catabolism.

█ NUCLEOTIDE AND ITS METABOLISM

Components of a nucleotide (Fig. 32.1): Nucleotides are made up of three components:

1. Base
2. Pentose
3. Phosphate

Base may be purine or pyrimidine. Pentose may be ribose or deoxyribose. Number of phosphate in a nucleotide may be 1, 2 or 3.

When base and pentose alone are linked, it is a nucleoside.

Difference in the purine and pyrimidine bases is as follow:
Purine base is double cyclical, heterocyclic structure and pyrimidine ring is single cyclical, heterocyclic structure.

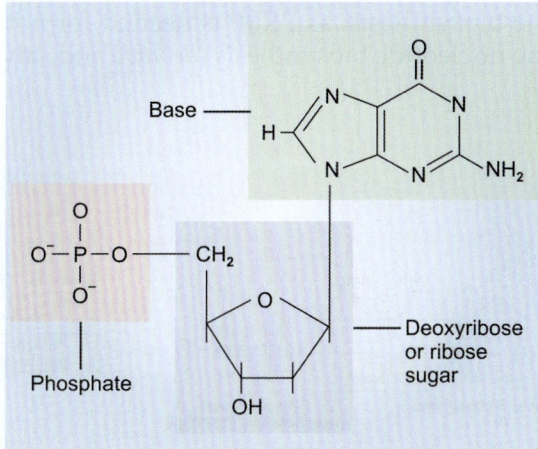

Fig. 32.1: Structure of a typical nucleotide

Significance of Nucleotide in a Cell Functioning

Nucleotides are not only required for polynucleotide (DNA, RNA) synthesis, they are also needed as the energy currency of the cell (ATP). They also have a role as coenzyme for various enzymes (NAD, NADP, FAD).

Unusual/Minor Bases (Purine/Pyrimidine)

There are certain purine and pyrimidine bases which are not abundantly found in the cell. They are:

• *Hypoxanthine:* 6-oxopurine
• *Xanthine:* 2,6-oxopurine
• *Uric acid:* 2,6,8-oxopurine
• Caffeine
• Dihydrouridine
• 5-methylcytosine

PURINE NUCLEOTIDE

Biosynthesis of Purine Nucleotides

Three processes contribute to biosynthesis of purine nucleotides:

1. *De novo* biosynthesis (synthesis from amphibolic intermediates)
2. Salvage pathway (phosphoribosylation of purine)
3. Phosphorylation of purine nucleosides (adenosine/ guanosine)

De novo Biosynthesis (Synthesis from Amphibolic Intermediates)

This pathway is mainly seen in liver and is cytosolic.

- Starting material is D-ribose-5-phosphate, which is converted to phosphoribosyl-pyrophosphate (PRPP) by PRPP synthetase.
- Synthesis of PRPP is not the committed step of *de novo* purine biosynthesis, as PRPP is needed for not only purine nucleotide biosynthesis (*de novo* and salvage),

it is also needed for pyrimidine nucleotide (*de novo* and salvage).

- PRPP glutamyl amidotransferase converts PRPP to 5-phospho-D-ribosyl amine. This is the first reaction uniquely committed to purine nucleotide *de novo* synthesis. PRPP glutamyl amidotransferase is the rate-limiting step of *de novo* purine nucleotide biosynthesis.
- Thereafter multiple reactions catalysed by different enzymes occur which form hypoxanthine ring (IMP) (Fig. 32.2A).
- Thus, the first purine nucleotide synthesized by this pathway is inosine monophosphate (IMP). The pathway then branches and two short reactions lead to the formation of AMP and GMP (Figs 32.2B).
  - AMP and GMP feedback regulate PRPP glutamyl amidotransferase.
  - AMP and GMP feedback regulate their formation from IMP.

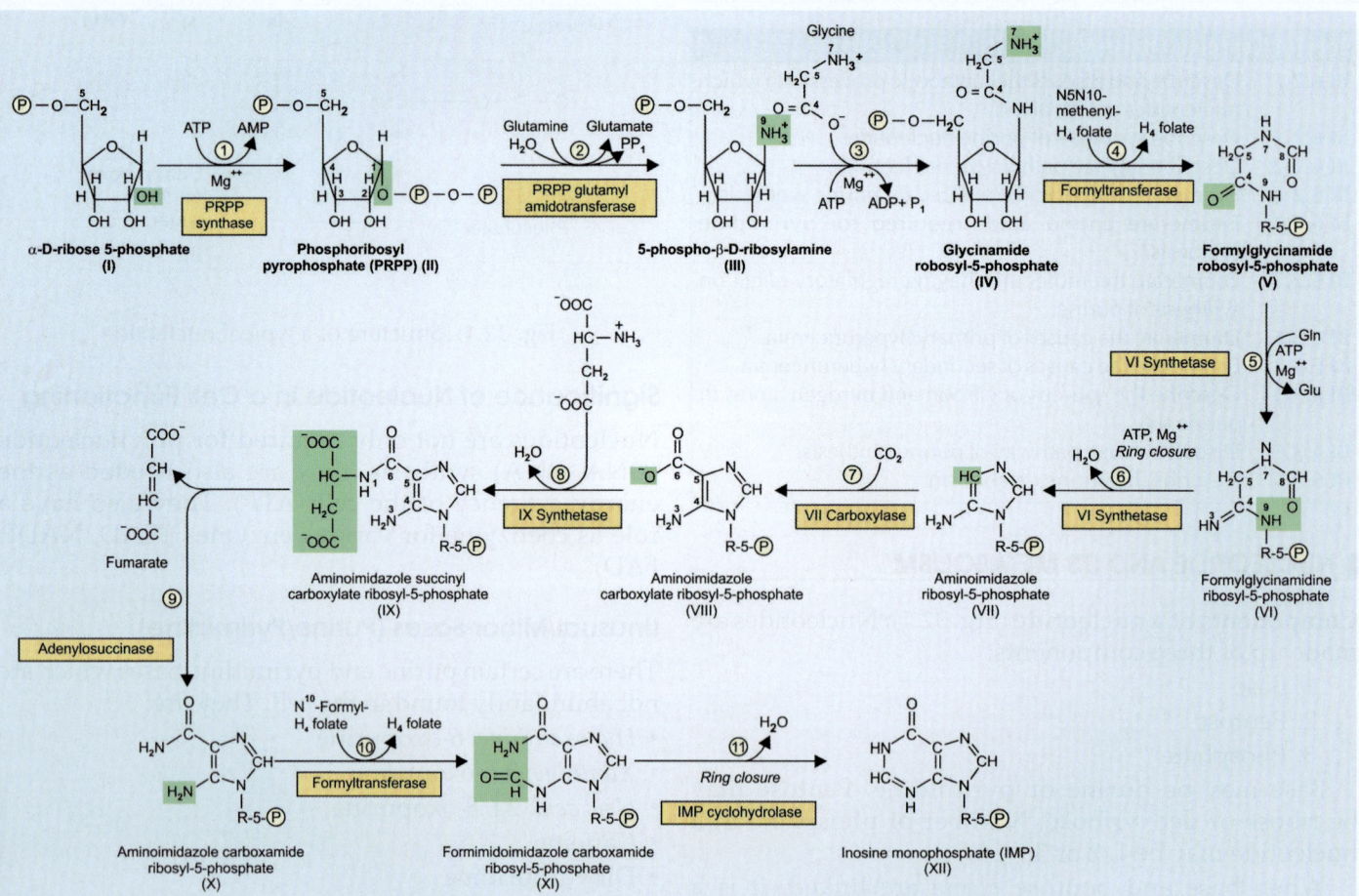

Fig. 32.2A: *De novo* biosynthesis of purine nucleotide

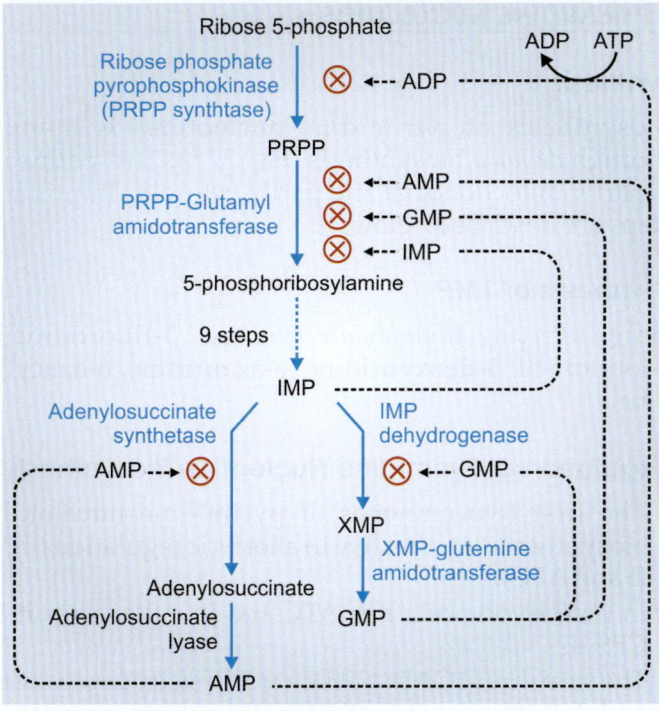

Fig. 32.2B: Purine nucleotide *de novo* biosynthesis

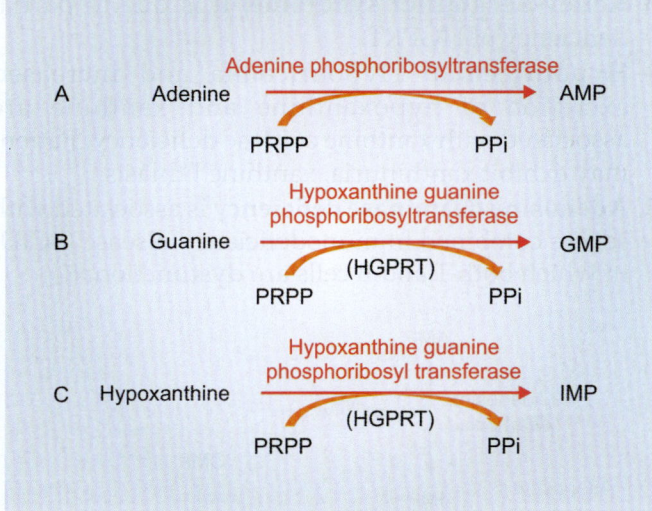

Fig. 32.3: Salvage pathway for purine nucleotide biosynthesis

Catabolism of Purine Nucleosides

- Human converts major purine nucleosides adenosine and guanosine to uric acid. This pathway occurs mainly in liver.
- Various steps of this catabolic pathway is shown in Fig. 32.4.

Salvage Pathway

In this pathway the available purine rings are reutilized to synthesize purine nucleotides.

It is rather a simpler process compared to *de novo* biosynthesis. This pathway is significant in those cells where *de novo* biosynthesis does not occur, e.g. brain and RBC.

Reaction of salvage pathway is as follow (Fig. 32.3):

- Adenine phosphoribosyltransferase transfers adenine on PRPP. Guanine and hypoxanthine are transferred on PRPP by HGPRT.

Regulation of Purine Nucleotide Biosynthesis

1. PRPP pool size regulates purine nucleotide bio-synthesis.

Important Note

- Xanthine oxidase is a molybdenum and iron containing enzyme, which is inhibited by allopurinol.
- In body fluids uric acid and its monosodium urate salt are present.

- Urate is far more soluble in water than uric acid. Urine at pH 5 can dissolve only about one-tenth as much urates (15 mg/dl) as urine at pH 7 (150–200 mg/dl). pH of normal urine typically is below 5.8. Urinary tract crystals thus are sodium urate anywhere proximal to the site of urine acidification, but these stones are uric acid at distal sites.
- Since most stones of urinary collecting system are composed of uric acid. Stone formation can be reduced by alkalinization of the urine.

Metabolic Disorders of Purine Catabolism

There are many disorders which are associated with defective catabolism of purine nucleotides (Fig. 32.4). They are described below:

1. **Gout:** In case of hyperuricemia, serum urate levels exceed the solubility limit. Resulting crystallization of sodium urate in soft tissues and joints forms deposits called tophi, causing an inflammatory reaction, acute gouty arthritis, which can progress to chronic gouty arthritis.

    Visualization of needle shaped, intensively negatively birefringent crystals of sodium urate in joint fluid under a polarizing light microscope is diagnostic of gout. The crystals appear yellow when their long axis is parallel to the plane of polarized light and they appear blue when they are perpendicular to plane polarized light.

2. **Lesch–Nyhan syndrome**
    - It is an X-linked recessive disorder, which is due to complete deficiency of enzyme 'HGPRT' (an enzyme of purine salvage pathway).
    - It is characterized by hyperuricemia, uric acid lithiasis and a syndrome of selfmutilation.

Section 9 ■ Nucleic Acids: Chemistry, Metabolism and Applied Aspects

32

3. **Kelley-Seegmiller syndrome:** It is due to partial deficiency of HGPRT.
4. **Hypouricemia:** Hypouricemia and increased excretion of hypoxanthine and xanthine are associated with xanthine oxidase deficiency. Patient may exhibit xanthinuria, xanthine lithiasis.
5. **Adenosine deaminase deficiency** is associated with severe combined immunodeficiency disease (SCID) in which both T and B cells are dysfunctional.

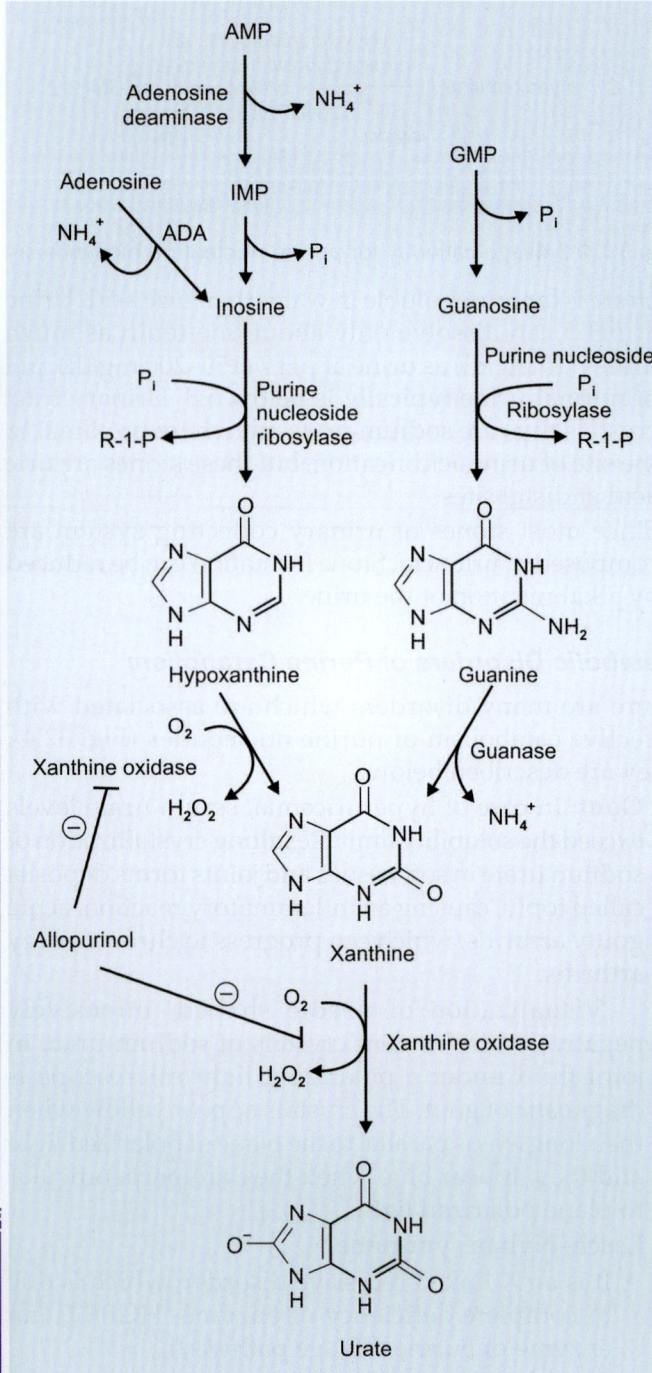

Fig. 32.4: Purine nucleotide catabolism

PYRIMIDINE NUCLEOTIDE

Synthesis

Biosynthesis of pyrimidine nucleotides is mainly through *de novo* biosynthesis (Fig. 32.5). This pathway is partly mitochondrial and partly cytosolic. Important steps are described below:

Synthesis of TMP

Drugs affecting thymidylate synthase: 5-fluorouracil, 5-iodouracil, 3-deoxyuridine, 6-azauridine, 6-azacytidine.

Regulation of Pyrimidine Nucleotide Biosynthesis

- The first two enzymes of pyrimidine nucleotide biosynthesis are sensitive to allosteric regulation (CPS II and ATC).
- In prokaryotic cell, it is ATC and in eukaryotes it is CPS II.
- The first three (CAD: CPS II + ATC + dihydroorotase) and last two enzymes of pathway are regulated at genetic level by coordinate repression and derepression.

Catabolism of Pyrimidines

The end products of pyrimidine catabolism are CO_2, NH_3, β-alanine and β-aminoisobutyrate (Fig. 32.6).

Overproduction is rarely associated with clinically significant abnormalities as all these products are water soluble. Excretion of aminoisobutyrate increases due to increased destruction of DNA.

Disorder associated with pyrimidine nucleotide metabolism:

Orotic aciduria: It is an autosomal recessive disorder.

Type I: Due to OPRTsae deficiency and ODC deficiency.

Type II: Due to ODC deficiency.

Cytidine and uridine feeding helps in orotic aciduria.

Drugs affecting Purine and Pyrimidine nucleotide metabolism

1. Structural analogue of base or nucleotide:
   - 6-mercaptopurine
   - 6-thioguanine
   - 5-fluorouracil
   - Cytosine arabinoside (Ara C)
   - Acyclovir (acycloguanosine)
   - Azidodoxy thymidine (AZT)
2. Antifolate:
   - Methotrexate

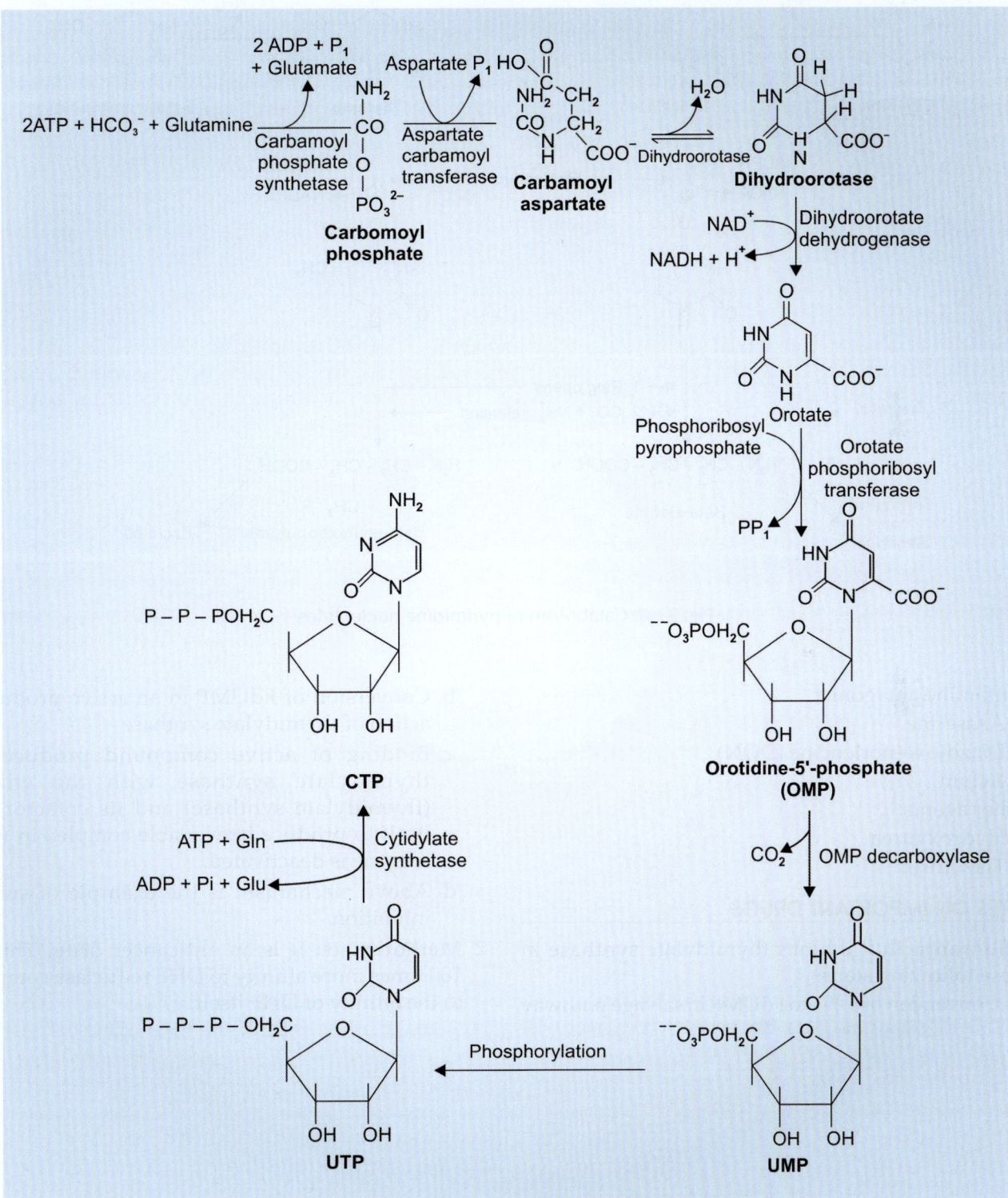

Fig. 32.5: *De novo* synthesis of pyrimidine nucleotide

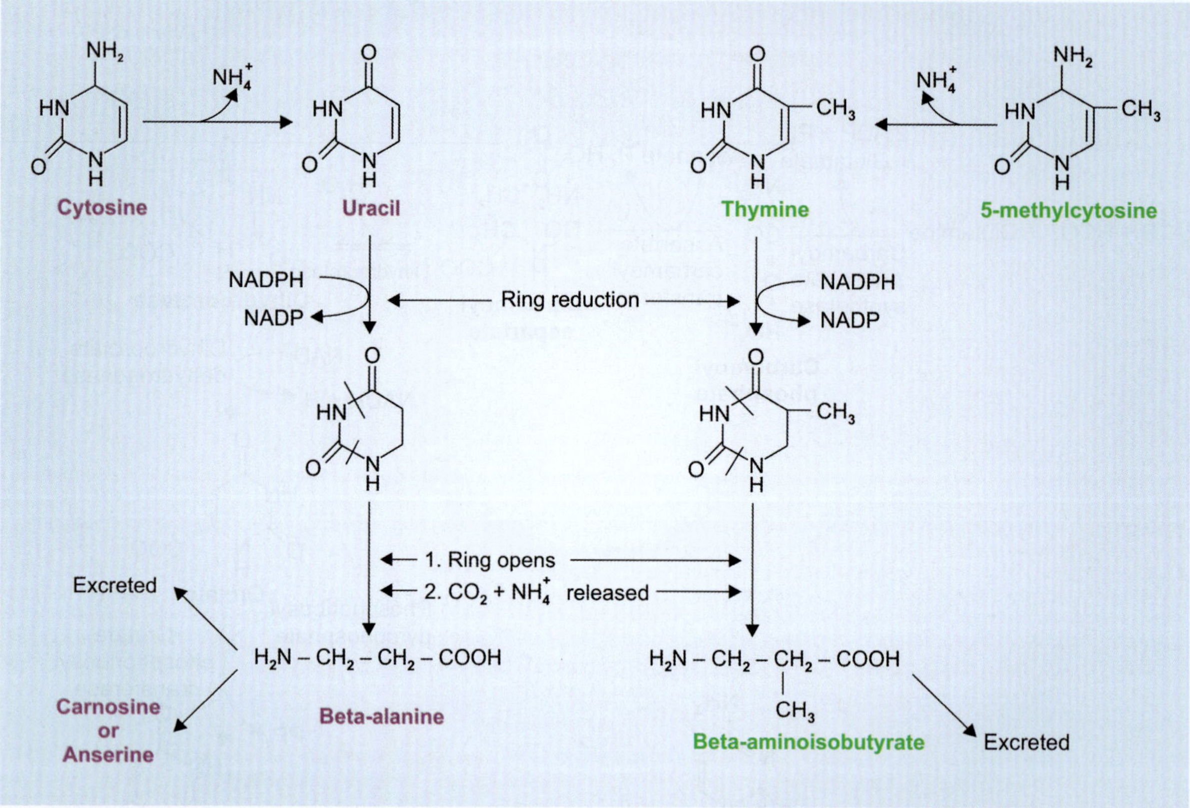

Fig. 32.6: Catabolism of pyrimidine nucleotides

3. Glutamine antagonist:
   - Azaserine
   - Diazo-oxo-norleucine (DON)
   - Acivin
4. Other agents:
   - Hydroxyurea
   - Tiazofurin

NOTES ON IMPORTANT DRUGS

1. **5-fluorouracil:** It inhibits thymidylate synthase in these following steps:
   a. Conversion of 5-FU to FdUMP in salvage pathway

   b. Conversion of FdUMP in an active product by action of thymidylate synthase
   c. Binding of active compound produced by thymidylate synthase with the enzyme (thymidylate synthase) and its cofactor THF itself to produce irreversible complex in which enzyme is deactivated.
   d. Above mechanism is the example of suicidal inhibition.

2. **Methotrexate:** It is an anticancer drug. This has 100 times more affinity to DHF reductase compared to the affinity of DHF itself.

33

Nucleic Acid I: Structural Organization of DNA and RNA

COMPETENCY BI 7.1

> At the end of this chapter learner should be able to describe the structure and functions of DNA and RNA and outline the cell cycle.

Specific Learning Objectives	
BI 7.1.1	Describe DNA double helix structure.
BI 7.1.2	Discuss difference between DNA and RNA.
BI 7.1.3	Describe DNA sequencing.
BI 7.1.4	Describe role of DNA.
BI 7.1.5	Describe role of RNA.
BI 7.1.6	Describe technique of DNA sequencing.

TYPES OF NUCLEIC ACIDS

1. Deoxyribonucleic acid (DNA)
2. Ribonucleic acid (RNA)
   Both DNA and RNA are made up of nucleotides.

DNA

- DNA is the long thread-like polymer made up of deoxynucleotides linked through 3′–5′ phosphodiester bond.
- DNA is the genetic material for both prokaryotes and eukaryotes.
- In prokaryotes, DNA is a double stranded structure and circular with no free ends.
- In eukaryotes, DNA is a double stranded structure and linear with free ends.
- Linear DNA is a polar molecule which has 5′ and 3′ polarity.
- 5′-end of DNA denotes the nucleotide having free 5′ phosphate and 3′-end denotes nucleotide with free 3′ hydroxyl group.
- In eukaryotes major amount of DNA is found in the nucleus, though <1% of DNA is found in mitochondria.
- In the double stranded DNA molecule, the genetic information resides in the sequence of nucleotides on one strand. This strand is known as template strand (also called noncoding strand).
- The opposite strand is considered as coding strand because it matches the RNA transcript that encodes the protein.

Watson and Crick Model of DNA

- Proposed in 1953 by James Watson and Francis Crick.
- It is a double stranded structure. Each strand possesses polarity and they are arranged in antiparallel direction.
- DNA backbone is made up of phosphodiester bond and bases are perpendicular to the helical axis.
- The two strands of DNA are coiled around a common axis.
- Helix is repeated at interval of 34Å.
- Each helix has 10 base pairs and so distance between adjacent bases on a strand is 3.4Å.
- Width of helix is 20 Å (2.0 nm).
- The two strands of double stranded helix are held in place by hydrogen bonds between the purines and pyrimidine bases.
- Adenine pairs with thymine with two hydrogen bonds and guanine pairs with cytosine with the help of three hydrogen bonds ($A = T$, $C \equiv G$).
- Major and minor grooves are present on double helix DNA (Figs 33.1a and b).

Chargaff's Rule

In a double stranded DNA, purine bases are equal to pyrimidine bases.

$$A + G = C + T$$

Ratio of total purine bases and pyrimidine bases is equal to one.

$$\frac{\text{Total number of purine bases in the DNA}}{\text{Total number of pyrimidine bases in the DNA}} = 1$$

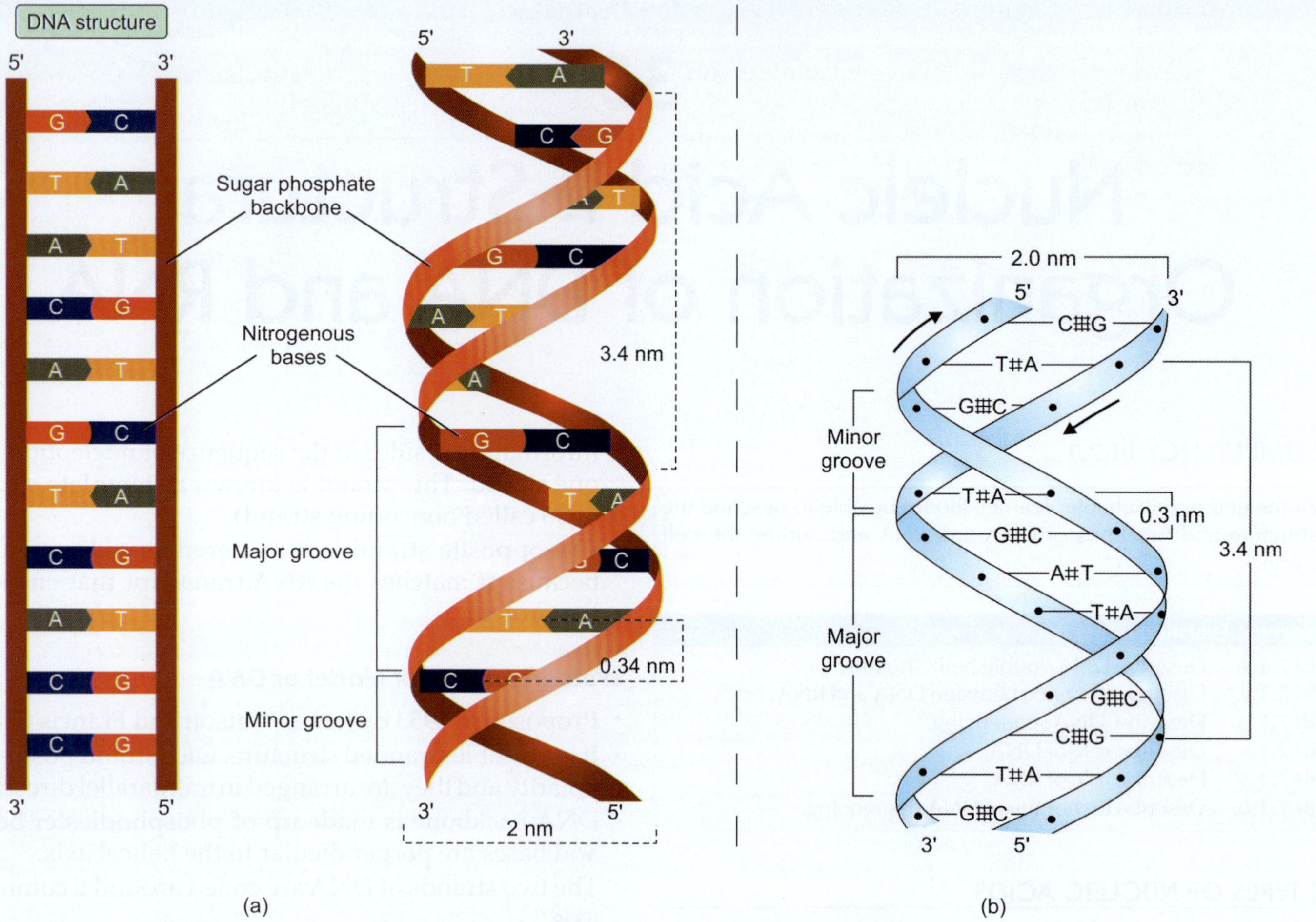

DNA structure

5' 3'

Sugar phosphate backbone

Nitrogenous bases

3.4 nm

Major groove

0.34 nm

Minor groove

3' 5'

2 nm

(a)

2.0 nm

5' 3'

C#G

T#A

G#C

Minor groove

T#A

G#C

0.3 nm

A#T

3.4 nm

T#A

Major groove

G#C

C#G

T#A

G#C

3' 5'

(b)

Figs 33.1a and b: Watson and Crick model of DNA

Supercoiling of DNA

- When two ends of DNA are fixed and are twisted around its own axis, supercoiling is produced (Fig. 33.2).
- When the twisting is done in right hand direction in B type DNA, positive supercoiling is produced and when twisting is done in left hand direction in B type DNA, negative supercoiling is produced.
- Most of the natural form of DNA supercoiling is left handed (negative).
- Supercoiling makes DNA more compact.
- Supercoiling affects gene expression (via affecting the transcription and replication).

Euchromatin and Heterochromatin

- Transcriptionally active chromatin stains less densely and is referred to as euchromatin.
- Transcriptionally inactive chromatin is densely packed during interphase as observed by electron microscopic studies and is referred to as heterochromatin.
- There are two types of heterochromatin—constitutive and facultative (Fig. 33.3).

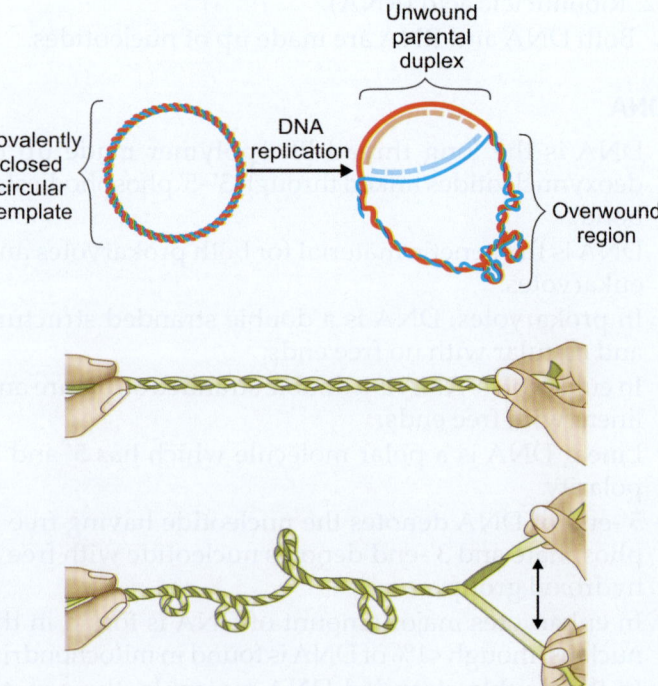

Fig. 33.2: Supercoiling of DNA

- Constitutive heterochromatin is always condensed and thus essentially inactive. It is found in the regions near the chromosomal centromere and at chromosomal ends (telomeres).
- Facultative heterochromatin is at times condensed (heterochromatin, but at other times it is actively transcribed and, thus uncondensed and appears as euchromatin.

- Similarly, there are two types of euchromatin—constitutive and facultative.
  - Constitutive euchromatin is always uncondensed and thus essentially active.
  - Facultative euchromatin is at times condensed (heterochromatin, but at other times it is actively transcribed and, thus uncondensed and appears as euchromatin).

Types of DNA

Though the model described by Watson and Crick was type B DNA, double stranded DNA exists in at least six forms (A, B, C, D, E and Z)

Table 33.1 shows important difference in various types of DNA.

Denaturation of DNA

- Strand separation is also known as melting/denaturation of DNA. Strands of a given DNA molecule separate over a temperature range. The midpoint of this temperature range is called the melting temperature (T_m).
- Increasing the temperature or decreasing the salt concentration leads to strand separation.
- 10-fold increase in monovalent cation increases T_m by 16.6°C.
- DNA rich in G-C pairs (having 3 hydrogen bonds) melts at a higher temperature than that rich in A-T pairs, which have 2 hydrogen bonds.

Histones

- These are basic proteins binding to DNA.
- These are of following types—H1, H2A, H2B, H3, H4.
- H2A and H2B are lysine rich and form dimer.
- H3 and H4 are arginine rich and form tetramer.
- All these combine to form a disc-like octamer.
- Covalent modification in histone may be acetylation, methylation, phosphorylation, ADP ribosylation, ubiquitination and sumoylation (Table 33.2).

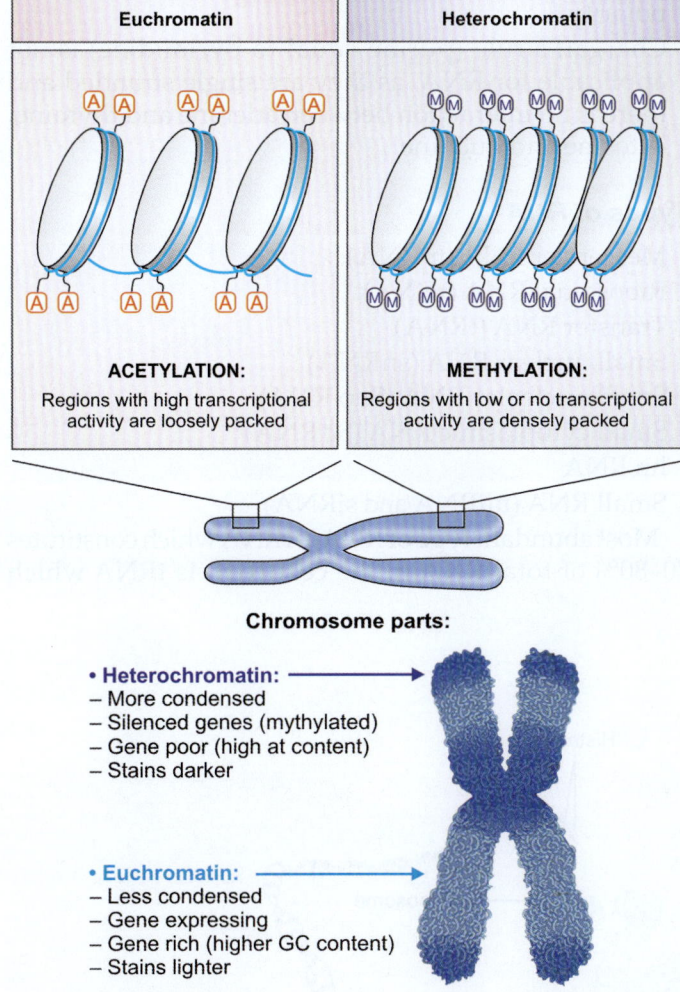

ACETYLATION:
Regions with high transcriptional activity are loosely packed

METHYLATION:
Regions with low or no transcriptional activity are densely packed

Chromosome parts:

- **Heterochromatin:**
  – More condensed
  – Silenced genes (mythylated)
  – Gene poor (high at content)
  – Stains darker

- **Euchromatin:**
  – Less condensed
  – Gene expressing
  – Gene rich (higher GC content)
  – Stains lighter

Fig. 33.3: Euchromatin and heterochromatin regions in chromosome

TABLE 33.1	Differences between various types of DNA		
Feature	B-DNA	A-DNA	Z-DNA
Type of helix	Right-handed	Right-handed	Left-handed
Helical diameter (nm)	2.37	2.55	1.84
Rise per base pair (nm)	0.34	0.29	0.37
Distance per complete turn (pitch) (nm)	3.4	3.2	4.5
Number of base pairs per complete turn	10	11	12
Topology of major groove	Wide, deep	Narrow, deep	Flat
Topology of minor groove	Narrow, shallow	Broad, shallow	Narrow, deep

TABLE 33.2	Possible roles of modified histones

1. Acetylation of histones H3 and H4 is associated with the activation or inactivation of gene transcription.

2. Acetylation of core histone is associated with chromosomal assembly during DNA replication.

3. Phosphorylation of histone H1 is associated with the condensation of chromosomes during the replication cycle.

4. ADP-ribosylation of histones is associated with DNA repair.

5. Methylation of histones is correlated with activation and repression of gene transcription.

6. Monoubiquitylation is associated with gene activation, repression, and heterochromatic gene silencing.

7. Sumoylation of histones (SUMO; small ubiquitin-related modifier) is associated with transcription repression.

Condensation of DNA to Chromosome

DNA is compacted to many fold (10,000-fold) to form final structure chromosome (Fig. 33.4).

Various levels of this condensation are:
1. Helix of double strand DNA (2 nm)
2. Nucleosome (11 nm)
3. Solenoid (6 nucleosomes per turn) (30 nm)
4. Supercoiled loop (250–400 nm)

Nucleosome

Double strand DNA wrapped around histone octamer constitutes a nuclesome.

RNA

- RNA is the polymer of ribonucleotides which are linked through 3'–5' phosphodiester bond.
- It is a single stranded molecule with 5' and 3'-end polarity.
- Chargaff's rule (purine equal to pyrimidine) is not applicable for RNA, as they are single stranded and there is no interaction between adenine and thymine, cytosine and guanine.

Types of RNA

- Messenger RNA (mRNA)
- Ribosomal RNA (rRNA)
- Transfer RNA (tRNA)
- Small nuclear RNA (snRNA)
- Small nucleolar RNA (Sno RNA)
- Small cytoplasmic RNA (Sc RNA)
- hn RNA
- Small RNA (miRNA and siRNA)

Most abundant type of RNA is rRNA which constitutes 70–80% of total RNA in the cell. Next is tRNA which

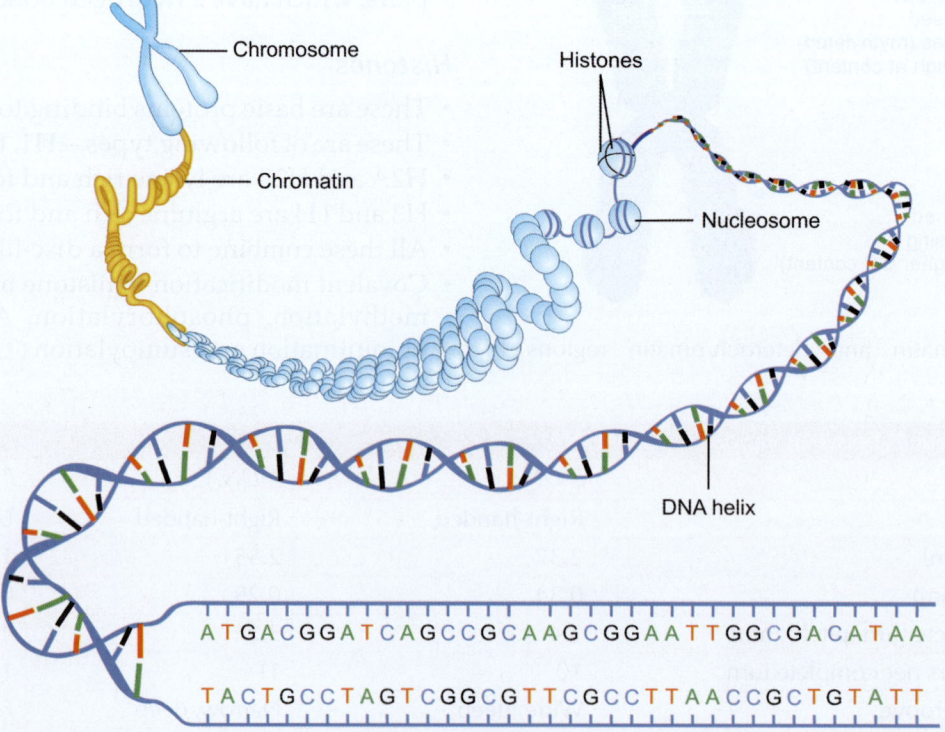

ATGACGGATCAGCCGCAAGCGGAATTGGCGACATAA

TACTGCCTAGTCGGCGTTCGCCTTAACCGCTGTATT

Fig. 33.4: Organisation of DNA into chromosome

is 15% of total RNA. mRNA constitutes only 5–10% of total RNA. Rest other types of above mentioned RNA constitute only minor fraction of total RNA.

Messenger RNA (mRNA)

- This is the most heterogeneous in size and stability and represents 5–10% of total eukaryotic cellular RNA.
- These are messengers conveying the information of a gene to the protein synthesizing machinery, where mRNA serves as a template on which a specific sequence of amino acids is polymerized to form specific protein molecule.

5′ cap: The 5′-terminal of mRNA is capped by a 7-methyl guanosine triphosphate. The cap is involved in the:

- Recognition of mRNA by the translating machinery.
- Stabilization of mRNA by preventing the attack of 5′-exonucleases.

3′ polyA tail: The 3′-hydroxyl terminal of mRNA molecules has a polymer of adenylate residues (polyA) 20–250 nucleotides in length. It seems to prevent an attack by 3′-exonucleases and also facilitates translation.

Sometimes mRNAs for example some histones mRNA do not contain polyA tail.

In mammalian cells, mRNA molecules present in the cytoplasm are formed by processing of a precursor molecule hnRNA (heteronuclear RNA) synthesized in nucleus. hnRNA consists of exons (coding portions), and introns (noncoding portions).

The intron RNA sequences are cleaved out and the exon sequences are appropriately spliced (joined) together in the nucleus before the resulting mRNA molecule appears in the cytoplasm for translation. This process is called splicing.

Ribosomal RNA (rRNA)

Ribosomal RNA present in various ribosomal subunits and helps in making of body of the ribosome (Fig. 33.5).

In addition to this role, rRNA is seen to be playing important role in binding of mRNA to the ribosome and facilitating the process of translation.

rRNA is also seen to have catalytic role (peptidyltransferase activity) which helps in protein synthesis. 23S rRNA and 28S rRNA of large subunits of the ribosome are having this catalytic activity.

Transfer RNA (tRNA) (also called soluble RNA)

- tRNA molecule serves as adapter molecules for the translation of mRNA into protein sequences.
- These vary in length from 74–95 nucleotides.

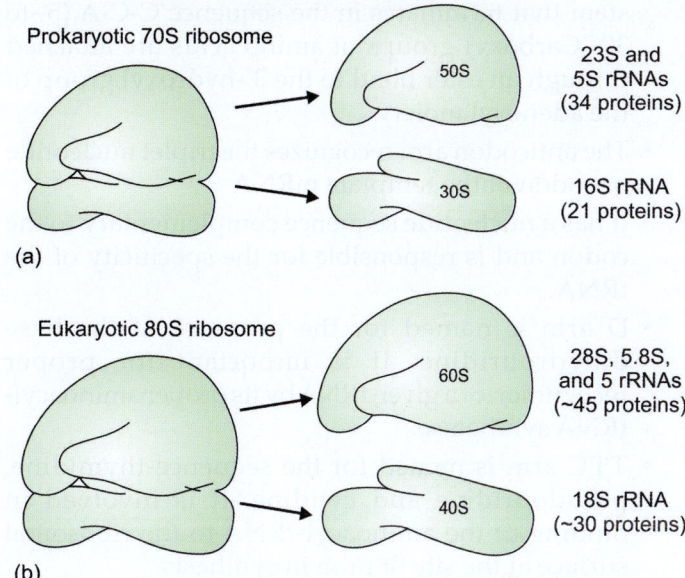

(a)

(b)

Fig. 33.5: Composition of subunits of eukaryotic and prokaryotic ribosomes

- Molecular weight is approximately 25,000.
- The primary structure allows extensive folding and intrastrand complementarity to generate a secondary structure that appears like a clover leaf.

Structure of a transfer RNA (Fig. 33.6): All tRNAs contain 4 main arms and 1 extra arm (total 5 arms).

- *Acceptor arm:* It is called acceptor arm because it is involved in accepting the amino acid at its 3′ end. The acceptor arm consists of a base paired

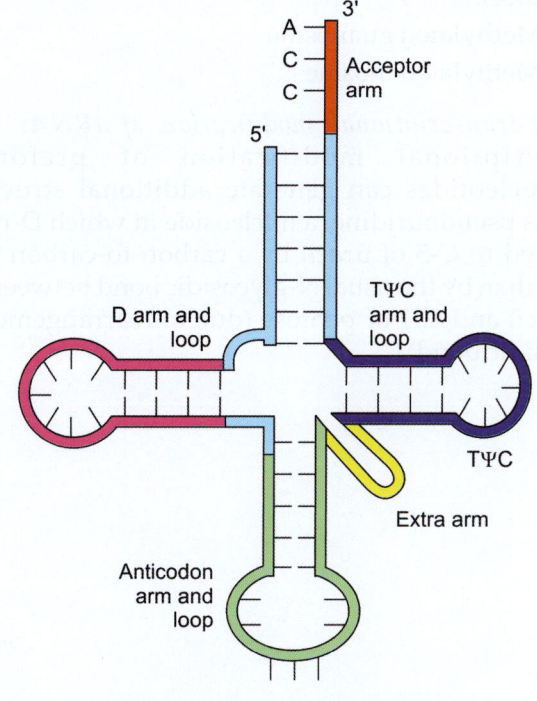

Fig. 33.6: Structure of tRNA

stem that terminates in the sequence C-C-A (5'-to 3'). Carboxyl groups of amino acids are attached through an ester bond to the 3'-hydroxyl group of the adenosyl moiety.

- The anticodon arm recognizes the triplet nucleotide or codon of the template mRNA.
- It has a nucleotide sequence complementary to the codon and is responsible for the specificity of the tRNA.
- D arm is named for the presence of the base dihydrouridine. It is important for proper recognition of a given tRNA by its proper aminoacyl-tRNA synthetase.
- TΨC arm is named for the sequence-thymidine, pseudouridine and cytidine. It is involved in binding of the aminoacyl-tRNA to the ribosomal surface at the site of protein synthesis.
- The extra arm is the most variable feature of tRNA and provides the basis for classification of tRNA into two classes:
    - *Class 1:* This class is predominant (75%). Here size of extra arm is small (3–5 bp).
    - *Class 2:* This class is less predominant (25%). Here size of extra arm is large (13–20 bp).

Unusual nucleosides found in tRNA are:
1. Ribothymidine
2. Pseudouridine
3. Dihydrouridine
4. Inosine
5. Methylated guanosine
6. Methylated inosine

Post-transcriptional modification of tRNA: Post-transcriptional modification of preformed polynucleotides can generate additional structures such as pseudouridine, a nucleoside in which D-ribose is linked to C-5 of uracil by a carbon-to-carbon bond rather than by the usual N-glycosidic bond between N-1 of uracil and C-1 of pentose (due to rearrangement of glycosidic bond).

Similarly, methylation by S-adenosylmethionine of an UMP of preformed tRNA results in formation of thymidine monophosphate (TMP).

tRNA and rRNA differ in their stability in prokaryotes and eukaryotes. tRNAs are quite stable in prokaryotes but somewhat less stable in eukaryotes. On the other hand, mRNAs are quite unstable in prokaryotes but generally stable in eukaryotic organisms (Table 33.3).

TABLE 33.3	Comparison of RNA in prokaryotes and eukaryotes	
RNA	*Eukaryotes*	*Prokaryotes*
tRNA	Less stable	More stable
mRNA	More stable	Less stable

Small Nuclear RNA (snRNA)

These small-sized RNAs are of various types and are significantly involved in rRNA and mRNA processing and gene regulation. Of the several snRNAs, U1, U2, U4, U5, and U6 (not U3) are involved in intron removal and the processing of mRNA precursors into mRNA.

The U7 snRNA is involved in production of the correct 3'-ends of histone mRNA which lacks a polyA tail.

Small RNA (miRNA and siRNA) (Table 33.4)

These are recently described types of RNAs.

TABLE 33.4	Comparison of small interference RNA (siRNA) and microRNA (miRNA)		
S. No.	*Particulars*	*siRNA*	*miRNA*
1.	Function	Gene regulation	Gene regulation
2.	Size in nucleotides	20–25	21–23
3.	Strands	Two complementary	Single
4.	Site of attachment to mRNA	Coding region	Noncoding region
5.	Effect on translation	Translation is blocked	Translation is blocked

Nucleic Acid II: DNA Replication (Prokaryotes and Eukaryotes)

COMPETENCY BI 7.2

At the end of this chapter learner should be able to describe the processes involved in replication and repair of DNA and the transcription and translation mechanisms.

Specific Learning Objectives

BI 7.2.1	Describe the replication process of DNA in prokaryotes.
BI 7.2.2	Discuss the differences between prokaryotic and eukaryotic DNA replication.
BI 7.2.3	Discuss Okazaki fragment.
BI 7.2.4	Describe DNA topoisomerases and its inhibitors.
BI 7.2.5	Discuss inhibitors of DNA replication in prokaryotes.

DNA replication is also known as DNA synthesis or DNA duplication.

Whether it is prokaryotic or eukaryotic DNA replication, it is always semiconservative.

Semiconservative replication means new set of DNA has one parent strand and one daughter strand.

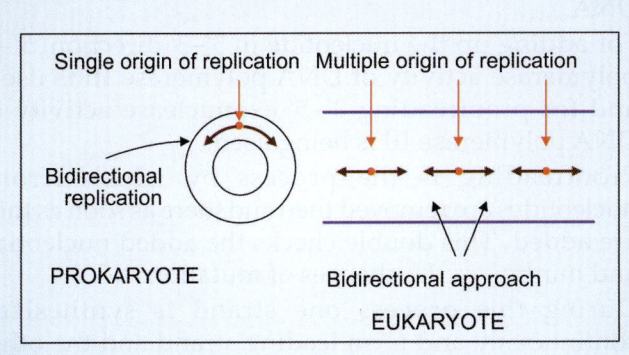

Fig. 34.1: Prokaryotic and eukaryotic DNA replication

DNA REPLICATION IN PROKARYOTES

- Prokaryotes have double stranded circular DNA.
- In prokaryotes, DNA replication begins at specific nucleotide sequence known as origin of replication 'ori'.
- In prokaryotes the origin of replication is single from where it proceeds in both the directions (bidirectional) (Fig. 34.1).

REPLICATION FORK

- This is formed at the region where DNA separates. It is a 'V' shaped structure during DNA replication (Fig. 34.2).
- This replication fork moves in both directions from the site of origins.
- A protein single strand binding protein (SSBP also known as helix destabilizing protein) is important for DNA separation.
- Enzyme helicase acts on DNA strand to unwind dsDNA in 5'–3' direction. Helicase requires ATP.
- Helicase associates with primase, so that primase may have access to template and may make RNA primer. Helicase and primase together form mobile complex known as primosome.
- During helix separation, the region of the DNA ahead of the replication fork develops positive supercoiling. A group of enzyme known as topoisomerase is responsible for removing the supercoil.

Number of enzymes and protein factors are needed for DNA replication in prokaryotes. They are enlisted in Table 34.1.

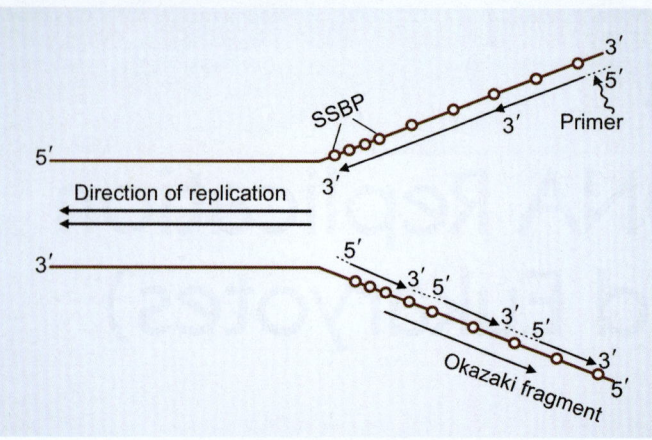

Fig. 34.2: DNA replication

TABLE 34.1	Enzymes and protein factors needed for DNA replication in prokaryotes
Enzymes/proteins	*Possible role*
DNA A protein	Open duplex DNA
DNA B protein	Helicase (unwind)
DNA C protein	Binding of DNA B protein at the origin
DNA G protein	Primase
Single strand binding protein (SSBP)	Binding of single strand
HU (histone-like)	Stimulates initiation
DNA topoisomerase I	Relieves torsional strain
DNA topoisomerase II (DNA gyrase)	Introduces negative supercoiling

Enzymes/proteins involved in prokaryotic DNA replication.

The whole process of DNA replication may be divided into three phases:
• Initiation
• Elongation
• Termination

Initiation

• DNA A protein recognizes the ORI site and leads to denaturation of DNA.
• Binding of DNA B protein occurs which leads to helicase activity and unwinding of DNA (replication fork is produced).
• SSBP stabilizes the separated strand and prevents their premature reannealing.
• Supercoiling produced by helicase activity is relieved by topoisomerase.
• Primase bindining occurs.
• 10-nucleotide long RNA primer is synthesized against parent strand by primase enzyme. Primase enzyme acts without proofreading.

Elongation

It is important to understand these few terms:
• **Chain elongation:** Rate at which polymerization occurs (number of nucleotides added per second).
• **Processivity:** Number of nucleotides added to the nascent chain before the polymerase disengages from the template.
• **Proofreading:** Identifies copying errors and corrects them.

Of all the DNA polymerases, DNA polymerase III catalyzes the highest rate of chain elongation and is the most processive.

Main enzyme of this phase of DNA replication is DNA polymerase. DNA polymerase is of following types:
• DNA polymerase I
• DNA polymerase II
• DNA polymerase III

Kornberg discovered DNA polymerase I and named it as Kornberg enzyme.

DNA polymerase I have following activity:
• 5'–3' polymerase activity
• 3'–5' exonuclease activity
• 5'–3' exonuclease activity

DNA polymerase II and III have following activity:
• 5'–3' polymerase activity
• 3'–5' exonuclease activity

5'–3' exonuclease activity is not seen in DNA polymerase II and III.
• During elongation parent strand of DNA is read in 3'–5' direction and correspondingly deoxynucleotides are added in 5'–3' direction by DNA polymerase III with simultaneous proofreading of newly synthesized DNA.
• For adding up the nucleotide in 5'–3' direction, 5'–3' polymerase activity of DNA polymerase III is used, and for proofreading 3'–5' exonuclease activity of DNA polymerase III is being used.
• Proofreading is the process by which wrong nucleotides are removed then and there as soon as they are added. This double checks the added nucleotide and minimizes the chances of mutation.
• During this process one strand is synthesized continuously and form leading strand and the other strand is synthesized discontinuously and known as Okazaki fragments.
• Okazaki fragments are 1000–2000 nucleotides long in prokaryotes.

Primer removal and gap filling: For removal of primer 5'–3' exonuclease activity of DNA polymerase I is utilized.

After removal of the RNA primer, the gap is filled with the help of 5'–3' polymerase activity of the DNA polymerase I. For this gap filling the receding Okazaki fragment acts as a primer.

Nick sealing: It is done by DNA ligase enzyme which seals the nick between the fragment synthesized by DNA polymerase I and DNA polymerase III. This enzyme uses energy from NADH in prokaryotes.

TERMINATION

'ter' sequence is bound by 'ter binding protein', which prevents further unwinding by helicase (DNA B) activity.

Topoisomerase

Two varieties of topoisomerases are known in prokaryotes:
- Type I DNA topoisomerase
- Type II DNA topoisomerase

DNA REPLICATION IN EUKARYOTES

DNA replication in eukaryotes is much more complex compared to prokaryotes. Salient differences in DNA replication in these species are enumerated in Table 34.2.

It is characterized by multiple origin of replication. At each point of replication, the DNA replication I bidirectional.

Autonomous replication sequence (ARS) is the AT rich sequence identified in yeast, is the site of origin of replication complex (ORC).

Steps of Eukaryotic DNA Replication

- DNA helicase
- Replication protein A
- DNA polymerase α
- Protein replication factor C (PRFC)
- Proliferating cell nuclear antigen (PCNA)
- Binding of DNA polymerase S (polymerase switching)

Eukaryotic DNA replication encounters a special problem of end shortening which is tackled by telomere addition.

TELOMERASE AND TELOMERE

- Telomerase is a ribonucleoprotein complex with a short strand of RNA and various proteins which are having reverse transcriptase activity, as an integral part of it (Fig. 34.3).

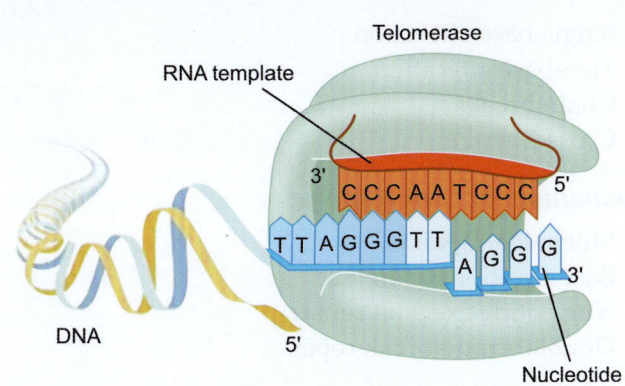

Fig. 34.3: Telomerase

- Telomerase is expressed in stem cell and most cancer cell but not in somatic cell.
- Telomerase uses RNA as a template and add GT rich hexa nucleotide 5'-TTAGGG-3' telomere repeat at the 3'-end of the DNA chain.
- Telomere finally terminates into a single stranded overhang that is roughly 150 nucleotides long.

Function of Telomere

- Provides arrangement by which progressive shortening of DNA while replication is avoided. During DNA replication 5'-end of new strand of DNA shorten by 100 bp with each replication. This telomere provides innocuous source of DNA whose decreasing length during each replication does not effect the functioning of the cell.
- Exposed ends of linear polynucleotide would participate in deleterious genetic recombination events.

Length of the Telomere

Telomere in the yeast is few hundred nucleotide long and in human it is several thousand nucleotide long.
- Telomere is critical for maintaining the stability of the genome. Progressive shortening of the telomere is avoided by persistent telomerase activity in tumor cell which is responsible for their immortality.
- Telomerase is not active in normal somatic cell.

During the S phase, the nuclear DNA is replicated completely once and only once.

Once, chromatin, has been replicated, it is marked (through DNA methylation), so as to prevent replication till it passes again through mitosis (parent strand is methylated).

DNA Repair

Damage to DNA by environmental, physical and chemical agents is of four types:

Section 9 ■ Nucleic Acids: Chemistry, Metabolism and Applied Aspects

34

a. Single base alteration
b. Two-base alteration
c. Chain breaks
d. Cross-linkage

Mechanism of DNA Repair

1. Mismatch repair
2. Base-excision repair
3. Nucleotide excision repair
4. Double strand break repair

Mismatch Repair

Mismatch repair corrects errors made when DNA is copied.

Specific proteins scan the newly synthesized DNA, using adenine methylation within a GATC sequence as the point of reference. The parent strand is methylated (N6 methyl adenine) and the newly synthesized strand is not. This difference allows the repair enzymes to identify the strand that contains the wrong nucleotide which requires replacement. If a mismatch or small loop is found, a GATC endonuclease cuts the strand bearing the mutation at a site corresponding to the GATC.

Now the gap is filled by DNA polymerase III activity followed by action of DNA ligase enzyme which seals the nick (Fig. 34.4).

HNPCC (hereditary nonpolyposis colon cancer) is due to defect in the mismatch repair system.

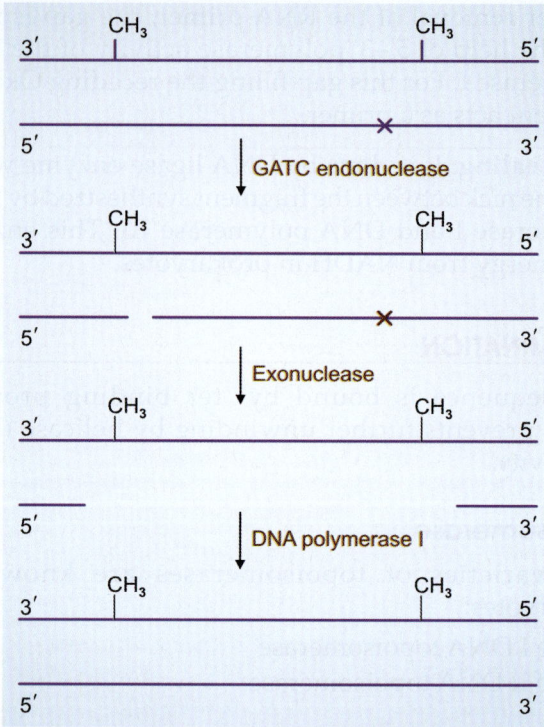

Fig. 34.4: Mismatch repair

Base Excision Repair

Base lost or altered rectified by base excision repair. Here defective base is excised first followed by occurrence of AP site (apurinic/apyrimidinic site).

TABLE 34.2	Similarities and differences in the mechanism of DNA replication of prokaryotes and eukaryotes	
Prokaryotes	**Eukaryotes**	
DNA is double stranded and circular molecule.	DNA is double stranded and linear molecule open at both its ends.	
Origin of replication at 'ORI' single origin of replication.	Origin of replication at AT rich 'ARS' sequence in yeast multiple origin of replication	
Replication proceeds bidirectionally.	Here too, replication proceeds bidirectionally	
RNA primer is needed which is approximately 50-nucleotide long	RNA primer is needed which is much small (approximately 9-nucleotides long)	
Number of nucleotides in Okazaki fragment is 1000–2000.	Number of nucleotides in Okazaki fragment is approximately 200.	
Rate of replication is faster (500 nucleotides added per second)	Rate of replication is slower (50 nucleotides added per second)	
Types of DNA polymerase: I, II, III	DNA polymerase in eukaryotes: α, β, γ, δ, ε	
	α: primase activity	β: gap filling
	δ: lagging	ε: leading
	γ: mitochondrial DNA	
DNA ligase is required and source of energy is NADH.	DNA ligase is required and source of energy is ATP.	
Drugs inhibiting prokaryotic DNA replication are ciprofloxacin, novobiocin.	Drugs inhibiting eukaryotic DNA replication are etoposide, adriamycin, camptothrecin	
	RNA primer removal by RNAase H and FEN-1.	

Following enzymes are needed for base excision repair:

- DNA-glycosylase
- Apurinic or apyrimidinic endonuclease (AP endo nuclease)

Deoxyribose phosphodiesterase

- DNA polymerase I to fill the gap
- DNA ligase

Then AP endonuclease recognizes the base missing and initiates the process of excision and gap filling.

Gap thus created is filled by DNA polymerase I (Fig. 34.5).

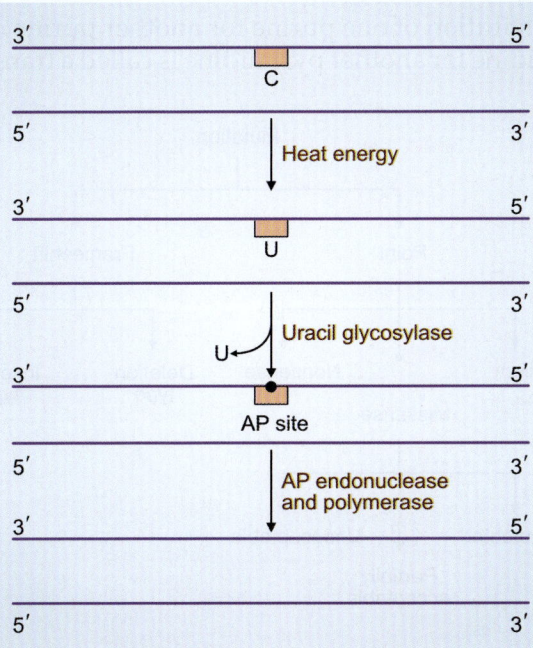

Fig. 34.5: Base excision repair

Nucleotide Excision Repair

UV light, which induces the formation of pyrimidine-pyrimidine dimers, and smoking, which causes formation of benzo (a) pyrene-guanine adducts are repaired by nucleotide excision repair.

Following enzymes are needed for NER:

- UV ray A,B,C excinuclease
- DNA polymerase I
- DNA ligase

In eukaryotic cells the enzyme (UV specific endonuclease also known as UVRABC excinuclease) cut between the third to fifth phosphodiester bond 3' from the lesion, and on the 5' side the cut is somewhere between the twenty-first and twenty-fifth bonds. Thus, a fragment of DNA 27–29 nucleotides long is excised (Fig. 34.6).

After the strand is removed, it is replaced, again by exact base pairing, through the activity of DNA polymerase I, and the ends are joined to the existing strands by DNA ligase.

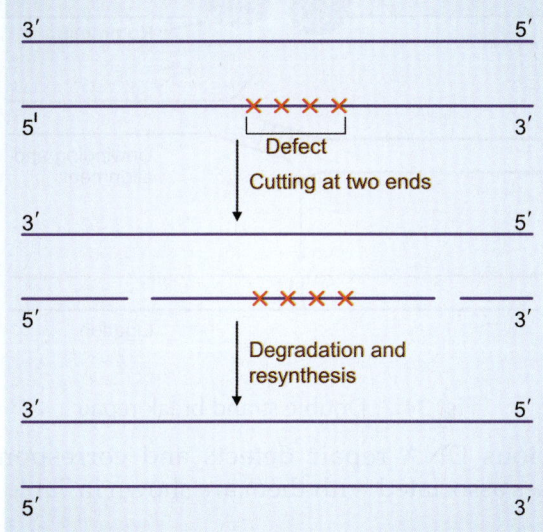

Fig. 34.6: Nucleotide excision repair

Xeroderma pigmentosum (XP): It is an autosomal recessive inherited disorder. It is due to defect in repair of damaged DNA, especially thymine dimers. Culture of cells from patients shows low activity of the nucleotide excision-repair processes. The most common form of this disease is due to absence of UV specific excinuclease.

Direct repair: Here pyrimidine dimer is cleaved by photochemical cleavage.

Following enzymes are needed for such kind of repair process:

- DNA photolyase
- N5N10 methyl THF
- FAD as a cofactor

Double Strand Break Repair

Double strand break repair is a part of the physiologic process of immunoglobulin gene rearrangement. It is also an important mechanism for repairing damaged DNA, which results due to ionizing radiation or oxidative free radical generation. Some chemotherapeutic agents destroy cells by causing double strand break or by preventing their repair.

Double strand breaks are repaired by one of the two systems:

1. Nonhomologous end joining repair
2. Homologous recombination repair

Nonhomologous end joining repair is the main system of DNA repair. The two proteins involved in the nonhomologous rejoining are Ku and DNA-dependent protein kinase (DNA-PK) (Fig. 34.7).

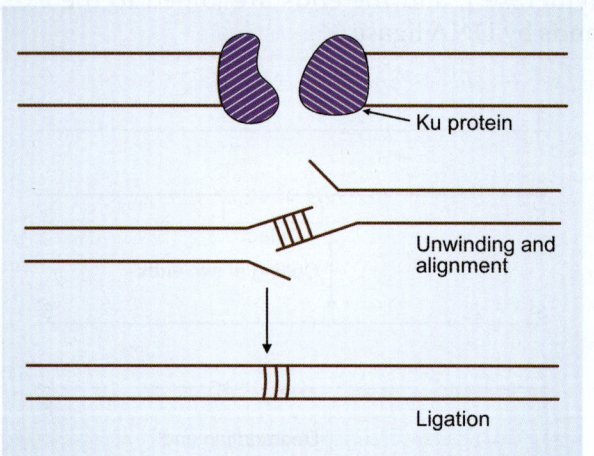

Fig. 34.7: Double strand break repair

Various DNA repair defects and corresponding diseases associated with them are shown in Table 34.3.

TABLE 34.3	Defect in DNA repair mechanism and disease associated with it
Defect in	*Diseases associated with it*
NER	Xeroderma pigmentosa (XP), trichothio-dystrophy (TTD), cockayne syndrome (Cs)
BER	MUTYH-associated polyposis (MAP]
Mismatch repair	Hereditary nonpolyposis colorectal cancer (HNPCC)
NHEJ repair	Severe combined immunodeficiency disease (SCID)/radiation sensitive SCID [IRS-SCID]
Homologous repair	Bloom syndrome (BS), breast cancer susceptibility 1 and 2 (BRCA-1, BRCA-2) Nismegen breakage syndrome (NBS) Werner syndrome (WS)

MUTATION

A mutation can be defined as a heritable change in DNA due to an alteration in the base sequence (Fig. 34.8).

Mutations occur at a rate of one in every 10^6 cell divisions. Factors increasing the rate of mutation are:
a. Viruses
b. Chemicals
c. UV light
d. Ionising radiations

1. Point Mutation

Alterations in any one single nucleotide base on the mRNA.

Substitution of one purine for another purine or one pyrimidine for another pyrimidine is called a transition.

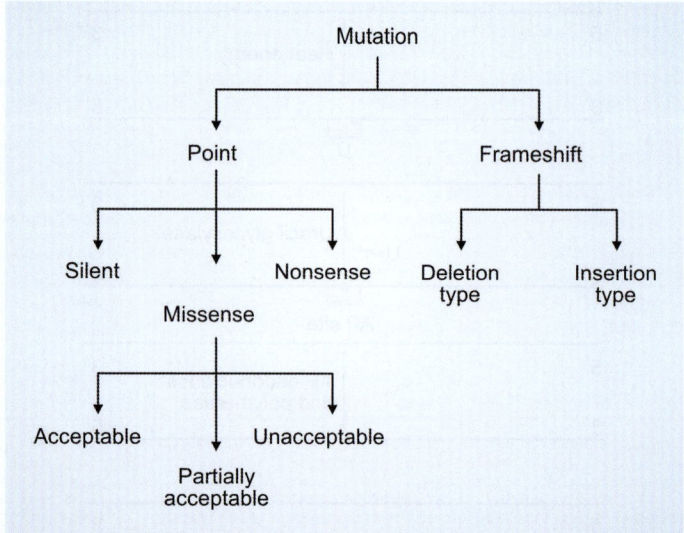

Fig. 34.8: Examples of various mutations

When conversion of a purine to a pyrimidine or vice versa occurs, the mutation is called a transversion.

TABLE 34.4	Point Mutations		Example	Change
Silent	Here change of codon results in another codon for same amino acid			
Missense		Acceptable	Hb A → Hb Hikari	β-chain 61 Lysine → Asparagine
		Partially acceptable	Hb A → HbS	β-chain 6 Glutamate → Valive
		Unacceptable	Hb A → HbM	α-chain 58 Histidine → Tyrosin
Nonsense	Here coding is changed to a stop codon after mutation		Boston hemoglobin	

Effect of point mutation may be (Table 34.4):

- **Silent mutation:** No change results, as the codon containing the changed base, still code for the same amino acids due to degeneracy of the codon.
- **Missense mutation:** The codon containing the changed base, code for another amino acid. New amino acid may be acceptable/partally acceptable or unacceptable.
- **Nonsense mutation:** The codon containing the changed base may become a termination codon, thus stopping the translation process prematurely.

2. Frameshift Mutation

Addition or deletion of one or more bases in the sequence may occur. If this does not happen in the multiple of three bases, it results in frameshift mutation, and the message read distal to mutation is garbled.

Other Mutations

a. *Suppressor mutation:* Some abnormal tRNA molecules (themselves the results of mutations), are capable of suppressing the effects of mutations in distant structural genes. These suppressor tRNA molecules, usually formed as the result of alterations in their anticodon regions, are capable of suppressing certain missense mutations, nonsense mutations, and frameshift mutations.

However, since the suppressor tRNA molecules are not capable of distinguishing between a normal codon and one resulting from a gene mutation, their presence in a cell usually results in decreased viability.

b. *Trinucleotide repeat expansion:* Sometimes sequence 3 bases which are repeated in tandem will be amplified in number, so that too many copies of the triplet occur. Such phenomenon is seen in:
  1. Huntington's disease
  2. Fragile X syndrome
  3. Myotonic dystrophy

Section 9 ■ Nucleic Acids: Chemistry, Metabolism and Applied Aspects

34

Nucleic Acid III: Transcription and Post-Transcriptional Modifications

At the end of this chapter learner should be able to describe the processes involved in replication and repair of DNA and the transcription and translation mechanisms.

Specific Learning Objectives	
BI 7.2.1	Describe the process of transcription of the gene.
BI 7.2.2	Discuss different types of RNA polymerase enzymes in eukaryotes.
BI 7.2.3	Discuss post-transcriptional modification of various RNA precursors.

TRANSCRIPTION (RNA SYNTHESIS)

Transcription is the process of synthesis of RNA from the DNA. It results in transfer of genetic information from DNA to RNA, which directs the synthesis of protein in the cell.

Transcription unit is defined as that region of DNA that extends between the promoter and the terminator.

The process of transcription is described under following headings:

- Factors required for transcription
- Initiation phase of transcription
- Elongation phase of transcription
- Termination phase of transcription
- Post-transcriptional modification

Transcription in prokaryotes and eukaryotes differs considerably in factors required, phases of transcription as well as post-transcriptional modifications.

The important differences in prokaryotic and eukaryotic trancriptions are enumerated in tabular column (Table 35.1).

PROKARYOTIC TRANSCRIPTION

- Process of transcription involves initiation, elongation and termination.
- Only a very small portion of genome is transcribed at a time.
- Unlike DNA replication, primer is not involved in transcription.
- No proofreading occurs during transcription in prokaryotes.

Enzyme involved in the Process of Transcription

In bacteria, single type of RNA polymerase is required for the synthesis of all types of RNA.

RNA polymerase of bacteria is made up of 5 subunits: Two α, one β, one β' and one sigma subunit.

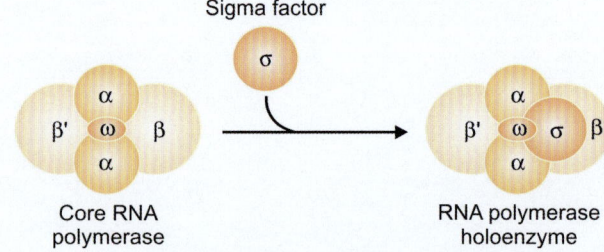

Fig. 35.1: RNA polymerase of prokaryotes

Four of the enzyme subunits (two α, one β, one β') constitute core enzyme. These components are having following activity subunit important for recognition of promoter element on the DNA for binding of RNA polymerase enzyme (Fig. 35.1).

Initiation Phase of Transcription

Promoter region: These are conserved consensus sequence where RNA polymerase binds the strand of the DNA.

In prokaryotic cell these are:

a. *Pribnow box:*
   - Located 8–10 nucleotides upstream
   - Sequence is 5'-TATAAT-3'.
b. *–35 sequence:*
   - Centered around 35 bases upstream from the initiation site
   - Sequence is 5'-TTGACA-3'.

Elongation Phase of Transcription

Once bound RNA polymerase covers large area (even the portion of gene is covered) (Fig. 35.2).

Termination Phase of Transcription

Termination in the prokaryotic transcription may be **rho factor dependent** or **rho factor independent**.

Rho-dependent: Termination of synthesis of RNA molecule is signaled by a sequence in the template strand of the DNA molecule, a signal that is recognized by a termination protein the rho factor. Rho factor is an ATP dependent RNA-DNA helicase that disrupts the nascent RNA/DNA complex. RNA polymerase then gets separates from DNA template (Fig. 35.3).

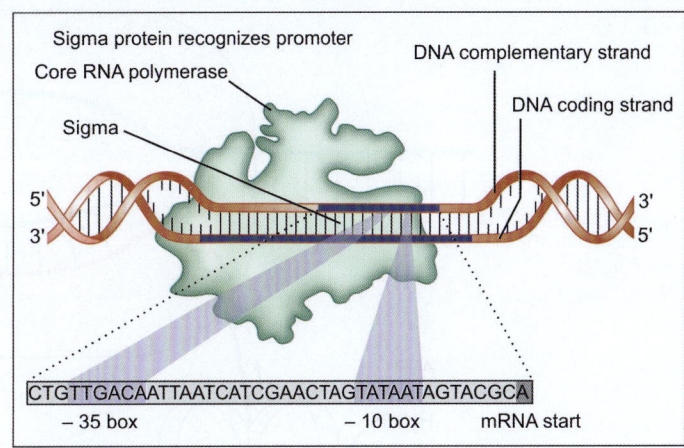

Fig. 35.2: Promoter of DNA and RNA polymerase covering large area of DNA

Rho-independent: In some cases bacterial RNA polymerase can directly recognize DNA-encoded termination signals without assistance by the rho factor. But for this kind of termination process, newly synthesized RNA should have two important structural features:

GC-rich region at the termination end of the RNA, which is capable of forming hairpin turn.

TABLE 35.1	Differences in prokaryotic and eukaryotic transcription
In prokaryotes	*In eukaryotes*
• Factors required for transcription:	• Factors required for transcription:
▪ Template strand of DNA	▪ Template strand of DNA
▪ Nucleotides: ATP, GTP, UTP, CTP	▪ Nucleotides: ATP, GTP, UTP, CTP
▪ RNA polymerase (only one subtype)	▪ RNA polymerase (three types):
	◆ RNA polymerase I
	◆ RNA polymerase II
	◆ RNA polymerase III
• Initiation phase of transcription. Promoter site	• Initiation phase of transcription. Promoter site:
▪ –10 region (pribnow box/TATAAT)	▪ –25 region (Hogness box/TATA box)
▪ –35 region: TTGACA	▪ –75 region: CAAT box (GGCAATCT)
▪ Not many initiation factors needed	• GC box
▪ Only sigma subunit needed	• Multiple initiation factors needed
• Elongation phase of transcription	
• Phosphodiester bond is formed and RNA synthesis occurs in 5'–3' direction	• Phosphodiester bond is formed and RNA synthesis occurs in 5'–3' direction
• No proofreading occurs while elongation	• No proofreading occurs while elongation
• Termination phase of transcription It may be rho-dependent or rho-independent	• Termination phase of transcription not well defined but believed to be similar to mechanism of rho-independent termination in prokaryotes.

Section 9 ■ Nucleic Acids: Chemistry, Metabolism and Applied Aspects

35

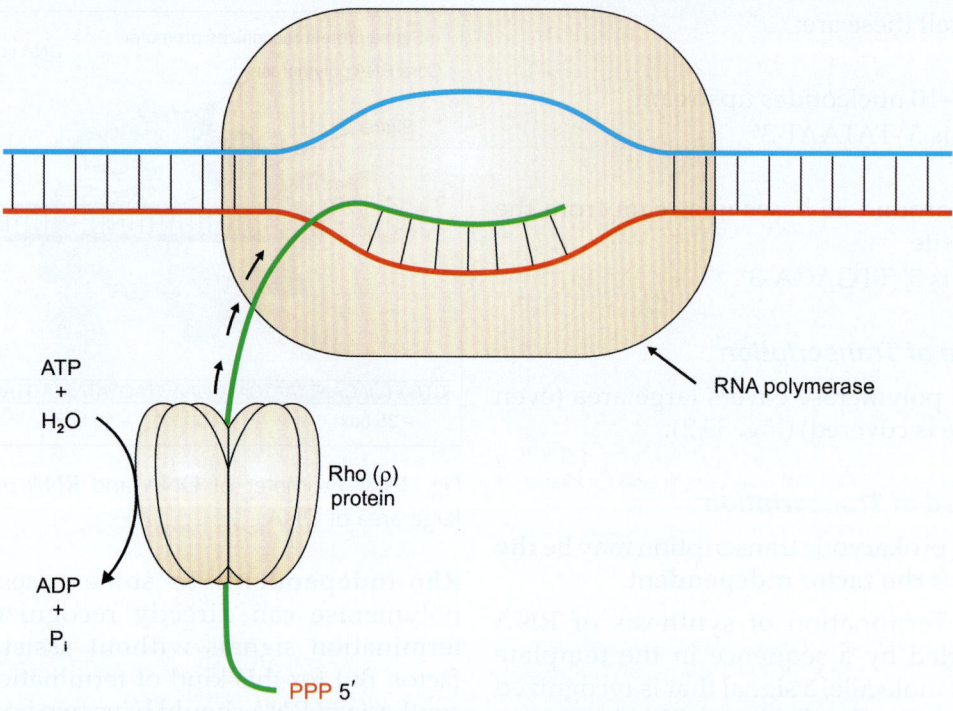

Fig. 35.3: Rho-dependent termination of prokaryotic transcription

A chain of U-nucleotide should be their beyond hairpin structure.

The binding between U and A is weak which facilitates separation of newly synthesized RNA from its DNA template (Fig. 35.4).

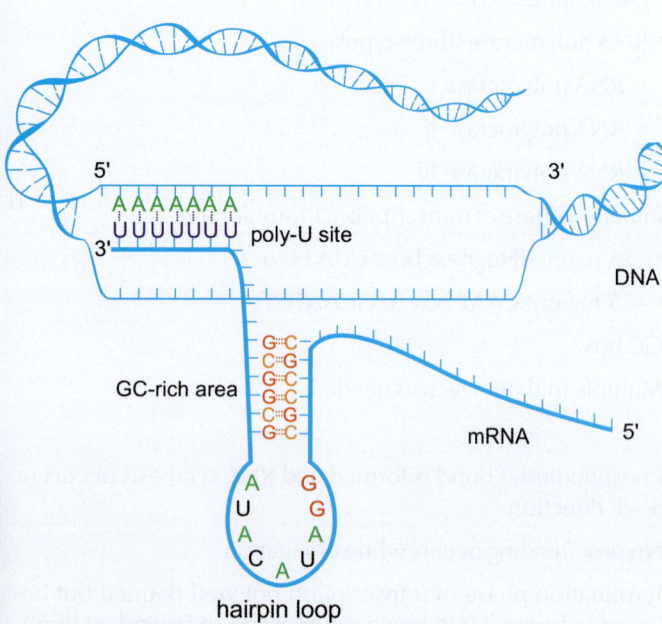

Fig. 35.4: Rho-independent termination of transcription

EUKARYOTIC TRANSCRIPTION

Eukaryotic transcription is more complex than prokaryotic transcription.

In addition to RNA polymerase enzyme, various transcription factors are also required for eukaryotic transcription process.

There are three distinct classes of the RNA polymerase enzyme in eukaryotic cell:

1. RNA polymerase I
2. RNA polymerase II
3. RNA polymerase III

Various types of RNAs produced by these respective RNA polymerases and their sensitivity to α-amanitin is shown in Table 35.2.

Process of transcription involves three phases:

1. Initiation
2. Elongation
3. Termination

Initiation

RNA polymerase scans the DNA sequence at a rate of 10^3 bp/s, until it recognizes certain specific regions of DNA to which it binds with higher affinity. This region is called promoter region and association of RNA polymerase with promoter region ensures accurate initiation of transcription.

TABLE 35.2	Mammalian RNA polymerases and their products		
Form of RNA polymerase	Sensitivity to α-amanitin	Major products	Site
I	Insensitive	rRNA (28S, 18S, 5.8S)	nucleolus
II	High sensitivity	mRNA, miRNA, snRNA	nucleus
III	Intermediate	tRNA, 5S rRNA, some snRNA	nucleus

Eukaryotic Promoters

a. **TATA box:** Most mammalian genes have a TATA box located 15–30 bp upstream from transcript start site (5′-TATAAA-3′), this is also known as Hogness box.

   TATA box binds the 30 KD TATA binding protein (TBP), within turn binds several other proteins called TBP-associated factors (TAFs).

   TBP and TAFs together are known as TFIID.

   Binding of TFIID to TATA box represents the first step in the formation of transcription complex on the promoter.

b. Sequences further upstream from the start site determine how frequently the transcription event will occur. Typical of these DNA elements are the GC box and CAAT box (Fig. 35.5).

Enhancer and repressor may either increase or decrease the rate of transcription initiation of eukaryotic genes. These elements may be found in variety of locations both upstream and downstream from transcript start site. These can exert their effect when located hundred or even thousand of bases away from transcription units located on the same chromosome.

Cis acting element: Promoter and enhancer elements are known as cis-acting element, as they are located on the same DNA molecule as their gene.

Trans-acting element: Various transcription factors are known as trans-acting elements, as they are synthesized from different chromosomes in the cytosol and get diffused within the nucleus to bind with various DNA. (Here one more thing should be clear to the student

that the promoter element is the cis-acting element and necessarily it should be present on the same strand of the DNA which has gene and that too only in upstream direction, while enhancer which is also the cis-acting element; location of it may be on either strand of the chromosome upstream or downstream direction.)

Elongation

Certain elongation factors help in elongation process, for which 5′–3′ polymerase activity of RNA polymerase enzyme is used.

   Three types of RNA polymerase enzymes are needed for synthesis of various types of RNA.

Termination

- Signals for the termination of transcription by eukaryotic RNA polymerase II are only poorly understood.
- It appears that the termination signals exist far downstream of the coding sequence of eukaryotic genes. For example, the transcription termination signal for mouse-globin occurs at several positions 1000–2000 bases beyond the site at which the poly(A) tail will eventually be added. Less is known about the termination process or whether specific termination factors similar to the bacterial factor are involved (Fig. 35.6).
- Phosphorylation of CTD (carboxy terminal domain) tail of the large subunit of the RNA polymerase II occurs in initiation and elongation phase.

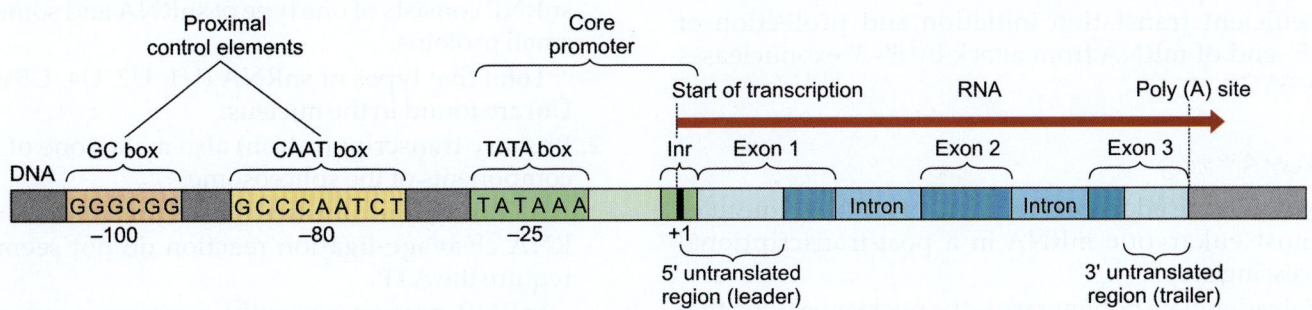

Fig. 35.5: Various promoters on DNA of eukaryotes

Section 9 ■ Nucleic Acids: Chemistry, Metabolism and Applied Aspects

35

The CTD of RNA Pol II

❑ The largest subunit of RNA polymerase II had a seven amino acid repeat at the C terminus called the carboxy-terminal domain (CTD).

❑ This sequence, Tyr-Ser-Pro-Thr-Ser-Pro-Ser, is repeated 52 times in the mouse RNA polymerase II

Fig. 35.6: Carboxy terminal domain of RNA polymerase II

Detailed Description

Nearly all RNA primary transcripts (mRNA, rRNA and tRNA precursors) undergo extensive processing between the time they are synthesized and the time at which they serve their ultimate functions.

mRNA is synthesized as large precursor hnRNA which undergoes following changes to ultimately convert itself to mRNA.

Post-transcriptional Modification of Primary Transcript to mRNA

Primary transcript of the mRNA consists of alternate exons and introns. Exons are amino acid coding portion and introns are intervening sequences which do not code for any amino acid.

There occur three processes during post-transcriptional modification of hnRNA:

a. 5′ capping
b. Poly A tailing
c. Splicing

a. 5′ capping

This is the first processing reaction for hnRNA. hnRNA is modified at the 5′-end by 7-methylguanosine cap structure. Guanosine triphosphate is attached at the 5′-end of the hnRNA by an unusual 5′–5′ triphosphate linkage with the help of a nuclear enzyme guanylyltransferase.

The 5′ cap of the RNA transcript is required both for efficient translation initiation and protection of the 5′-end of mRNA from attack by 5′–3′ exonucleases (Fig. 35.7).

b. Poly A Tailing

Poly A tails are added to the 3′-end of mRNA molecules in most eukaryotic mRNA in a post-transcriptional processing step.

Polyadenylate polymerase is the nuclear enzyme that adds a poly A tail using ATP as a substrate. Poly A tail

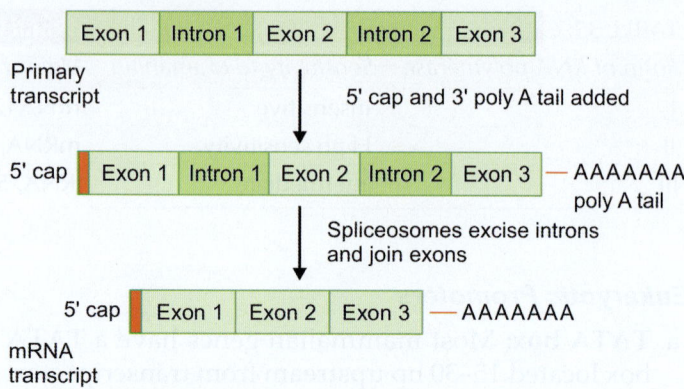

Fig. 35.7: Splicing of primary transcript

is subsequently extended to 80–250 A residues. This tail appears to protect the 3′-end of mRNA from 3′–5′ exonuclease attack and also facilitates its exit from the nucleus.

Role of poly A tailing in initiation of protein synthesis: Experiments in yeast have revealed that the 3′ poly A tail and its binding protein, PAB1, are required for efficient initiation of protein synthesis. Further studies showed that the poly A tail stimulates recruitment of the 40S ribosomal subunit to the 5′-end of mRNA through a complex set of interactions. This helps explain how the cap and poly A tail structures have a synergistic effect on protein synthesis.

Some mRNAs do not have poly A tailing. For example histone mRNA and mRNA of some interferon do not possess poly A tail.

c. Splicing

It is the process by which introns are removed and exons are joined together. For this process to occur a special multicomponent complex known as spliceosome, is required.

Spliceosome: Fig. 35.8 shows make-up of spliceosome.

1. Specialized RNA-protein complex termed as small nuclear ribonucleoproteins (snRNP) proteins. Each snRNP consists of one type of snRNA and some 50 small proteins.

   Total five types of snRNA (U1, U2, U4, U5 and U6) are found in the nucleus.

2. Primary transcript (intron) also makes one of the components of the spliceosome.

   ATP is required for assembly of the spliceosome. RNA cleavage-ligation reaction do not seem to require the ATP.

   snRNP protein correctly positions exon and intron segments for necessary splicing reaction.

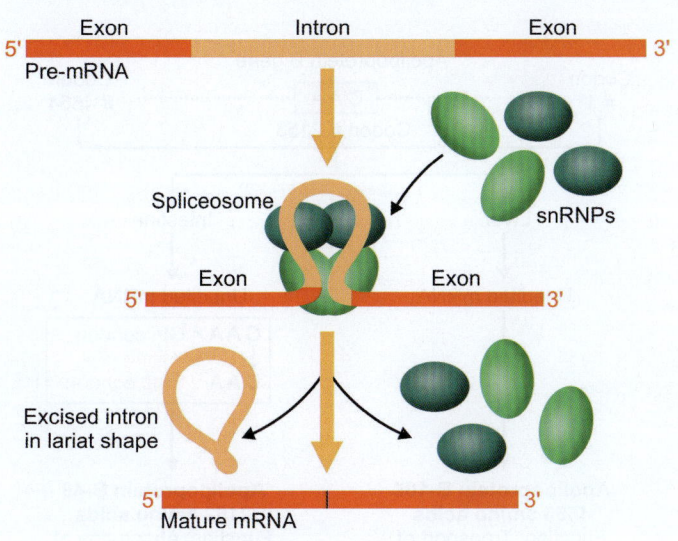

Fig. 35.8: Spliceosome

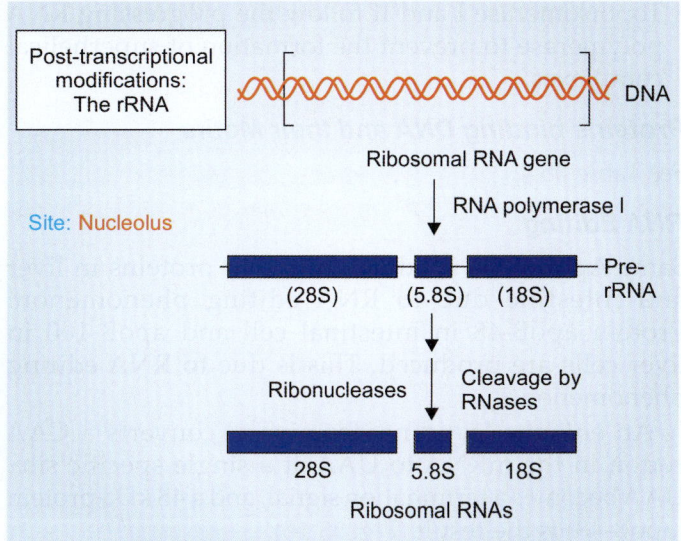

Fig. 35.9: Post-transcriptional modification of rRNA

Introns are removed in the form of lariat/loop structure which is formed between 5' PO$_4$ group and 2' OH group of some internal nucleotide. The 5' and 3' exons are ligated to form a continuous sequence. (Few eukaryotic mRNA primary transcript do not contain intron regions, e.g. primary transcript of histone protein).

Alternate splicing: Alternative patterns of mRNA splicing result from tissue-specific adaptive and developmental control mechanisms. In this kind of splicing reaction, there occurs ligation of adjacent exons in one cell and ligation of exons situated far away in other cell resulting in varied expression of same gene in two different cells.

Faulty splicing: Thalassemia, a disease in which β-globin gene of hemoglobin is underexpressed due to a nucleotide change at an exon-intron junction, precluding removal of the intron and therefore leading to diminished or absent synthesis of the β-chain protein.

Post-transcriptional Modification of rRNA

Preribosomal RNA of both prokaryotes as well as of eukaryotes undergo processing.

In eukaryotes all of the ribosomal RNA molecules (except the 5S rRNA, which is independently transcribed by RNA polymerase III) are processed from a single 45S precursor RNA molecule (transcribed by RNA polymerase I) in the nucleolus.

The preribosomal RNA are cleaved by ribonucleases to yield intermediate sized pieces of rRNA, which is further trimmed to produce required RNA species (Fig. 35.9).

Post-transcriptional Modification of tRNA

tRNAs are often synthesized as precursor tRNA, with extra sequences at both 5'- and 3'-ends. A small fraction of tRNAs contains introns in the anticodon loop.

Following post-transcriptional processes occur in the primary transcript of the tRNA:

1. Ribonuclease P is an example of endonuclease which removes approximately 16 nucleotides of the RNA at the 5'-end of the tRNA.
2. The 3'-end of the tRNA is processed by one or more nucleases, including the exonuclease RNase D.
3. Addition of CCA terminal at the 3'-end of the tRNA, is cytoplasmic post-transcriptional phenomenon.
4. Removal of intron segment from the anticodon loop.
5. *Modification of bases:* Pseudouridine, dihydrouridine, methyl guanosine, ribothymidine are all modified bases.

Table 35.3 summarises major differences in prokaryotic and eukaryotic post-transcriptional modiciations of various RNAs.

Important Points to Remember

- In both prokaryotes and eukaryotes, a purine ribonucleotide is usually the first nucleotide to be polymerized in the RNA molecule.
- 5' triphosphate of this first nucleotide is maintained in prokaryotes but removed in the process of cap formation in eukaryotic mRNA.
- RNA polymerase has an 'unwindase' activity which opens DNA double helix.

Section 9 ■ Nucleic Acids: Chemistry, Metabolism and Applied Aspects

35

- Topoisomerase I and II follow the progressing RNA polymerase to prevent the formation of superhelical complexes.

Proteins binding DNA and their Motifs

See Table 35.4.

RNA Editing

Same ApoB gene produces different proteins in liver and intestine due to RNA editing phenomenon. Protein apoB-48 in intestinal cell and apoB-100 in liver cells are produced. This is due to RNA editing phenomenon.

An enzyme 'cytidine deaminase' converts a CAA codon in the mRNA to UAA at a single specific site. UAA becomes a termination signal, and a 48 kDa protein (apoB-48) is the result (Fig. 35.10).

GENETIC CODE

The four nucleotides found in the DNA are organized into three-letter code word called codons, and the collection of these codons makes up the genetic code.

Out of total 64 codons, 3 codons do not code for any amino acids and are termed nonsense codons (termination codons, stop codons)—UAA, UAG and UGA.

Remaining 61 codons code for 20 amino acids . Thus, multiple codons decode the same amino acide, e.g. six different codons specify serine. This is termed as *degeneracy of genetic code*. Methionine and tryptophan have only one codon (Fig. 35.11).

However, for a specific codon, only a single amino acid is indicated, this is termed as *unambiguous* nature of the genetic code.

The reading of genetic code during the process

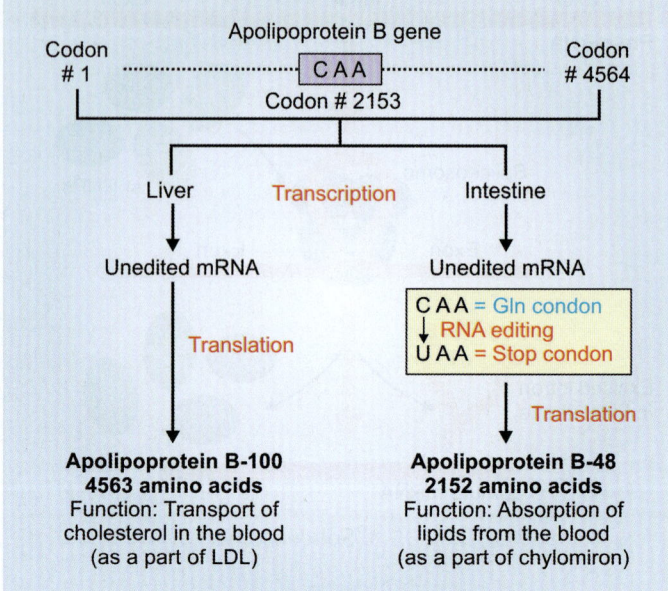

Fig. 35.10: RNA editing (formation of ApoB-100 and ApoB-48 from same gene by RNA editing phenomenon)

of protein synthesis does not involve any overlap of codons. Thus, the genetic code is *nonoverlapping*.

There is *no punctuation* between codons.

The genetic code is *universal* except for the following 4 codons which are read differently by mitochondrial tRNA from the cytoplasmic tRNA (Table 35.5).

WOBBLE HYPOTHESIS

The degeneracy of the genetic code resides mostly in the last nucleotide of the codon triplet, suggesting that the pairing of codon and anticodon can 'wobble' at this

TABLE 35.3	Post-transcriptional modifications of various types of RNA in prokaryotes and eukaryotes	
• Post-transcriptional modifations in prokaryotes	• Post-transcriptional modifations in eukaryotes

• **mRNA:** In prokaryotes, mRNA is not undergoing post-transcriptional modification, it is functional immediately after its synthesis, i.e it is translated simultaneously as it is transcribed.	• Here extensive post-transcriptional modifications takes place in hnRNA as to convert it to mRNA.
	• Following are the steps:
	  ▪ 5' capping
	  ▪ Splicing
	  ▪ 3' tailing

• **rRNA and tRNA:** They are generated after cleavage and other modifications of nascent RNA chain. Prokaryotes have gene for 16S, tRNA, 23S and 5S rRNA, which are consequently present on DNA which is transcribed in a common RNA precursor.	• Even rRNA and tRNA undergo extensive posttranscriptional modifications.
• CAA terminal is added at the 3'-end of all tRNA	
• Modification of rRNA bases by methylation	
• UMP is modified to produce ribothymidylate and pseudouridylate.	

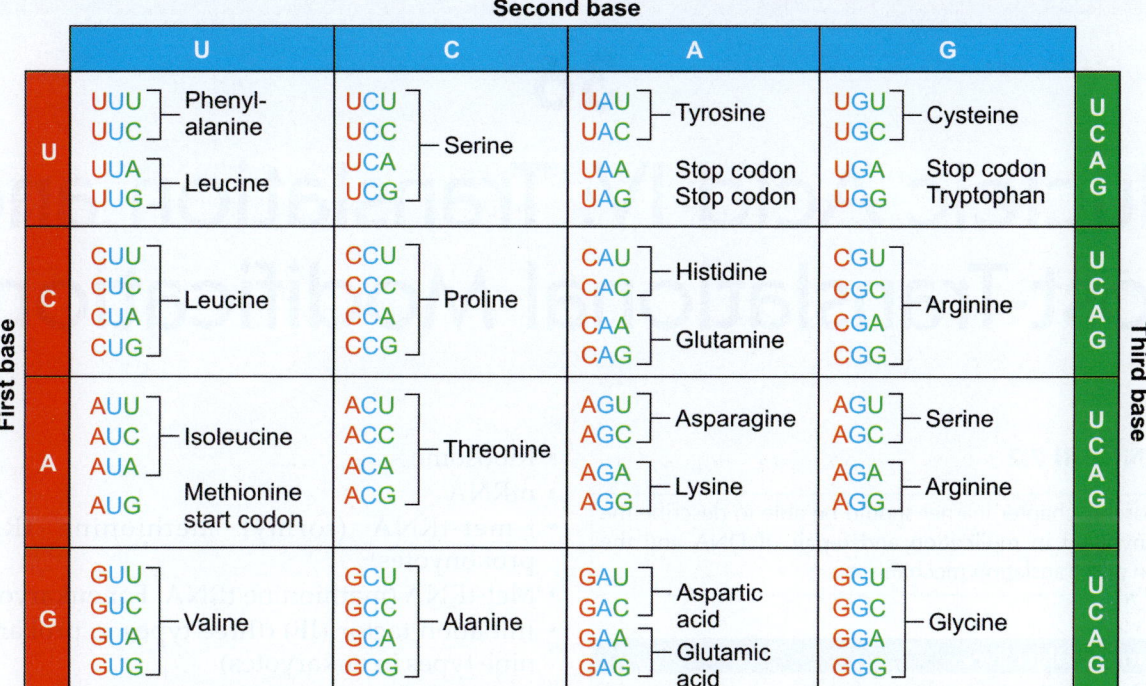

Fig. 35.11: Genetic code

TABLE 35.4	Examples of transcription regulatory proteins that contain the various binding motifs	
Binding motif	*Organism*	*Regulatory protein*
Helix-turn-helix	E. coli	Lac repressor
	Phage	CAP
	Mammals	cl, cro, and tryptophan and 434 repressors homeobox proteins
Zinc finger	E. coli	Gene 32 protein
	Yeast	Gal4
	Drosophila	Serendipity, hunchback
	Xenopus	TFIIIA
	Mammals	Steroid receptor family, Sp1
Leucine zipper	Yeast	GCN4
	Mammals	C/EBP, fos, Jun, Fra-1, CRE binding protein, c-*myc*, n-*myc*, I-*myc*

specific nucleotide pairing site. This is called 'wobble phenomenon' (Fig. 35.12).

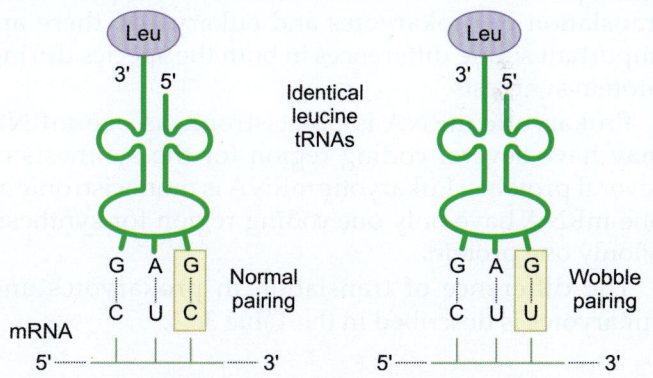

Fig. 35.12: Wooble hypothesis

For example as shown in Table 35.6, if tRNA has guanosine nucleotide at its 5'-end of anticodon loop, this guanine base of guanoside nucleotide 'GMP' can pair with cytosine or uracil bases at 3'-end of codon on mRNA.

TABLE 35.5	Exception to rule of universality	
Codon	*Mitochondrial tRNA*	*Cytoplasmic tRNA*
AUA	Methionine	Isoleucine
UGA	Tryptophan	Stop codon
AGA	Stop codon	Arginine
AGG	Stop codon	Arginine

TABLE 35.6	Example of wobbling
tRNA 5'-anticodon base	*mRNA 3'-codon base*
A	U
C	G
G	C or U
U	A or G
I	A or C or U

Section 9 ■ Nucleic Acids: Chemistry, Metabolism and Applied Aspects

35

Nucleic Acid IV: Translation and Post-Translational Modifications

COMPETENCY BI 7.2

At the end of this chapter learner should be able to describe the processes involved in replication and repair of DNA and the transcription and translation mechanisms.

Specific Learning Objectives	
BI 7.2.1	Describe the process of translation.
BI 7.2.2	Discuss inhibitors of translation.

Synthesis of polypeptide chain from the mRNA is known as translation.

In spite of mechanistic similarity in the process of translation of prokaryotes and eukaryotes, there are important subtle differences in both the species during protein synthesis.

Prokaryotic mRNA is polycistronic as one mRNA may have several coding region for the synthesis of several proteins. Eukaryotic mRNA is monocistronic as one mRNA have only one coding region for synthesis of only one protein.

The difference of translation in prokaryotes and eukaryotes is described in the Table 36.1.

▌ DESCRIPTION OF TRANSLATION

Reader is suggested to read the following description of mechanism of translation keeping in mind the difference for prokaryotics and eukaryotics translation mentioned in Table 36.1.

Translation can be divided into three phases:
1. Initiation
2. Elongation
3. Termination

Initiation

Following materials are needed for initiation phase of translation process:

- Ribosome
- mRNA
- f-met-tRNA (formyl methionine tRNA: For prokonyotes)
- Met-tRNA (methionine tRNA: For eukaryotes)
- Initiation factor (IF) (three types in prokaryotes and nine types in eukaryotes)

TABLE 36.1	Main differences in the process of translation of prokaryotes and eukaryotes	
Features	Prokaryotes	Eukaryotes
Initiating amino acid	Formyl methionine	Methionine
Ribosome	70S	80S
Start codon	AUG preceded by purine rich sequence 6–10 bp upstream (Shine Dalgarno sequence)	AUG preceded by 5'cap (7 methyl guanosine)
Initiation factor	Three types	Nine types
Elongation factor	EFG (translocase)	eEF2
Peptidyltransferase activity	23S rRNA	28S rRNA
Termination signal	RF1, RF2, RF3	Single type: eRF

In this phase, all the components of the translational machinery are assembled. It includes association of two ribosomal subunits, incorporation of mRNA to be translated, aminoacyl-tRNA at the P site, GTP and the initiation factors.

Initiation can be divided into four steps (Fig. 36.1):
1. *Dissociation of the ribosome* into its 40S and 60S subunits (eIF-3 and eIF-1A binds with 40S subunits and prevents its premature re-association).
2. *Formation of 43S preinitiation complex:* Binding of a ternary complex consisting of met-tRNA, GTP,

and eIF-2 to the 40S ribosome to form 43S pre-initiation complex.

3. *Formation of 48S initiation complex :* Binding of mRNA to the 43S preinitiation complex to form a 48S initiation complex. In prokaryotes Shine Dalgarno sequence present on mRNA shows complimentary to 16S rRNA of small subunit of ribosome.

4. *Formation of 80S initiation complex* of the 48S initiation complex with the 60S ribosomal subunit to form the 80S initiation complex. At this point, the met-tRNAi is on the P site of the ribosome, ready for the elongation cycle to commence.

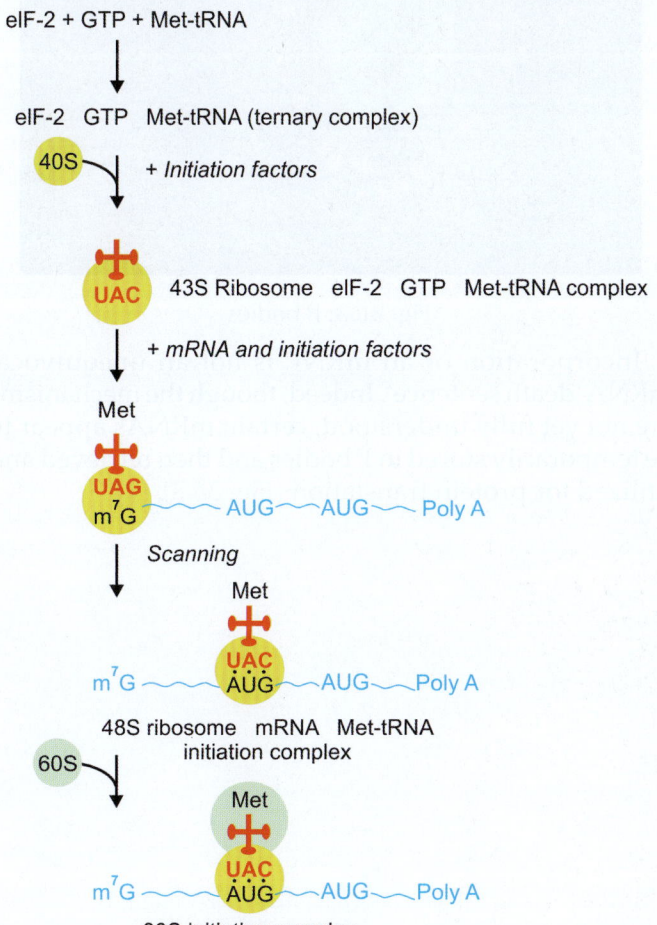

Fig. 36.1: Protein synthesis (formation of 80S initiation complex)

There are two mechanisms by which ribosome recognizes the nucleotide sequence that initiates translation:

The 4F complex is particularly important in controlling the rate of protein translation.

4F is a complex consisting of 4E which binds to the m^{7}G cap structure at the 5'-end of the mRNA, and 4G which serves as a scaffolding protein.

In addition to binding 4E, 4G binds to eIF-3, which links the complex to the 40S ribosomal subunit. It also binds 4A and 4B, the ATPase-helicase complex that helps unwind the RNA.

4E is responsible for recognition of the mRNA cap structure, a rate-limiting step in translation.

Elongation

Elongation is a cyclic process on the ribosome in which one amino acid at a time is added to the nascent peptide chain. Elongation involves several steps. These steps are (Fig. 36.2):

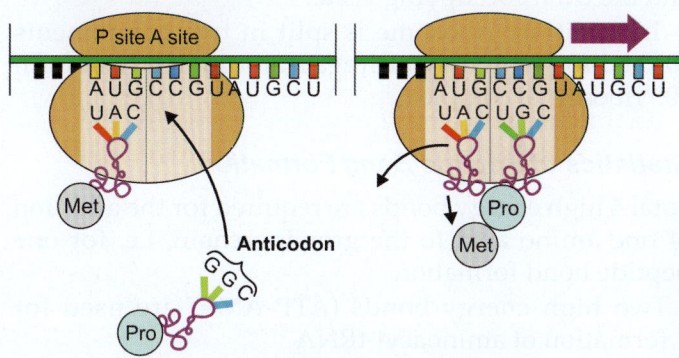

Fig. 36.2: Elongation of polypeptide

1. Binding of aminoacyl-tRNA to the A site.
2. Peptide bond formation (this reaction is catalyzed by a peptidyltransferase, a component of the 28S RNA of the 60S ribosomal subunit in the eukaryotes or 23S RNA of 50S subunit in prokaryotes).
3. Translocation of the ribosome on the mRNA (it needs EFG in prokaryotes and eEF2 in eukaryotes).

Charging of tRNA

Addition of correct amino acid at the acceptor arm of the tRNA is the function of enzyme aminoacyl tRNA synthetase found in the cytosol of the cell. This enzyme uses terminal two phosphate from the ATP. In addition, this enzyme is responsible for editing or proofreading activity which removes wrongly added amino acid from the tRNA. Thus, this enzyme is responsible for maintaining the fidelity of the protein synthesis (Table 36.2).

Termination

Termination occurs when either UAA, UAG or UGA is encountered at the A site of the ribosome.

In prokaryotes, three releasing factors—RF-1, RF-2, RF-3 are responsible for release of polypeptide chain. Whereas in eukaryotes, it is carried out by a single release factor eRF, a GTP driven protein. This factor,

TABLE 36.2	Inhibitors of protein synthesis

- Tetracycline prevents the binding of aminoacyl tRNA to A site
- Chloromycetin and macrolide bind to 23S rRNA, which has a role in peptide bond formation (class of antibiotics).
- Puromycin structural analogue of tyrosine tRNA
- Cycloheximide Inhibits peptidyltransferase in 60s ribosomal subunit.
- Diphtheria toxin catalyses ADP-ribosylation of eEF-2 in mammalian cells and inactivates it.

in conjunction with GTP and the peptidyltransferase promotes the hydrolysis of the bond between the peptide and the tRNA occupying P site.

In addition, ribosome is split in two components 60S and 40S subunits which again are modified and form 80S ribosomal complex.

Statistics of Peptide Bond Formation

Total 4 high energy bonds are required for the addition of one amino acid to the growing chain, i.e. for one peptide bond formation.

- Two high energy bonds (ATP-AMP) are used for formation of aminoacyl-tRNA.
- One high energy bond (GTP-GDP) is used for binding aminoacyl-tRNA to A site and one high energy bond (GTP-GDP) for translocation step in which ribosome advances three nucleotides forward towards 3'-end of mRNA.

■ 'P' BODIES

P bodies are sites of translation repression and mRNA decay. P bodies are small dense compartments found in the cytosol that incorporate mRNAs as mRNPs. Over 35 distinct proteins have been suggested to reside exclusively and extensively within P bodies. These proteins are mRNA decapping enzymes, RNA helicases and RNA exonucleases, components involved in miRNA function and mRNA quality control.

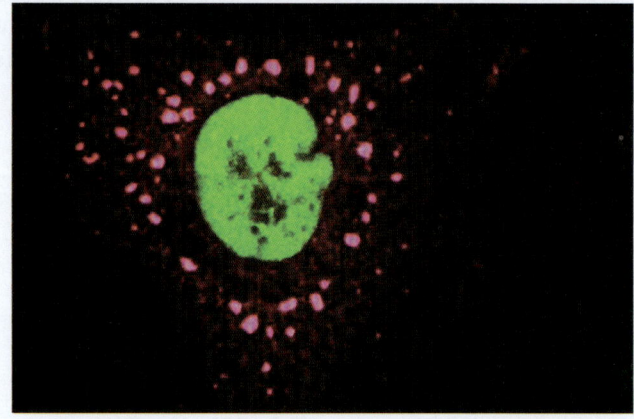

Fig. 36.3: P bodies

Incorporation of an mRNP is not an unequivocal mRNA 'death sentence'. Indeed, though the mechanisms are not yet fully understood, certain mRNAs appear to be temporarily stored in P bodies and then retrieved and utilized for protein translation (Fig. 36.3).

Gene Expression and Regulation

COMPETENCY BI 7.3

At the end of this chapter learner should be able to describe gene mutations and basic mechanism of regulation of gene expression.

Specific Learning Objectives	
BI 7.3.1	Describe various types of mutations.
BI 7.3.2	Discuss regulation of gene in prokaryotes and in eukaryotes.

LAC OPERON MODEL

- Jacob and Monod in 1961 described lac operon model. In this model they explained the regulation of lactose metabolism by an induction or derepression process.
- The structural genes for three enzymes, along with the lac promoter and lac operator are physically associated to constitute the lac operon.
- Expression of the normal lacI gene of the lac operon is constitutive, it means that the expression of it is at constant rate, resulting in the formation of the subunits of the lac repressor.
- Lac repressor molecule consists of four identical subunits with molecular weights of 37,000 Da and it has high affinity for the operator locus.
- The operator locus is a region of double-stranded DNA, which is 27 base pairs long with a two-fold rotational symmetry and an inverted palindrome.

- When attached to the operator locus, the LacI repressor molecule prevents transcription of the distal structural genes, lacZ, lacY, and lacA by interfering with the binding of RNA polymerase to the promoter.
- Thus, the lacI repressor molecule is a negative regulator, it means that in its presence (and in the absence of inducer), expression from the lacZ, lacY, and lacA genes is very low.
- The lacI repressor molecule have a high affinity for the inducer.
- Binding of the inducer to repressor molecule induces a conformational change in the structure of the repressor and causes its dissociation from operator DNA, thus derepressing the lac operon.
- Inducer in this case is al-lactose which is a metabolite of the lactose.

The lac operon is therefore controlled by two distinct, ligand-modulated DNA binding trans factors; one that acts positively (cAMP-CRP complex) to facilitate productive binding of RNA polymerase to the promoter and one that acts negatively (lacI repressor) that antagonizes RNA polymerase promoter binding.

Maximal activity of the lac operon occurs when glucose levels are low (high cAMP with CAP activation) and lactose is present (lacI is prevented from binding to the operator in presence of lactose). (Fig. 37.1)

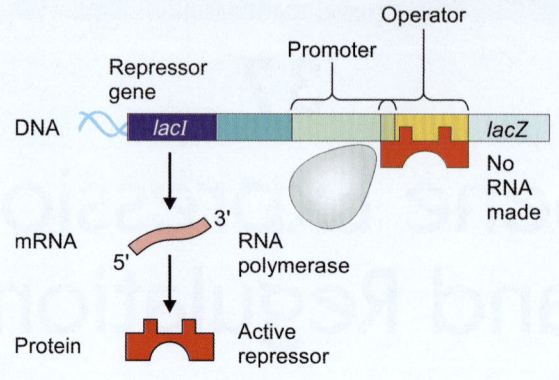

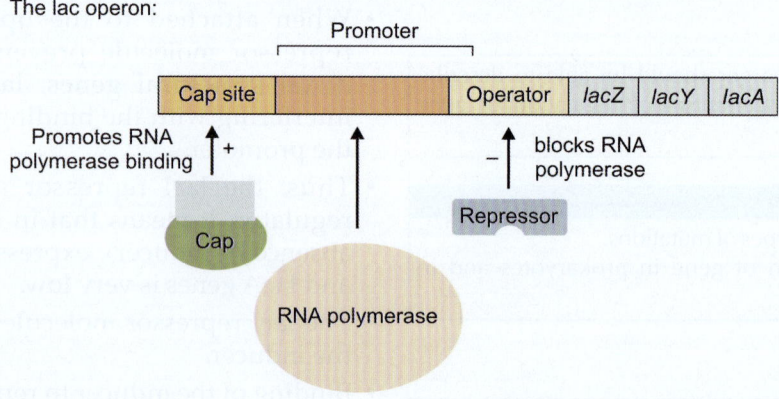

Fig. 37.1: Lac operon model

38

Technologies in Genetics

COMPETENCY BI 7.4

At the end of this chapter learner should be able to describe applications of molecular technologies like recombinant DNA technology, PCR in the diagnosis and treatment of diseases with genetic basis.

Specific Learning Objectives	
BI 7.4.1	Describe the basic principles underlying the recombinant DNA technology.
BI 7.4.2	Discuss various blotting techniques.
BI 7.4.3	Describe PCR and is various types.
BI 7.4.4	Discuss application of PCR.

RECOMBINANT DNA TECHNOLOGY (GENETIC ENGINEERING)/DNA CLONING

The process whereby a gene or a DNA fragment of one species is transferred to the DNA of other species is known as recombinant DNA technology or genetic engineering.

Preparation of chimeric DNA molecules, (e.g. molecules containing both human and bacteria DNA sequences in a sequence independent fashion) is the essence of recombinant DNA research.

It is important to understand the concept of restriction endonuclease enzyme and chimeric DNA molecule before we understand recombinant DNA technology.

A. Restriction Enzyme

- This enzyme was first isolated in 1970 by Hamilton Smith who named it as beta Hind-1.
- It was seen to destroy the genetic material of bacteriophages, and hence restrict their growth in the bacterial cell. This is the reason, they were called restriction endonuclease.
- Restriction endonuclease enzyme thus is a protective enzyme for the bacterial cell.

- Todays date more than 800 restriction endonuclease have been discovered, all of them are named according to the species from which they have been isolated.
- These enzymes have tendency to recognise certain palindromic sequences in the DNA, i.e. the sequence which has twofold rotational symmetry (Fig. 38.1).

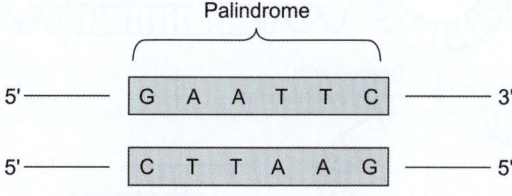

Palindrome

Fig. 38.1: Palindrome

- Palindromic sequence is also called inverted repeat. It is a segment of double stranded DNA, where nucleotide sequence is same in 5'–3' direction on both the strands. Generally, the size of palindromic sequence is 4–7 bp long.
- Restriction endonuclease enzyme are present in the cell along with site-specific DNA methylases, which methylate the host DNA rendering it an unsuitable substrate for digestion by the restriction enzyme.
- Activity of restriction endonuclease enzyme on DNA results either blunt end or overlapping (sticky/cohesive/staggered) end production (Fig. 38.2).
- Sticky ends are particularly useful in constructing hybrid or chimeric DNA molecules.

Restriction map: As the palindromic sequences are 4–7 bp long, when a DNA from a species is made to react with the given restriction endonuclease enzyme, DNA is converted to number of pieces all of which shows similar ends. When electrophoresis is done for all these pieces on agarose gel or PAGE, a characteristic pattern is produced and this is called restriction map.

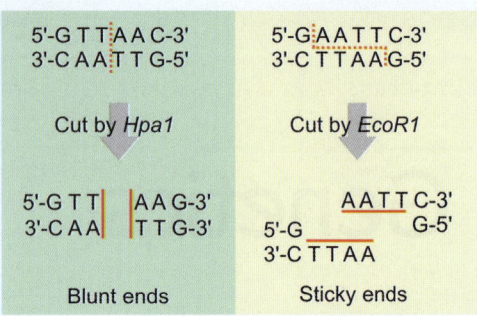

Fig. 38.2: Blunt and sticky ends of DNA produced by action of restriction endonuclease

B. Chimeric DNA Molecule/Recombinant DNA Molecule

Ligation of foreign gene in the vector DNA creates chimeric DNA molecule (Fig. 38.3).

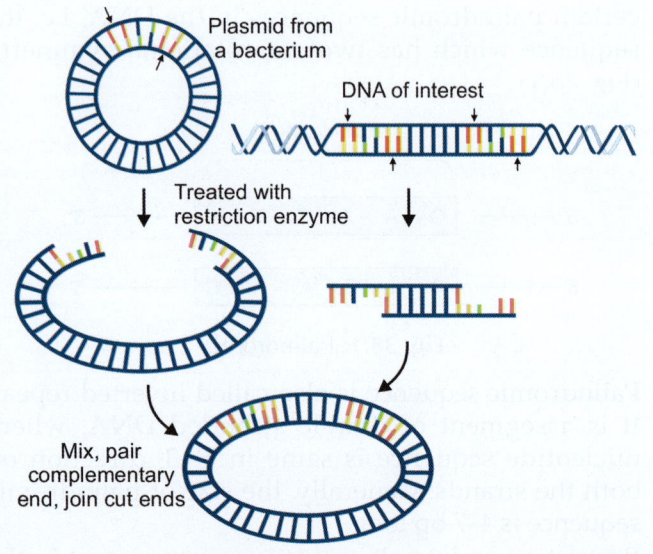

Fig. 38.3: Chimeric DNA

Restriction enzymes and DNA ligase are used to prepare chimeric DNA molecules.

Sticky-end ligation is technically easy but sticky ends of a vector may reconnect with themselves resulting in no net gain. To circumvent these problems, an enzyme that generates blunt ends can be used. Blunt ends can be ligated directly, however ligation is not directional. Two alternatives thus exist:

a. New ends are created using the enzyme terminaltransferase and synthetic sticky ends are added. If poly d(G) is added to the 3'-ends of the vector and poly d(C) is added to the 3'-ends of the foreign DNA using terminaltransferase, the two molecules now can anneal only to each other, thus circumventing the problems listed above. This procedure is called homopolymer tailing.

b. Synthetic blunt ended duplex oligonucleotide sequence having recognition element for a specific restriction endonuclease is ligated to blunt ended DNA. These chimeric DNA/recombinant vectors are now introduced into the host cells which provide enzymatic machinery for DNA replication.

Vectors for Preparation of Chimeric DNA Molecule

A vector is the carrier which is used to transfer the gene from human to bacteria.

Types
1. Plasmids
2. Bacteriophages, e.g. lambda phage
3. Cosmids
4. Bacterial artificial chromosome (BAC)
5. Yeast artificial chromosome (YAC)
6. P-1 vectors

Various vectors accommodate different sized DNA fragments. Table 38.1 illustrates the capacity of each vector.

Plasmid is a small circular duplex DNA molecule whose natural function is to confer antibiotic resistance to the host bacterium.

It has a special characteristic that it replicates in the host cell independently.

Cosmids: Combine the best features of plasmid and phage. Cosmid are plasmid that contain the DNA sequences required for packaging lambda DNA into the phage particle (cos site).

Expression vector: A vector in which the gene introduced by recombinant DNA technology actually synthesizes the protein is known as expression vector.

Such vectors are now commonly used to produce proteins by genetic engineering techniques.

For preparation of expression vector many other elements in addition to foreign gene are also inserted in to the vector. These are as follows:

a. Promoter element
b. Bacterial ribosomal binding sequence (RBS)

TABLE 38.1	Cloning capacities of common cloning vectors
Vector	DNA insert size (kb)
Plasmid pBR322	0.01–10
Lambda charon 4A	10–20
Cosmids	35–50
Bacterial artificial chromosome (BAC) P1 vector	50–250
Yeast artificial chromosome (YAC)	500–3000

c. cDNA insert (and not the genomic DNA) must be used. Cloned cDNA is inserted into bacterial genome in lacZ gene.

Steps of Recombinant DNA Technology *(Fig. 38.4)*

1. Preparation of specific gene (either isolation via use of restriction endonuclease or preparation of cDNA by mRNA using reverse transcriptase enzyme).
2. Preparation of chimeric/recombinant DNA molecule using DNA ligase enzyme.
3. Transfection of recombinant vector into the bacterial cell (assisted by electroporation/osmotic stress)
4. Selection of transfected bacterial cell using the characteristic of plasmid that provides antibiotic resistance to the bacterial cell.
5. Cloning of bacteria having recombinant plasmid.
6. Selection of correct colonies using labelled DNA/oligonucleotide probe.
7. Isolation of either recombinant vector from the bacterial cell, whose number are now amplified or isolation of desired protein from the host bacterial cell if the vector which was used initially was an expression vector.

List of important enzymes used in recombinant DNA technology:

1. Alkaline phosphatase (ALP)
2. DNA ligase
3. DNA polymerase I
4. DNAase I
5. Exonuclease III
6. Reverse trascriptase
7. Terminaltransferase

Application of Recombinant DNA Technology *(Fig. 38.4)*

1. *In medical diagnosis:* Sickle cell anemia.
2. *Gene therapy:* Detail will be discussed shortly.
3. Commercial preparation of proteins and hormones. Following are produced:
   • Recombinant human insulin
   • Recombinant human growth hormone
   • Recombinant hepatitis B, HPV vaccine

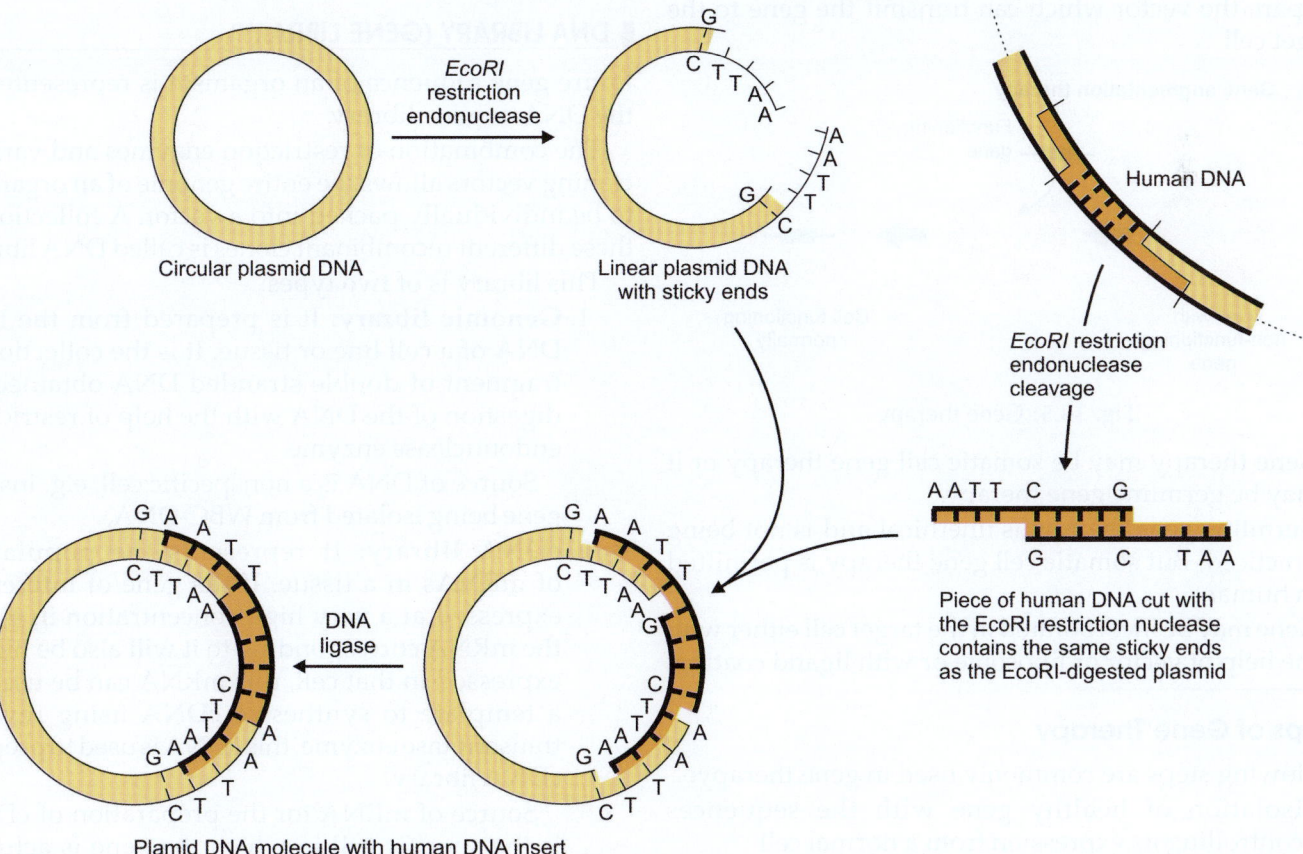

Fig. 38.4: Recombinant DNA technology and formation of chimeric vector

Section 9 ■ Nucleic Acids: Chemistry, Metabolism and Applied Aspects

38

- Recombinant enzyme (acid α-glucosidase)
- Clotting factor VIII, IX and tPA
- Interferon, interleukins

4. *Basic application:* Site directed mutagenesis, knock out mice.
5. DNA vaccine preparation.
6. Enhancement of genetic engineering.

GENE THERAPY

It is the process by which a defective gene is either repaired or is replaced by a normal gene so that the normal functioning gene is produced. Sometimes gene therapy involves introduction of the normal gene in the cell without any attempt to rectify or replace the defective gene.

- Accordingly gene therapy may be done in any of the following approaches:
  - Gene replacement
  - Gene correction
  - Gene augmentation (Fig. 38.5)

Gene therapy is one application of recombinant DNA technology, as the process of recombination is done to prepare the vector which can transmit the gene to the target cell.

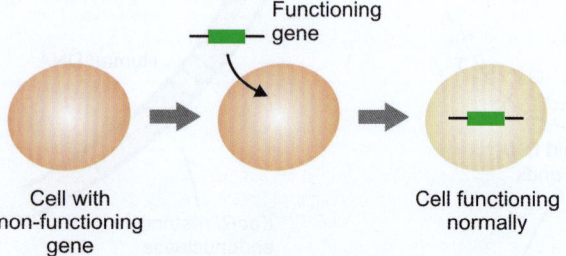

Gene augmentation therapy

Fig. 38.5: Gene therapy

- Gene therapy may be somatic cell gene therapy or it may be germline gene therapy.
- Germline gene therapy is unethical and is not being practiced. But somatic cell gene therapy is permitted in human.
- Gene may be incorporated in the target cell either with the help of vector or liposome or with ligand coating.

Steps of Gene Therapy

Following steps are commonly used in gene therapy:
a. Isolation of healthy gene with the sequences controlling its expression from a normal cell
b. Gene is incorporated in the vector using recombinant DNA technology.
c. Delivery of vector to the target cell

- Most advanced vector used in gene therapy is retrovirus.
- Delivery of gene to the target cell may be done using liposome, where gene is solublized in the aqueous compartment of the liposome. Fusion of liposome membrane to the plasma membrane will deliver the gene to the target cell.
- Gene to be delivered may be coated with the ligand and receptors present on the target cell which identify these ligand bind the ligand, coated gene and phagocytose them.

Achievement of Gene Therapy

Following diseases gene therapy has shown promising results:
1. Hemophilia A and B
2. Duchene muscular dystrophy
3. Familial hypercholesterolemia
4. Cystic fibrosis
5. Severe combined immunodeficiency (SCID)
6. Leber's hereditary optic neuropathy (LHON)
   (*Mnemonic:* HDFC Serve Long)

DNA LIBRARY (GENE LIBRARY)

Entire gene sequence of an organism is represented in the DNA or gene library.

The combination of restriction enzymes and various cloning vectors allows the entire genome of an organism to be individually packed into a vector. A collection of these different recombinant clones is called DNA library.

This library is of two types:
1. **Genomic library:** It is prepared from the total DNA of a cell line or tissue. It is the collection of fragment of double stranded DNA obtained by digestion of the DNA with the help of restriction endonuclease enzyme.

   Source of DNA is a nonspecific cell, e.g. insulin gene being isolated from WBC-DNA.

2. **cDNA library:** It represents the population of mRNAs in a tissue. If the gene of interest is expressed at a very high concentration in a cell, the mRNA corresponding to it will also be highly expressed in that cell, this mRNA can be used as a template to synthesize cDNA using reverse transcriptase enzyme, this cDNA is used to prepare cDNA library.

   Source of mRNA for the preparation of cDNA is the specific cell in which the gene is actually expressed.

For commercial production of proteins at large scale by recombinant DNA technology, the preferred source of neuclotide sequence is cDNA library rather than genomic library.

NUCLEOTIDE PROBES

- These are generally pieces of DNA (sometimes RNA known as riboprobe) labelled with either radioisotope or nonradioactive material.
- These probes are used to recognize a sequence of nucleotide which is complimentary to the sequence of probe in various genetic techniques.
- Size of the probe varies from 15 bp to several hundred kilo base pair.
- The process by which the probes are synthesized is known as nick translation.

Nick Translation (Fig. 38.6)

- It is the process by which labelled probe is produced.
- DNA is nicked and is repaired.

1. DNAse treatment nicks DNA

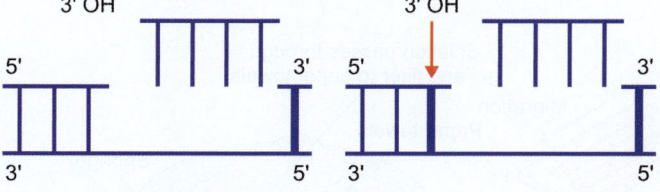

2. 5' to 3' exonuclease activity of DNA polymerase 1 removes nucleotide from 5' phosphate terminus

3. 5' to 3' polymerase activity of DNA polymerase 1 simultaneously incorporates nucleotides at the 3' hydroxyl terminus

New DNA strand

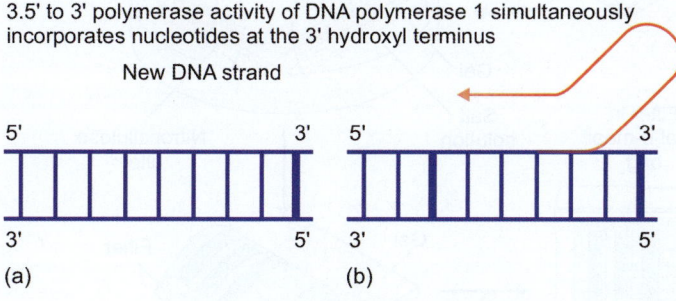

(a)   (b)

Fig. 38.6: Nick translation

- During repair DNA polymerase I, which is having 5'–3' exonuclease activity as well as 5'–3' polymerase activity is used and also 32P labelled dCTP is required for the synthesis of DNA in the nick.

- This labelled DNA fragment which is synthesized acts as a probe.

BLOTTING TECHNIQUE

Visualization of a specific DNA or RNA fragment among the many thousands of 'contaminating' molecules requires the convergence of a number of techniques, collectively termed as blot transfer/blotting technology.

A. Southern Blotting Technique

- Proposed by EM Southern in 1970.
- Purpose of this technique is to identify the presence or absence of particular nucleotide sequence in the given DNA sample.
- Following steps are involved in this technique (Fig. 38.7):
  - Extraction of the genomic DNA from a cell
  - Action of restriction enzyme to convert it into a mixture of DNA fragments
  - Electrophoretic separation of DNA fragments on Agarose or polyacrylamide gel. DNA being negatively charged, migrates toward the anode; smaller fragments move the most rapidly (Fig. 38.7).
  - After a suitable time, the DNA within the gel is denatured by exposure to mild alkali (0.5 N NaOH).
  - Transfer of DNA fragment to nitrocellulose or nylon paper, resulting in an exact replica of the pattern on the gel, by the blotting technique (either manual or electrical blotting)
  - *Fixation:* Transferred DNA fragment is bound to the paper by exposure to heat at 80°C for one hour.
  - Hybridization of the probe: Nitrocellulose replica is soaked in the neutral solution of the probe at suitable temperature to allow hybridization of the probe to its complimentary sequence.
  - *Washing:* After thorough washing to remove excess unbound probe, the paper is exposed to X-ray film, which is developed to reveal several specific bands corresponding to the DNA fragment that recognize the sequences in the cDNA probe.

B. Northern Blot

- It is conceptually similar to Southern blotting technique.
- Purpose of this blotting is to quantitate the gene expression in a cell.
- Gene expression analysis is done via quantifying the mRNA transcript of that gene .
- Following steps are involved in northern blotting technique (Fig. 38.8):

Section 9 ■ Nucleic Acids: Chemistry, Metabolism and Applied Aspects

38

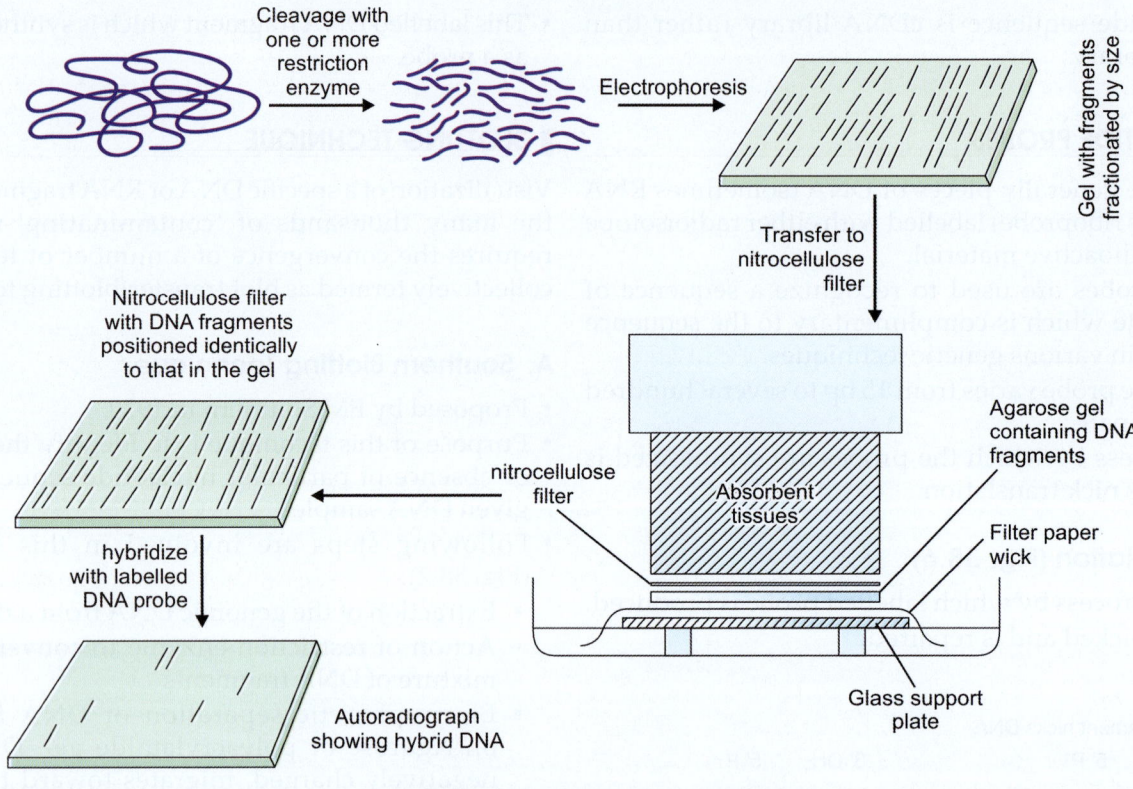

Fig. 38.7: Steps of southern blot

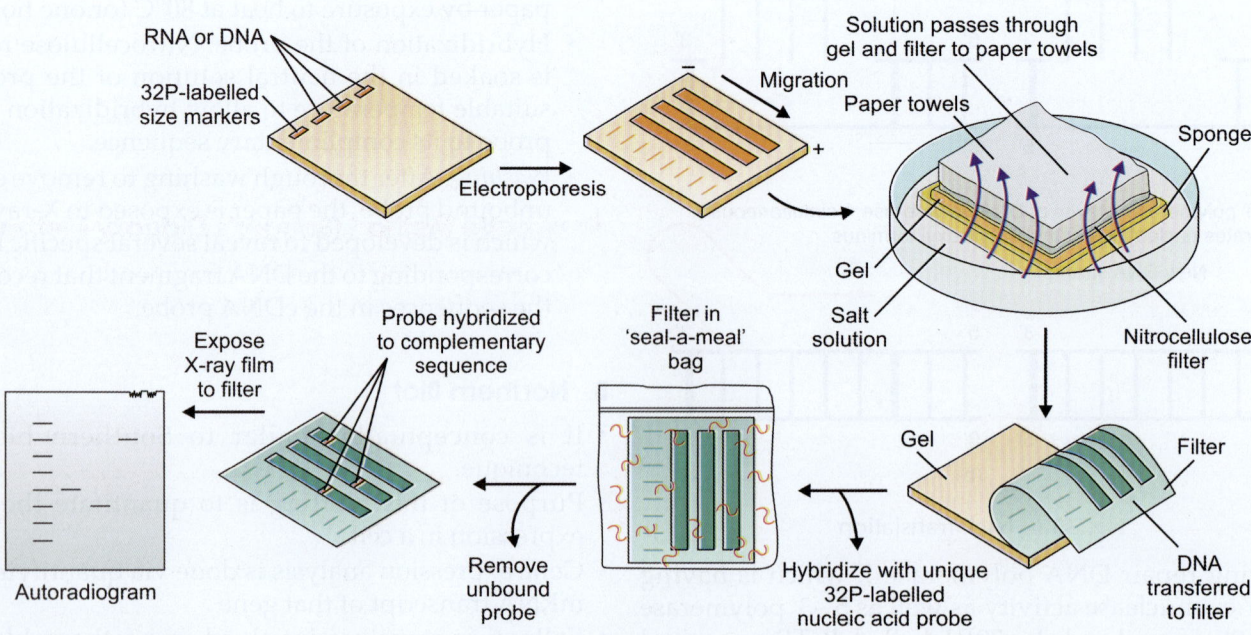

Fig. 38.8: Steps of northern blot

- Extraction of the RNA from a cell
- Preparation of cDNA from these RNAs.
- Electrophoretic separation of cDNA on Agarose or polyacrylamide gel
- After a suitable time, the cDNA within the gel is denatured by exposure to mild alkali (0.5 N NaOH)
- Transfer of cDNA fragment to nitrocellulose or nylon paper, resulting in an exact replica of the pattern on the gel, by the blotting technique (either manual or electrical blotting)
- *Fixation:*Transferred cDNA fragment is bound to the paper by exposure to heat at 80°C for one hour
- *Hybridization of the probe:* Nitrocellulose replica is soaked in the neutral solution of the probe at suitable temperature to allow hybridization of the probe to its complimentary sequence.
- *Washing:* After thorough washing to remove excess unbound probe, the paper is exposed to X-ray film, which is developed to reveal several specific bands corresponding to the cDNA fragment as the specific probe which is used to bind the cDNA specifically.
- Quantification of the probe on nitrocellulose paper helps identifying the expression of the gene in that cell at given time and place.

C. Western Blot

- In this technique proteins are identified.
- Principle of this technique is immunological.
- Proteins are electrophoresed and transferred to special paper that avidly binds macromolecules and then probed with a specific antibody or other probe molecule.

D. Southwestern Blotting

- In this technology DNA binding characteristic of the protein is analysed.
- A protein blot similar to that shown above under 'Western' blotting is exposed to labelled nucleic acid, and protein-nucleic acid complexes formed are detected by autoradiography.

FLUORESCENCE *IN SITU* HYBRIDIZATION (FISH)

'*In situ* hybridization' is a process where a radioactive probe is added to a metaphase spread of chromosomes on a glass slide. The exact area of hybridization is localized by layering photographic emulsion over the slide and, after exposure, lining up the grains with some histologic identification of the chromosome.

Fluorescence *in situ* **h**ybridization (FISH), which utilizes fluorescent rather than radioactively labelled

probes, is a very sensitive technique that is also used for this purpose (Fig. 38.9).

In this process, DNA is not isolated from the cell and the process of hybridization occurs within the cell (*in situ*). As the fluorescent dye known as fluoresence iso thiocyanate (FIT) is used to tag the probe for FISH technology, this process is known as fluorescence *in situ* hybridization. It is done in following steps:

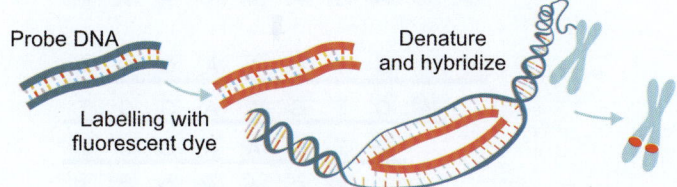

Fig. 38.9: Fluorescence *in situ* hybridization (FISH)

- Preparation of a slide of intact cell in which chromosome is located
- Treatment with colchicine to arrest the cell in metaphase
- Denaturation under controlled condition
- Layering of the probe
- Washing of excess unbound probe
- Examination of the cell under electron microscope to find out the fluorescent band which denotes the site of the gene on the chromosome.

DNA SEQUENCING

To analyse the nucleotide sequence of a segment of specific DNA molecule, large number of identical DNA molecules are made by cloning the fragment of interest. Two methods are:

1. Enzymatic method by Sanger
2. Chemical cleavage approach by Maxam and W. Gilbert

Enzymatic Method (Sanger's Dideoxy Method)

Out of the above mentioned two methods, Sanger's method is the method of choice as it can sequence long stretch of the DNA (400 bases) relative to Maxam and Gilbert method which can sequence only 250 base stretch of the DNA (Fig. 38.10).

DNA polymerase I is used to copy a particular sequence of a single stranded DNA. A primer is added along with the four deoxy NTPs (radio actively labelled).

The incubation mixture also contains a 2',3'-dideoxy analogue of one of them to terminate the synthesis of DNA abruptly at various points.

The incorporation of this analogue blocks further growth of the new chain because it lacks the 3'-hydroxyl

38

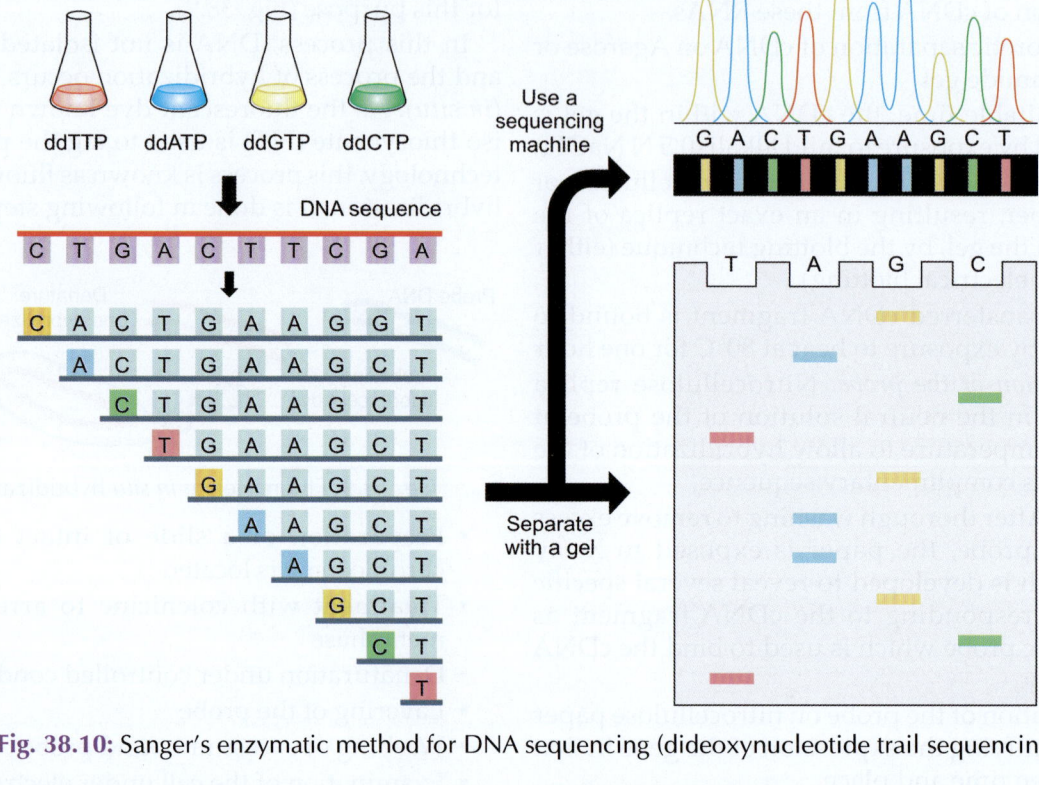

Fig. 38.10: Sanger's enzymatic method for DNA sequencing (dideoxynucleotide trail sequencing)

terminus needed to form the next phosphodiester bond formation in the elongating chain.

Hence, fragments of various lengths are produced in which the dideoxy analogue is at the 3'-end. Four such sets of chain-terminated fragments (one for each dideoxy analog) are then electrophoresed and the base sequence of the new DNA is read from the autoradiogram of the four lanes.

Chemical Cleavage Method by Maxam and Gilbert

This method starts with a DNA that is labelled at one end of one strand with 32P. The labelled DNA is then broken preferentially at one of the four nucleotides in such a way that an average of one break is made per chain. Each broken chain yields a radioactive fragment extending from the 32P label to one of the positions of that base and such fragments are produced for every position of the base.

The fragments in each mixture are then separated by PAGE, which can resolve DNA molecules differing in length by just one nucleotide.

The autoradiogram of a gel produced from four different chemical cleavages displays a pattern of bands from which the sequence can be read directly.

▌POLYMERASE CHAIN REACTION (PCR)

- PCR is a method of amplifying a target sequence of DNA *in vitro*.
- It is a sensitive, selective and extremly rapid means of amplifying a desired DNA sequence. It allows the DNA in a single cell, hair follicle or sperm to be amplified and analyzed.
- DNA sequences as short as 50 bp and as long as 10 kb can be amplified.
- For the purpose of PCR, DNA is divided into target sequence and flanking sequence.
- Information about the nucleotide sequence of the flanking region is must as the primer is to be prepared according to that for initiating the PCR.

Following steps are involved in each cyclical reaction:

a. **Denaturation:** Double stranded DNA is melted (separated) using heat at 95°C for 15 seconds.

b. **Annealing:** Primer is annealed by reducing the temperature to 50°C for 2 minutes.

c. **Polymerization:** Taq polymerase (derived from *Thermus aquaticus*) is used to polymerise the DNA at temperature of 72°C for variable number of minutes (this duration depends upon the length of the target sequence).

Above said steps a, b, c are repeated for set number of cycles for achieving the exponential amplification of DNA segments of defined length (Fig. 38.11).

E. coli DNA polymerase was used in earlier PCR reactions and because of its thermolabile nature it was destroyed, and repeated addition of the enzyme in each cycle was needed. Substitution of a heat stable DNA polymerase from '*Thermus aquaticus*' an organism that lives and replicates at 70–80°C, obviates this problem and has allowed for automation of the reaction.

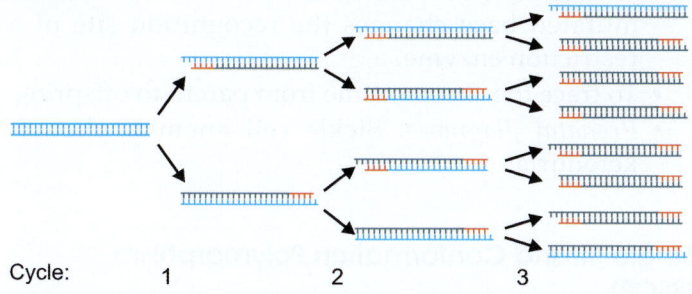

Cycle: 1   2   3

Fig. 38.11: Polymerase chain reaction

Application of PCR

a. In forensic medicine (DNA received from the crime scene is amplified by PCR and is studied)

b. To detect infectious agents (early diagnosis of tuberculosis, HIV, CMV)

c. To make prenatal genetic diagnosis (to amplify the foetal genetic material received from amino-centesis)

d. In the diagnosis of genetic disorders like sickle cell anemia, beta thalassemia and cystic fibrosis

e. To study evolution, using DNA from archeological samples (fossil study)

Types of PCR

1. **Reverse transcriptase PCR (RT PCR):** In this type of PCR, RNA is the starting material. Reverse transcriptase enzyme acts on RNA to convert it to the DNA which is subsequently used for PCR.

    The process of PCR is same as discussed above except that the starting material is the RNA and not the DNA. Additionally, the DNA polymerase which is used is derived from *Thermus thermophilus* organism. Tth polymerase has additional reverse transcriptase activity and hence is preferred for reverse transcriptase PCR.

2. **Real time PCR:** In this type of PCR, a fluorescent dye known as 'real time reportier' is used to tag the primer, this helps in quantitative detection of number of virus present in the sample.

Following are the examples of certain real time reportier: SYBR green dye, TaqMan dye and molecular beacon.

3. **Nested PCR:** In this type of PCR, specificity of amplification is enhanced by using new set of primer in each phase of the PCR. New set of primer is complimentary to the template DNA sequence which is downstream to the first primer, i.e nested between the original set of primer. It is a successful technique to amplify the specific sequence of the DNA but requires more detailed knowledge of the sequence to be amplified.

4. **Invert PCR:** In this type of PCR, the flanking region of the DNA is converted to target region and target region is converted to flanking region. This is done for those DNA fragments for which the sequence of outer flanking region for the construction of primer is not known.

5. **Rapid amplification of cDNA ends (RACE) PCR:** Sometimes called one sided PCR or anchored PCR. It is done to amplify the ends of mRNA, the sequence of which is not known. To conduct this type of PCR, knowledge of the center of the transcript is must.

6. **Multiplex PCR:** In this type of PCR multiple, unique primer set within a single PCR run is used to amplify multiple segments of the gene. It is used for detection of deletion mutation of a specific gene sequence. In this technique, prior knowledge of the gene sequence is must.

RESTRICTION FRAGMENT LENGTH POLYMORPHISM (RFLP)

- An inherited difference in the pattern of restriction enzyme digestion is known as a restriction fragment length polymorphism, or RFLP.
- Principle of this technique is polymorphism.

Polymorphism

- Detectable, accepable, inherited or acquired change in the sequence of the nucleotide in the DNA of different individuals is known as polymorphism.
- Polymorphism differs from mutation in the sense polymorphism is a commonly occurring pheno-menon (>1% of population have such changes in the nucleotide). Mutation is less common phenomenon.
- Polymorphism is of two types:
    1. Single base change in the DNA (SNP)
    2. Variable number of tandem repeat (VNTR)

Section 9 ■ Nucleic Acids: Chemistry, Metabolism and Applied Aspects

38

(a) Single Base Change in the DNA (SNP)

The alteration of one nucleotide base may abolish the recognition element of a specific restriction endonuclease enzyme. Not only this, a SNP may even create a recognition site of a specific restriction endonuclease enzyme.

In either case the length of the DNA fragment produced by respective restriction endonuclease enzyme will be different from normal DNA, which can be detected by DNA hybridization (Fig. 38.12).

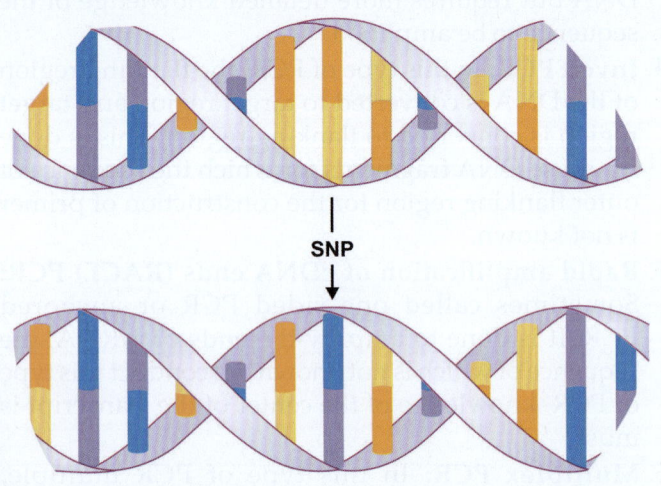

SNP

Fig. 38.12: Single nucleotide polymorphism (SNP)

(b) Variable Number of Tandem Repeat (VNTR)

These are certain short sequences of the DNA which are scattered throughout in the genome and are arranged in tandem order (Fig. 38.13).

The number of this tandem repeat varies from one individual to another. Variable number of this tandem repeat is responsible for different fragments length of the DNA in different individuals. This helps in preparation of DNA fingerprinting.

RFLP is done in following steps:
1. DNA is cleaved into fragments using restriction endonuclease enzyme
2. Electrophoresis is done to separate the DNA fragments.
3. Southern blotting is done to transfer the DNA fragments to the nitrocellulose paper.
4. Hybridization of the probe to the desired DNA fragment.

Application of RFLP:
- RFLP can be used for detection of mutation, if the mutated base changes the recognition site of a restriction enzyme.
- To trace the chromosome from parent to offspring
- *Prenatal diagnosis:* Sickle cell anemia, phenylketonuria.

Single Strand Conformation Polymorphism (SSCP)

- If the base change is not changing the restriction site, that time RFLP can not be done to detect the base change, that time SSCP could be done to find out the base change.
- Basic principle of SSCP is that movement of smaller DNA fragment (<400 base pairs) on the electrophoresis is partially dependent on their conformation. Single base change usually modifies the conformation of the DNA sequence sufficiently enough to cause the mobility shift on the electrophoresis through a nondenaturing PAGE (Fig. 38.14).
- SSCP requires prior knowledge of the sequence of the gene or gene fragment of interest, while RFLP analysis requires only restriction map analysis of the DNA.

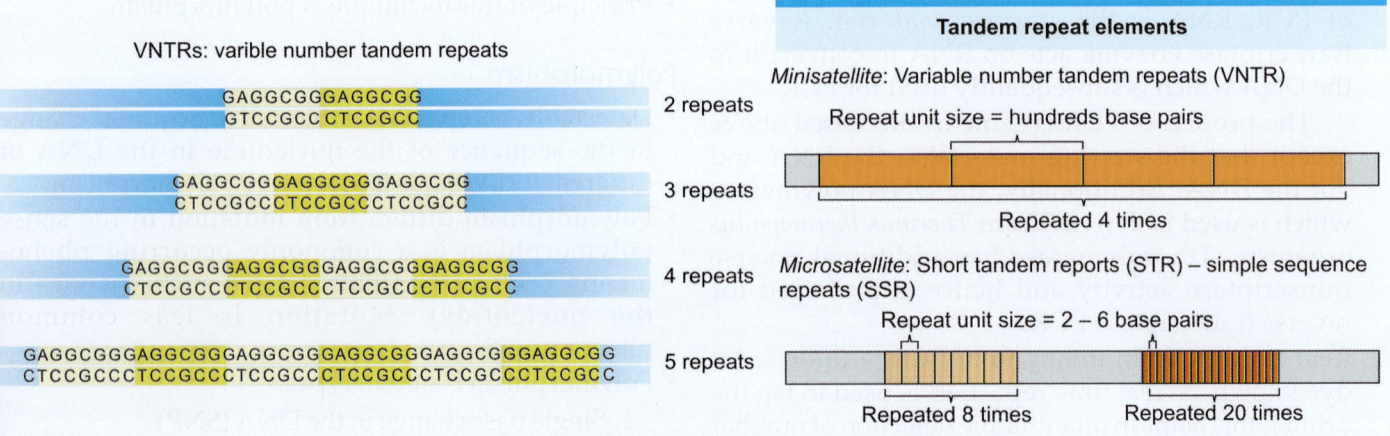

Fig. 38.13: VNTR

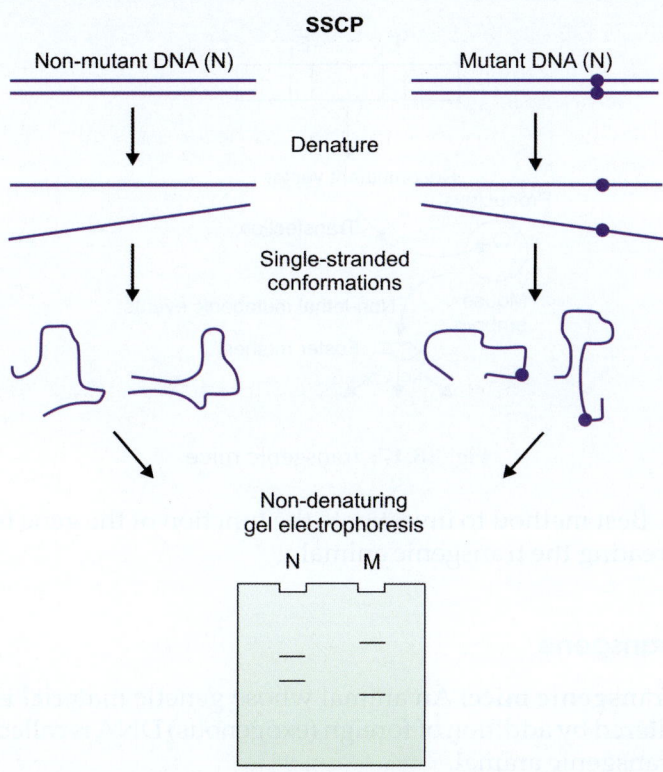

Fig. 38.14: Single strand conformation polymorphism (SSCP)

Chromosomal Walking

It will define the gene arrangement in the long stretch of the DNA. In chromosome walking, a fragment representing one end of a long piece of DNA is used to isolate another, that overlaps but extends the first. Steps of chromosomal walking is illustrated in Fig. 38.15.

Site Directed Mutagenesis of a Single Nucleotide

It is done to evaluate the role of one nucleotide at a selected site within the DNA so as to evaluate the role of specific amino acid in a protein.

This method also permits creation or destruction of a restriction endonuclease site at specific location.

Microarray

- This technique is used for analysing a DNA sample for the presence of gene variation or mutation (genotyping), and may also be used for determining the pattern of mRNA production (gene expression analysis).
- Major advantage of this technique is that it analyses thousands of gene at the same time.
- A microchip (DNA chip) is required which contains thousand of gene coated in number of wells (Fig. 38.16).

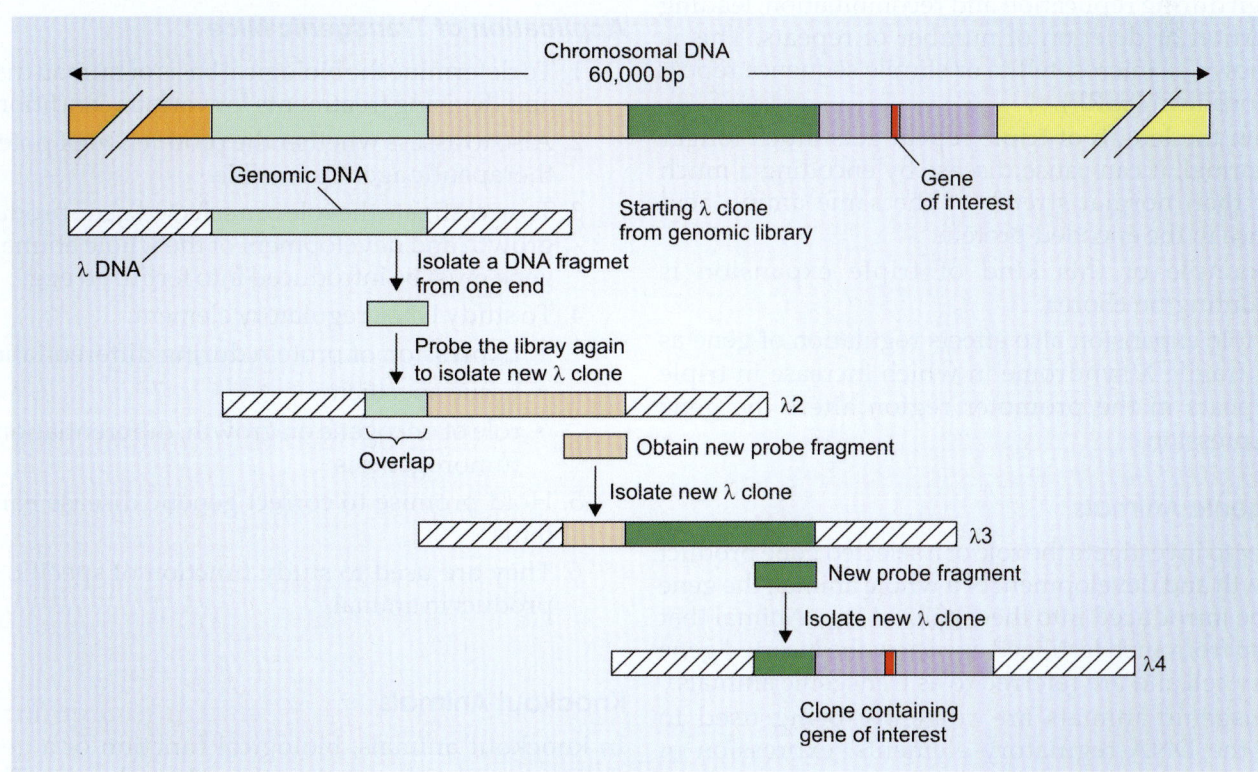

Fig. 38.15: Chromosome walking

Section 9 ■ Nucleic Acids: Chemistry, Metabolism and Applied Aspects

38

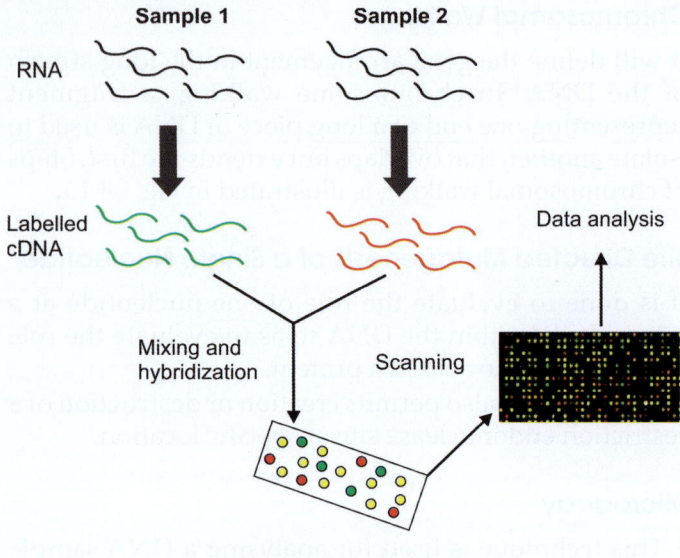

Fig. 38.16: Microarray

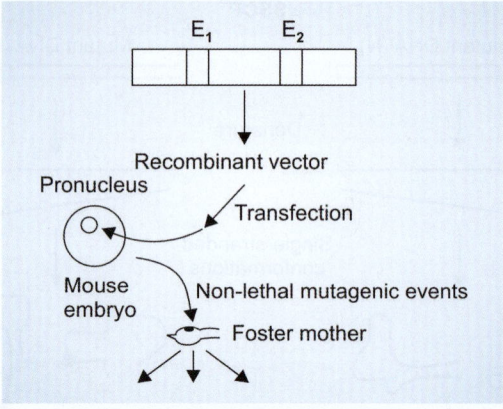

Fig. 38.17: Transgenic mice

- For genotype analysis cellular sample is genomic DNA and for the expression analysis population of mRNA of a cell which is converted to cDNA and is tagged with a fluorescent dye is used.

Triple Expansion

Genome contains many stretches of repeating 2, 3, 4 or 5 nucleotide sequence. These simple repeats have higher than average mutation rate because they can occasionly misalign during replication and recombination, leading to insertion or deletion of number of repeats. This is also known as microsatellite or simple sequence repeat polymorphism (SSRP).

When the length of triple repeat gets much longer than normal, it can cause disease by encoding a much longer than normal stretch of the same amino acid sequence in the encoded protein.

- Example of this kind of triple expansion is Huntington chorea.
- Triple expansion also effects regulation of gene as in fragile X syndrome in which increase in triple repeats in the promoter region alters the gene expression.

Transgenic Animals

In order to investigate the role of a selected gene product in growth and development of a whole animal, the gene must be introduced into the fertilized egg. Animal that develop from such fertilized egg carry the inserted gene in every cell and are referred to as transgenic animals.

Transgenic animals are currently being used to study the DNA regulatory elements, expression of protein during differentiation, tissue specificity, role of oncogene.

Best method to investigate the function of the gene is creating the transgenic animal.

Transgene

Transgenic mice: An animal whose genetic material is altered by addition of foreign (exogenous) DNA is called transgenic animal.

The DNA that is introduced is called as transgene and overall technology is known as 'transgene technology or transgenesis' (Fig. 38.17).

Application of Transgenic Mice

1. To determine the biological basis of human disease and devising treatments for various condition.
2. Also to assess whether the production of potential therapeutic agent is feasible.
3. To investigate the role of a selected gene product in growth and development of the whole animal, the gene must be introduced into fertilized egg.
4. To study DNA regulatory element:
   - Expression of protein during differentiation.
   - tissue specificity
   - role of oncogene on growth, differentiation and tumorogenesis
5. Hold promise to correct genetic disease early in fetus.
6. They are used to study function of specific gene product in animal.

Knockout Animals

In knockout animals, biological function of a gene is determined by destroying the selected gene. This is possible only if the loss of the gene is nonlethal.

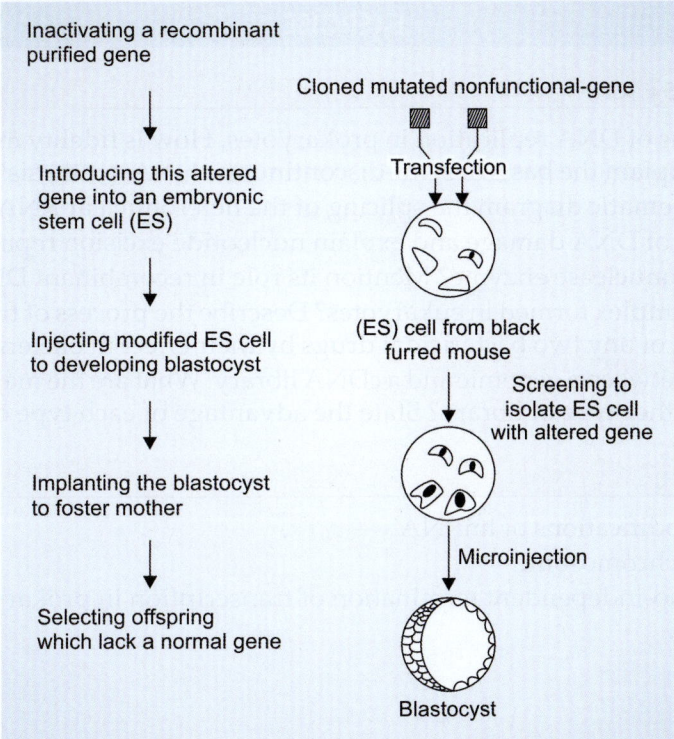

Inactivating a recombinant
purified gene

Cloned mutated nonfunctional-gene

Introducing this altered
gene into an embryonic
stem cell (ES)

Transfection

(ES) cell from black
furred mouse

Injecting modified ES cell
to developing blastocyst

Screening to
isolate ES cell
with altered gene

Implanting the blastocyst
to foster mother

Microinjection

Selecting offspring
which lack a normal gene

Blastocyst

Fig. 38.18: Technique of preparing knock out mice (null mice)

Fig. 38.18 illustrates the salient steps involved in producing knock out mice.

Embryonic stem cells (ES) are isolated which have altered gene in them and then are being microinjected in blastocyst.

EXERCISE

LONG QUESTIONS (10 MARKS EACH)

Q 1. Discuss the mechanisms of DNA replication in prokaryotes. How is fidelity maintained during the process of DNA replication? Explain the basis of semi-discontinuous DNA synthesis.

Q 2. Explain with a neat schematic diagram the splicing of the heteronuclear RNA to m-RNA.

Q 3. Describe various types of DNA damage and explain nucleotide excision repair mechanism in detail.

Q 4. What is restriction endonuclease enzyme? Mention its role in recombinant DNA technology.

Q 5. How is 80S initiation complex formed in eukaryotes? Describe the process of translation in eukaryotes. Also explain the mechanism of any two bactericidal drugs by their effect in bacterial protein synthesis.

Q 6. Explain the difference between a genomic and a cDNA library. What are the major differences in the structure of a gene cloned into either type of library? State the advantage of each type of clone.

SHORT NOTES (5 MARKS EACH)

Q 1. Post-transcriptional modifications of hnRNA

Q 2. DNA packing into the chromosome

Q 3. Rho-dependent and Rho-independent termination of transcription in prokaryotes

Q 4. Various types of DNAs

Q 5. Southern blotting

Q 6. Mitochondrial DNA

Q 7. Telomerase

Q 8. Draw a neat diagram of t-RNA, indicating its binding sites

Q 9. Recombinant DNA technology with its significance in medicine

Q 10. Watson-Crick model of DNA

Q 11. Gene therapy for the treatment of hereditary disorders

Q 12. Lac operon

Q 13. Biochemical basis of action and clinical importance of two nucleotides

Q 14. Analogue as therapeutic agents

SHORT NOTES (2.5 MARKS EACH)

Q 1. Application of DNA recombinant technology in medicine

Q 2. Recombinant vector

Q 3. RNA polymerase in eukaryotes

Q 4. DNA polymerases in prokaryotes and eukaryotes

Q 5. Genetic code

Q 6. DNA fingerprinting

Q 7. DNA ligase and its biological significance

Q 8. Reverse transcriptase

Q 9. Proofreading

Q 10. Ribozyme

Q 11. Nucleotide of biological importance

Q 12. Peptide bond formation and translocation during protein synthesis

Q 13. Xeroderma pigmentosa

MULTIPLE CHOICE QUESTIONS

38.1 One strand of a double stranded DNA is found to have 20A, 25G, 30C, 22T. How many of each base is found in complete double stranded DNA?

a. A= 40, G=50, C=60, T=44
b. A= 44, G=60, C=50, T=40
c. A= 45, G=45, C=52, T=52
d. A= 42, G=55, C=55, T=42

38.2 Prokaryotic promoter of transcription situated 35 bp upstream is:

a. TATA box
b. Goldberg hogness box
c. CAAT box
d. TGG box

38.3 Normal role of micro RNA is:

a. Gene regulation
b. RNA splicing
c. Translation initiation
d. Conformational change of DNA

38.4 Using written convention, which one of the following sequences is complementary to TGGCAGCCT?

a. ACCGTCGGA
b. ACCGUCGGA
c. AGGCTGCCA
d. TGGCTCGGA

38.5 CG-rich islands in DNA is used for:

a. Acetylation
b. Methylation
c. tRNA synthesis
d. DNA replication

38.6 Mitochondrial codons are an exception for the property of 'universality' of codons. For example, initiation codon in mammals is AUG, which codes for methionine. But in mitochondria, methionine is coded by some other codon. Which among the following is that initiation codon?

a. AAG
b. AUG
c. AUA
d. AGA

38.7 Chargaff rule states that:

a. A + G = T + C
b. A/T = G/C
c. A = U = T = G = CT
d. A + T = G + C

38.8 Which of the following statements about nucleotide metabolism is not correct?

a. An early step in purine biosynthesis is the formation of PRPP (phosphoribosyl 1-pyrophosphate).
b. Inosine monophosphate (IMP) is a precursor of both AMP and GMP.
c. Orotic acid is an intermediate in pyrimidine nucleotide biosynthesis.
d. Humans catabolize uridine and pseudouridine by analogous reactions.

38.9 The initiator tRNA is placed within the active 80S complex at which of the three canonical ribosomal 'sites' during protein synthesis?

a. E site
b. P site
c. A site
d. Any of the above sites

38.10 Which of the following is the correct sequence of events in gene repair mechanisms in patients without a mutated repair process?

a. Nicking, excision, replacement, sealing, recognition
b. Nicking, recognition, excision, sealing, replacement
c. Nicking, sealing, recognition, excision, replacement
d. Recognition, nicking, excision, replacement, sealing

38.11 Aminoacyl-tRNA synthetases must be capable of recognizing which of the following?

a. A specific tRNA and a specific amino acid
b. A specific tRNA and the 40S ribosomal subunit
c. A specific amino acid and the 40S ribosomal subunit
d. A specific amino acid and the 60S ribosomal subunit

Section 9 ■ Nucleic Acids: Chemistry, Metabolism and Applied Aspects

38

38.12 Which sequences extend between the 5'-methylguanosine cap present on eukaryotic mRNAs to the AUG initiation codon?
  a. Last exon
  b. Last intron
  c. 3'-UTR
  d. 5'-UTR

38.13 All but one of the following histones are found located within the superhelix formed between DNA and the histone octamer; this histone is:
  a. Histone H2B
  b. Histone H3
  c. Histone H1
  d. Histone H4

38.14 Which component of the DNA duplex causes the molecule to have a net negative charge at physiological pH?
  a. Deoxyribose
  b. Ribose
  c. Phosphate groups
  d. Chlorine ions

38.15 How many high energy phosphate-bond equivalents are utilized in the process of activation of amino acid for protein synthesis?
  a. Zero
  b. 1
  c. 2
  d. 4

38.16 Most aminoacyl-tRNA synthetase possess an activity that is shared with DNA polymerases. This activity is the:
  a. Endonucleolytic
  b. Helicase
  c. Proteolytic
  d. Proofreading

38.17 RNA polymerase II promoters are located on which side of the transcription unit?
  a. 3'-downstream
  b. Nearest the C-terminus
  c. Nearest the N-terminus
  d. 5'-upstream

38.18 Which among the following is a feature of non-competitive inhibition?
  a. Increased V_{max}
  b. Decreased V_{max}

  c. Increased K_m
  d. Decreased K_m

38.19 The material which is not involved in protein translation in eukaryotes is:
  a. RNA polymerase
  b. Aminoacyl-tRNA
  c. Ribosomes
  d. Peptidyltransferase

38.20 All of the given statements are true, except:
  a. Heterochromatin is the relatively uncondensed portions of DNA
  b. Histones are positively charged because of the high content of basic amino acids in them
  c. Methylation of DNA will increase the condensed portions
  d. Euchromatin represents the transcriptionally active portions of the DNA

38.21 Which arm binds the aminoacyl-tRNA to the ribosomal surface?
  a. Acceptor arm
  b. Anticodon arm
  c. DHU arm
  d. Pseudouridine arm

38.22 Denaturation of DNA in PCR is carried out by heating to a temperature of:
  a. 40°C
  b. 60°C
  c. 76°C
  d. 94°C

38.23 In an embryo that lacked nucleoli, the synthesis of which type of RNA would be most directly affected?
  a. tRNA
  b. rRNA
  c. mRNA
  d. 5S RNA

38.24 Abnormal base in tRNA is:
  a. Dihydrouracil
  b. Orotic acid
  c. Methylxanthine
  d. Cystine

38.25 Which of the following enzymes is used in recombinant DNA technology?
a. Restriction endonuclease
b. Pyridoxine dehydrogenase
c. RNA polymerase II
d. DNA ligase

38.26 Restriction fragment length polymorphisms (RFLPs), which are used in the diagnosis of genetic diseases, are observed on:
a. Northern blots
b. Western blots
c. Southern blots
d. Eastern blots

38.27 Replication occurs during:
a. G1 phase
b. S phase
c. G2 phase
d. M phase

38.28 Which of the following enzymes can be described as a DNA-dependent RNA polymerase?
a. DNA ligase
b. Primase
c. DNA polymerase III
d. DNA polymerase I

38.29 Degeneracy of the genetic code denotes the existence of:
a. Multiple codons for a single amino acid.
b. Codons consisting of only two bases.
c. Base triplets that do not code for any amino acid.
d. Different systems in which a given triplet codes for different amino acids.

38.30 Aminoacyl-tRNA is required for all, except:
a. Hydroxyproline
b. Methionine
c. Cystine
d. Lysine

38.31 All are true about nucleotide excision repair, except:
a. Removal of damaged bases occurs only on one strand of the DNA.
b. It removes thymine dimmers generated by UV light.
c. Requires ligase and polymerase.
d. Only the damaged nucleotides are removed.

38.32 True statement regarding base excision repair is:
a. Used only for the bases which are deaminated
b. Uses enzyme called DNA glycosylase which generates abasic sugar site
c. Removes about 10–15 nucleotides
d. Recognizes a bulk lesion

38.33 Which RNA contains unusual purines and pyrimidines?
a. tRNA
b. rRNA
c. mRNA
d. snRNA
e. hnRNA

38.34 Ribosome consists of which all types of RNA?
a. 5S rRNA
b. 23S rRNA
c. 18S rRNA
d. 16S rRNA
e. 5.8S rRNA

38.35 End product of purine metabolism is:
a. Alanine
b. Uric acid
c. Prostaglandins
d. Allantoin

38.36 Allopurinol prevents the conversion of:
a. IMP to GMP
b. Adenosine to inosine
c. Xanthine to uric acid
d. dUMP to dTMP

38.37 A child presented with aggressive behavior, joint pain, decreased urine output and self-mutilating behavior. Enzyme deficient may be:
a. Adenosine deaminase
b. HGPRTase
c. APRTase
d. Acid maltase

38.38 Euchromatin is the region of the DNA that is relatively:
a. Uncondensed
b. Condensed
c. Overcondensed
d. Partially condensed

Section 9 ■ Nucleic Acids: Chemistry, Metabolism and Applied Aspects

38

38.39 Mitochondrial DNA is:
a. Closed circular
b. Nicked circular
c. Linear
d. Open circular

38.40 Which of the following types of the RNA has maximum modified bases?
a. mRNA
b. tRNA
c. rRNA
d. snRNA

38.41 Complementary RNA sequence of 5′-AGTCTGACT-3′ is:
a. 3′-UCAGACUGA 5′
b. 5′-UCAGACUGA 3′
c. 5′-UGACACUGA-3'
d. 3′-UGAGACCGA-5'

38.42 Stop codon is:
a. UAG
b. UCA
c. UAC
d. AUG

38.43 Which of the following compounds is an analogue of hypoxanthine?
a. Arabinoside C
b. Allopurinol
c. Ribose phosphate
d. 5-phosphoribosylpyrophosphate (PRPP)

38.44 Binding of protein to DNA is regulated by:
a. Copper
b. Zinc
c. Selenium
d. Nickel

38.45 Stop codons are:
a. UAA
b. UAG
c. UGA
d. UAC
e. UCA

38.46 Which among the following statements are true regarding DNA repair mechanisms?
a. Pyrimidine dimers are removed by nucleotide excision repair
b. Mismatch repair mechanism has high fidelity
c. Chemotherapy can lead to double-stranded breaks in DNA
d. Homologous recombination repair has highest fidelity and DNA preservation rate
e. Mismatch repair cannot overcome deletions

38.47 Transcription factor binds to:
a. DNA strand
b. Promoter region
c. Poly (A) tail
d. RNA polymerase
e. DNA polymerase

38.48 Which bonds are broken during DNA replication?
a. Hydrogen bonds
b. Glycosidic bonds between glucose and phosphate
c. Bonds between bases
d. Bonds between phosphate groups
e. Bonds between sugar

38.49 The snRNAs not the part of major spliceosome include:
a. U1
b. U2
c. U3
d. U4
e. U5

38.50 Restriction fragment length polymorphism (RFLP) was used in order to identify the five different spices of staphylococci in a surgical ICU. Which of the following sites does the restriction enzyme act?
a. TAGATA–ATCTAT
b. ATGGAC–TACGTG
c. AATATA–TATAAT
d. GATATC–CTATAG

38.51 Peptidyltransferase is an example of:
a. Enzyme
b. Catalyst
c. Elongation factor
d. Ribozyme

38.52 DNA microarrays allow detection of gene mutations using:
a. Polymerase chain reaction

b. Cloning

c. Southern blotting

d. Hybridization

38.53 Which of the following DNA element negatively regulates transcription initiation?

a. Origins of replication

b. Promoters

c. Enhancers

d. Repressors

38.54 DNA polymerase requires which of the following biomolecules for its activity?

a. Thioredoxin

b. Thioredoxin reductase

c. dUTP

d. A templete

38.55 Processing of RNA occurs in:

a. Nucleus

b. Nucleolus

c. Cytosol

d. Blood plasma

38.56 Okazaki fragment is formed during synthesis of:

a. dsDNA

b. ssDNA

c. mRNA

d. tRNA

38.57 For telomerase, all are the correct statements, except:

a. The RNA component acts as a template for the synthesis of a segment of the DNA.

b. It adds telomere to the 5′-end of the DNA strand.

c. Provides the mechanism for replicating the ends of the linear chromosome.

d. It recognises the G-rich single strand of the DNA.

38.58 True regarding DNA replication:

a. Occurs in M phase of cell cycle

b. Sister chromatids are formed

c. Follow base pair rule

d. Semiconservative

e. Single strand break

38.59 Base excision repair:

a. Is used only for bases that have been deaminated

b. Uses enzymes called DNA glycosylases to generate an abasic sugar site

c. Removes about 10–15 nucleotides

d. Requires the action to *E. coli* DNA polymerase III

38.60 Xeroderma pigmentosum is caused due to a group of closely related abnormalities in:

a. Mismatch repair

b. Base excision repair

c. Nucleotide excision repair

d. SOS repair

38.61 DNA repair defect is seen in:

a. Xeroderma pigmentosum

b. Bloom's syndrome

c. Ataxia-telangiectasia

d. Retinoblastoma

38.62 The correct sequence of cell cycle is:

a. G0-G1-S-G2-M

b. G0-G1-G2-S-M

c. G0-M-G2-S-G1

d. G0-G1-S-M-G2

38.63 Splicing activity is a function of:

a. mRNA

b. snRNA

c. rRNA

d. tRNA

38.64 The sigma subunit of prokaryotic RNA polymerase:

a. Binds the antibiotic rifampicin

b. It is inhibited by α-amanitin

c. Specifically recognizes the promoter site

d. It is a part of the core enzyme.

38.65 Methylation of bases in DNA usually:

a. Facilitates the binding of transcription factor to the DNA

b. Makes a difference in the activity only if it occurs in an enhancer region

c. Inactivates DNA for transcription

d. Results in increased production of product in whatever gene it is methylated

38.66 rRNA is mainly produced in:

a. Nucleus

b. Nucleolus

c. Ribosome

d. Endoplasmic reticulum

38.67 In conversion of DNA to RNA, enzyme required is:

a. DNA polymerase

b. DNA ligase

c. RNA polymerase

d. Primase

38.68 RNA polymerase does not require:

a. Template (dsDNA)

b. Activated precursor (ATP, GTP, UTP, CTP)

c. Divalent metal ion (Mn⁺⁺, Mg⁺⁺)

d. Primer

38.69 Gene transmitted but not translated is:

a. Glycosyltransferase

b. tRNA

c. Keratin

d. Histone

38.70 Poly A tailing translates into:

a. Polyproline

b. Polylysine

c. Polyalanine

d. Polyglycine

38.71 Shine-Dalgarno sequence in the bacteria mRNA is near:

a. AUG codon

b. UAA codon

c. UAG codon

d. UGA codon

38.72 Termination process of protein synthesis is performed by:

a. Releasing factor

b. Stop codon

c. Peptidyltransferase

d. UAA codon

e. AUG codon

38.73 Base substitution mutation can have following molecular consequences, except:

a. Changes one codon for an amino acid to the another codon for the same amino acid

b. Changes one codon for an amino acid to the another codon for some other amino acid

c. Reading frame changes downstream to the mutant site

d. Codon for one amino acid is changed into a translation termination codon

38.74 Mutation of which of the following sequences will result in problem in polyadenylation process?

a. CAAT

b. TATAT

c. AAUAAA

d. GGGCG

38.75 UAC to UAG:

a. Nonsense mutation

b. Frameshift mutation

c. Deletion

d. Missense mutation

38.76 Restriction enzymes type II:

a. Methylate specific DNA sequences

b. Cleave specific palindromic DNA sequences

c. Help in protein digestion

d. Keep the nascent protein unfolded

38.77 The following methods can be used to detect the point mutation in the beta globin gene that causes sickle cell anemia, except:

a. PCR with allele specific oligonucleotide hybridization

b. Southern blot analysis

c. DNA sequencing

d. Northern blot analysis

38.78 For PCR which of the following is not required?

a. Taq polymerase

b. d-NTP

c. Primer

d. Radiolabelled DNA probe

38.79 SYBR green dye is used for:

a. HPLC

b. PCR

c. ELISA

d. Immunofluorescence

38.80 Purpose of gene therapy is:

a. Replacement of abnormal gene by normal gene

b. Replacement of normal gene by abnormal gene
c. Knock out of abnormal gene
d. Introduction of viral gene

38.81 DNA fingerprinting was found by:
a. Watson
b. Galton
c. Jeffrey
d. None of the above

38.82 PCR detects:
a. Antigen
b. Antibody
c. Nucleic acid
d. All of the above

38.83 Correct statement about restriction fragment gene:
a. Detected by southern blot
b. Detected by northern blot
c. Used for identification of gene for genomic mapping
d. RFLP is a DNA variation sequence

38.84 True about DNA methylation:
a. Alters gene expression
b. Genetic code remains intact
c. Role in carcinogenesis
d. Protective mechanism against cleavage by restriction endonuclease

38.85 Oncogene can be best studied by:
a. Transfection
b. Transduction

c. Transformation
d. Conjugation

38.86 Gene therapy methods are:
a. Electroporation
b. Intranuclear injection
c. Site-directed mutagenesis
d. Retrovirus

38.87 Poly (A) tail is translated into:
a. Polylysine
b. Polyalanine
c. Polyarginine
d. Polycysteine

38.88 True about transition mutations is/are:
a. They are conservative mutations
b. Pyrimidine replaced by purine and purine replaced by pyrimidine
c. Purine replaced by purine and pyrimidine replaced by pyrimidine
d. Basic composition of gene product is not altered

38.89 Intron is not found in which DNA?
a. Nuclear DNA
b. Mitochondrial DNA
c. B DNA
d. Z DNA

38.90 For mitochondrial gene, true statement is:
a. Paternally inherited
b. Maternally inherited
c. Mandelian inheritance
d. Mitochondrial myopathy

Section 9 ■ Nucleic Acids: Chemistry, Metabolism and Applied Aspects

38

ANSWERS

38.1 (d) A= 42, G=55, C=55, T=42

- A corresponds to T and C corresponds to G.
- That gives total of each base is found in complete double stranded DNA as A= 42, G=55, C=55, T=42

38.2 (d) TGG box

- Bacterial promoter situated 35 bp upstream to the starting site of transcription is TGG box
- Promoters are short conserved sequences in the coding strand of DNA that specifies the start of transcription

Bacterial promoters:
- Pribnow box
  Situated 10 bp upstream
- TGG box
  Situated 35 bp upstream

Eukaryotic promoters :
- Goldberg hogness box
  Situated 25 bp upstream
- CAAT box
  Situated 70 bp upstream
  GC-rich region

38.3 (a)   Gene regulation

- Micro-RNA and siRNA are both involved in negative gene regulation
- Differences between miRNA and siRNA

miRNA	siRNA
• Involved in negative gene regulation	• Involved in negative gene regulation
• Small size (21–25 nucleotide large)	• Small size (21–25 nucleotide large)
• Derived from single stranded RNA	• Derived from double stranded RNA
• miRNA binds the 3' untranslated region (UTR) of the mRNA and thus prevents the expression of the mRNA	• siRNA binds nonspecific area of the mRNA and this duplex is degraded in the P bodies

38.4 (c) AGGCTGCCA

- Since the DNA is polar, with one end having 5'-PO$_4$ group and the other end 3'-OH group.
- Convention dictates that base sequences are written in a 5'-to-3' direction, much like amino acids are written in an amino end to carboxyl end direction.
- Thus, the complement to 5'-AGCT-3' is 5'-AGCT-3' when written conventionally and 3'-TCGA-5' when written in a truly complementary way.

38.5 (b)   Methylation

- Epigenetic changes are nonmutational changes where gene expression is regulated.
- Methylation of bases in the DNA is one of the epigenetic change, the other type of epigenetic change is covalent modification of histone proteins.
- Cytosine is the usual base (in CpG island) of the DNA which undergoes methylation. This epigenetic change is seen to be associated with suppression of certain genes.
- Histone undergoes following covalent modifications: Ubiquitinylation, phosphorylation, methylation and acetylation [Pneumo: UPMA]

38.6 (c)   AUA

- Each codon consists of a **sequence of 3 nucleotides**
- In mammalian cells, AUG **codes for methionine (initiation** colon)
- Stop codons are: UGA, UAG and UAA.

  In mitochondria:
  ◇ AUA codes for methionine (mitochondrial initiation codon)
  ◇ UGA codes for tryptophan
  ◇ AGA and AGG serve as chain terminators
    ♦ In prokaryotes, AUG, the initiation codon codes for formyl methionine
    ♦ The Shine-Dalgarno (SD) sequence, is a ribosomal binding site in prokaryotic mRNA, generally located around 8 bases upstream of the start codon AUG. The Shine-Dalgarno sequence helps recruit the ribosome to the mRNA to initiate protein synthesis by aligning it with the start codon.
    ♦ **Features of genetic code:**
    ✪ *Degenerate:* There are 61 codons for 20 amino acids
    ✪ This implies multiple codons decode the same amino acid
    ✪ *Unambiguous:* Given a specific codon, only a single amino acid is indicated
    ✪ Nonoverlapping
    ✪ No punctuation
    ✪ Universal

38.7 (a)   A + G = T + C

Chargaff's rule states that in a double stranded DNA fragment, total number of purine nucleotide is equal to total number of pyrimidine nucleotide.

38.8 (d) Humans catabolize uridine and pseudouridine by analogous reactions.

No enzyme in humans catabolizes pseudouridine which is hence excreted unchanged in the urine.

38.9 (b) P site

38.10 (d) Recognition, nicking, excision, replacement, sealing

38.11 (a) A specific tRNA and a specific amino acid

38.12 (d) 5'-UTR

38.13 (c) Histone H1

38.14 (c) phosphate groups

38.15 (c) 2

38.16 (d) Proofreading

Aminoacyl-tRNA synthetase is a cytosolic enzyme which has proofreading activity.

38.17 (d) 5'-upstream

38.18 (b) Decreased V_{max}

- A noncompetitive inhibitor has no effect on K_m but decreases V_{max}.
- V_{max}: Maximum velocity
- K_m: The substrate concentration at which the enzyme attains half of the V_{max}.

	Competitive inhibition	Noncompetitive inhibition
Acting on	Active site	May or may not
Structure of inhibitor	Substrate analogue	Unrelated
Inhibition	Reversible	Generally irreversible
Excess substrate	Inhibition relieved	No effect
K_m	Increased	No change
V_{max}	No change	Decreased
Significance	Drug action	Toxicological

38.19 (a) RNA polymerase

- RNA polymerase enzyme is involved in transcription process, not in translation process.
- Aminoacyl-tRNA is needed during the process of translation to carry the amino acid at the surface of the ribosome for the attachment in the elongating polypeptide chain.

- Ribosome is the organelle on which the protein synthesis takes place.

38.20 (a) Heterochromatin is the relatively uncondensed portions of DNA

Heterochromatin

- Transcriptionally inactive DNA
- Condensed
- Formed by histone deacetylation and DNA methylation
- Has very high methyl cytosine content
- Two types:
  ◇ *Constitutive:* Always occurs in condensed form; seen in centromere and ends of telomere.
  ◇ *Facultative:* At times condensed and at other times actively transcribed.

38.21 (d) Pseudouridine arm

Pseudouridine arm (TΨC)

TΨC stands for thymidine, pseudouridine, cytosine, involved in the binding of aminoacyl tRNA to the ribosomal surface.

38.22 (d) 94°C

Polymerase Chain Reaction

- It is a test tube method for amplifying a selected DNA sequence
- The method can be used to amplify DNA sequences from any source—bacterial, viral, plant or animal.
- PCR utilizes DNA polymerase to repetitively amplify targeted portions of DNA requirements.
- DNA to be amplified
- Primer RNA
- Deoxynucleotides
- DNA polymerase (Taq polymerase)

PCR Steps

1. Primer construction:
   - It is not necessary to know the nucleotide sequence of the target DNA
   - But it is necessary to know the nucleotide sequence of short segments on each side of target DNA-flanking sequences
2. Denature the DNA:
   - The DNA to be amplified is heated to separate the double stranded target DNA into single strands.
   - This is done by heating at 92–96°C for 10 minutes.
3. Annealing of primers to ssDNA:
   - The separated strands are cooled and allowed to anneal to the two primers (one each strand).

38

◆ Temperature : 45°C for 4 minutes

4. Chain extension:
   ◆ DNA polymerase and deoxyribonucleoside triphosphates are added to the mixture to initiate the synthesis of two new chains complementary to the original DNA
   ◆ Taq polymerase (from thermusaquaticus) is used
   ◆ At 72°C for variable time

Generally, cycles are repeated for 20–30 times.

38.23 (b) rRNA

In nucleoli, rRNA genes are transcribed to produce the 45S rRNA precursor, which is trimmed, modified, and complexed with proteins to form ribosomal subunits. Therefore, the synthesis of rRNA would be most directly affected. The embryo probably would not survive.

38.24 (a) Dihydrouracil

- The transfer RNAs show extensive internal base pairing and acquire clover leaf-like structure.
- They contain a significant proportion of unusual bases.
- These include dihydrouracil (DHU), pseudouridine and hypoxanthine.
- Many bases are methylated; this occurs in the nucleus.
- The 5′-end often has a phosphorylated guanosine.

38.25 (a) Restriction endonuclease

- Werner Arber showed that certain enzymes of bacteria restrict the entry of phages into host bacteria. Hence, the name restriction endonucleases. Hamilton Smith in 1970 isolated the first restriction enzyme beta Hindi.
- Daniel Nathans in 1971 for the first time applied this restriction enzyme to cut SV 40 DNA. All the three scientists received Nobel prize in 1978.
- The restriction endonucleases are named after the species and strains of bacteria and the order of discovery. For example, the enzyme EcoRI is isolated from *Escherichia coli* RY13 strain.
- The Roman numeral 'I' indicates the order' discovery of an enzyme from that species. Restriction enzymes are isolated from bacteria. Bacterial DNA is not broken by RE, because restriction sites are protected by site-specific methylation.

38.26 (c) Southern blots

- Restriction fragment length polymorphisms are obtained from DNAs that differ in the location of restriction enzyme sites due to differences in the sequence of the bases.
- Following digestion with restriction enzymes, the resulting DNAs are electrophoresed and the resulting fragments are resolved by length. In Southern blots (named after the originator), DNA is electrophoresed.
- In northern blots, RNA is run on the electrophoretic gels. In western blots, protein is electrophoresed and usually identified immunochemically.

38.27 (b) S phase

- The sequence of cell cycle is, G0-G1-S-G2-M is mitosis phase, where cell division occurs.
- Before cell division, nuclear division should occur.
- For nuclear division to occur, we require the synthesis of two dsDNA from single dsDNA (i.e. replication has to occur). This occurs during S phase/synthetic phase.

38.28 (b) Primase

- Primase is a DNA-dependent RNA polymerase located in the primosome at the replication fork of DNA.
- Primase initiates DNA synthesis by synthesizing a 10-base RNA primer. The DNA-RNA helix formed binds DNA polymerase III, which synthesizes a DNA fragment (the Okazaki fragment) in a 5′ to 3′ direction.
- When the RNA primer of the previous Okazaki fragment is met, DNA polymerase I replaces III and digests the RNA primer, replacing it with appropriate DNA bases.
- When the RNA primer is completely removed, DNA ligase synthesizes the last phosphodiester bond, thereby sealing the space. What is left is a new lagging strand extended by the new Okazaki fragment with the 10-base RNA primer at its 5′-end.
- Reverse transcriptase is a DNA polymerase that uses RNA as a template found in retroviruses as well as normal eukaryotic cells. Unlike DNA polymerase I and III, which proofread for errors during normal synthesis, reverse transcriptase has no proofreading capabilities.
- Hence, it has an exceedingly high error rate that contributes to the high rate of mutation in retroviruses like HIV.

38.29 (a) Multiple codons for a single amino acid.
- This is the definition of degeneracy, although sometime tRNA reads only the first two bases of a triplet (wobble), and sometime unusual bases occur in anticodons.
- Base triplets denote the stop (nonsense) codons.

38.30 (a) Hydroxyproline
- Hydroxyproline is a derived amino acid and there is no tRNA available to transport derived amino acids: Hydroxyproline and hydroxylysine are two examples of derived amino acids for which there is no tRNA available.

38.31 (d) Only the damaged nucleotides are removed.
- Cuts are made several nucleotides on either side of the damaged base. The intact strand acts as a template strand for the repair. Many lesions are removed by this nucleotide excision repair.
- Ultraviolet-induced thymine dimmers are only one example of such lesions. To fill the gap, polymerase and ligase activity is required.

38.32 (b) Uses enzyme called DNA glycosylase which generates abasic sugar site
- This is the first step of base excision repair. Bases modified by deamination, methylation, or by other chemical modification are removed by this kind of repair system.

38.33 (a) tRNA
- tRNA has numerous modified bases.
- It has up to 25% of post-translationally modified or hypermodified bases.

Following are the examples:

Uracil derivatives	Pseudouridine Dihydrouridine Ribothymidine 4-thiouridine
Cytosine derivatives	3-methyl cytidine N4-acetyl cytidine Lysidine
Adenine derivatives	1-methyladenosine N6-isopentenyladenosine Inosine
Guanine derivatives	N7-methylguanosine N2N2-dimethyl guanosine (Wyosine)

38.34 (a) 5S rRNA and (b) 23S rRNA
- Prokaryotic 30S subunits of ribosome contain 16S rRNA.

- Prokaryotic 50S subunits of ribosome contain 5S rRNA, 23S rRNA.
- Eukaryotic 40S subunits of ribosome contain 18S rRNA.
- Eukaryotic 60S subunits of ribosome contain 5S rRNA, 5.8S rRNA, 28S rRNA.

38.35 (b) Uric acid
- In human and higher primates, uric acid is the final oxidation (breakdown) product of purine metabolism and is excreted in urine.
- Allantoin is a natural end product of purine metabolism in most mammals other than humans. It is produced by action of uricase enzyme on uric acid.

38.36 (c) Xanthine to uric acid
- **Xanthine oxidase** is involved in the conversion of the purine bases to uric acid. It catalyzes the oxidation of hypoxanthine to xanthine and also xanthine to uric acid.
- **Allopurinol is used in the treatment of gout,** which is caused by the precipitation of uric **acid crystals in the joints**.

38.37 (b) HGPRTase
- Child is presenting with joint pain which may be due to hyperuricemia. Child is also manifesting neurological symptoms like aggressive behavior and self mutilation. This child may be suffering from **complete deficiency of HGPRT** which is **Lesch-Nyhan syndrome**.
- **Partial deficiency of HGPRT** is **Kelly-Seegmiller syndrome**. The only feature of which is hyperuricemia. Neruological symptoms are absent.

38.38 (a) Uncondensed
Chromatin is made up of euchromatin and heterochromatin regions. Euchromatin is the uncondensed region of the DNA and heterochromatin is the densely condensed region of the DNA.

Binding of the DNA to the basic protein histone makes DNA more condensed (heterochromatin).

Acetylation of the histone protein converts the heterochromatin DNA to the euchromatin DNA. This is due to more electronegativity imparted to the histone protein which thus converts dense packed DNA to loose packed euchromatin region.

38.39 (a) Closed circular

38.40 (b) tRNA

Pseudouridine and thymidine are two modified bases found in the tRNA.

38.41 (a) 3′-UCAGACUGA 5′

38.42 (a) UAG

38.43 (b) Allopurinol

38.44 (b) Zinc

38.45 (a) UAA, (b) UAG, (c) UGA

Stop codons are:

UGA (opal)

UAG (amber)

UAA (ochere)

Point to note

Sometimes UGA codes for selenocysteine, but those mRNA, UGA of which codes for selenocysteine contain selenocysteine insertional element.

UAG codes for pyrrolysine.

38.46 (a) Pyrimidine dimers are removed by nucleotide excision repair

(b) Mismatch repair mechanism has high fidelity and

(c) Chemotherapy can lead to double-stranded breaks in DNA

Summary of DNA repair mechanisms.

So, maximum fidelity is with mismatch repair, base excision repair and nucleotide excision repair.

Least fidelity is with NHEJ.

Disorders associated with defect in DNA repair mechanism

DNA repair	
Defect in	*Diseases associated with*
Mismatch repair	HNPCC (hereditary nonpolyposis colon cancer)
Nucleotide excision repair	Xeroderma pigmentosum Cockayne's syndrome (defective transcription coupled repair/TCR)
NHEJ	SCID
Homologous repair	Bloom syndrome, Werner syndrome, breast cancer

38.47 (a) DNA strand and (b) Promoter region

Target of transcriptional regulators (Mol Bio: McLennan 4th ed).

1. Chromatin structure
2. Interaction with TFIID through specific TAFIIs

3. Interaction with TFIIB
4. Interaction or modulation of the TFIIH complex activity leading to differential phosphorylation of the CTD of RNA polymerase II.

38.48 (a) Hydrogen bonds and (c) Bonds between bases

Helicase activity leads to dissociation of hydrogen bonds between bases so that the parent strands go apart.

During proofreading the phosphodiester bond is broken, where the bond between phosphate and pentose sugar is broken.

38.49 (c) U3

Each spliceosome is composed of 5 small nuclear RNAs (snRNAs) and some associated protein factors. The snRNAs making up the major spliceosome include U1, U2, U4, U5 and U6.

38.50 (d) GATATC–CTATAG

- In molecular biology, restriction fragment length polymorphism, or RFLP, is a technique that exploits variations in homologous DNA sequences.
- It refers to a difference between samples of homologous DNA molecules from differing locations of restriction enzyme sites, and to a related laboratory technique by which these segments can be illustrated.
- In RFLP analysis, the DNA sample is broken into pieces (and digested) by restriction enzymes and the resulting restriction fragments are separated according to their lengths by gel electrophoresis.

Restriction Enzyme

- Restriction enzymes are DNA-cutting enzymes.
- A palindromic sequence is a sequence made up of nucleic acids within double helix of DNA and/or RNA that is the same when read from 5′-to-3′ on one strand and 5′-to-3′ on the other complementary strand. It is also known as a palindrome or an inverted or reverse sequence.
- Restriction enzymes cleave at the palindromic sites.
- Usually the palindromic sequence will be 4–6 nucleotides length.

38.51 (d) Ribozyme

Ribozymes are RNA having catalytic activity.

Following are the examples of ribozymes:

1. Peptidyltransferase
2. Telomerase
3. Phosphodiesterase
4. RNase P

38.52 (d) Hybridization

'A DNA microarray (also commonly known as gene chip, DNA chip, for biochip) is a collection of microscopic DNA spots attached to a solid surface. The core principle behind microarrays is hybridization between two DNA strands, the property of complementary nucleic acid sequences to specially pair with each other by forming hydrogen bonds between complementary nucleotide base pairs'.

38.53 (d) Repressors

- Transcription begins when RNA polymerase recognizes and binds to specific promoter sequences on the DNA molecule found very close to the RNA synthesis start site.
- Therefore, to regulate transcription initiation, the interaction between an RNA polymerase protein and its promoter DNA sequence must be controlled.
- Enhancers are regions of DNA that increase the transcriptional activity of a gene. Three types of proteins regulate transcription initiation, including specificity factors, repressors, and activators.
- Specificity factors regulate the specificity of an RNA polymerase for a given promoter or set of promoters. A repressor binds to a specific DNA region and induces negative regulation by blocking RNA polymerase binding or movement along DNA strands.
- An activator offers positive regulation by binding to sites adjacent to the promoter region on DNA and enhancing RNA polymerase binding and activity. Origins of replication are regions of DNA that are the start sites for copying DNA during DNA replication.

38.54 (d) A template

- DNA polymerase binds to template, and the template determines the sequence of the newly synthesized DNA using Watson-Crick base pairing.
- Thioredoxin and thioredoxin reductase are necessary for the conversion of ribonucleotides to deoxyribonucleotides.
- dUTP is not a physiological substrate for DNA polymerase.
- dUTP is converted to dUMP, which is a substrate for the thymidylate synthase reaction.

38.55 (b) Nucleolus

In the nucleolus 45S rRNA is cleaved into smaller component like 5.8S rRNA, 18S rRNA and 28S rRNA. This cleavage is the only post-transcriptional modification of rRNA.

38.56 (a) dsDNA

Okazaki fragment is a small stretch of DNA with the RNA primer attached at one of its ends. It is synthesized while the dsDNA is undergoing replication, because synthesis of DNA is a directional process, and always the reading of DNA parent strand occurs in 3'–5' direction and synthesis of daughter strand in 5'–3' direction.

During replication of single strand DNA, there is no formation of Okazaki fragment.

38.57 (b) It adds telomere to the 5'-end of the DNA strand.

Telomerase

- It is a ribonucleoprotein complex with a short strand of RNA (3'-CCCAATCCC-5') and various proteins which are having reverse transcriptase activity.
- It adds 6 nucleotides telomere repeat at the 3'-end of the DNA chain. Telomere is G-rich sequence: TTAGGG.

Telomerase binds to the end of 3'-end, with part of telomerase RNA hydrogen bonded to last a few nucleotide of the chromosome.

Telomere finally terminates into a single-stranded overhang that is roughly 150-nucleotide long.

Telomere is critical for maintaining the stability of the genome. Progressive shortening of the telomere is avoided by telomerase activity.

38.58 (b) Sister chromatids are formed; (c) Follow base pair rule; (d) Semiconservative; and (e) Single strand break

DNA replication is a semiconservative process which occurs in S phase of cell cycle. Sister chromatids are synthesized following base pair rule.

Single and double strand breaks are needed to relieve supercoiling.

38.59 (b) Uses enzymes called DNA glycosylases to generate an abasic sugar site

38.60 (c) Nucleotide excision repair

Xeroderma pigmentosum (XP): It is an **autosomal recessive** inherited disorder. It is due to **defect in repair of damaged DNA especially thymine dimers**. Culture of cells from patients shows low activity of the nucleotide excision repair processes. **The most**

Section 9 ■ Nucleic Acids: Chemistry, Metabolism and Applied Aspects

38

common form of this disease is due to absence of UV specific excinuclease.

38.61 (a) Xeroderma pigmentosum; (b) Bloom's syndrome; and (c) Ataxia-telangiectasia

Diseases associated with DNA repair mechanism are:

1. Xeroderma pigmentosum (defective nucleotide excision repair)
2. Cockayne syndrome (defective nucleotide excision repair)
3. Fanconi's anemia (defect in DNA crosslink repair)
4. Hereditary polyposis colon cancer (Lynch syndrome) (defect in mismatch repair)
5. Ataxia-telangiectasia and Bloom's syndrome are also due to DNA repair mechanism defect.

38.62 (a) G0-G1-S-G2-M

Duration in each phase

G1	2 hours to 12 hours (variable)
S	6 hours (fixed)
G2	4 hours (fixed)
M	2 hours (fixed)

38.63 (b) snRNA

snRNA has **phosphodiesterase activity** (an example of ribozyme), which is essential for making a nick at the 5'-end of the intron region of the hnRNA for removal of the intron.

snRNA is an important component of the spliceosome, a machinery responsible for splicing of hnRNA converting to the mRNA.

Other example of ribozyme is **peptidyltransferase**.

38.64 (c) Specifically recognizes the promoter site

- Prokaryotic RNA polymerase enzyme consists of core enzyme + sigma factor
- Core enzyme has following subunits: 2 alpha, one beta, one beta prime, one omega subunit (beta subunit is catalytic)
- Sigma subunit helps in tight attachment of core complex to the promoter region.

Mammalian RNA polymerase enzyme

Class of enzyme	Sensitivity to α-amanitin
I(A)	Insensitive
II(B)	Sensitive to low concentration of α-amanitin (so highly sensitive)
III(C)	Sensitive to high concentration of α-amanitin (so less sensitive)

α-amanitin is derived from Amanita phalloides.

Option a: Rifampicin binds beta subunit of prokaryotic RNA polymerase.

Option b: α-amanitin inhibits eukaryotic RNA polymerase I and III.

Option d: Core enzyme has α, α, β, β', ω subunits. Sigma subunit is a part of holoenzyme.

38.65 (c) Inactivates DNA for transcription

Methylated DNA is the inactive form of the DNA.

Options (a) and (d) say that the methylation enhances the rate of transcription which is a wrong statement.

Alteration in enhancer region may make a difference, but alteration in the promoter region would certainly make the difference.

38.66 (b) Nucleolus

rRNA is mainly produced in the nucleolus by RNA polymerase I, there itself it is cleaved into smaller fragments like 5.8S rRNA, 18S rRNA, 28S rRNA.

5S rRNA is produced in the nucleus by RNA polymerase III. This variety of rRNA makes only the small component of total rRNA.

38.67 (c) RNA polymerase

Only correct enzyme here for transcription is RNA polymerase.

38.68 (d) Primer

RNA polymerase should bind the promoter region of DNA template and it needs all.

Four nucleotides are needed for RNA synthesis (ATP, GTP, UTP, CTP).

In addition, Mn^{++}, Mg^{++} are also needed.

Primer is needed for DNA synthesis and not for RNA synthesis.

38.69 (b) tRNA

tRNA helps in translation process by transferring the amino acid for the process of translation. tRNA itself is not translated. Glycosyltransferase, keratin, histone are proteins which are the result of translation process.

38.70 (b) Polylysine (Mnemonic: Poly ly for lysine)

AAA is the codon for lysine, so poly (A) tail gets translated into polylysine.

38.71 (a) AUG codon

Shine-Dalgarno sequence is present in prokaryotic polycistronic mRNA 6 to 10 bp upstream to AUG codon. This sequence is having complementarity to 3'-end of 16S rRNA.

This complementarity helps in localization of ribosome on the mRNA.

In eukaryotes the corresponding sequence is Kozak consensus sequence.

38.72 (a) Releasing factor; (b) Stop codon; (c) Peptidyltransferase and (d) UAA codon

Termination of polypeptide chain synthesis occurs when a stop codon is encountered at the 'A' site. At this stage no tRNA binds the 'A' site and instead releasing factors bind the 'A' site. With the help of H_2O, peptidyltransferase, and the GTP, they release the newly synthesized polypeptide chain from the 'P' site.

38.73 (c) Reading frame changes downstream to the mutant site

Reading frameshifting occurs in deletion or insertion type of mutation. Base substitution mutation (point mutation) results in change of amino acid to either the same amino acid/other amino acid or sometimes the changed amino acid after mutation results in appearance of the stop codon.

There occurs no shifting of the reading frame in this type of mutation.

Shifting of reading frame occurs in deletion or insertion type of mutation.

38.74 (c) AAUAAA Mutation of this sequence will result in difficulty of polyadenylation process.

38.75 (a) Nonsense mutation

As we can seen in the question, UAC is changed to stop codon, it is a nonsense mutation.

38.76 (b) Cleave specific palindromic DNA sequences

Restriction enzymes identify the palindromic sequences on the DNA and cut the DNA strand at certain specific site.

There are three class of restriction enzymes.

38.77 (d) Northern blot analysis

Methods to detect the mutation are :
1. Southern blotting
2. DNA sequencing
3. PCR with oligonucleotide hybridization
4. RFLP
5. Microarray
6. SSCP (single strand conformational polymorphism)

38.78 (d) Radiolabelled DNA probe

Materials needed for PCR process are:
- DNA
- Primer set (forward and reverse)
- Deoxynucleotide (dAMP, dGMP, dCMP dTMP)
- Mg^{++}, Mn^{++}
- Buffer to maintain the pH

38.79 (b) PCR

SYBR green dye is used for quantifying the PCR product.

38.80 (a) Replacement of abnormal gene by normal gene

38.81 (c) Jeffrey

38.82 (c) Nucleic acid

38.83 (a) Detected by southern blot; (c) Used for identification of gene for genomic mapping; and (d) RFLP is a DNA variation sequence

Southern blotting technology is used to identify the restriction fragment, where a particular probe is used to identify the presence or absence of restriction fragment and thus helps in identification of polymorphism/mutation (RFLP).

38.84 (a) Alters gene expression; (c) Role in carcinogenesis; and (d) Protective mechanism against cleavage by restriction endonuclease

38.85 (a) Transfection

38.86 (a) Electroporation; (b) Intranuclear injection; (c) Site-directed mutagenesis; and (d) Retrovirus

Section 9 ■ Nucleic Acids: Chemistry, Metabolism and Applied Aspects

38

38.87 (a) Polylysine

Poly (A) tail is translated into the polylysine tail. As AAA is the codon for lysine amino acid.

38.88 (c) Purine replaced by purine and pyrimidine replaced by pyrimidine

(c) Transition is when purine nucleotide is replaced by purine nucleotide and pyrimidine nucleotide is replaced by pyrimidine nucleotide.

When purine nucleotide is replaced by pyrimidine nucleotide and pyrimidine nucleotide is replaced by purine nucleotide it is called as transversion.

38.89 (b) Mitochondrial DNA

Histone DNA and mitochondrial DNA do not have intron.

38.90 (b) Maternally inherited and (d) Mitochondrial myopathy

Heme and Hemoproteins

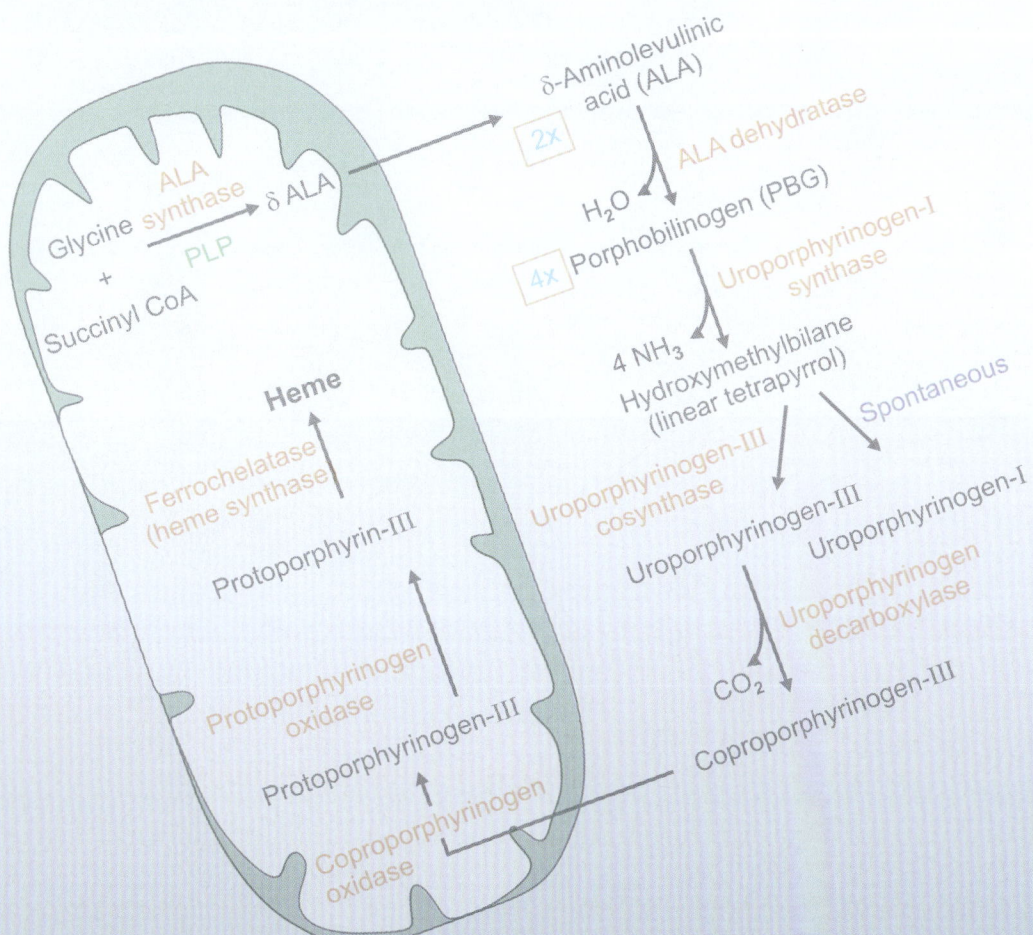

Heme Metabolism

COMPETENCY BI 6.11

At the end of this chapter learner should be able to describe the functions of heme in the body and describe the processes involved in its metabolism and describe porphyrin metabolism.

Specific Learning Objectives

BI 6.11.1 Enumerate various functions of heme in our body.

BI 6.11.2 Discuss various aspects of heme metabolism.

BI 6.11.3 Define porphyria and classify them.

BI 6.11.4 Discuss the impact of lead on heme metabolism.

Heme proteins are a group of specialized proteins which have heme as tightly bound prosthetic group (Fig. 39.1).

Examples of heme proteins are:

- Hemoglobin
- Myoglobin
- Cytochrome *c*
- Cytochrome P450
- Catalase
- Peroxidase
- Tryptophan pyrrolase
- Nitric oxide synthase
- Guanylyl cyclase
- Heme is a complex of protoporphyrin IX and ferrous iron (Fe^{++}). It is a tetrapyrrole where 4 pyrrole rings are named as I, II, III and IV. The rings are attached with the help of methenyl bridges.
- 6 electrons of Fe^{++} interact in following ways: Four e^- with porphyrin's nitrogens, fifth e^- interacts with imidazole nitrogen of proximal histidine and sixth e^- interacts with the oxygen atom of the oxygen molecule. Table 39.1 shows differences between porphyrinogens and porphyrins.
- Hemoglobin is a tetramer consists of two identical dimers—2α and 2β (HβA).
- The two polypeptide chains in each dimer are held together by strong hydrophobic interaction.

- Dimers are having weak ionic and hydrogen bonds between them, so two dimers are able to move with respect to each other (Fig. 39.2).
- In deoxygenated form hemoglobin is found in the T(taut/tense) form. T form is low oxygen affinity form of the hemoglobin.
- In oxygenated form, hemoglobin is found in the R (relaxed) form. R form is more oxygen affinity form of the hemoglobin.

METABOLISM OF HEME

Synthesis of Heme

- Synthesis of heme takes place in two organs—bone marrow cell and hepatic cell.
- 85% of heme synthesis occurs in bone marrow cell and 15% of heme synthesis occurs in liver.
- The complex heme molecule is synthesized from two simple precursors, glycine and succinyl coenzyme A (Fig. 39.3).

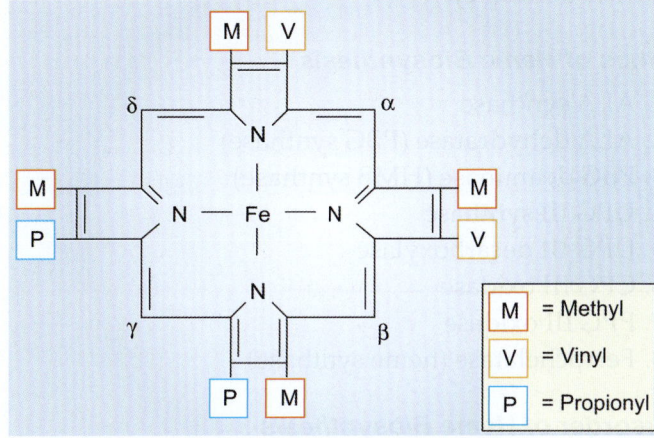

Fig. 39.1: Structure of heme: Tetrapyrrole ring of heme with iron in the center

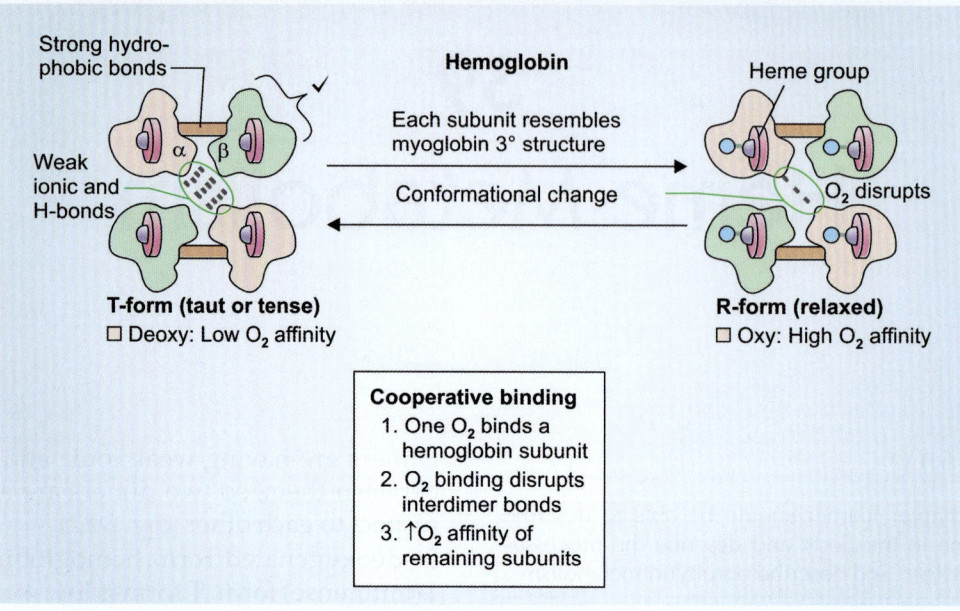

Fig. 39.2: Hb Tetramer

- Synthesis of heme begins in the mitochondria and ends in the mitochondria with some intermediate steps occurring in cytosol.
- ALA synthase is the rate-limiting enzyme of hepatic biosynthesis of heme.
- Repression-derepression mechanism is involved in the regulation of heme biosynthesis. Heme is a corepressor which combines with aporepressor molecule to form a repressor molecule which is capable of repressing the gene of ALA synthase.
- At the time of heme deficiency this repressor molecule is not formed and gene of ALA synthase is derepressed leading to synthesis of ALA synthase which fulfills heme deficiency.

Steps of Heme Biosynthesis

1. ALA synthase
2. ALA dehydratase (PBG synthase)
3. PBG deaminase (HMB synthase)
4. UPG III synthase
5. UPG III decarboxylase
6. CPG III oxidase
7. PPG III oxidase
8. Ferrochelatase (heme synthase)

Disorder of Heme Biosynthesis

Porphyrias

- Group of disorders due to abnormalities in the pathway of biosynthesis of heme.

These can be genetic or acquired.
- **Six major types** of porphyrias are described resulting from decreased activities of enzymes in the pathway of heme biosynthesis. They are:
    1. Acute intermittent porphyria (AIP)
    2. Congenital erythropoietic porphyria (CEP)

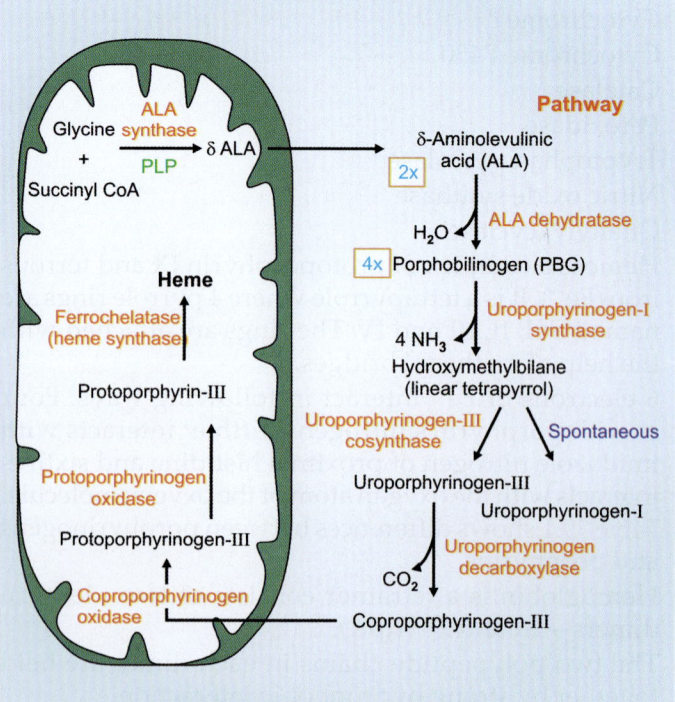

Fig. 39.3: Heme synthesis

3. Porphyria cutanea tarda (PCT)
4. Hereditary coproporphyria (HCP)
5. Variegated porphyria (VP)
6. Protoporphyria (PP)

In general, porphyrias are inherited in autosomal dominant manner, with the exception of congenital erythropoietic porphyria, which is inherited in the autosomal recessive mode.

Porphyrias may also be classified on the basis of the organs or cells that are predominantly affected, in following two categories:

  a. *Erythropoietic:* Bone marrow cells are predominantly affected.

  b. *Hepatic:* Hepatic cells are predominantly affected.

Erythropoietic porphyria includes:
• Congenital erythropoietic porphyria (CEP)
• Protoporphyria (PP)

Hepatic porphyria includes:
• Acute intermittent porphyria (AIP)
• Porphyria cutanea tarda (PCT)
• Hereditary coproporphyria (HCP)
• Variegated porphyria (VP)
• Plumboporphyria

Porphyrias may also be classified on the the basis of clinical symptoms: Cutaneous and neurological porphyria (Figs 39.4a and b).

• *Pure cutaneous:* PCT, CEP, PP
• *Pure neurological:* AIP
• *Both cutaneous and neurological:* HCP and VP

Heme Degradation/Catabolism

After breakdown of scencent RBC, heme is converted to biliverdin and then to bilirubin in reticuloendothelial cell of liver, spleen and bone marrow. This bilirubin is conjugated and excreted.

1. Conversion of heme to biliverdin is catalyzed by heme oxygenase. This reaction is catalysed by heme

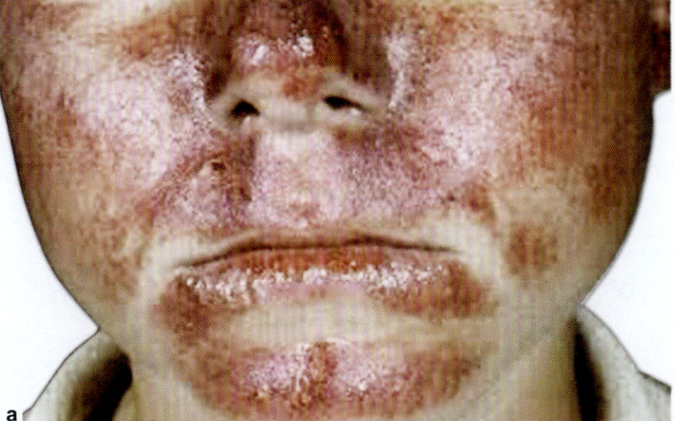
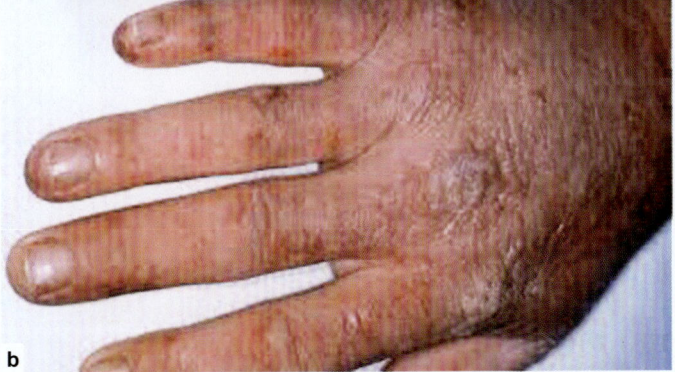

Figs 39.4a and b: Porphyria—cutaneous manifestation

oxygenase which produces carbon monoxide. This is the only reaction which produces carbon monoxide in human cell (Fig. 39.5).

2. Biliverdin is reduced by (NADPH) to bilirubin by enzyme biliverdin reductase.
3. Bilirubin is transported to the liver bound to serum albumin.
4. In the liver, bilirubin is conjugated with glucuronic acid by enzyme uridine diphosphate (UDP)-glucuronyltransferase. The bilirubin diglucuronide that is formed is soluble and is secreted into the bile.
5. Bilirubin diglucuronide is hydrolyzed to free bilirubin in the bowel, there it is reduced to urobilinogens.

Section 10 ■ Heme and Hemoproteins

39

TABLE 39.1	Differences between porphyrinogens and porphyrins	
Porphyrinogens	*Porphyrins*
Colourless	Coloured
Contain six extra hydrogens, so it is also called reduced porphyrins.	Porphyrinogens gets auto-oxidized to their respective porphyrins. This reaction is catalyzed by light.
Do not absorb at 400 nm wavelength light.	Show characteristic absorbance at 400 nm (regardless of side).
Do not emit fluorescence, when illuminated by UV light.	Porphyrins dissolved in strong mineral acids emit a strong red fluorescence, when illuminated by UV light.
Pyrrole rings are joined by methylene bridges (–CH$_2$–).	Pyrrole rings are joined by methenyl bridges (–HC=).

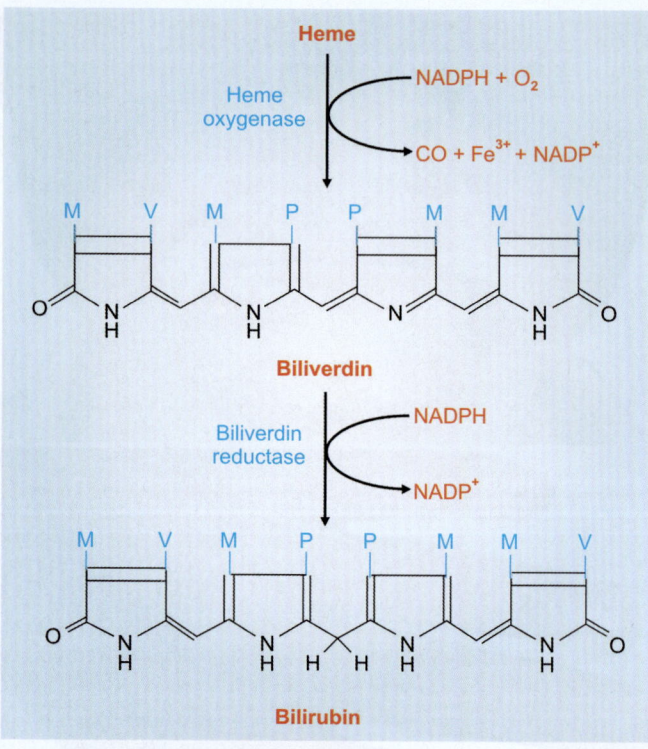

Heme

Heme oxygenase

$NADPH + O_2$

$CO + Fe^{3+} + NADP^+$

M   V   M   P   P   M   M   V

Biliverdin

Biliverdin reductase

NADPH

$NADP^+$

M   V   M   P   P   M   M   V

Bilirubin

Fig. 39.5: Heme catabolism

Urobilinogen is the colourless substance which is oxidized to urobilin which is excreted in feces.

Glycosylated Hemoglobin (HbA1c)

Hb is nonenzymatically glycosylated when blood glucose enters the erythrocytes. About 5% fraction of total Hb is glycosylated when blood glucose is within normal limits. Since the mean life of an erythrocyte is 120 days, HbA1c level reflects the average blood glucose concentration over the preceding 12 weeks.

Hemoglobin and Myoglobin

COMPETENCY BI 6.12

At the end of this chapter learner should be able to describe the major types of hemoglobin and its derivatives found in the body and their physiological/pathological relevance.

Specific Learning Objectives

BI 6.12.1 Enumerate various types of normal hemoglobin.
BI 6.12.2 Discuss abnormal hemoglobin.
BI 6.12.3 Describe various hemoglobinopathies.

Hemoglobin: It is a heme protein.

Myoglobin: Myoglobin is the heme protein found in heart and skeletal muscles. It consists of single polypeptide chain that is similar to beta subunit polypeptide chain of the hemoglobin molecule.

O_2 Dissociation Curve

• When the % saturation of Hb or Mb with the O_2 is plotted at y-axis against the partial pressure of the oxygen (pO_2) at the x-axis, the curve obtained is known as oxygen dissociation curve (ODC) (Fig. 40.1).

• ODC is hyperbolic for myoglobin and it is sigmoidal for hemoglobin.

• P50 is partial pressure of the oxygen at which the saturation of hemoglobin or myoglobin is 50%.

• P50 for myoglobin is 1 mmHg.

• P50 for hemoglobin is 26 mmHg.

• Sigmoidal shape for hemoglobin ODC is due to cooperative binding of O_2 with the hemoglobin subunits.

Cooperative binding means O_2 binding at one of the heme groups increases the O_2 affinity for other remaining heme groups in the same hemoglobin molecule. This is also known as heme-heme interaction. This heme-heme interaction (cooperative binding) occurs to the extent that the affinity of hemoglobin for the last oxygen bound is approximately 300 times greater than its affinity for the first oxygen bound.

Steep upward slope in the region of 20–30 mmHg in oxygen dissociation curve of the hemoglobin is due to this cooperative phenomenon (Fig. 40.2).

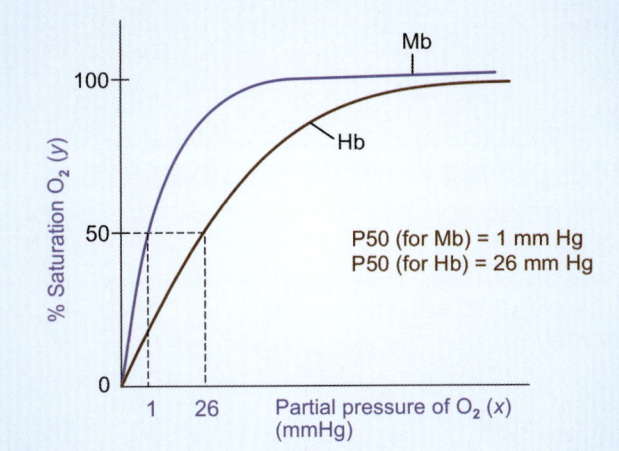

Fig. 40.1: O_2 dissociation curve

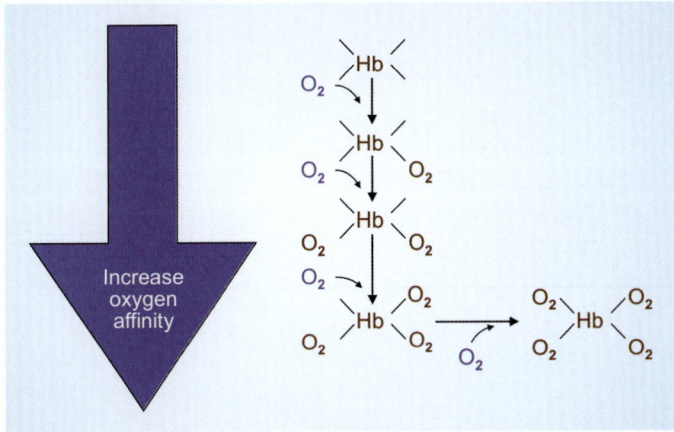

Fig. 40.2: Cooperative binding of oxygen to the hemoglobin molecule

Various allosteric effectors for O_2 binding to the Hb are pO_2, pH, pCO_2 and 2,3-bisphosphoglyserate (BPG).

2,3-BPG: It decreases the O_2 affinity of the hemoglobin by binding to the deoxyhemoglobin but not to oxyhemoglobin. This binding of 2,3-BPG stabilizes taut configuration of deoxyhemoglobin.

2,3-BPG binds the pocket formed by two beta globin chains, in the center of deoxyhemoglobin tetramer.

Bohr's effect: A shift to right of the ODC at low pH and increase in pCO_2 is known as Bohr's effect. This effect is due to the fact that the deoxy form of the hemoglobin has greater affinity for the protons.

Factors causing shift to right of the ODC:
- Low pH
- High CO_2
- High 2,3-BPG
- High temperature

Factors causing shift to left of the ODC:
- High pH
- Low CO_2
- Low 2,3-BPG
- Low temperature

MULTIPLE CHOICE QUESTIONS

40.1 Which of the following is not a heme protein?
  a. Myoglobin
  b. Cytochrome *c*
  c. Catalase
  d. Albumin

40.2 A 10-year-old boy presented with abdominal pain, muscle weakness and fatigue. On investigations, serum lead levels were found increased in blood. Activity of which of the following enzymes in the liver is increased?

  a. ALA synthase
  b. Ferrochelatase
  c. PGB deaminase
  d. Heme oxygenase

40.3 Ferrous of heme is bound to:
  a. Proximal histidine
  b. Distal histidine
  c. Tyrosine of alpha chain
  d. None of the above

ANSWERS

40.1 (d) Albumin

Following is the list of heme proteins:
- Hemoglobin
- Myoglobin
- Catalase
- Peroxidase
- Nitric oxide synthase
- Guanylyl cyclase

40.2 (a) ALA synthase

- This is a case of lead poisoning. Lead inhibits ALA dehydratase enzyme leading to plumboporphyria.
- Pb also competes with Fe^{++} to get incorporated in the center of tetrapyrrole ring and impairs the heme synthesis.
- Lack of heme 'derepress' ALA synthase (rate-limiting enzyme of heme biosynthesis) and hence the activity of ALA synthase is increased in liver.

40.3 (a) Proximal histidine

Heme is a complex of protoporphyrin IX and ferrous ion (Fe^{++}).

Iron can form six bonds, four with porphyrin nitrogen, fifth with the proximal histidine residue of the globin chain and sixth with one atom of oxygen molecule.

Section 10 ■ Heme and Hemoproteins

40

Oxidative Stress and Cancer

Mitosis

Prophase
Metaphase
Anaphase
Telophase
Cytokinesis

Second growth phase

Growth and preparation for division

First growth phase

Growth and normal metabolic roles

M

G_2 G_1

S

Interphase

DNA Replication

Synthesis phase

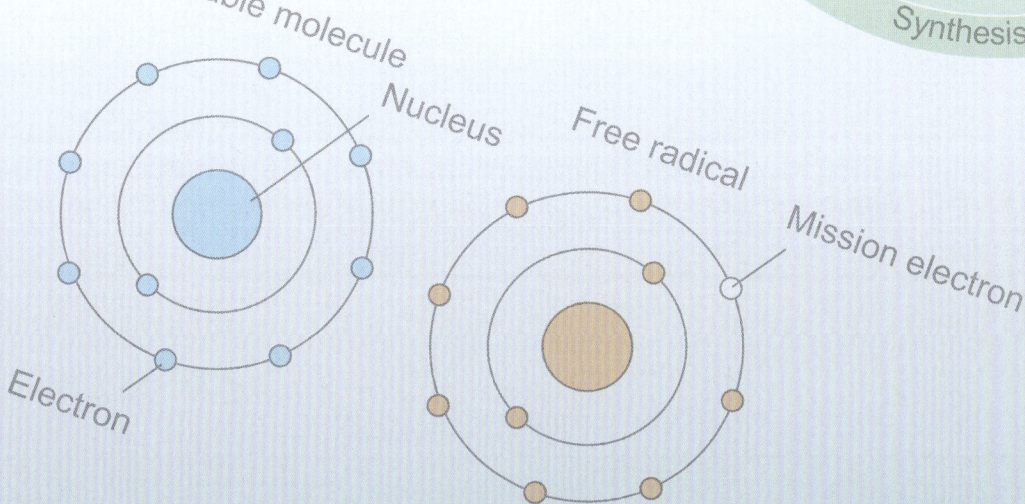

Stable molecule

Nucleus

Free radical

Mission electron

Electron

11

Oxidative Stress and Cancer

41

Free Radicals

Free radical is the molecule or molecular fragment which is having one or more unpaired (free) electron in the outer orbital.

Free radical is having the tendency to start a chain reaction as it removes the electron from other molecule in an attempt to fulfill its own orbit (Fig. 41.1).

Free radical and reactive oxygen species (ROS) terminology are interchangeably used.

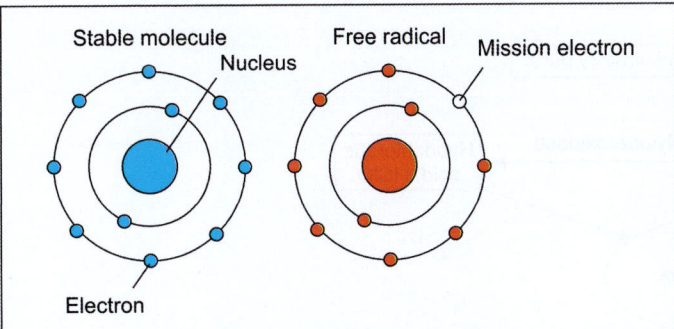

Fig. 41.1: Free radical

REACTIVE OXYGEN SPECIES (ROS)

These are highly reactive form of oxygen which make havoc in the biological system. These result from partial reduction of oxygen.

Transfer of 4 e^- to the O_2 will result in complete reduction and formation of H_2O moleclule in the electron transport chain. Partial reduction of O_2 molecule will result in the formation of ROS.

Examples of ROS are:
1. Superoxide anion radical (O_2^-)
2. Hydro-peroxy-radical (HOO^-)
3. Hydrogen peroxide (H_2O_2)
4. Hydroxyl radical (OH^-)
5. Lipid peroxy radical (ROO)
6. Singlet oxygen ($1O_2$)
7. Nitric oxide (NO)
8. Peroxy nitrite ($ONOO^-$)

Out of various free radicals, the **hydroxyl radical (OH^-) is undoubtedly the most dangerous free radical** because it is involved in lipid peroxidation and generation of other toxic radical.

Hydrogen peroxide (H_2O_2), though a ROS, is not a free radical, but it is converted to hydroxyl free radical either by **Fenton reaction or Haber–Weiss reaction** (Fig. 41.2).

Sites of production of ROS are:
- Mitochondria (leakage from ETC)
- Peroxisome
- Endoplasmic reticulum (cytochrome P450)
- Phagocytes (during respiratory burst)

Generation of free radicals occurs in following manner:
- Leak from electron transport chain
- Xanthine oxidase
- NADPH oxidase (during phagocytosis)

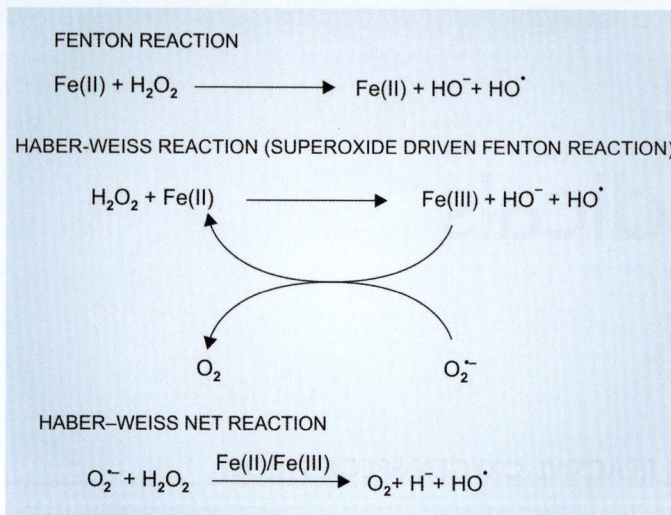

Fig. 41.2: Fenton reaction and Haber–Weiss reaction

- Heme oxidation
- Synthesis of prostaglandin
- Peroxisomal generation of H_2O_2 and O_2
- Drug metabolism
- Cigarette smoking

Respiratory Burst

To deal with the microbial infection, phagocyte produces toxic oxygen radical in a reaction catalysed by NADPH oxidase in a process known as respiratory burst.

Superoxide and hypochlorous ion produced during respiratory burst is the final effector of microbial killing.

NADPH oxidase is found at the WBC cell membrane. Genetic deficiency of this enzyme will lead to chronic granulomatous disease (CGD).

This is the example of beneficial effect of free radical in biological system (Fig. 41.3).

Damage Produced by Free Radical

A. **On biomolecules**
   1. *On protein:* Free radical oxidizes sulphydryl group of certain proteins and affect their function. In addition free radical will cause fragmentation, crosslinking and aggragation of proteins destroying their function.
   2. *On lipids:* Polyunsaturated fatty acids are specially prone to undergo free radical damage. Membrane lipid peroxidation occurs in chain reaction under initiation, elongation and propagation phase.
   3. *On nucleic acid:* DNA are prone to be damged by free radicals.

B. **Free radical and disease**
   1. Atherosclerosis via oxidised LDL
   2. Cataract
   3. Cancer
   4. Diabetes mellitus
   5. Rheumatoid arthritis
   6. Respiratory distress syndrome
   7. Retinopathy of prematurity
   8. Male infertility

CELLULAR DEFENCE AGAINST FREE RADICAL (DETOXIFICATION OF FREE RADICAL)

Antioxidant

Antioxidants are body's defence mechanism. There are many substances which act as antioxidants. They are classified according to their mechanism of action (enzymatic/nonenzymatic)

A. **Enzymatic antioxidants**
   1. *Superoxide dismutase (SOD):* Mammals have three different isoenzymes of superoxide dismutase

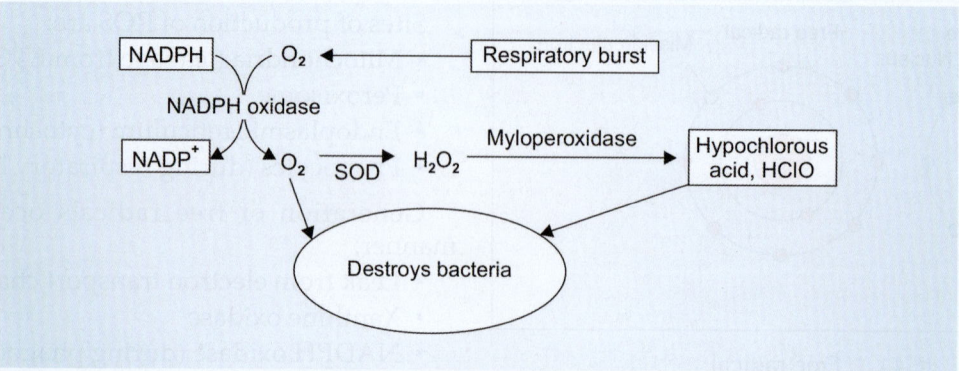

Fig. 41.3: Respiratory burst

that catalyse the conversion of superoxide to hydrogen peroxide. H_2O_2 are though toxic, they are much less toxic compared to superoxides (Fig. 41.4).

- Cytosolic (Cu/Zn containing)
- Extracellular (Cu/Zn containing)
- Mitochondrial (Mn containing)

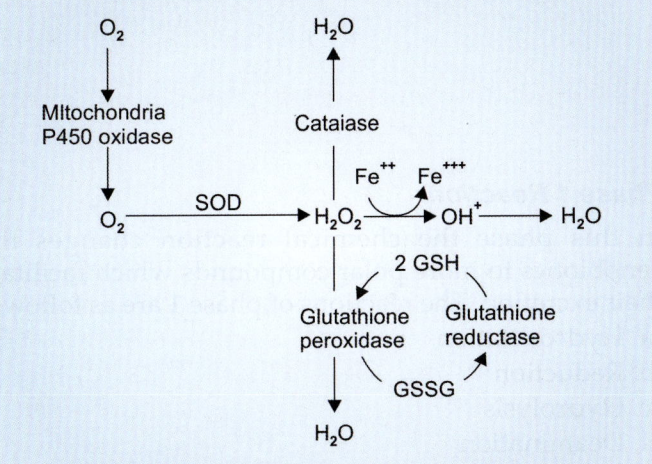

Fig. 41.4: Superoxide dismutase (SOD)

2. *Catalase:* Hydrogen peroxide is removed by catalase, a heme containing enzyme present in highest concentration in the peroxisome, and to a lesser extent in the mitochondria and the cytosol (Fig. 41.5).

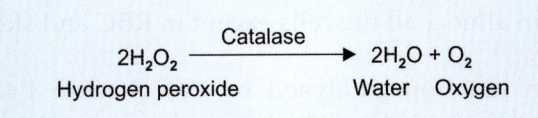

$$2H_2O_2 \xrightarrow{\text{Catalase}} 2H_2O + O_2$$

Hydrogen peroxide   Water   Oxygen

Fig. 41.5: Catalase

3. *Glutathione peroxidase:* It is a selenium containing enzyme. It requires reduced glutathione for detoxifying H_2O_2, during this process reduced glutathione is converted to oxidized glutathione. Glutathione reductase enzyme in turn converts oxidized glutathione to reduced form with the help of NADPH (Fig. 41.6).

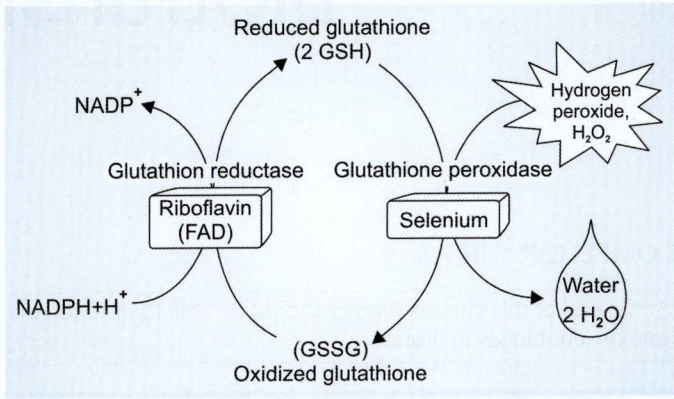

Fig. 41.6: Glutathione peroxidase

B. **Nonenzymatic antioxidants**
1. Vitamin E (tocopherol)
2. Vitamin C (ascorbic acid)
3. Beta carotenoids
4. Lycopene
5. Selenium (works in collaboration with vitamin E and glutathione)
6. Coenzyme Q10
7. Lipoic acid
8. Curcuminoids (turmeric)
9. Catechins (green tea)
10. Uric acid
11. Ceruloplasmin
12. Transferrin
13. Bilirubin
14. Albumin

42

Biotransformation

At the end of this chapter learner should be able to describe the role of xenobiotics in disease.

Specific Learning Objectives

BI 7.5.1	Describe detoxification of xenobiotics.
BI 7.5.4	Discuss various phases of detoxification with suitable example.

XENOBIOTICS AND THEIR BIOTRANSFORMATION

What is Xenobiotics?

Xenos means strange (foreign). All the chemicals which are foreign to the cell are called xenobiotics. Examples are drugs, pollutants, food additives, pesticides, cosmetics etc.

These xenobiotics poses strong risk to various biomolecules like DNA, RNA, protein etc. in the cell, hence need to be tackled effectively.

Biotransformation

Process by which xenobiotics are changed from one chemical form to other by series of enzymatic reactions is called biotransformation. It results in either entoxification or detoxification of the xenobiotics.

During entoxification, reactions of biotrans-formation convert the drug to more active metabolite but majority number of times the purpose of biotransformation is to convert the drug/xenobiotic to less active/inactive products which are more soluble and excretable. The latter phenomenon is known as detoxification.

Main organ involved in the process of biotransformation is the liver. Overall reaction of biotransformation may be conveniently divide into two phases.

Phase 1 Reaction

In this phase the chemical reaction changes the xenobiotics to more polar compounds which facilitate their excretion. The reactions of phase 1 are as follows:

a. Hydroxylation
b. Reduction
c. Hydrolysis
d. Deamination
e. Desulphation
f. Epoxidation
g. Peroxygenation

Hydroxylation is the most important reaction of phase 1. Enzymes called cytochrome P450 or mono-oxygenase are involved in the reaction of hydroxylation.

Cytochrome P450: These are groups of enzymes found in all species ranging from bacteria to mammals, they are found in almost all the cells except in RBC and skeletal muscle.

Main reaction catalysed by cytochrome P450 is hydroxylation reaction which is rendering hydrophobic compounds to hydrophilic compounds.

Cytochrome P450 is also called mixed function oxidase as it oxidizes two different substrates at a time. Out of the two substrates needed by these cytochrome P450, one substrate is incorporating oxygen atom and other substrate is donating hydrogen atom as to convert another atom of oxygen molecule to water.

Cytochrome P450 are also known as mono-oxygenase enzyme because it incorporates single atom of oxygen in the substrate.

Nitro compounds are reduced to their amines and aldehydes, and ketones are reduced to alcohols.

Hydrolysis reaction breaks the toxic compound into smaller molecules with the help of water. Example of such compounds are aspirin, atropine, xylocaine, acetanilide, procaine.

Phase 2 Reactions

In this phase there occurs conjugation of xenobiotics by various compounds which are rendering them more soluble and excretable.

In most of the cases, phase 2 reactions follow the phase 1 reaction, but in rare circumstances phase 2 reaction directly modifies the xenobiotics without crossing the phase 1 reaction.

Various conjugating agents of phase 2 reactions are as follows:

a. *Glutathione:* Conjugation of cyclophosphamide
b. *Glycine:* Conjugating with benzoic acid to produce hippuric acid.
c. *Glucuronic acid:* Bilirubin conjugation.
d. *Sulphation:* 3'-adenosine 5'-phosphosulphate (PAPS) serves as sulphate donor.
e. *Acetylation*
f. *Methylation*

Sometimes conjugation of glutathione constitutes phase 3 reaction.

EXERCISE

SHORT NOTES (5 MARKS EACH)

Q 1. Metabolism of xenobiotics
Q 2. Conjugation reactions in xenobiotic metabolism
Q 3. Role of cytochrome P450 in detoxification of xenobiotics.
Q 4. Phase 2 of detoxification

43

Cancer Biochemistry

COMPETENCY BI 10.1

At the end of this chapter learner should be able to describe the cancer initiation, promotion oncogenes and oncogene activation. Also focus on P53 and apoptosis.

Specific Learning Objectives
BI 10.1.1 Define cancer and its stages.
BI 10.1.2 Describe etiological agents of cancer, mutagens, physical carcinogens and oncogenic viruses.
BI 10.1.3 Discuss cancer initiation, promotion of cancer.
BI 10.1.4 Describe oncogenes and proto-oncogenes. Enumerate factors activating proto-oncogenes.
BI 10.1.5 Explain apoptosis and discuss the role of P53 in the process of apoptosis.

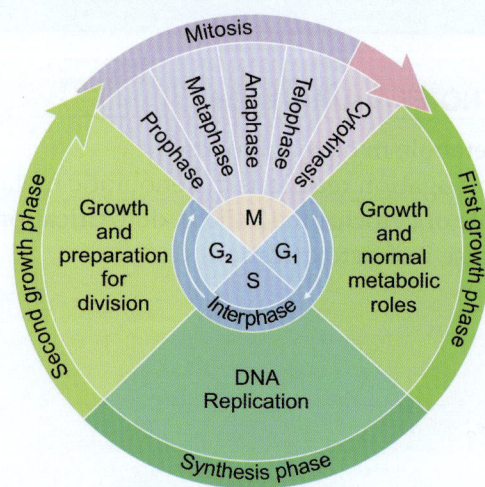

Fig. 43.1: Cell cycle

CELL CYCLE

Total duration of cell cycle of a normal cell is 18–24 hours. Steps of cell divison in a normal cell can be divided into four phases as follows:

1. **G1 phase**
2. **S phase:** This is the phase in which duplication of DNA takes place. This phase lasts for 10–12 hours.
3. **G2 phase**
4. **M phase:** It is the smallest phase of cell divison. This phase lasts for only 1 hour in a fibroblast which divides once in 24 hours (Figs 43.1 and 43.2).

Difference in Cell Cycle of a Normal and a Tumor Cell

In tumor cell, total duration of cell cycle remains more or less same as that of normal cell, but in a normal cell only 1% of cell is in dividing phase and remaining are in rest phase. In a cancerous cell, this percentage is increased considerably to an extent of 2–5% (depending upon the severity of malignancy) in dividing phase and remaining in rest phase.

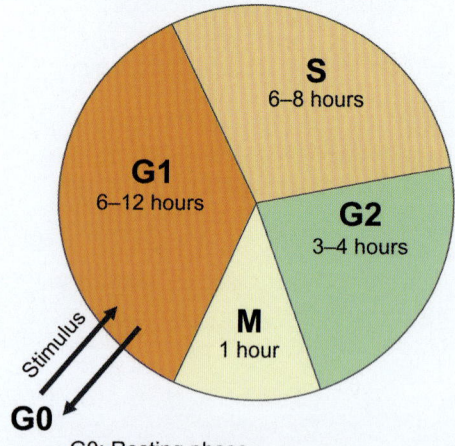

Eukaryotic replication cycle
(Times for cells growing in culture)

G0: Resting phase
G1: Growth and metabolism
S: DNA replication
G2: Growth of structural elements
M: Mitosis

Fig. 43.2: Duration of each phase of cell cycle

CANCER

It is the state of abnormal and aberrant growth of cells of the body resulting in the formation of tumor mass. Cancer cells are characterized by following features :

1. Uncontrolled growth
2. Invasion to the local tissue
3. Tendency to metastasis

Mutagens

Agents causing mutagenesis (cancer transformation) are known as mutagens. These may be of following types:

a. Radiant energy
b. Chemicals
c. Viruses

a. **Radiant energy :** Ultraviolet rays, X-rays, γ-rays may cause mutation and hence will lead to mutagenesis.

b. **Chemicals:** Many chemicals like benzene, asbestos, aflatoxin-B1, cigarette smoking, tobacco, food additives, colouring agents may cause cancer.

c. **Viruses**

Ames Test

This test is done to find out whether a suspected mutagen possess mutagenecity or not.

In this test an artificial strain of *Salmonella typhimurium* which has a mutated gene which is incapable of synthesizing histidine is used.

A carcinogen will change His– to His+ (reverse mutation). So, in a medium where a filter impregnated with the carcinogen is placed, growth of colony of *S. typhimurium* will be seen around this filter paper suggesting that the carcinogen has mutated His gene to His+ gene.

If no colony is seen around the filter paper, it suggests that the suspected carcinogen is in fact not a carcinogen at all and hence His– gene remained as His– and *S. typhimurium* could not grow.

Antimutagens

These are substances which either prevent the occurrence of cancerous condition or reverse the precancerous conditions. Examples are:

1. Vitamin A
2. Vitamin E
3. Vitamin C
4. Tubers
5. Leafy vegetables
6. Beans
7. Turmeric (curcumin)

ONCOGENE AND ANTIONCOGENE

Oncogenes are expressed in small letters, and antioncogenes are expressed in capital letters (Table 43.1).

Oncogene

Oncogenes are derived from proto-oncogene. Proto-oncogenes are normal constituents of the cell and play very important role in normal cell functioning. It is abnormal overexpression of these genes which results in malignant transformation. Proto-oncogenes have following roles in a normal cell:

1. They produce various growth factors, e.g. PDGF from sis gene needed for normal wound healing.
2. They produce receptor for growth factors, e.g. erb-B produces receptor for EGF.
3. Product of some oncogenes like src is capable of phosphorylating a specific tyrosine residue of some specific receptors, which results in various effect on cellular functioning. Example of such receptors are receptors of EGF, insulin, PDGF.

Mechanism of Activation of Proto-oncogene to Oncogene

There are many factors which are responsible for conversion of proto-oncogene to oncogene. They all lead to over-expression of proto-oncogene, resulting in uncontrolled growth of the cell and malignant transformation.

a. **Promoter insertion during viral infection:** Insertion of viral promoter region in the upstream portion of a gene upregulates it (Fig. 43.3).

b. **Enhancer insertion:** Upstream or downstream insertion of viral enhancer element in the DNA near the gene enhances its expression (Fig. 43.4).

TABLE 43.1	Product and functions of proto-oncogenes	
Proto-oncogene	*Product*	*Function*
sis gene	PDGF	Normal wound healing
erb-B	Receptor for EGF	Binding of EGF
src	Protein capable of phosphorylating a specific tyrosine residue of some specific receptors	Various effect on cellular functioning

Section 11 ■ Oxidative Stress and Cancer

43

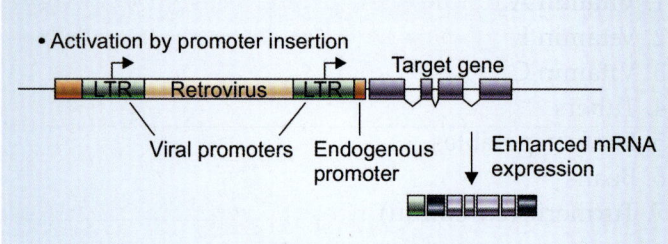

Fig. 43.3: Promoter insertion

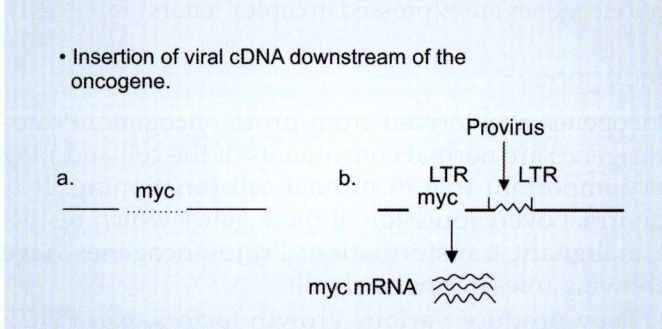

Fig. 43.4: Enhancer insertion both (a) and (b) are examples of insertional mutagenesis

c. **Chromosomal translocation:** In this mechanism a piece of a chromosome is transferred to other which positions on enhancer element near the gene. This mechanism is similar to enhancer insertion except that chromosomal translocation, rather than integration of provirus is responsible for placing the proto-oncogene under the influence of an enhancer. Examples are:
   i. Burkitt's lymphoma (Fig. 43.5)
   ii. Philadelphia chromosome in CML (Fig. 43.6)

d. **Gene amplification:** Here abnormal multiplication of gene occurs resulting in many copies. Example is methotrexate administration in a tumor cell which will amplify the gene of dihydrofolate reductase (DHF reductase) 400 times.

   This kind of gene amplification will occur in many oncogenes and also in gene involved in tumor drug resistance.

e. **Point mutation:** ras gene point mutation is a good example of the fact that how a point mutation results in tumor formation.

   A protein known as P21 which has GTPase activity is produced by ras gene which terminates the activity of adenylyl cyclase. Due to mutation, ras gene results in production of abnormal P21 production which has rather reduced GTPase activity, resulting in continued activity of adenylyl cyclase.

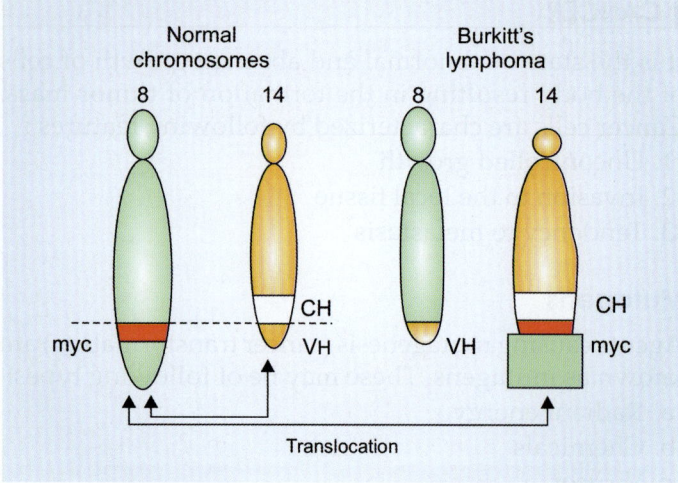

Fig. 43.5: Burkitt's lymphoma

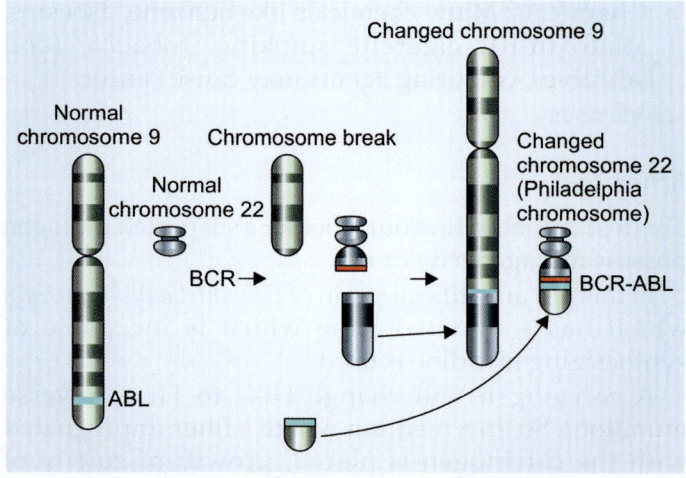

Fig. 43.6: Philadelphia chromosome

Antioncogene (Onco-suppressor Gene/Tumor-suppressor Gene)

These are genes which are responsible for suppression of oncogenesis (cancer suppression). Deletion or mutation of these genes results in carcinogenesis. Antioncogenes are represented in capital letters. Examples are:
1. Retinoblastoma (RB)
2. Wilm's tumor (WT)
3. Familial adenomatous polyposis (FAP)
4. P53
5. Familial breast cancer (BRCA-1)
6. Von-Hippel-Lindau gene (VHL)

P53

P53 is a onco-suppressor gene that is found at the short arm of chromosome 17. Nomenclature is so because this gene is responsible for the synthesis of a phosphoprotein whose molecular weight is 53,000 Da.

P53 is also called guardian of genome. P53 prevents oncogenesis by following method:

1. During DNA damage, this gene upregulates gene for P21 protein, which blocks cell division via inhibiting G1-cdK unless the damage is repaired.
2. If the damage of the DNA is beyond repair, then the cell is directed towards apoptosis.

3. It can complex with number of transforming proteins generated by bacteria, e.g. T antigen of SV 40, E6 of HPV-16.
4. Activates expression of genes that suppress cell proliferation.

Differences between Oncogene and Antioncogene

See Table 43.2.

TABLE 43.2	Differences between oncogene and tumor suppressor gene (antioncogene)
Oncogene	Antioncogene
Mutation in one of the two alleles is sufficient.	Mutation of both the alleles is must.
'Gain of function' in a protein which promotes cell divison.	'Loss of function' in a protein which is responsible for suppression of aberrant growth.
Somatic cell affected, so not inherited.	Germ cell or somatic cell may get affected, so may be inherited or not.
Some tissue preference	Strong tissue preference

EXERCISE

SHORT NOTES (5 MARKS EACH)

Q 1. Oncogenes and tumor suppressor genes
Q 2. Frame shift mutation with example
Q 3. Tumor markers
Q 4. Proto-oncogene
Q 5. Cell cycle
Q 6. Minerals
Q 7. Absorption of iron in the body and causes of iron deficiency in our country.
Q 8. Importance of calcium in body and calcium homeostasis
Q 9. Mechanism of iron absorption and transport in the body
Q 10. Iron homeostasis
Q 11. Fluorosis
Q 12. Selenosis

44

Tumor Marker

COMPETENCY BI 10.2

At the end of this chapter learner should be able to describe various biochemical tumor markers and the biochemical basis of cancer therapy.

Specific Learning Objectives

BI 10.2.1 Define tumor markers and their diagnostic importance.

BI 10.2.2 Describe important anticancer agents and biochemical basis of their mechanism of action.

A tumor marker is a substance which is secreted from tumor cell. It is defined as 'a substance sometimes found in increased amount in blood, body fluid, or tissue that may suggest the presence of a type of a cancer'.

In general, they represent re-expression of substances produced normally by embryogenically related tissues.

An ideal tumor marker should be specific for a given type of cancer and also it should be sensitive enough to detect small tumors for early diagnosis and screening.

Most tumor markers are neither specific nor sensitive.

Potential Use of Tumor Markers

These tumor markers may be used for following:
1. Screening of general population
2. Differential diagnosis of a disease
3. Clinical staging of cancer
4. Prognostic indicator of disease progression
5. Evaluation of success of treatment
6. Detection of recurrence of cancer
7. Localization of tumor using radiolabel antibody against tumor marker.

Classification of Tumor Markers

- *Oncofetal antigens:* AFP, CEA
- *Tumor associated antigens:* CA125, CA19-9, CA15-3, CA72-4, CA50

- *Hormones:* β-hCG, calcitonin
- *Receptors:* ER, PR, EGFR
- *Enzymes and isoenzymes:* PSA, PAP, NSE, PALP
- *Serum and tissue proteins:* -β2 microglobulin, monoclonal immunoglobulin/para-proteins, GFAP, protein S-100, ferritin, fibrinogen.
- *Other biomolecules:* Polyamines
- *Oncogenes:* ras, myc, ABL-BCR
- *Tumor supressor genes:* BRCA-1, P53, RB

Prostate-specific Antigen

- 32 kDa single chain glycoprotein.
- Produced by epithelial cell of the prostate gland
- It is a protease and circulates in the plasma in bound form to alpha-1 antitrypsin.

Clinical Application

- Early detection of prostate cancer (elevated in 70% of patients of prostate cancer)
- Staging of prostate cancer
- Monitoring of treatment
- Normal level of total PSA is <4 ng/L.

Alkaline Phosphatase

- *Regan isoenzyme (related to placental ALP):* It is raised in 15% cases of carcinoma lung , liver and gut.
- *Leukocyte ALP:* Raised in lymphoma,CML.

Neuron-specific Enolase

- Found in neuronal tissue, cells of neuroendocrine system and APUD tissues.
- Detection for small cell cancer lung, neuroblastoma, pheochromocytoma, carcinoid syndrome.
- Normal level is <9 µg/ml.

Calcitonin

- Produced by parafollicular C cells of thyroid gland
- Raised in medullary cancer thyroid
- Normal level is 5–12 μg/ml.

Human Chorionic Gonadotropin

- hCG is a glycoprotein synthesized by normal syncytiotrophoblast.
- It has two subunits—α and β.
- α subunit is similar to FSH, LH and TSH. β subunit is specific for hCG.
- Secreted by syncytiotrophoblast of the placenta.
- Raised in hyadatiform mole, choriocarcinoma and germ cell tumors.
- Normal level is <20 IU/L in male and nonpregnant female.
- >1,00,00 IU/L indicates trophoblastic tumor.

Alpha Fetoprotein

- Produced by fetal yolk sac and liver
- It is fetal albumin having similarity to adult albumin.
- Raised in hepatocellular and germ cell tumor, neural tube defect
- Normal value is <15 ng/L.

Carcinoembryonic Antigens

- Single chain glycoprotein
- Marker of colorectal, gastrointestinal, lung and breast cancer
- Found in embryonic tissue
- Increased in cirrhosis, emphysema, rectal polyp, ulcerative colitis also.

CA125

- Glycoprotein having molecular weight of 10 million
- Marker of ovarian, endometrial carcinoma
- Useful to monitor response to therapy, detecting residual tumor cell postsurgery, metastasis, recurrence.
- Normal level is <35 U/ml.

CA19-9

- Glycolipid
- Synthesized by gastric, pancreatic, colonic, biliary and salivary epithelium
- Marker of pancreatic and colorectal cancer

Bence Jones Proteins

- Light chain of immunoglobulin
- Raised in multiple myeloma

C-peptide

- Raised in insulinoma

Estrogen/Progesterone Receptor

- Found on breast cancer cell
- Indicator of hormonal therapy with tamoxifen.

Beta-2 Microglobulin

- Increased in multiple myeloma and CLL.

Thyroglobulin

- It is synthesized by thyroid gland and is increased in various cancers of thyroid.

Oncofetal Antigen

There are certain genes which are expressed and synthesize the protein in fetal life alone. They are repressed in adult life, only to re-express at the time when such cells are affected by malignancy.

These proteins produced by such type of genes are known as oncofetal antigen. Important examples are:
1. Alpha fetoprotein (α-FP) in hepatoma
2. CEA in colon cancer

Section 11 ■ Oxidative Stress and Cancer

44

Index

Q

R

S